HEPATOBILIARY AND PANCREATIC SURGERY

A Companion to Specialist Surgical Practice

Series Editors
O. James Garden
Simon Paterson-Brown

HEPATOBILIARY AND PANCREATIC SURGERY

FOURTH EDITION

Edited by

O. James Garden
BSc MB ChB MD FRCS(Glasg) FRCS(Ed)
FRCP(Ed) FRACS(Hon) FRCSC(Hon)

Regius Professor of Clinical Surgery
Clinical and Surgical Sciences (Surgery)
University of Edinburgh;
Honorary Consultant Surgeon
Royal Infirmary of Edinburgh
Edinburgh, UK

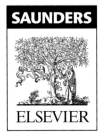

SAUNDERS

ELSEVIER

Edinburgh   London   New York   Oxford   Philadelphia   St Louis   Sydney   Toronto   2009

SAUNDERS
ELSEVIER

First edition 1997
Second edition 2001
Third edition 2005
Fourth edition 2009

ISBN 9780702030147

British Library Cataloguing in Publication Data
A catalogue record for this book is available from the British Library

Library of Congress Cataloging in Publication Data
A catalog record for this book is available from the Library of Congress

Notice
Knowledge and best practice in this field are constantly changing. As new research and experience broaden our knowledge, changes in practice, treatment and drug therapy may become necessary or appropriate. Readers are advised to check the most current information provided (i) on procedures featured or (ii) by the manufacturer of each product to be administered, to verify the recommended dose or formula, the method and duration of administration, and contraindications. It is the responsibility of the practitioner, relying on their own experience and knowledge of the patient, to make diagnoses, to determine dosages and the best treatment for each individual patient, and to take all appropriate safety precautions. To the fullest extent of the law, neither the Publisher nor the Editors assumes any liability for any injury and/or damage to persons or property arising out of or related to any use of the material contained in this book.

The Publisher

ELSEVIER your source for books,
journals and multimedia
in the health sciences
www.elsevierhealth.com

Working together to grow
libraries in developing countries
www.elsevier.com | www.bookaid.org | www.sabre.org

ELSEVIER   BOOK AID International   Sabre Foundation

The Publisher's policy is to use paper manufactured from sustainable forests

Printed in China

Commissioning Editor: Laurence Hunter
Development Editor: Elisabeth Lawrence
Project Manager: Andrew Palfreyman
Text Design: Charlotte Murray
Cover Design: Kirsteen Wright
Illustration Manager: Gillian Richards
Illustrators: Martin Woodward and Richard Prime

Contents

Contents

Contributors

Jacques Belghiti, MD
Professor of Surgery and Head of Department
Department of Hepato-Bilio-Pancreatic Surgery and
Transplantation
Hôpital Beaujon
Paris, France

Willem A. Bemelman, MD, PhD
Professor of Surgery
Department of Surgery
Academic Medical Center
Amsterdam, The Netherlands

Philippus C. Bornman, MB, ChB, MMED(Surg),
FRCS(Ed), FCS(SA), FRCS(Glasg)
Professor of Surgery
University of Cape Town and
Grooteschuur Hospital
Cape Town, South Africa

John A.C. Buckels, CBE, MD, FRCS
Professor of Hepatobiliary and Transplant
Surgery
Liver Unit
Queen Elizabeth Hospital
Birmingham, UK

Olivier R.C. Busch, MD, PhD
Gastrointestinal Surgeon
Department of Surgery
Academic Medical Center
Amsterdam, The Netherlands

C. Ross Carter, MD, FRCS, (Gen Surg)
Consultant Pancreaticobiliary Surgeon
West of Scotland Pancreatic Unit
Glasgow Royal Infirmary
Glasgow, UK

Kevin C.P. Conlon, MCh, MBA, FRCSI,
FACS, FRCS, FTCD
Professor of Surgery
Department of Surgery
University of Dublin Trinity College
Adelaide & Meath Hospitals
Dublin, Ireland

Saxon Connor
Consultant General Surgeon
Department of Surgery
Christchurch Hospital
Christchurch, New Zealand

Cornelius H.C. Dejong, MD, PhD
Professor of Hepatopancreatobiliary Surgery
Department of Surgery
University Hospital Maastricht
Maastricht, The Netherlands

Euan J. Dickson, MD, FRCS(Glasg)
Consultant Surgeon West of Scotland
Pancreatico-Biliary Unit
Glasgow Royal Infirmary
Glasgow, UK

Olivier Farges, MD, PhD
Professor of Surgery
Hôpital Beaujon
Université Paris VII
Paris, France

Stuart J. Forbes, MD, FRCP
Professor of Transplantation and Regenerative Medicine
Centre for Inflammation Research
Queens Medical Research Institute
University of Edinburgh
Edinburgh, UK

Niels A. van der Gaag, MD, PhD
Surgical Resident
Department of Surgery
Academic Medical Center
Amsterdam, The Netherlands

Steven Gallinger, MD, MSc, FRCS
Professor of Surgery
Mount Sinai Hospital
Toronto, Ontario, Canada

O. James Garden, MB, ChB, MD,
FRCS(Glas), FRCS(Ed), FRCP(Ed),
FRACS(Hon), FRCSC(Hon)
Regius Professor of Clinical Surgery
Clinical and Surgical Sciences (Surgery)
University of Edinburgh; Honorary
Consultant Surgeon
Royal Infirmary of Edinburgh
Edinburgh, UK

Dirk J. Gouma, MD, PhD
Professor of Surgery
Chair of the Department of Surgery
Academic Medical Center
Amsterdam, The Netherlands

Contributors

Geoffrey H. Haydon, MB, ChB, MD, FRCP(Ed)
Consultant Hepatologist
Liver Unit
Queen Elizabeth Hospital
Birmingham, UK

William Jarnagin, MD
Professor of Surgery, Chief, HPB Service
Department of Surgery
Memorial Sloan-Kettering Cancer Center
New York, NY, USA

Iqbal Z. Khan, MB, BS, MRCSI, FRCSI
Department of Surgery
University of Dublin, Trinity College, Adelaide &
Meath Hospital
Dublin, Ireland

Shishir K. Maithel, MD
Fellow Surgical Oncology and HPB Surgery
Department of Surgery
Memorial Sloan-Kettering Cancer Center
New York, NY, USA

Colin J. McKay, MD, FRCS
Senior Lecturer in Surgery
West of Scotland Pancreatic Unit
Glasgow Royal Infirmary
Glasgow, UK

Lynn Mikula, MD, MSc
Resident, General Surgery
University of Toronto ,Toronto, Ontario, Canada

Carol-Anne Moulton, MB, BS, FRACS, MEd
Assistant Professor of Surgery
Division of General Surgery
University of Toronto, Toronto, Ontario, Canada

Leslie K. Nathanson, MB, ChB, FRACS
Consultant Surgeon
Royal Brisbane and Women's Hospital
Brisbane, Australia

Simon P. Olliff, MRCP, FRCR
Consultant Radiologist
Department of Radiology
Queen Elizabeth Hospital
Birmingham, UK

Derek A. O'Reilly, PhD, FRCS
Consultant Hepatobiliary and Pancreatic Surgeon
Department of Surgery
North Manchester General Hospital
Manchester, UK

Rowan W. Parks, MD, FRCSI, FRCS(Ed)
Reader in Surgery and Honorary Consultant
Department of Clinical and Surgical Sciences
Royal Infirmary of Edinburgh
Edinburgh, UK

Graeme J. Poston, MB, BS, MS, FRCS
Consultant Hepatobiliary Surgeon
Department of Surgery
University Hospital Aintree
Liverpool, UK

Richard T. Schlinkert, MD, FACS
Department of General Surgery
Professor of Surgery
Mayo Clinic College of Medicine
Mayo Clinic Arizona
Phoenix, AZ, USA

Steven M. Strasberg, MD, FACS, FRCS(C), FRCS(Ed)
Pruett Professor of Surgery and
Section of Hepatobiliary-Pancreatic Surgery
Washington University in Saint Louis
St Louis, MO, USA

Benjamin N.J. Thomson, MB, BS, FRACS
Consultant Hepatobiliary Surgeon
Department of Surgical Oncology
Peter MacCallum Cancer Centre;
Department of General Surgery
Royal Melbourne Hospital
Melbourne, VIC, Australia

Stephen J. Wigmore, BSc(Hons), MB, BS, MD, FRCS(Ed)
Professor of Transplantation Surgery
Clinical and Surgical Sciences (Surgery)
Royal Infirmary of Edinburgh
Edinburgh, UK

Series preface

Since the publication of the first edition in 1997, the *Companion to Specialist Surgical Practice* series has aspired to meet the needs of surgeons in higher training and practising consultants who wish contemporary, evidence-based information on the subspecialist areas relevant to their general surgical practice. We have accepted that the series will not necessarily be as comprehensive as some of the larger reference surgical textbooks which, by their very size, may not always be completely up to date at the time of publication. This Fourth Edition aims to bring relevant state-of-the-art specialist information that we and the individual volume editors consider important for the practising subspecialist general surgeon. Where possible, all contributors have attempted to identify evidence-based references to support key recommendations within each chapter.

We remain grateful to the volume editors and all the contributors of this Fourth Edition. Their enthusiasm, commitment and hard work has ensured that a short turnover has been maintained between each of the editions, thereby ensuring as accurate and up-to-date content as possible. We remain grateful for the support and encouragement of Laurence Hunter and Elisabeth Lawrence at Elsevier Ltd. We trust that our aim of providing up-to-date and affordable surgical texts has been met and that all readers, whether in training or in consultant practice, will find this fourth edition an invaluable resource.

O. James Garden MB, ChB, MD, FRCS(Glas), FRCS(Ed), FRCP(Ed), FRACS(Hon), FRCSC(Hon)

Regius Professor of Clinical Surgery, Clinical and Surgical Sciences (Surgery), University of Edinburgh, and Honorary Consultant Surgeon, Royal Infirmary of Edinburgh

Simon Paterson-Brown MB, BS, MPhil, MS, FRCS(Ed), FRCS

Honorary Senior Lecturer, Clinical and Surgical Sciences (Surgery), University of Edinburgh, and Consultant General and Upper Gastrointestinal Surgeon, Royal Infirmary of Edinburgh

Editor's preface

This Fourth Edition of *Hepatobiliary and Pancreatic Surgery* builds on the strong foundations laid by successive contributors since the First Edition appeared in 1997. It would be a challenge to ensure that every specific area of the subspecialty could be covered and I have not sought to duplicate in any detail those areas of the specialty which will be covered more comprehensively, for example, in *Endocrine Surgery* or *Transplantation*. Trainee surgeons may feel that they will be able to obtain greater depth of knowledge in those areas where there is some subspecialty overlap by referring to these texts in paper or electronic form! All chapters have been substantially updated. The increasing tendency to work within multidisciplinary teams and our continuing attempts to push out the boundaries in resectional surgery led me to incorporate chapters on 'Liver function and liver failure', 'Non-colorectal hepatic metastases' and 'Non-adenocarcinoma of the pancreas'. I have purposely sought to broaden further the international feel and content of this edition and am grateful to all the contributors for keeping to their brief and tight deadlines. For those who struggled to do this, I hope that they will forgive my heavy editorial hand where this has been necessary to produce a uniform style.

Acknowledgements

I remain grateful to colleagues at Elsevier who have ensured that the quality and appearance of this edition have been enhanced. I trust that the addition of colour and reformatting of the text layout will produce an even easier read.

Despite the increasing editorial reliance on electronic media, I remain most grateful to our departmental secretaries for their continuing support. My children, Stephen and Katie, have grown up and almost left home during the production of successive editions. I remain grateful for the tolerant support of my wife, Amanda.

O. James Garden
Edinburgh

Evidence-based practice in surgery

Critical appraisal for developing evidence-based practice can be obtained from a number of sources, the most reliable being randomised controlled clinical trials, systematic literature reviews, meta-analyses and observational studies. For practical purposes three grades of evidence can be used, analogous to the levels of 'proof' required in a court of law:

1. **Beyond all reasonable doubt.** Such evidence is likely to have arisen from high-quality randomised controlled trials, systematic reviews or high-quality synthesised evidence such as decision analysis, cost-effectiveness analysis or large observational datasets. The studies need to be directly applicable to the population of concern and have clear results. The grade is analogous to burden of proof within a criminal court and may be thought of as corresponding to the usual standard of 'proof' within the medical literature (i.e. $P < 0.05$).

2. **On the balance of probabilities.** In many cases a high-quality review of literature may fail to reach firm conclusions due to conflicting or inconclusive results, trials of poor methodological quality or the lack of evidence in the population to which the guidelines apply. In such cases it may still be possible to make a statement as to the best treatment on the 'balance of probabilities'. This is analogous to the decision in a civil court where all the available evidence will be weighed up and the verdict will depend upon the balance of probabilities.

3. **Not proven.** Insufficient evidence upon which to base a decision, or contradictory evidence.

Depending on the information available, three grades of recommendation can be used:

a. Strong recommendation, which should be followed unless there are compelling reasons to act otherwise.

b. A recommendation based on evidence of effectiveness, but where there may be other factors to take into account in decision-making, for example the user of the guidelines may be expected to take into account patient preferences, local facilities, local audit results or available resources.

c. A recommendation made where there is no adequate evidence as to the most effective practice, although there may be reasons for making a recommendation in order to minimise cost or reduce the chance of error through a locally agreed protocol.

Strong recommendation

Evidence where a conclusion can be reached **'beyond all reasonable doubt'** and therefore where a **strong recommendation** can be given.

This will normally be based on evidence levels:

- **Ia.** Meta-analysis of randomised controlled trials
- **Ib.** Evidence from at least one randomised controlled trial
- **IIa.** Evidence from at least one controlled study without randomisation
- **IIb.** Evidence from at least one other type of quasi-experimental study.

Expert opinion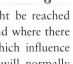

Evidence where a conclusion might be reached **'on the balance of probabilities'** and where there may be other factors involved which influence the recommendation given. This will normally be based on less conclusive evidence than that represented by scalpel icons:

- **III.** Evidence from non-experimental descriptive studies, such as comparative studies and case–control studies
- **IV.** Evidence from expert committee reports or opinions or clinical experience of respected authorities, or both.

Evidence in each chapter of this volume which is associated with either a strong recommendation or expert opinion is annotated in the text by either a **scalpel** or **pen-nib** icon as shown above. References associated with **scalpel** evidence will be highlighted in the reference lists, along with a short summary of the paper's conclusions where applicable.

Liver function and failure

Cornelius H.C. Dejong
Stuart J. Forbes
Stephen J. Wigmore

Overview of liver functions and evolution

The liver is the largest solid organ in the human body. It has a unique structure with a dual blood supply, being approximately one-third from the hepatic artery and two-thirds from portal venous blood. Within the liver substance blood flows through sinusoids between plates of hepatocytes to drain into central veins, which in turn join the hepatic veins draining into the vena cava. The liver is a major site of protein synthesis exporting plasma proteins to maintain oncotic pressure and coagulation factors. Acute phase proteins which act as antiproteases, opsonins and metal ion carriers are synthesised by the liver in response to injury or infection. Numerous immune cells populate the liver and the resident tissue macrophages, the Kupffer cells, form an important component of the innate immune system. Nutrients are extracted from portal blood by the liver and processed, and the liver acts as an important reservoir for glycogen. Waste products are either modified in the liver for excretion by the kidneys or are excreted into bile. Many drugs are taken up by the liver and metabolised, giving either active metabolites or inactive metabolites for excretion. In man, as in many vertebrates, the liver's capacity for metabolism and clearance far exceeds what is required for day-to-day life. It is possible that in evolutionary terms this ability offers a survival advantage in terms of survival of poisoning, starvation or trauma.

Symptoms of liver failure: acute and chronic

In the acute setting, liver failure can present with a number of symptoms, but it is important to note that not all of these may be present at the same time. Typically, a patient with acute liver failure after surgery, transplantation or in acute poisoning will be confused or slow as a result of encephalopathy, which may progress to loss of consciousness and a need to protect the airway by intubation and mechanical ventilation. Patients are often not immediately jaundiced, but jaundice may develop over the course of several days. Patients may be hypoglycaemic and the requirement for intravenous infusion of dextrose is a sinister development and an indicator of severe acute liver failure. Coagulopathy may develop with evidence of bruising or bleeding from line sites or surgical scars. Severe acute liver failure can be assessed using the King's College Hospital criteria, which were designed to predict mortality in paracetomol- and non-paracetomol-dependent acute liver failure.[1] Later, this scoring system was adopted in the UK to determine criteria indicating likely benefit from liver transplantation. In the surgical patient, the development of acute liver failure is usually more gradual and less dramatic; a useful scoring system for liver dysfunction in the acute setting is given in Box 1.1.

Box 1.1 • Definition of postoperative hepatic dysfunction based on results from blood tests and clinical observation

Total serum bilirubin (μmol/L)

≤20
21–60
>60

Prothrombin time (seconds above normal)

<4
4–6
>6

Serum lactate (mmol/L)

≤1.5
1.6–3.5
>3.5

Encephalopathy grade

No
1 and 2
3 and 4
0
1
2

Severity of hepatic dysfunction

None (0), mild (1–2), moderate (3–4), severe (>4)

Adapted from Schindl MJ, Redhead DN, Fearon KC et al. The value of residual liver volume as a predictor of hepatic dysfunction and infection after major liver resection. Gut 2005; 54:289–96. With permission from the BMJ Publishing Group Ltd.

Common causes of acute liver failure: hepatic insufficiency following liver resections

Liver resection is the only treatment with the potential to cure patients with cancers that have originated in the liver itself (primary liver cancer) or that have originated elsewhere and have subsequently spread to the liver (metastatic liver cancer). Equally, it is a preferred therapy in patients with tumours in the liver that are benign, but with the potential of malignant transformation (uncertain benign primary liver tumours). Liver resection of even major parts of the liver (up to 70%) is feasible, because the liver has a remarkable capacity to regenerate. Within 6–8 weeks following 60–70% hepatectomy, the liver has regained nearly its original size and weight.

The most common cause of metastatic liver cancers is primary colorectal cancer, and it is estimated that in the West there is a yearly incidence of 300 new cases of liver metastases from colorectal origin

per million population. The current estimate is that this should lead to about 100–150 patients per million eligible for liver resection for this indication. To this should be added the patients with primary benign and malignant liver tumours, and hence about 150–200 liver resections should probably be performed per million population each year.

Ever since the first liver resection by Langenbuch in 1887, this procedure has remained a major undertaking and even in the recent past, liver resection was still a dangerous surgical procedure with a high mortality of 20–30% in the 1970s. This was mainly due to excessive intraoperative bleeding but, over the subsequent decades, the procedure has become increasingly safe due to improvements in surgical and anaesthetic techniques. At present, mortality rates are reported to be well below 5%. Currently, the single most important cause of lethal outcome following surgical removal of major parts of the liver is liver failure. For this reason, many researchers and clinicians have attempted to design methods to identify patients at risk of liver failure (and hence mortality) following liver resection. The development of such a method has been hampered by several factors, as outlined below.

The critical point determining lethal outcome following liver resection has been a failure of the residual liver to function properly. Therefore, focus in this research area has always been in identifying a single liver function test that singles out those patients that have a liver with limited function. This has proven exceedingly difficult, and hence such a test is not available for a number of reasons.

First, as outlined above, the liver has a remarkable capacity to regenerate very rapidly, which underlines that there is tremendous overcapacity of several liver functions. In this context, it is known that it is entirely safe in most instances to resect 50% of the liver, because the residual half liver will simply take over all vital liver functions such as clearing bacteria, urea synthesis and synthesis of crucial proteins. From this, it has been estimated that a crucial liver function such as urea synthesis has an overcapacity of 300%, which implies that a static preoperative liver function test will be unable to assess this particular function. An alternative and innovative strategy would be to give a challenge to the liver and measure the ability of the liver to respond or cope – a dynamic test.

The critical minimum residual liver volume has been estimated to be ~25% after resection.[2]

The second crucial problem has been that there is only a poor correlation between volume and function. However, it is still unclear why some patients with smaller hepatic remnants do not develop liver failure whilst some with greater residual volumes do. These observations suggest, however, that peri- and intraoperative events superimposed on the innate hepatic capacity to withstand injury play a role. Hepatic insufficiency in this situation may arise either if not enough liver volume is left after partial hepatectomy or if the residual volume does not function properly. A functional limitation may arise, for example, in patients that have received aggressive chemotherapy in order to reduce the number and size of metastases prior to surgical treatment by liver resection. One of the factors contributing to defective defence may be preoperative fasting,[3] but equally prior chemotherapy and pre-existent steatosis may play a role.

A third important aspect is that during liver surgery deliberate hypotension and temporary hepatic blood inflow occlusion (the so-called Pringle manoeuvre) are used by many surgeons to reduce blood loss during liver surgery (15 minutes ischaemia, 5 minutes reperfusion (15/5 Pringle)). Other surgeons do not use this manoeuvre, assuming that it causes oxidative stress and ischaemia/reperfusion (I/R) injury.[4,5] There is little doubt that this procedure does cause oxidative stress and I/R injury; however, the consequence of this is variable. In a situation where defence mechanisms against oxidative stress are deficient it may adversely affect liver function. In this situation hepatic steatosis may constitute an additional predisposing factor to damage by ischaemia/reperfusion.

Ischaemia/reperfusion is, on the other hand, the basis of ischaemic preconditioning, a process in which temporary clamping and release of the liver blood flow has been shown to be beneficial in terms of increasing resistance to subsequent injury.[6]

In this situation it is assumed that defence mechanisms against oxidative stress are adequate and are indeed enhanced by short-term I/R injury.[7]

The above three factors explain why it has been exceedingly difficult hitherto to design a proper liver function test that reliably singles out those patients at risk of liver failure following liver resection. The term 'liver function' is a rather crude denominator for a range of functions that includes ammonia detoxification, urea synthesis, protein synthesis and breakdown, bile synthesis and secretion, gluconeogenesis and detoxification of drugs, bacteria and bacterial toxins.

Chronic liver failure

The clinical signs of chronic liver failure are often insidious and can also be related to the type of disease. Cirrhosis is associated with a failure of hepatic function and the consequences of increased hepatic vascular resistance. Metabolic impairment is manifest by jaundice, coagulopathy, impaired ammonia clearance and encephalopathy, hypoalbuminaemia and oedema. The presence of increased vascular resistance is associated with the development of splenomegaly, ascites and gastro-oesophageal or abdominal wall varices. The slow progression of many chronic liver diseases, over years, implies a gradual almost incremental loss of liver cell mass or function. There are many causes of liver failure, including hepatitis B and C virus, autoimmune diseases such as primary biliary cirrhosis, primary sclerosing cholangitis and autoimmune hepatitis, alcoholic liver disease, Wilson's disease, α_1-antitrypsin deficiency and others. All are associated with chronic or repeated cell injury and attempts at repair. The fibrosis and scarring associated with this regeneration and repair lead to the clinical condition termed cirrhosis, with a typically small shrunken irregular liver and an increased risk of cancer.

The Child–Pugh score for chronic liver disease[8] has served as a useful means of categorising patients based on the severity of their liver disease. It employs five clinical measures of liver disease and each measure is scored 1–3, with 3 indicating the most severe derangement (Table 1.1).

Table 1.1 • Child–Pugh score for chronic liver disease[8]

Measure	1 point	2 points	3 points	Units
Bilirubin (total)	<34 (<2)	34–50 (2–3)	>50 (>3)	µmol/L (mg/dL)
Serum albumin	>35	28–35	<28	g/L
INR	<1.7	1.71–2.20	>2.20	No unit
Ascites	None	Suppressed with medication	Refractory	No unit
Hepatic encephalopathy	None	Grade I–II (or suppressed with medication)	Grade III–IV (or refractory)	No unit

Metabolic liver function

The liver plays a central role in fat, carbohydrate and protein metabolism, as well as in acid–base homeostasis. In the context of liver failure, disturbances of fat metabolism are probably not crucially important. With respect to carbohydrate metabolism, it is well known that the liver plays a central role in the conversion of lactate to glucose. Part of this lactate is formed due to anaerobic metabolism of, amongst others, glucose in skeletal muscle. This metabolic route of glucose to lactate (muscle) and then back to glucose (liver) is very important for glycaemic homeostasis and is called the Cori cycle. Failure of the liver will be witnessed by lactic acidosis and hypoglycaemia.

Next to its role in carbohydrate metabolism, the liver plays a central function in nitrogen homeostasis. Hepatic synthesis and breakdown of proteins, amino acids and detoxification and clearance of nitrogenous waste products of amino acid and protein metabolism in other organs is of central importance. For example, the gut uses the amino acid glutamine as a fuel for enterocytes, which give rise to the production of waste end-products of intestinal metabolism, like ammonia. This ammonia is then transported by the portal vein to the liver, where it is detoxified by the formation of urea.

Liver failure gives rise to multiple abnormalities in nitrogen metabolism, some of which are thought to play a crucial role in the characteristic syndrome of hepatic encephalopathy that accompanies liver failure. Hepatic encephalopathy is a reversible neuropsychiatric syndrome, with a probably multifactorial cause.[9] The current belief is that ammonia is one of the key components in the aetiology of hepatic encephalopathy[10] because liver failure is usually associated with moderate to severe hyperammonaemia. Hyperammonaemia leads to increased brain uptake of ammonia, followed by detoxification of ammonia in the brain by coupling to glutamate to form glutamine. This process consumes glutamate (an important excitatory neurotransmitter) and leads to the formation of glutamine, which acts as an osmolite causing brain oedema.

One other well-known metabolic abnormality during liver failure is an imbalance in plasma amino acids, notably the ratio between the branched chain amino acids (BCAAs) and the aromatic amino acids (AAAs).

> Some 30 years ago, Fischer and colleagues published their 'unified hypothesis on the pathogenesis of hepatic encephalopathy',[11] based on the observation that, during hepatic failure, plasma levels of BCAAs were decreased and the AAAs were increased.[11–13]

These changes in plasma levels were thought to be caused by increased BCAA catabolism in muscle and decreased AAA breakdown in the failing liver.[14] A reduction in the insulin–glucagon ratio in this situation may play a key role in disturbing the balance between anabolism and catabolism. Accumulation of AAAs in the circulation in combination with the increased breakdown of BCAAs, particularly in skeletal muscle, would according to this hypothesis give rise to a decrease in the BCAA to AAA ratio, the so-called Fischer ratio. The increase in plasma AAAs in combination with increased blood–brain barrier permeability for neutral amino acids has been suggested to contribute to an increased influx of AAAs in the brain, since they compete for the same amino acid transporter. This, in turn, would lead to imbalances in neurotransmitter synthesis and accumulation of false neurotransmitters such as octopamine in the brain, which may contribute to hepatic encephalopathy.[15]

Measuring liver volume

Advances in imaging have permitted the development of in vivo imaging of the liver. Three-dimensional models of the liver can be constructed from computed tomography (CT) scans or other cross-sectional imaging modalities, such as magnetic resonance imaging (MRI). The volume of the liver can then be calculated based on known separation of image slices combined with planar mapping of cross-sectional areas. In addition, such 3-D computer models can be simulated to map the effects of surgery by performing virtual hepatic resection, and studies have demonstrated that there is a good correlation between computer modelling and actual resection weight of surgical liver specimens (**Fig. 1.1**).[2,16]

This technology is useful as a research tool because it allows liver function to be put into the direct context of the volume of functioning liver tissue. In addition, this technology is useful for predicting the need for reconstruction of venous territories of the liver in split liver transplantation. Usually, liver volumetry is performed on software directly linked to the hardware MRI or CT. In recent years, however, stand-alone software has become available, which makes it possible to perform hepatic volumetry remote from the radiological hardware. Examples of such software are the freely downloadable program ImageJ (for Windows-based PCs) and OsiriX (for Apple Macintosh). Our group has recently shown that the ImageJ software is very useful in measuring liver volumes in patients referred with a CT scan already made in the referring centre[17] (**Figs. 1.2 and 1.3**).

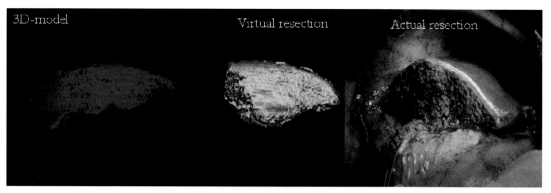

Figure 1.1 • Three-dimensional reconstruction of the liver preoperatively (red) showing tumours (green). Computer prediction of residual liver volume based on virtual hepatectomy of 3-D model (yellow) and actual photograph of resection showing residual liver segments. Reproduced from Schindl MJ, Redhead DN, Fearon KC et al. The value of residual liver volume as a predictor of hepatic dysfunction and infection after major liver resection. Gut 2005; 54:289–96. With permission from the BMJ Publishing Group Ltd.

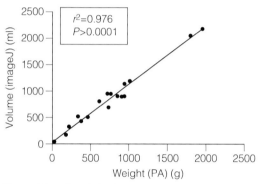

Figure 1.2 • Correlation between volume of resection calculated with ImageJ and actual measured weights of the resection specimens ($n = 15$, Pearson's test).[14] Reproduced with permission from World J Surg.

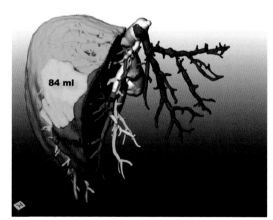

Figure 1.3 • Mapping the territory of the right hepatic lobe drained by the middle hepatic vein. The numbers represent the volumes of the territories at risk if segment 5 and 8 tributaries of the middle hepatic vein were not reconstructed in a potential right lobe living donor liver transplant. Image reproduced with permission of MeVis imaging technologies, Bremen, Germany. (Kindly provided by H. Lang and A. Radtke, Plainz, Germany.)

Blood tests of liver function

As part of many blood chemistry analyses it is possible to request liver function tests. These tests refer to the transaminases, alkaline phosphatase, γ-glutamyl transferase and bilirubin. These tests are not truly measures of function but do give an indication of processes going on within the liver. Aspartate aminotransferase and alanine aminotransferase are hepatocyte enzymes which are released in conditions in which hepatocytes are damaged or killed, such as ischaemic injury, hepatitis, severe sepsis and in response to cancer. Liver-specific alkaline phosphatase is expressed predominantly in the biliary epithelium and is elevated in conditions such as cholangitis or biliary obstruction. γ-Glutamyl transferase is expressed by both hepatocytes and biliary epithelium, and can also be induced by high alcohol consumption.

Biochemical markers of true liver function vary depending on whether acute or chronic liver failure or injury is being considered (Table 1.2).

Table 1.2 • Blood tests useful to assess function in acute and chronic liver injury

	Acute	**Chronic**
Albumin	–	+++
Prothrombin time	+++	+++
Bilirubin	+	+++
Lactate	++	–
Glucose requirement	++	–
Ammonia	+	+

Tests of liver function measuring metabolite clearance

Various tests have been developed to predict liver function. All of these have, over the years, been proven to have insufficient sensitivity and specificity to predict liver function and outcome on the level of the individual patient. The tests currently in common use, e.g. the indocyanine green (ICG) clearance test, lidocaine clearance test, the aminopyrine breath test, the galactose elimination test, and the combination of serum transaminases, bilirubin and clotting factors, are all static tests that only provide point estimates of liver function. None of these tests challenges the liver to demonstrate its full functional capacity. The most commonly used test for liver function prior to liver resections is the ICG clearance test.

Indocyanine green (ICG)

ICG is a compound that is used widely to measure liver function. It is rapidly cleared from blood by hepatocytes and is excreted into bile. ICG clearance can be measured as 'disappearance' from the blood or can also be measured as accumulation in bile. Liver dysfunction is demonstrated as a slower rate of clearance from the blood and is usually expressed as percentage retention at 5 or 15 minutes after injection. Continuous measurement of ICG clearance can also be performed which offers the potential improvement in accuracy of measurement of area under the clearance curve (**Fig. 1.4**).

A disadvantage of the ICG clearance test is that it is not a true liver function test, but more a blood flow-dependent clearance test. The fact that this test has not found its way into general practice in a more widespread fashion provides circumstantial evidence that it is not good enough. Equally, this test does not provide information on the capacity of the liver to increase its function following a challenge.

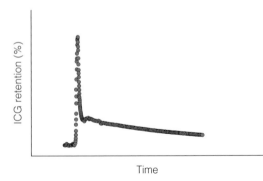

Figure 1.4 • Typical ICG clearance curve for a subject with healthy liver function.

Lidocaine (MEG-X)

Lidocaine, also known as monoethylglycinexylidide (MEG-X), is a local anaesthetic that is taken up by the liver and undergoes biotransformation by a cytochrome P450 enzyme, CYP1A2. The rate of disappearance of lidocaine from plasma correlates with liver function; however, measurement of lidocaine is more complex than that of ICG.

Aminopyrine breath test

The aminopyrine breath test was the first breath test that has been proposed for the assessment of liver function in patients with liver disease. The test uses $^{13}C_2$-aminopyrine, which is a stable, non-radioactive, isotopically labelled compound eliminated almost exclusively by the liver. Following oral intake, the compound is taken up by the gut and then transported to the liver, where it is metabolised by microsomal cytochrome P450 function. This metabolism will liberate $^{13}CO_2$, which can be measured non-invasively in exhaled air. This test is not readily available at the bedside and requires fairly sophisticated apparatus to measure stable isotopic enrichment in the exhaled air. Induction of microsomal metabolism by various drugs may constitute a problem.

Urea synthesis

In the recent past, we have explored the feasibility of measuring urea synthesis using stable isotopes and relating this to liver volume in patients undergoing liver resection.[18] This study was conducted against the background of the notion that liver failure is almost always accompanied by hyperammonaemia, related to a presumed failure of hepatic urea synthesis. Using stable isotopically ^{13}C-labelled urea, urea synthesis was measured before and after major hepatic resection, and liver volumes before and after resection with CT scans.

Major hepatic resection did not affect total body ureagenesis, because the synthesis of urea per gram of residual liver went up and increased 2.6-fold.[18] Therefore, it is unlikely that urea synthesis is a limiting factor in the initial aetiology of liver failure and this test is not likely to contribute to predicting which patient's liver will fail following liver resection.

Glutathione synthesis

Unfortunately, most of the above tests focus on very specific functions or pathways. None of them assesses the main hepatic protection system against many diverse forms of stress and intoxications: the intracellular content and synthesis of glutathione (GSH). It is generally accepted that GSH plays a key role in the protection of the liver against many forms of stress, ischaemia and toxic compounds such as paracetamol. Unfortunately, there is currently no adequate test to assess hepatic GSH synthesis and metabolism in vivo in humans, even though such a test would be of great clinical importance. We have previously explored the feasibility of measuring GSH synthesis in vivo during liver surgery in humans using stable isotopically labelled $^2H_2$-glycine, a component of GSH (γ-glutamyl-cysteinyl-glycine), but this approach was not suitable, because part of the deuterium label of glycine was lost (unpublished data). Future research will have to focus on designing a test that is both dynamic and which focuses on the GSH system, making it possible to determine liver function correlated to the liver's volume, and assess a person's risk of developing liver failure upon liver resection.

Measuring liver blood flow

Blood flow in the splanchnic area, particularly the gut and liver, can be measured in a number of ways. These can basically be either invasive (i.e. intraoperative) or non-invasive. During surgery, when the abdomen is opened, blood flow can be measured in the portal vein and in the main hepatic artery. Portal vein blood flow measurements provide predominantly information on the flow across the intestines. By summing up the blood flow in the hepatic artery and the portal vein, total hepatic blood flow can be calculated. Theoretically, this could also be achieved by measuring hepatic venous outflow, but this is impractical in humans because of the short common outflow tract of the three hepatic veins.

Such measurements of hepatic and portal arterial blood flow can be obtained using 6–8 mm and 12–14 mm handle ultrasonic flow probes respectively (Transonic Systems, Kimal PLC, Uxbridge, UK). Essentially, the vessels have to be dissected free for this flow measurement and the 3/4 circular probe is applied to the vessel. These probes are believed to provide the most accurate technique for assessing flow in relatively small vessels. However, there is considerable variability in measurement related to Doppler ultrasound signal strength and coupling with the vessel wall. Also, there are likely to be changes in diameter of the artery, in particular related to its handling during surgery. The advantage is that repeated measurements can be obtained and that the surgeon can operate this application without help from a radiologist. Likewise, post-resection blood flow measurements can be taken before closure of the abdomen, typically 1–2 hours after the first measurement. This gives an impression of blood flow across the residual liver following major resections.

During liver surgery, organ blood flow can also be measured by means of colour Doppler ultrasound scanning (e.g. Aloka Prosound SSD 5000; Aloka Co, Ltd, Tokyo, Japan). A 5 MHz probe is used to trace the vessels and calculate the cross-sectional area. Then, time-averaged mean velocities of the bloodstream are measured at the point where the cross-sectional area of the portal vein and hepatic artery is taken. For accurate velocity measurements, care must be taken to keep the angle between the ultrasonic beam direction and blood flow direction below 60°. The cross-sectional area of the vessel is calculated by drawing an area ellipse at the same point as where the velocity was measured. Portal venous and hepatic arterial blood flows can then be measured proximal to their hilar bifurcations. In the case of an accessory hepatic artery, both arteries should obviously be measured.[19,20] In our experience, this method gives roughly the same values as the ultrasonic flow measurement described above. Theoretically, it is possible to perform such flow measurements preoperatively or postoperatively using a percutaneous approach, although the measurement in the hepatic artery requires a skilled ultrasonographer.

In recent years, technical improvements in hardware and software applications for MRI have made it possible to measure blood flow in the portal vein and hepatic artery in a non-invasive manner. By linking this method of flow measurement to hepatic volumetry using MRI, blood flow per volume unit of liver can be calculated.[21,22] Our limited personal experience with MRI blood flow measurement would suggest that there is a need for quite substantial improvements in the technique.

A further technique which is emerging is the use of near-infrared spectroscopy. This technique measures absorption of near-infrared wavelength light and from this can be calculated tissue oxygenation, since haemoglobin oxygenation status alters absorption of this wavelength light. This technique is more useful for estimating tissue oxygenation and perfusion at a sinusoidal level, but could potentially be combined with other measures to estimate liver blood flow.[23]

Effect of major liver resection on hepatic blood flow

Direct measurement of hepatic artery and portal vein blood flow before and after liver resection reveals interesting results. When expressed as absolute values portal blood flow does not change whereas hepatic artery blood flow falls. Typically, portal vein flow is approximately 840 mL/min and post-resection 805 mL/min. Using this method, hepatic artery flow pre-resection is about 450 mL/min and post-resection 270 mL/min. When these flows are expressed in relation to the preoperative liver volume and residual postoperative liver volume, it can be seen that the blood flow per gram of liver tissue increases in portal flow from a mean 0.55 mL/min per g liver to 1.09 mL/min per g liver and the hepatic artery flow remains relatively constant (**Fig. 1.5**). In experimental research, pressure measurements can also be obtained using radial artery invasive monitoring to estimate hepatic artery pressure and direct portal vein pressure measurement using a small needle coupled to a pressure transducer similar to that used for measuring central venous pressure. The combination of flow and pressure measurement then allows calculation of hepatic sinusoidal resistance (**Fig. 1.5**).

The effect of major liver resection on innate immunity

The liver forms an important part of the innate immune system by producing acute-phase proteins and other opsonins, proteins which bind to bacteria facilitating their phagocytosis. In addition, 85% of the reticuloendothelial system is located in the liver (Kupffer cells) and clearly surgical resection will involve a reduction of this cell mass.

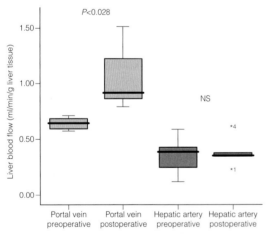

Figure 1.5 • Directly measured blood flow intraoperatively in six patients during major hepatic resection. Measurements were taken from the main portal vein and the main hepatic artery simultaneously using multichannel Transonics ultrasound flow probes. During the liver resection one branch of each of the portal vein and hepatic artery are ligated. The post-resection blood flow measurement has been taken just before closure of the abdomen, typically 1–2 hours after the first measurement. Results are expressed per gram of liver tissue.

It is not unreasonable to expect that major liver resection might result in some impairment of innate immunity. Our group has previously demonstrated that major liver resection is associated with increased frequency of infection as well as increased likelihood of objective evidence of liver function impairment.[2]

In a separate study, our group has also shown that major liver resection is associated with a temporary defect in the ability of the reticuloendothelial system to clear albumin microspheres which were used as a surrogate for bacteria.

> This study demonstrated that loss of approximately 50% of liver volume such as might occur during a right hepatectomy was associated with impairment of reticuloendothelial cell clearance equivalent to that of non-surgical patients with Child C chronic liver disease.[24]

The liver also synthesises and exports many acute-phase proteins involved in innate immunity or homeostasis. C-reactive protein, for example, binds to phosphoryl choline moieties of encapsulated bacteria and acts as an opsonin, promoting phagocytosis. Mannan-binding lectin, complement fragments and α_1-acid glycoprotein (orosomucoid) can also act as opsonins. Transferrin and caeruloplasmin are important in the binding and carriage of free metal ions and α_1-antitrypsin and α_1-antichymotrypsin act as antiproteases. Liver failure or liver surgery may be associated with a reduction in synthesis of some of these acute-phase proteins (mannan-binding lectin, haptoglobin, α-fetuin and fibronectin) whereas the concentrations of others may be increased despite a reduction in functional liver tissue (C-reactive protein, liver fatty acid-binding protein; unpublished data). The exact significance of these changes is unclear but may contribute to a global impairment in innate immunity in the injured liver.

Liver regeneration

The liver is unique in that it is the only organ in the adult that is capable of regenerating or renewing itself to restore the ratio between pre-injury liver volume and body weight. Knowledge of the capacity for the liver to regenerate is presumed to be ancient and is the basis for the punishment meted out by Zeus to Prometheus, who according to Greek mythology was chained to a rock and had his liver eaten daily by a vulture (only for it to regenerate overnight). This continued for several years until the vulture was finally killed by

Heracles, who also released Prometheus. While the speed of liver regeneration is exaggerated in this myth it is true that it is an extremely rapid process. In the context of surgery liver regeneration happens very rapidly, with most of the cell division required for regeneration occurring within 72 hours of injury. Full liver function and volume are usually restored within 6–12 weeks. In chronic injury or in the presence of fibrosis, liver regeneration can be chaotic with repeated insults causing scarring, and nodular regeneration with disordered architecture leading to cirrhosis.

Molecular signals for hepatic regeneration

At a cellular level liver regeneration depends on the coexistence of three key factors: changes in the microenvironment of the liver cell supporting growth, the ability of differentiated hepatocytes to proliferate and inhibition of processes, linking injury to programmed cell death.

Stimuli for liver regeneration stimulate transcription factors which turn on a variety of genes expressing growth factors. Although not direct growth factors, the hormones insulin and adrenaline potentiate the effects of growth factors on hepatocyte regeneration. All elements of the liver are required to regenerate; however, the coordination of these processes is complex. Removal of the stimulus for regeneration by growth to pre-injury capacity and transforming growth factor-β act as brakes which slow regeneration of liver elements (**Fig. 1.6**).

Recently, it has been suggested that platelets and their serotonin content play an important role in the mouse in liver regeneration following resection.[25,26]

Barriers to hepatic regeneration include cirrhosis and fibrosis and ongoing liver injury such as might occur with biliary obstruction or sepsis.

Cell populations involved in liver regeneration

Histology of normal liver regeneration following resection or acute injury shows the presence of high mitotic rates in mature hepatocytes. Normally, these cells are mitotically quiescent but can move into S phase extremely rapidly. For example, following 70% hepatectomy in a rat approximately 30–40% of hepatocytes are seen to be undergoing mitosis within 48 hours of surgery and indeed the liver will regain its normal size within 10 days. The situation is more complex in chronically injured liver (e.g. cirrhotic liver); here, the hepatocytes are less able to undergo mitosis and are frequently in cell cycle arrest. Furthermore, the accumulation of excess scar tissue deposited in cirrhosis contributes to the inability of the liver to respond to injury and regenerate effectively. In this setting a second population of cells becomes activated and can contribute to parenchymal regeneration. These intrahepatic cells are located in the canal of Hering (the most distal branch of the biliary tree); termed hepatic progenitor cells (HPCs), they are bipotential and are capable of giving rise to both biliary and hepatocyte populations. This response is seen in chronic or severe injury and sometimes appears as a ductular reaction. Although it is now recognised that the HPCs can regenerate the liver in chronic liver disease, whether these progenitor cells are capable of responding to the acute demands of major hepatic resection is as yet unknown. It is also worth noting that there is an increasing recognition that intrahepatic stem cells are a likely source of a significant proportion of liver cancers. The role of circulating extrahepatic cells in liver regeneration has received interest recently and the potential bone marrow origin of hepatocytes has been suggested. However, if this phenomenon occurs at all, it is extremely rare. The bone marrow does, however, supply macrophages and myofibroblasts that are involved in the liver's scarring response to injury. There has been recent interest in the use of bone marrow population to

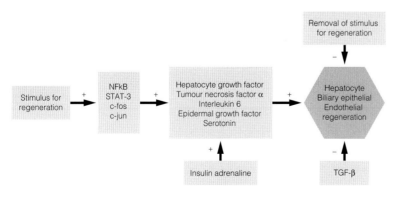

Figure 1.6 • Schematic of some of the factors known to regulate liver regeneration.

stimulate liver regeneration in both animal models and clinical studies (see later), and this is likely to be an area of future development.

Consequences of surgery

Unfortunately, at present it is unclear what the key mechanisms of liver failure are, and why the liver usually regenerates but sometimes progresses into liver failure. It is believed that ischaemia/reperfusion (I/R) injury plays an important role in the sequence of events leading to liver failure. Hepatic resections are major surgical procedures, often leading to significant blood loss. In order to reduce blood loss, central venous pressure is reduced during liver surgery and hepatobiliary surgeons frequently occlude hepatic blood inflow temporarily (Pringle manoeuvre). Obviously, all these factors may contribute to I/R injury in the liver. A key component of I/R injury is the generation of oxygen free radicals. The latter can induce ischaemic necrosis and caspase-dependent apoptosis, and may contribute to failure of vital metabolic synthetic pathways. However, it remains to be investigated which one of these plays a key role during liver failure. In this context, it has been proposed that the balance between hepatocyte regeneration and apoptosis can be tipped towards either side by hepatic defence mechanisms against oxygen free radical damage. Also, oxygen free radicals play a role in determining whether apoptosis or ischaemic necrosis occurs in the liver. Apparently, the equilibrium between oxygen free radicals and their scavengers plays a pivotal role in determining whether regeneration or decay occurs. Glutathione (GSH) is the principal oxygen free radical scavenger in the liver and the principal defence mechanism against I/R damage. Hepatic GSH levels decrease following I/R damage, inflammation and nutritional deprivation. It seems conceivable that a reduction in liver volume following surgery contributes to insufficient hepatic free radical scavenging capacity as a consequence of reduced GSH synthesis. I/R injury may aggravate this situation.

Small for size syndrome

The original descriptions of small for size syndrome described a condition arising in split liver transplantation characterised by the development of ascites, portal hypertension and liver dysfunction in an otherwise healthy transplanted portion of liver. The underlying cause for this syndrome is believed to relate to blood flow and the failure of a small liver volume to cope with often very high blood flows of patients with previous chronic liver disease undergoing transplantation. The validity of this hypothesis was supported by the observation that partial diversion of portal blood flow in to the graft using a portocaval shunt could limit

or prevent the development of small for size syndrome. Subsequently, other manoeuvres have also been effected such as ligation or embolisation of the splenic artery, which works in the same way by reducing portal vein flow.

In patients undergoing even very major liver resection it is rare to develop small for size syndrome. Some patients do, however, develop ascites, jaundice and a chronic liver dysfunction, and it is more likely that this syndrome is more dependent on a failure to regenerate rather than excessive blood flow.

Hepatic steatosis

Fat infiltration of the liver is an increasing problem with increased prevalence of obesity and the metabolic syndrome (obesity and type 2 diabetes). Macroscopically the liver may appear enlarged, pale or yellow coloured with rounded edges. Microscopically the liver can have microsteatosis (small fat droplets within every hepatocyte) or macrosteatosis (regional infiltration of hepatocytes with large fat droplets) (see **Fig. 1.7**).

Assessment of steatosis

Assessment of hepatic steatosis is notoriously difficult. Experienced surgeons can estimate liver fat by judging the size, rounded or sharp edges of the liver and its appearance. Even using colour as an estimate is prone to error, as can be seen in **Fig. 1.8**.

The gold standard for hepatic fat assessment is histology. Trucut or wedge biopsies can be assessed by a pathologist and a reliable estimate of the percentage fat content produced. In addition, useful information including the distribution – macrosteatosis or microsteatosis – and the presence of fibrosis or inflammation can be provided.

Chemotherapy-induced liver changes

Increased usage of chemotherapy in the neoadjuvant context has revealed changes in the liver associated with chemotherapy, particularly oxaliplatin

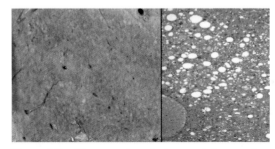

Figure 1.7 • Macroscopic and microscopic images of steatotic liver.

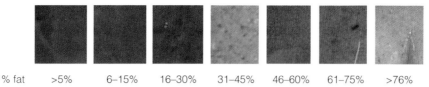

| % fat | >5% | 6–15% | 16–30% | 31–45% | 46–60% | 61–75% | >76% |

Figure 1.8 • Physical appearance of livers with varying fat content confirmed by histology to demonstrate the poor correlation between colour and objective measurement of fat content.

and irinotecan. These range from a soft, fragile pale liver to steatosis, steatohepatitis and sinusoidal dilatation. Surgery should be deferred until 6 weeks after chemotherapy and studies, although conflicting, suggest that tolerance of major liver resection may be reduced and complications more frequent in individuals who have received chemotherapy. A study by Mehta and colleagues[27] showed that oxaliplatin-based chemotherapy was associated with increased blood loss and prolonged hospital stay.

Portal vein embolisation

Morbidity and mortality after hepatectomy has constituted a limitation of the number of patients eligible for resection, and currently only 8% of patients with colorectal hepatic metastases are candidates for curative liver resection. Liver function is correlated with liver volume, and consequently hepatic insufficiency in this situation may arise because not enough functional liver volume is left after surgical removal of part of the liver. Interestingly, following removal of part of the liver, the residual liver usually regenerates to the point where the preoperative liver weight–body weight ratio is regained. This notion has led to the belief that if it were possible to increase preoperatively the volume of the future residual liver, it would be possible to perform more extensive liver resections and hence cure more patients. It has long been recognised that interruption of one part of the liver portal blood flow usually leads to hypertrophy of normally vascularised liver. This has been learned from the treatment of Klatskin tumours, which have a tendency of invading the portal vein, causing ipsilateral atrophy and contralateral hypertrophy. This concept has subsequently been harnessed by manoeuvres such as embolising the right portal vein prior to surgical resection. This leads to hypertrophy of the left liver lobe prior to surgery and facilitates the subsequent safe extensive resection of the right liver (extended right hepatectomy) 6 weeks later (**Fig. 1.9**). This phenomenon has been harnessed to maximise the residual functional liver volume of patients who are predicted to have a small remnant liver volume. This approach is fully based on the concept that, in the normal liver, volume is correlated to function and hence liver failure occurs when residual liver volume is too small. A completely different and novel approach would be to improve liver function per volume unit of liver. Limitations to portal vein embolisation (PVE)-induced hypertrophy include pre-existing hepatic fibrosis or cirrhosis and technical or anatomical inability to completely obstruct a major portal vein branch.

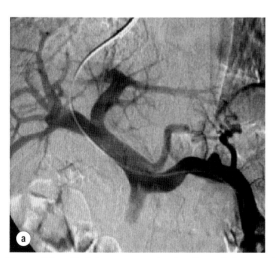 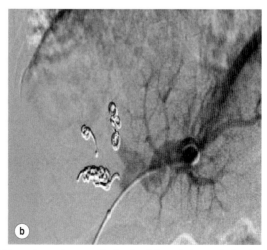

Figure 1.9 • Portal venograms showing the main left and right branches prior to embolisation **(a)**, and after embolisation of the right portal vein **(b)**.

Technique

The most common technique of PVE is to puncture a branch of the vein using a percutaneous approach. A venogram is obtained to demonstrate all of the relevant branches and then the branch to be embolised is cannulated and coils and embolic material delivered to obstruct portal flow. A check angiogram can be performed to demonstrate success of the technique. Usually either a left or right main branch is occluded. To obtain hypertrophy of segments 2 and 3 in large right-sided tumours, it is not sufficient to embolise just the right portal vein and it is recommended that the two (usually) branches supplying segment 4 should also be embolised. Patients usually tolerate PVE remarkably well, presumably because of the dual blood supply of the liver and complications are uncommon. Significant hypertrophy can be achieved, as can be seen in **Fig. 1.10**.

Therapy for liver failure

N-Acetyl cysteine

Glutathione depletion is a major problem in patients with paracetamol (acetaminophen) toxicity. *N*-Acetyl cysteine has been used for many years as a treatment for early paracetamol poisoning. It is thought to act by replenishing glutathione stores and by providing alternative thiol groups to which damaging reactive oxygen species can bind. The realisation that reactive oxygen species can be generated by conditions other than paracetamol poisoning such as sepsis and ischaemia/reperfusion has led to *N*-acetyl cysteine being used in a more general way to support patients with early evidence of liver dysfunction or failure.

Nutritional support in liver failure

The role of nutritional support in acute liver failure is uncertain largely because of a lack of evidence in the world literature. Enteral nutrition is known to preserve gut barrier function and thus might be considered to be beneficial in the context of liver failure. In addition, the provision of energy might be considered beneficial in the context of glycogen storage failure, and to fuel the regeneration of liver tissue and recover function. The limited ability of the failing liver to handle nitrogen and synthesise urea (potentially exacerbating encephalopathy) would argue against excessive provision of proteins unless these were in a form where they did not contribute to the circulating ammonia load.

Artificial extracorporeal liver support

Many patients who take toxic doses of paracetamol never develop liver failure; others demonstrate evidence of liver impairment which resolves spontaneously. Indeed, it is a small minority of patients who develop irretrievable liver failure and either require liver transplantation or die. The realisation that liver failure in the acute setting was often reversible if the organism could be kept alive stimulated different approaches to replace or reproduce liver functions to act either as a bridge to recovery or as a bridge to transplantation. Clearly such systems could also have a role in supporting the patient who develops severe liver dysfunction following liver resection.

Detoxification systems

Molecular adsorbents recirculation system (MARS)

Recently, experience is accumulating with MARS during liver failure. These systems have been shown to normalise certain of the metabolic abnormalities induced by hepatic failure. Thus, a low Fischer ratio can be corrected by recirculating albumin dialysis.[28] The MARS system removes both water-soluble and protein-bound toxins.[29] Because the system preferentially removes AAAs compared with BCAAs, the Fischer ratio significantly increases, predomi-

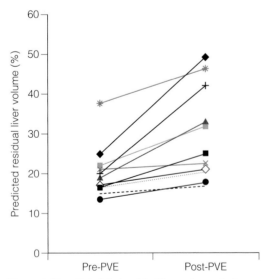

Figure 1.10 • Calculated residual liver volumes before and after portal vein embolisation (PVE) in patients scheduled to undergo major liver resection.

nantly by the removal of AAAs in a small series of patients.[28,30–32] MARS has been shown to be useful in fulminant hepatic failure, by attenuating the increase in intracranial pressure which plays a major role in this situation.[29] There may also be an effect on survival and improvement of degree of hepatic encephalopathy in patients with acute or chronic liver failure.[31,33] Equally, the system has been tested on artificial neuronal networks showing a normalisation of abnormal signals if the medium (plasma derived from rats with liver failure) was pretreated with MARS. The role of MARS in a more chronic situation of mild hepatic encephalopathy, when correction of an abnormal Fischer ratio would likely be more important if this were a major pathogenetic factor, is still largely unknown and deserves further study.[34] A recent editorial suggests that the role of MARS and bioartificial liver support systems should be limited to carefully designed clinical trials.[35] It is currently uncertain how hepatic excretory assist devices, such as MARS, compare with bioartificial liver assist devices, which in addition to their excretory functions also have biosynthetic capacity.[31]

Bioartificial liver systems

The knowledge that patients with acute liver failure are likely to recover if they can be supported for sufficient time to allow liver regeneration was the impetus behind the development of bioartificial liver systems. A number of largely experimental models have been built and some have even been used to support a small number of patients. All work on the same principle of 'dialysing' the patient's blood though a cartridge containing hepatocytes. The design of bioartificial liver systems is challenging and the large surface area of hepatocytes needed to be effective is difficult. Engineering scaffolds of membranes or tubules has been the most popular approach. In normal liver, hepatocytes are polarised and have an epithelial surface. However, it is still to be determined how to recreate this polarity and its absolute importance has yet to be defined. One of the major problems with these systems is what type of cells to use and a variety of different approaches has been taken. Animal hepatocytes perform many of the same functions as human hepatocytes, although some of the proteins produced are obviously different. Human immortalised cell lines are an attractive proposition and some of the more differentiated cell lines can replicate many of the normal hepatocyte functions. Hepatocytes grow better in association with non-parenchymal cells; however, the creation of co-cultures in reactors produces its own problems. Cells must maintain viability or be able to be replenished to provide liver support over a prolonged period of time. In addition, very sick patients require a short time period to set up the support system, and the reactor must be easy to use by critical care nurses, safe from contamination and not overly expensive. For all of these reasons, bioartificial liver systems remain a tantalising prospect which has yet to break through into routine clinical practice.

Liver transplantation

Irreversible acute or chronic liver failure is amenable to treatment by liver transplantation. It is extremely uncommon for patients who have undergone liver resection to subsequently require or proceed to liver transplantation. The most obvious reason for this is that many patients who undergo liver resection do so for metastatic or primary liver cancer and transplantation would be contraindicated because of the risk of immunosuppression and aggressive recrudescence of the tumour. A number of patients with bile duct injury have progressed to transplantation usually in a chronic setting following the development of biliary stricture, cholangitis and secondary biliary cirrhosis. Similarly a number of patients who have undergone a 'cancer resection' for what turned out to be a benign biliary stricture perhaps as part of primary sclerosing cholangitis fail to regenerate their livers and may progress to transplantation.

Cell therapy for liver failure: general principles

A number of key principles have operated as key drivers for the development of cell therapies for clinical treatment of liver failure. Firstly, it is recognised that the injured liver usually provides a rich environment stimulating tissue regeneration and the liver can normally 'heal' itself. Secondly, in animal models there is evidence that stem cells or non-parenchymal cells can support regeneration of hepatocytes. Thirdly, it is recognised that the difference between liver failure and compensated liver function in terms of cellular functional equivalents is probably very small. Finally, it would be preferable to support the liver by techniques that were within the body rather than using extracorporeal devices. This desire has stimulated research into therapeutic application of cell or stem cell transplantation.

The dual goals of stem cell therapy in the context of acute liver failure or injury are to promote rapid recovery of hepatocyte function and to allow regeneration of liver tissue without excessive scarring.

Haemopoetic stem cell therapy for liver disease in humans

There are several reports in the scientific literature of bone marrow (BM) stem cell therapy in patients with advanced liver disease. It was first reported that BM stem cells could increase the liver's ability to regenerate in patients who were undergoing hepatic resection for various liver cancers sited in the right lobe. Here the patients underwent embolisation of the right branch of the portal vein prior to surgery to stimulate compensatory hypertrophy of the left lobe. Autologous CD133-positive BM stem cells were injected into the blood vessels that supply the left liver lobe shortly after the surgery[36] and accelerated regeneration of the non-embolised section of the liver was seen compared with control patients. However, it must be stated that this was a small non-randomised study. The second report[37] used BM stem cells in patients with liver cirrhosis. CD34-positive stem cells were isolated from the patients' own blood following granulocyte colony-stimulating factor (GCSF)-induced haematopoietic stem cell mobilisation and were re-injected into the blood supply to the liver – preliminary evidence appeared to show that improvement in liver function in three out of five of the patients occurred during this therapy. In the third study, patients with liver cirrhosis had mononuclear cells isolated from

their own BM during general anaesthesia.[38] These cells were re-injected into the patient's blood stream and again the patient's liver function appeared to improve. Although these studies are very encouraging, they are preliminary, of small numbers and non-randomised. Furthermore, in none of these studies were the cells marked to enable identification either by radiological tracking or in biopsies of the liver tissue. Therefore, a number of important questions are unanswered. It is not certain that these cells definitely settled in the liver over a period of time, whether some of the cells engrafted other organs in the body and by what mechanisms the cells were having their positive effects within the recipient's livers.

Future developments

The ability to exert greater control in modulating liver volume and function in the surgical patient would be a major advantage. Preoperative functional enhancement might expand the group of patients who would be amenable to surgery, while postoperative intervention might be useful in liver resection, transplantation and acute liver failure as a means of rescuing a failing liver. The potential to use autologous stem cells derived from bone marrow to stimulate liver regeneration has enormous potential if its positive effects are seen in larger randomised studies.

Key points

- Conventional measures of liver function are poor and take no account of liver volume.
- Liver resection leaving a residual liver volume of <25% is associated with a high risk of liver dysfunction and infection.
- In patients with chronic liver disease smaller resections can be dangerous.
- The combination of liver dysfunction and sepsis can be fatal.
- Preoperative portal vein embolisation and newer regenerative strategies may improve the safety of liver surgery.

References

1. O'Grady JG, Alexander GJ, Hayllar KM et al. Early indicators of prognosis in fulminant hepatic failure. Gastroenterology 1989; 97:439–45.

2. Schindl MJ, Redhead DN, Fearon KC et al. The value of residual liver volume as a predictor of hepatic dysfunction and infection after major liver resection. Gut 2005; 54:289–96.

   The first paper providing strong evidence of an association between residual liver volume and clinical infection.

3. van Hoorn EC, van Middelaar-Voskuilen MC, van Limpt CJ et al. Preoperative supplementation with a carbohydrate mixture decreases organ dysfunction-associated risk factors. Clin Nutr 2005; 24:114–23.

4. Kretzschmar M, Kruger A, Schirrmeister W. Hepatic ischemia–reperfusion syndrome after partial liver resection (LR): hepatic venous oxygen saturation, enzyme pattern, reduced and oxidized glutathione,

procalcitonin and interleukin-6. Exp Toxicol Pathol 2003; 54:423–31.

5. Garcea G, Gescher A, Steward W et al. Oxidative stress in humans following the Pringle manoeuvre. Hepatobil Pancreat Dis Int 2006; 5:210–14.

6. Clavien PA, Yadav S, Sindram D et al. Protective effects of ischemic preconditioning for liver resection performed under inflow occlusion in humans. Ann Surg 2000; 232:155–62.

The first randomised clinical trial demonstrating benefit in clinical markers from ischaemic preconditioning of the liver in patients undergoing liver resection.

7. Patel A, van de Poll MC, Greve JW et al. Early stress protein gene expression in a human model of ischemic preconditioning. Transplantation 2004; 78(27):1479–87.

8. Pugh RN, Murray-Lyon IM, Dawson JL et al. Transection of the oesophagus for bleeding oesophageal varices. Br J Surg 1973; 60:646–9.

9. Albrecht J, Jones EA. Hepatic encephalopathy: molecular mechanisms underlying the clinical syndrome. J Neurol Sci 1999; 170:138–46.

10. Shawcross D, Jalan R. The pathophysiologic basis of hepatic encephalopathy: central role for ammonia and inflammation. Cell Molec Life Sci 2005; 62:2295–304.

11. James JH, Ziparo V, Jeppsson B, Fischer JE. Hyperammonaemia, plasma aminoacid imbalance, and blood–brain amino acid transport: a unified theory of portal-systemic encephalopathy. Lancet 1979; 2:772–5.

Explanation of the relationship between the urea cycle and hepatic encephalopathy.

12. Fischer JE, Yoshimura N, Aguirre A et al. Plasma amino acids in patients with hepatic encephalopathy. Effects of amino acid infusions. Am J Surg 1974; 127:40–7.

13. Soeters PB, Fischer JE. Insulin, glucagon, aminoacid imbalance, and hepatic encephalopathy. Lancet 1976; 2:880–2.

14. Fischer JE, Rosen HM, Ebeid AM et al. The effect of normalization of plasma amino acids on hepatic encephalopathy in man. Surgery 1976; 80: 77–91.

15. Fischer JE, Baldessarini RJ. False neurotransmitters and hepatic failure. Lancet 1971; 2:75–80.

16. Wigmore SJ, Redhead DN, Yan XJ et al. Virtual hepatic resection using three-dimensional reconstruction of helical computed tomography angioportograms. Ann Surg 2001; 233:221–6.

17. Dello SA, van Dam RM, Slangen JJ et al. Liver volumetry plug and play: do it yourself with ImageJ. World J Surg 2007; 31:2215–21.

18. van de Poll MC, Wigmore SJ, Redhead DN et al. Effect of major liver resection on hepatic urea-genesis in humans. Am J Physiol Gastrointest Liver Physiol. 2007; 293:G956–62.

Clinical experimental study demonstrating the relationship between liver volume and urea synthesis in patients undergoing varying degrees of liver resection.

19. van de Poll MC, Ligthart-Melis GC, Boelens PG et al. Intestinal and hepatic metabolism of glutamine and citrulline in humans. J Physiol. 2007; 581:819–27.

20. van de Poll MC, Siroen MP, van Leeuwen PA et al. Interorgan amino acid exchange in humans: consequences for arginine and citrulline metabolism. Am J Clin Nutr 2007; 85:167–72.

21. Barbaro B, Manfredi R, Bombardieri G et al. Correlation of MRI liver volume and Doppler sonographic portal hemodynamics with histologic findings in patients with chronic hepatitis C. J Clin Ultrasound 2000; 28:461–8.

22. Nanashima A, Shibasaki S, Sakamoto I et al. Clinical evaluation of magnetic resonance imaging flowmetry of portal and hepatic veins in patients following hepatectomy. Liver Int 2006; 26:587–94.

23. El-Desoky AE, Seifalian A, Cope M et al. Changes in tissue oxygenation of the porcine liver measured by near-infrared spectroscopy. Liver Transpl Surg 1999; 5:219–26.

24. Schindl MJ, Millar AM, Redhead DN et al. The adaptive response of the reticuloendothelial system to major liver resection in humans. Ann Surg 2006; 243:507–14.

25. Lesurtel M, Graf R, Aleil B et al. Platelet-derived serotonin mediates liver regeneration. Science 2006; 312:104–7.

26. Clavien PA, Petrowsky H, DeOliveira ML et al. Strategies for safer liver surgery and partial liver transplantation. N Engl J Med 2007; 356:1545–59.

27. Mehta NN, Ravikumar R, Coldham CA et al. Effect of preoperative chemotherapy on liver resection for colorectal liver metastases. Eur J Surg Oncol 2008; 34:782–6.

28. Loock J, Mitzner SR, Peters E et al. Amino acid dysbalance in liver failure is favourably influenced by recirculating albumin dialysis (MARS). Liver 2002; 22(Suppl 2):35–9.

29. Tan HK. Molecular adsorbent recirculating system (MARS). Ann Acad Med Singapore 2004; 33:329–35.

30. Awad SS, Swaniker F, Magee J et al. Results of a phase I trial evaluating a liver support device utilizing albumin dialysis. Surgery 2001; 130:354–62.

31. Mitzner S, Loock J, Peszynski P et al. Improvement in central nervous system functions during treatment of liver failure with albumin dialysis MARS – a review of clinical, biochemical, and electrophysiological data. Metab Brain Dis 2002; 17:463–75.

32. Steczko J, Bax KC, Ash SR. Effect of hemodiabsorption and sorbent-based pheresis on amino acid levels in hepatic failure. Int J Artif Organs 2000; 23:375–88.

33. Boyle M, Kurtovic J, Bihari D et al. Equipment review: the molecular adsorbents recirculating system (MARS). Crit Care 2004; 8:280–6.

34. Hassanein TI, Tofteng F, Brown RS Jr et al. Randomized controlled study of extracorporeal albumin dialysis for hepatic encephalopathy in advanced cirrhosis. Hepatology 2007; 46:1853–62.

35. Ferenci P, Kramer L. MARS and the failing liver – Any help from the outer space? Hepatology. 2007; 46:1682–4.

36. am Esch JS 2nd, Knoefel WT, Klein M et al. Portal application of autologous CD133+ BM cells to the liver: a novel concept to support hepatic regeneration. Stem Cells 2005; 23:463–70.

37. Gordon MY, Levicar N, Pai M et al. Characterisation and clinical application of human CD34+ stem/progenitor cell populations mobilised into the blood by G-CSF. Stem Cells 2006; 24:1822–30.

38. Terai S, Ishikawa T, Omori K et al. Improved liver function in liver cirrhosis patients after autologous bone marrow cell infusion therapy. Stem Cells 2006; 24:2292–8.

2

Hepatic, biliary and pancreatic anatomy

Steven M. Strasberg

This chapter will provide the basic anatomical foundation for performing liver, biliary and pancreatic surgery. Surgically unimportant anatomical features are omitted, but anatomical distortions due to pathological processes are included. A key point of hepato-pancreato-biliary (HPB) surgical anatomy is that whilst there is a **prevailing pattern** of anatomy, variations from those most commonly found, termed **anomalies**, are frequent. Every surgical operation in this area should be conducted with this fact in mind.

Liver

Overview of hepatic anatomy and terminology

Modern hepatic anatomy is concerned mainly with internal vascular and biliary structures rather than surface markings. Ramifications of the hepatic artery and bile ducts are regular and virtually identical. The portal vein on the left side of the liver is a vessel with unusual morphology, consequent to its need to perform different functions in the foetus. Consequently the Brisbane 2000 Terminology of Hepatic Anatomy and Resections of the International Hepatobiliary Pancreatic Association[1] used in this chapter is primarily based on hepatic artery and bile duct ramifications.

Divisions of the liver based on the hepatic artery

The primary (first-order) division of the proper hepatic artery is into the right and left hepatic arteries (**Fig. 2.1**). These branches supply arterial

inflow to the **right and left hemilivers or livers** (**Fig. 2.2**). The plane between the two distinct zones of vascular supply is called a watershed. The border or watershed of the first-order division is called the **midplane of the liver**. It intersects the gallbladder fossa and the fossa for the inferior vena cava (Fig. 2.2). The right liver usually has a larger volume than the left liver (60:40), although this is variable.

The second-order divisions (**Figs. 2.1** and **2.3**) of the hepatic artery supply four distinct zones of the liver. Each is referred to as a **section**. The right liver is divided into the **right anterior section** and the **right posterior section**. These sections are supplied by the right anterior sectional hepatic artery and a right posterior sectional hepatic artery Fig. 2.1). The plane between these sections is the **right intersectional plane**. The right intersectional plane does not have any surface markings to indicate its position. The left liver is divided into a **left medial section** and a **left lateral section** (Fig. 2.3), and is supplied by a left medial sectional hepatic artery and a left lateral sectional hepatic artery (Fig. 2.1). The plane between these sections is referred to as the left intersectional plane. It does have surface markings indicating its position – the umbilical fissure and the line of attachment of the falciform ligament to the anterior surface of the liver.

The third-order divisions of the hepatic artery divide the right and left hemilivers into **segments** (Sg) 2–8 (**Figs. 2.1** and **2.4**). Each of the segments has its own feeding segmental artery. The left lateral section is divided into Sg2 and Sg3. The pattern or ramification of vessels within the left medial section does not permit subdivision of this section into

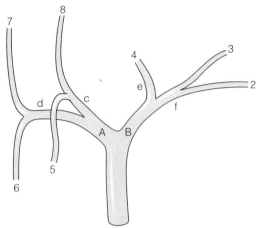

Figure 2.1 • Ramification of the hepatic artery in the liver. The prevailing pattern is shown. The first-order division of the proper hepatic artery shown in purple is into the right **(a)** and left **(b)** hepatic arteries, which supply right and left hemilivers (Fig. 2.2) respectively. The second-order divisions of the hepatic arteries supply the four sections (Fig. 2.3). The third-order division supplies the segments (Fig. 2.4). Since the left medial section and segment 4 are the same the artery is shown as being both sectional and segmental. The caudate lobe is supplied by branches from **(a)** and **(b)**. Bile duct anatomy and nomenclature is similar to that of the hepatic artery. © Washington University in St Louis.

segments, each with its own arterial blood supply. Therefore the left medial section and Sg 4 are synonymous. However, segment 4 is arbitrarily divided into superior (4a) and inferior (4b) parts without an exact anatomical plane of separation based on internal ramification of vessels. The right anterior section is divided into two segments, Sg5 and Sg8. The right posterior section is divided into Sg6 and Sg7. The planes between segments are referred to as **intersegmental planes**. The ramifications of the bileducts are identical to that described for the arteries, as are the zones of the liver drained by the respective ducts.

Segment 1 (caudate lobe) is a distinct portion of the liver, separate from the right and left hemilivers (**Fig. 2.5**). It is appropriately referred to as a lobe since it is demarcated by visible fissures. It consists of three parts: the bulbous left part (Spiegelian lobe), which grips the left side of the vena cava and is readily visible through the lesser omentum; the paracaval portion, anterior to the vena cava; and the caudate process, on the right, merging indistinctly with the right hemiliver. It is situated posterior to the hilum and the portal veins. Lying anterior and superior to the paracaval portion are the hepatic veins which limit its upper extent (Fig. 2.5). It receives its vascular supply from both right and left hepatic arteries (and portal veins). Caudate bile ducts drain into both right and left hepatic ducts.[2,3] The caudate lobe is drained by several short caudate veins of variable number and size, that enter

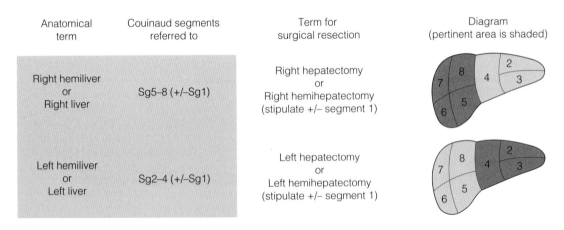

Anatomical term	Couinaud segments referred to	Term for surgical resection	Diagram (pertinent area is shaded)
Right hemiliver or Right liver	Sg5–8 (+/–Sg1)	Right hepatectomy or Right hemihepatectomy (stipulate +/– segment 1)	
Left hemiliver or Left liver	Sg2–4 (+/–Sg1)	Left hepatectomy or Left hemihepatectomy (stipulate +/– segment 1)	

Border or watershed: The border or watershed of the first-order division which separates the two hemilivers is a plane which intersects the gallbladder fossa and the fossa for the IVC and is called the midplane of the liver.

Figure 2.2 • Nomenclature for first-order division anatomy (hemilivers or livers) and resections. © Washington University in St Louis.

Second-order division
(second-order division based on bile ducts and hepatic artery)

Anatomical term	Couinaud segments referred to	Term for surgical resection	Diagram (pertinent area is shaded)
Right anterior section	Sg 5,8	Add (-ectomy) to any of the anatomincal terms as in Right anterior sectionectomy	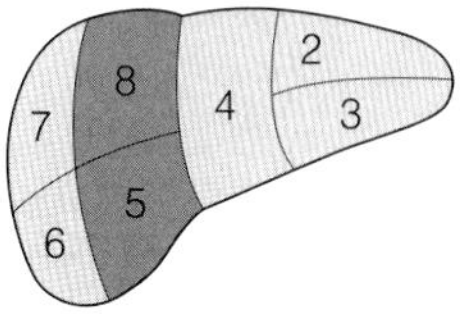
Right posterior section	Sg 6,7	Right posterior sectionectomy	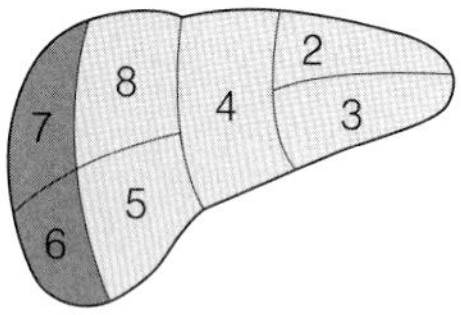
Left medial section	Sg 4	Left medial sectionectomy or Resection segment 4 (also see third order) or Segmentectomy 4 (also see third order)	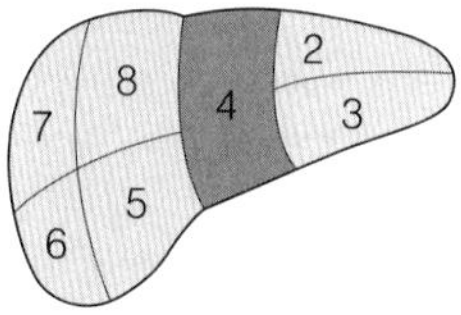
Left lateral section	Sg 2,3	Left lateral sectionectomy or Bisegmentectomy 2,3 (also see third order)	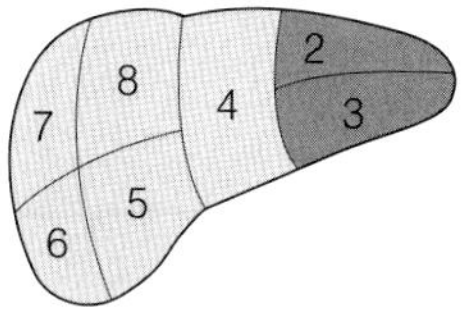

Other sectional liver resections

	Sg 4–8 (+/–Sg1)	Right trisectionectomy (preferred item) or Extended right heptectomy or Extended right hemihepatectomy (stipulate +/– segment 1)	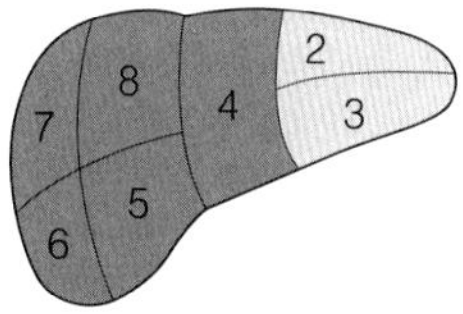
	Sg 2,3,4,5,8 (+/–Sg1)	Left trisectionectomy (preferred term) or Extended left hepatectomy or Extended left hemihepatectomy (stipulate +/– segment 1)	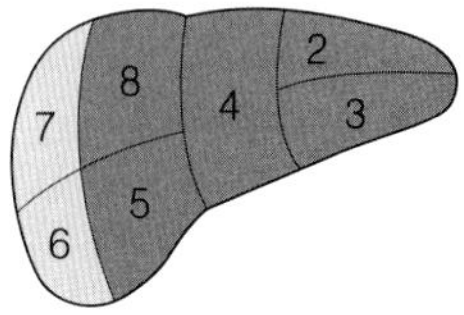

Border or watershed: The borders or watersheds of the sections are planes referred to as the right and left intersectional planes. The left intersectional plane passes through the umbilical fissure and the attachment of the falciform ligament. There is no surface marking of the right intersectional plane.

Figure 2.3 • Nomenclature for second-order division anatomy (sections) and resections including extended resections.
© Washington University in St Louis.

Third-order division

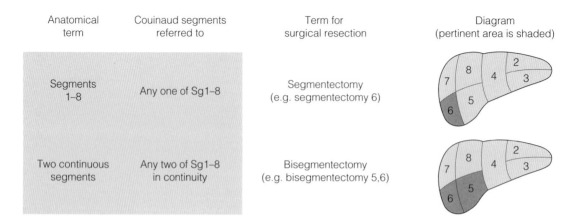

Anatomical term	Couinaud segments referred to	Term for surgical resection	Diagram (pertinent area is shaded)
Segments 1–8	Any one of Sg1–8	Segmentectomy (e.g. segmentectomy 6)	
Two continuous segments	Any two of Sg1–8 in continuity	Bisegmentectomy (e.g. bisegmentectomy 5,6)	

Border or watershed: The borders or watersheds of the segments are planes reffered to as intersegmental planes.

Figure 2.4 • Nomenclature for third-order division anatomy (segments) and resections. © Washington University in St Louis.

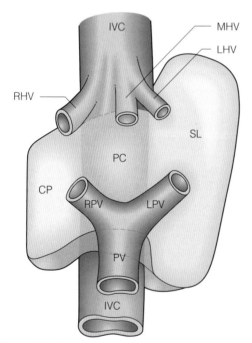

Figure 2.5 • Schematic representation of the anatomy of the caudate lobe. The caudate lobe consists of three parts: the caudate process (CP), on the right; the paracaval portion anterior to the vena cava (PC); and the bulbous left part (Spiegelian lobe, SL). IVC, inferior vena cava; PV, portal vein; LHV, MHV, RHV, left hepatic, middle hepatic and right hepatic veins respectively. © Washington University in St Louis.

the inferior vena cava (IVC) directly from the caudate lobe. On occasion, caudate veins are quite short and wide, and therefore must be isolated and divided cautiously.

Resectional terminology

The terminology of hepatic resections is based upon the terminology of hepatic anatomy, and resection of one side of the liver is called a hepatectomy or hemihepatectomy (Fig. 2.2). Therefore, resection of the right side of the liver is right hepatectomy or hemihepatectomy. Resection of a liver section is referred to as a sectionectomy (Fig. 2.3). Resection of the liver to the left side of the umbilical fissure would be referred to as a left lateral sectionectomy. The other sectionectomies are named accordingly, e.g. right anterior sectionectomy. Resection of the whole right liver plus Sg4 is referred to as a right trisectionectomy (Fig. 2.3). Similarly, resection of the left hemiliver plus the right anterior section is referred to as a left trisectionectomy.

Resection of one of the numbered segments is referred to as a segmentectomy (Fig. 2.4). Resection of the caudate lobe can be referred to as a caudate lobectomy or resection of Sg1. It is always appropriate to refer to a resection by the numbered segments. For instance, it would be appropriate to call a left lateral sectionectomy a resection of Sg2 and Sg3.

Surgical anatomy for liver resections

Hepatic arteries and liver resections

In the prevailing anatomical pattern, the coeliac artery terminates to divide into splenic and common hepatic arteries. Rarely, the hepatic artery arises directly from the aorta. The common hepatic artery runs for 2–3 cm anteriorly and to the right to ramify into gastroduodenal and proper hepatic arteries. The proper hepatic artery enters the hepatoduodenal ligament and normally runs for 2–3 cm along the left side of the common bile duct and terminates by dividing into the right and left hepatic arteries, the right immediately passing behind the common hepatic duct. The four sectional arteries arise from the right and left arteries 1–2 cm from the liver. While this is the commonest pattern, variations from this pattern are also very common (**Fig. 2.6**). The surgeon is wise not to make assumptions regarding hepatic arteries based on size or position, but rely instead on complete dissection, trial occlusions and radiological support. When an artery appears unusually large it is especially important to dissect until identification is unquestionable.

'Replaced' arteries are surgically important anomalies. 'Replaced' means that the artery supplying a particular volume of liver is in an unusual location and also that it is the sole supply to that volume of liver. 'Aberrant' means the structure is in an unusual location. While the definition of 'aberrant' does not state whether the structure provides sole supply, it is usually considered to be synonymous with 'replaced' in respect to these arteries. 'Accessory' refers to an artery which is additional, i.e. is present in addition to the normal structure and as a result is **not** the sole supply to a volume. Consequently, ligation of an accessory artery does not result in ischaemia.

In about 25% of patients, part or all of the liver is supplied by a replaced (or aberrant) artery. The **replaced right hepatic artery** arises from the superior mesenteric artery. It runs from left to right behind the lower end of the common bile duct to emerge and course on its right posterior border. It may supply a segment, section or the entire right hemiliver. Rarely, this artery supplies the entire liver and then it is called a **replaced hepatic artery**. The **replaced left hepatic artery** arises from the left gastric artery and courses in the lesser omentum in conjunction with vagal branches to the liver (hepatic nerve). As with the right artery it may supply a segment, section (usually the left lateral section), hemiliver or very rarely the whole liver. Sometimes left hepatic arteries arising from the left gastric artery are actually accessory rather than replaced, and exist in conjunction with normally situated left hepatic arteries. Knowledge of these particular arterial variations is of importance not only in hepatobiliary surgery including transplantation, but in gastric surgery and pancreatic surgery. Transection of the left gastric artery at its origin during gastrectomy may cause ischaemic necrosis of the left hemiliver if a replaced left artery is present; the same may occur on the right side as a result of injury to a replaced right artery. Also, these vessels need to be preserved and perfused during donor hepatectomy. Sometimes there is no proper hepatic artery because the entire liver is supplied by right or left replaced arteries, or both. This anomaly may be suspected when on opening the peritoneum at the base of the right side of the hepatoduodenal ligament the portal vein is immediately apparent instead of the hepatic artery. Replaced arteries may confer an advantage during surgery. For instance, when a replaced left artery supplies the left lateral section it is possible to resect the entire proper hepatic artery when performing a right trisectionectomy for hilar cholangicarcinoma. The replaced right artery is sometimes invaded by pancreatic head tumours and is in danger of injury during pancreato-duodenectomy.

In performing hepatectomies by the standard technique of isolating individual structures instead of pedicles it is critical to correctly identify the particular artery(ies) supplying the volume

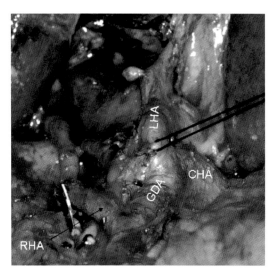

Figure 2.6 • A most dangerous arterial anatomy. The right hepatic artery (RHA) arises from the gastroduodenal artery (GDA). There is no proper hepatic artery. The left hepatic artery (LHA) could easily be mistaken for the proper hepatic artery. Ligation of the GDA would lead to arterial devascularisation of the right liver. Note early branching of the RHA into anterior and posterior sectional branches. © Washington University in St Louis.

of liver to be resected. One important anatomical point is that an artery located to the right side of the bile duct always supplies the right side of the liver, but arteries found on the left side of the bile duct may supply either side of the liver. Therefore, when using the individual vessel ligation method it is important to be aware of the position of the common hepatic duct. A trial occlusion of an artery with an atraumatic clamp should always be performed in order to be sure that there is a good pulse to the side of the liver to be retained.

Bile ducts and liver resections

Prevailing pattern and important variations of bile ducts draining the right hemiliver

Normally, only a short portion, about 1 cm, of the right hepatic duct is in an extrahepatic position. The prevailing pattern of bile duct drainage from the right liver is shown in **Figure 2.7a**. The segmental ducts from Sg6 and Sg7 (called **B6, B7**) unite to form the **right posterior sectional bile duct** and the segmental ducts from Sg5 and Sg8 (**B5, B8**) unite to form the **right anterior sectional bile duct** (**Fig. 2.7a**). The sectional ducts unite to form the **right hepatic duct**, which unites with the left bile duct at the **confluence** to form the common hepatic duct.

There are two important sets of biliary anomalies on the right side of the liver. The first, a common anomaly, involves insertion of a right sectional duct into the left bile duct. The right posterior sectional duct inserts into the left hepatic duct in 20% of persons (**Fig. 2.7b**) and the right anterior bile duct does so in 6% (**Fig. 2.7c**). A right sectional bile duct inserting into the left hepatic duct is in danger of injury during left hepatectomy. During this procedure the left hepatic duct should be divided close to the umbilical fissure to avoid injury to a right sectional duct (Fig. 2.7b, 'correct'). If the left hepatic duct is divided at its termination at the normal site of confluence of the right and left hepatic ducts, the right sectional duct may be injured and require reconstruction (Fig. 2.7b, 'incorrect'). Also, because of the frequency of this anomaly it is the author's practice to perform intraoperative cystic duct cholangiography or preoperative magnetic resonance cholangiography (MRCP), if a prior cholecystectomy has been done, whenever performing a left hepatectomy.

The second important anomaly is insertion of a right bile duct into the biliary tree at a lower level than the prevailing site of confluence (**Fig. 2.7d**). Low union may affect the main right bile duct, a sectional right duct (usually the anterior one), a segmental duct or a subsegmental duct. The duct will unite with the common hepatic duct below the prevailing site of confluence, or in about 2% of persons first unite with the cystic duct and then with the common hepatic duct. The latter anomaly places the aberrant duct at great risk for injury during laparoscopic cholecystectomy.

The right **posterior** sectional duct normally hooks over origin of the right **anterior** sectional portal vein ('Hjortsjo's Crook'),[4] where it is in danger of being injured if the right anterior sectional pedicle is clamped too close to its origin (**Fig. 2.8**).

Prevailing pattern and important variations of bile ducts draining the left hemiliver

The prevailing pattern of bile duct drainage from the left liver is shown in **Fig. 2.9a**. It is present in only 30% of individuals such that variations are present in the majority of individuals. In the prevailing pattern, the segmental ducts from Sg2 and Sg3

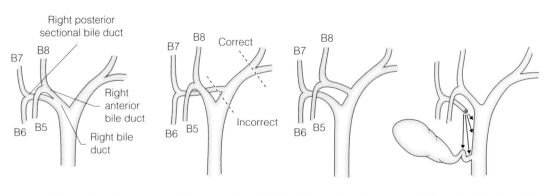

Prevailing pattern of right bile ducts

Separate entry of right anterior and right posterior sectional ducts (no right duct)

Shifting of entry of a right bile duct inferiorly

Figure 2.7 • Prevailing pattern **(a)** and important variations **(b–d)** of bile ducts draining the right hemiliver (see text). © Washington University in St Louis.

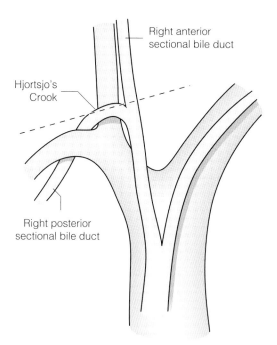

Figure 2.8 • Hjortsjo's Crook. Note that the right posterior sectional bile duct (RPSBD) crosses the origin of the right anterior sectional portal vein. RASBD, right anterior sectional bile duct. © Washington University in St Louis.

(**B2, B3**) unite to form the **left lateral sectional bile duct**. This duct passes behind the umbilical portion of the portal vein and unites with the duct from Sg4 (**B4**; also called the left medial sectional duct since section and segment are synonymous for this volume of liver). The union of these ducts to form the left hepatic duct occurs about one-third of the distance between the umbilical fissure and the midplane of the liver. The left hepatic duct continues from this point for 2–3 cm along the base of Sg4 to its confluence with the right hepatic duct. Note that it is in an extrahepatic position and that it has a much longer extrahepatic course than the right bile duct. The extrahepatic position of the left hepatic duct is a key anatomical feature, which makes this section of duct the prime site for high biliary-enteric anastomosis. The left hepatic duct runs at a variable angle. In some individuals, it is almost horizontal but in others it runs sharply upward. It is much easier to expose a long length of duct in the former type.

The main anomalies of the left ductal system involve variations in site of insertion of B4 (**Fig. 2.9b**), multiple ducts coming from B4 (**Fig. 2.9c**), and primary union of B3 and B4 with subsequent union of B2 (**Fig. 2.9d**). B4 may join the left lateral sectional duct to the left or right of its point of union in the prevailing pattern (Fig. 2.9b); in the former case the insertion of B4 is at the

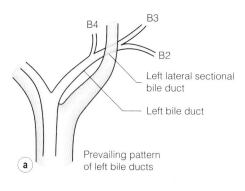

Left lateral sectional bile duct

Left bile duct

(a) Prevailing pattern of left bile ducts

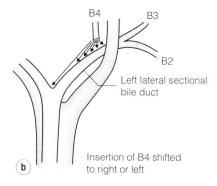

Left lateral sectional bile duct

(b) Insertion of B4 shifted to right or left

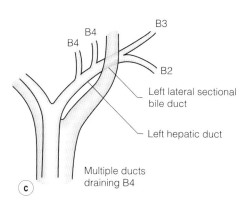

Left lateral sectional bile duct

Left hepatic duct

(c) Multiple ducts draining B4

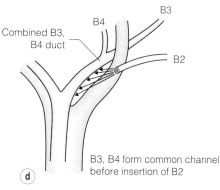

Combined B3, B4 duct

(d) B3, B4 form common channel before insertion of B2

Figure 2.9 • Prevailing pattern **(a)** and important variations **(b–d)** of bile ducts draining the left hemiliver. © Washington University in St Louis.

umbilical fissure and in the latter the insertion may occur at any place to the right of the prevailing location up to the point where the left hepatic duct normally unites with the right hepatic duct. In the latter instance, which according to Couinaud is present in 8% of individuals, there is no left hepatic duct. Instead there is a confluence of three ducts – the left lateral sectional duct, B4 and the right hepatic duct – to form the common hepatic duct. These variations are important in split liver transplantation and in repair of biliary injuries.

The bile duct to Sg3 has been used to perform biliary bypass (segment 3 cholangiojejunostomy) and can be isolated by following the superior surface of the ligamentum teres down to isolate the portal pedicle to Sg3.

Prevailing pattern of bile ducts draining the caudate lobe (Sg1)

Normally two or three caudate ducts enter the biliary tree. Their orifices are usually located posteriorly on the left duct, right duct or right posterior sectional duct.

Portal veins and liver resections

On the right side of the liver, the portal vein divisions correspond to those of the hepatic artery and bile duct, and they supply the same hepatic volumes. Therefore, there is a right portal vein which supplies the entire right hemiliver (**Fig. 2.10**). It divides into two sectional and four segmental veins, as do the arteries and bile ducts. On the left side of the liver, however, the left portal vein is quite unusual because of the fact that its structure was adapted to function in utero as a conduit between the umbilical vein and the ductus venosus, whilst postnatally the direction of flow is reversed. The left portal vein consists of a **horizontal or transverse portion**, which is located under Sg4, and a **vertical part or umbilical portion**, which is situated in the umbilical fissure (Fig. 2.10). Unlike the right portal vein, neither portion of the left portal vein actually enters the liver, but rather they lie directly on its surface. Often the umbilical portion is hidden by a bridge of tissue passing between left medial and lateral sections. This bridge of liver tissue may be as thick as 2 cm or only be a fibrous band. The junction of the transverse and umbilical portions of the left portal vein is marked by the attachment of a stout cord – the ligamentum venosum. This structure, the remnant of the foetal ductus venosus, runs in the groove between the left lateral section and the caudate lobe, and attaches to the left hepatic vein/IVC junction.

Ramification of the left portal vein (**Figs. 2.10** and **2.11**)

The transverse portion of the left portal vein sends only a few small branches to Sg4. Large branches

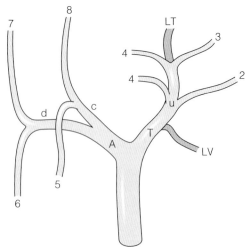

Figure 2.10 • Ramification of the portal vein in the liver. The portal vein divides into right (A) and left (T) branches. The branches in the right liver correspond to those of the hepatic artery and bile duct (Fig. 2.1). The branching pattern on the left is unique. The left portal vein has transverse (T) and umbilical portions (U). The transition point between the two parts is marked by the attachment of the ligamentum venosum (LV). All major branches come off the umbilical portion (see text). The vein ends blindly in the ligamentum teres (LT). © Washington University in St Louis.

from the portal vein to the left liver arise exclusively beyond the attachment of the ligamentum venosum – that is, from the umbilical part of the vein.[5] These branches come off both sides of the vein – those arising from the right side pass into Sg4 and those from the left supply Sg2 and Sg3. There is usually only one branch to Sg2 and Sg3, but often there is more than one branch to Sg4. The left portal vein terminates in the

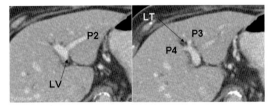

Figure 2.11 • Ramification of the left portal vein as seen on two computed tomography (CT) films. Note the branches to segments 2–4 and the ligamentum teres (LT). An arrow points to site of origin of the ligamentum venosum (LV), where the transverse portion becomes the umbilical portion of the vein, proving conclusively that the branch to segment 2 is not part of a terminal division of the transverse portion of the vein as might be concluded from cast studies (also see Ref. 5). © Washington University in St Louis.

ligamentum teres at the free edge of the left liver. Note that the umbilical portion of the portal vein has a unique pattern of ramification. The pattern is similar to an air-conditioning duct that sends branches at right angles from both of its sides to supply rooms (segments) – tapering as it does so, finally to end blindly (in the ligamentum teres). Other vascular and biliary structures normally ramify by dividing into two other structures at their termination and not by sending out branches along their length.

Although the divisions of the portal vein are unusual for the embryonic reasons described above, it is uncommon to have variations from this pattern. Probably the most common variation is absence of the right portal vein. In these cases the right posterior and right anterior sectional veins originate independently from the main portal vein. Under these circumstances the anterior sectional vein is usually quite high in the porta hepatis and may not be obvious. An unsuspecting surgeon may divide the posterior sectional vein thinking that it is the right portal vein and become confused when the anterior sectional vein is come upon during hepatic transection.

A rare but potentially devastating anomaly is the absent extrahepatic left portal vein (**Fig. 2.12**). The apparent right vein is really the main portal vein, a structure which enters the liver, gives off branches to the right liver and then loops back within the liver substance to supply the left side. The vein looks like a right vein in terms of position, but is larger. Transection results in total portal vein disconnection from the liver. This anomaly should always be sought on imaging as right hepatectomy is not usually possible when it is present. The presence of the transverse portion of the left vein at the base of Sg4, which then enters the umbilical fissure, precludes the presence of this anomaly.

The portal vein branches to Sg4 may be isolated in the umbilical fissure on the right side of the umbilical portion of the left portal vein. The veins here are associated with the bile ducts and the arteries passing to Sg4, i.e. they enter sheaths as they go into the liver substance. Isolation in this location may provide extra margin when resecting a tumour in Sg4 that impinges upon the umbilical fissure. Normally, the branches to Sg4 are isolated after dividing the parenchyma of the liver of Sg4 close to the umbilical fissure, an approach that is used to avoid injury to the umbilical portion of the left portal vein. Injury to this vein could of course deprive Sg2 and Sg3 of portal vein supply as well as Sg4. For instance, if this occurs when performing a right trisectionectomy, the only portion of the liver to be retained would be devascularised of portal vein flow. However, isolation of these structures within the umbilical fissure does provide an extra margin of clearance on tumours and can be done safely if care is taken to ascertain the position of the portal vein. Likewise, it is possible to isolate the portal vein branches going into Sg2 and Sg3 in the umbilical fissure and to extend a margin when resecting a tumour in the left lateral section. For the same reasons given above, caution must be taken when doing this in order not to injure the umbilical portion of the portal vein. It is usually necessary to divide the bridge of liver tissue between the left medial and lateral sections to access the portal vein in this location. Note that arteries and bile ducts passing to the left lateral section are in danger of being injured as one isolates the most posterior-superior portion of the bridge. The peritoneum at the base of the bridge may be opened in a preliminary step to facilitate passage of an instrument behind the bridge which is divided by cautery.

Hepatic veins and liver resection

(Fig. 2.13)

Three large hepatic veins run in the midplane of the liver (middle hepatic vein), the right intersectional plane (right hepatic vein) and the left intersectional plane (left hepatic vein). The left hepatic vein actually begins in the plane between Sg2 and Sg3 and travels in that plane for most of its length. It becomes quite a large vein even in that location. About 1 cm from its termination in the IVC, it enters the left intersectional plane (the same plane as the umbilical portion of the left portal vein), where it receives the umbilical vein from Sg4 (**Figs. 2.13** and **2.14**). It is important not to confuse the 'umbilical portion of

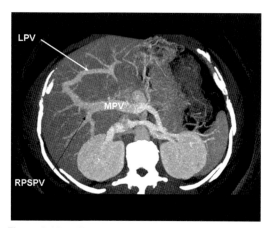

Figure 2.12 • Absent extrahepatic left portal vein, a rare and very dangerous anomaly. Three-dimensional reconstruction of CT scan. Note that the main portal vein (MPV) enters right liver, gives off right posterior sectional portal vein (RPSPV) and some branches to the right anterior section, then proceeds to the left as an internal left portal vein (LPV). © Washington University in St Louis.

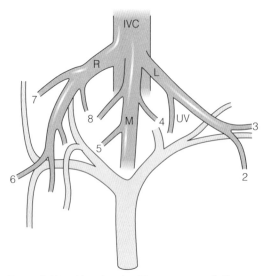

Figure 2.13 • Hepatic veins. There are normally three hepatic veins, right (R), middle (M) and left (L). Note the segments drained. UV is the umbilical vein, which normally drains part of Sg4 into the left hepatic vein. The latter is proof that the terminal portion of the left vein lies in the intersectional plane of the left liver. © Washington University in St Louis.

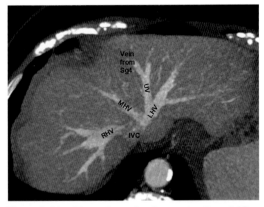

Figure 2.14 • Three-dimensional reconstruction of CT scan showing prevailing pattern of the umbilical vein (UV). The UV receives tributaries from Sg4 and Sg3 and travels in the plane of the umbilical fissure to join the left hepatic vein (LHV). The LHV then continues in the same plane for 1–2 cm before joining the middle hepatic vein and entering the IVC. This demonstrates that a major hepatic vein can lie in the same plane as a major portal vein (left portal vein) which also lies in this plane. The pattern shown in this figure is the prevailing pattern but the UV is not usually this prominent. MHV, middle hepatic vein; RHV, right hepatic vein. © Washington University in Saint Louis.

the left portal vein' with the 'umbilical vein', which is a tributary of the left hepatic vein that normally drains the most leftward part of Sg4.[6,7] The short left hepatic vein lies in the left intersectional plane between the point where it receives the **umbilical vein** from Sg4 and the IVC, a distance of only about 1 cm. The left and middle hepatic veins normally fuse at a distance of about 1–2 cm from the IVC, so that when viewed from within the IVC there are only hepatic vein openings. Rarely, hepatic veins join the IVC above the diaphragm.

In about 10% of individuals, there is more than one large right hepatic vein. In these persons, in addition to the right superior hepatic vein (normally called the right hepatic vein), which enters the IVC just below the level of the diaphragm, there is a right inferior hepatic vein, which enters the IVC 5–6 cm below this level. In the presence of this vein, resections of Sg7 and Sg8 may be performed, including resection of the right superior vein, without compromising the venous drainage of Sg5 and Sg6.

The caudate lobe is drained by its own veins – several short veins that enter the IVC directly from the caudate lobe. When performing a classical right hepatectomy caudate veins are divided in the preliminary portion of the dissection. As dissection moves up the anterior surface of the vena cava to isolate the right hepatic vein, one encounters a bridge of tissue lateral to the IVC referred to as the 'inferior vena caval ligament'.[8] This bridge of tissue usually consists of fibrous tissue but occasionally of liver and connects the posterior portion of the right liver to the caudate lobe behind the IVC. It limits exposure of the right side of the IVC at a point just below the right hepatic vein and must be divided in order to isolate the right hepatic vein. This must be done with care as the ligament may contain a large vein and forceful dissection of the ligament may also result in injury to the right lateral side of the IVC. Isolation of the right hepatic vein is also aided by clearing the areolar tissue between the right and middle hepatic veins down to the level of the IVC when exposing these veins from above.

Another approach to right hepatectomy is to leave division of the caudate and right hepatic veins until after the liver is transected. In this case a clamp may be passed up along the anterior surface of the vena from below to emerge between the right and middle hepatic veins. Once an umbilical tape is passed the liver may be hung to facilitate transection ('hanging manoeuvre').[9] This is possible since caudate veins usually lie lateral to the midplane of the vena cava, as noted above.

The left and middle veins can also be isolated prior to division of the liver. There are several ways to achieve this anatomically. One method is to divide all the caudate veins as well as the right hepatic vein. This exposes the entire anterior surface of the retrohepatic vena cava and leaves the liver attached to the vena cava only by the middle and left hepatic veins, which are then easily isolated. This is suitable when performing a right hepatectomy or extended right hepatectomy, especially when the caudate lobe is also to be resected. The advantage of having control of these veins during operations on the right liver is that total vascular occlusion is possible without occlusion of the IVC and haemodynamically the effect is not much different from occlusion of the main portal pedicle alone (Pringle manoeuvre).

In performing a left hepatectomy, the right hepatic vein is conserved and a different anatomical approach to isolation of the left and middle hepatic veins is required. They may be isolated from the left side by dividing the ligamentum venosum where it attaches to the left hepatic vein, then dividing the peritoneum at the superior tip of the caudate lobe and gently passing an instrument on the anterior surface of the vena cava to emerge between the middle and right veins and/or between the left and middle veins. Again, care needs to be taken when performing this manoeuvre in order to avoid injury to the structures.

Isolation of the vena cava above and below the hepatic veins is also a technique which should be in the armamentarium of every surgeon performing major hepatic resection. It is not usually necessary when performing standard liver resections but surgeons should be familiar with the anatomical technique of doing so. Isolation of the vena cava superior to the hepatic veins is done by dividing the left triangular ligament and the lesser omentum, being careful to first look for a replaced left hepatic artery. Next the peritoneum on the superior border of the caudate lobe is divided and a finger is passed behind the vena cava to come out just inferior to the crus of the diaphragm. The crus of the diaphragm makes an easily identified column on the right side. This column passes across the right side of the vena cava and dissection of the space inferior to this column and behind the vena cava facilitates passage of the finger from the left side to the right side in the space behind the vena cava. Isolation of the vena cava below the liver is more straightforward, but one should be aware of the position of the adrenal vein. In some cases, it is necessary to isolate the adrenal vein if bleeding persists after occlusion of the vena cava above and below the liver.

Finally, the surgeon should be aware that, during transection of the liver, large veins will be encountered in certain planes of transection. For instance, in its passage along the midplane the middle hepatic vein usually receives two large tributaries, one from Sg5 inferiorly and the other from Sg8 superiorly (Fig. 2.12). Both are encountered routinely in performing right hepatectomy. The venous drainage of the right side of the liver is highly variable and additional large veins, including one from Sg6, may also enter the middle hepatic vein.

The plate/sheath system of the liver

The system of fibrous plates and sheaths which lies on the ventral surface of the liver and extends into it is of great importance in liver surgery. The plate/sheath system can be understood by first imagining a shirt with the front cut away to leave only the back and the sleeves (**Fig. 2.15**, inset).[10] If the shirt were made of fibrous tissue the back of the shirt would be a plate and the sleeves would be sheaths. The true plate/sheath system is more complex as there are four plates (hilar, cystic, umbilical and arantian) and several sheaths[3] (Fig. 2.15). The hilar plate is the most important plate in liver surgery. It is a mostly flat structure, which lies principally in the coronal plane, posterior to the main bilo-vascular structures in the porta hepatis. However, its upper border is curved, so that it has the shape of a toboggan when viewed in the sagittal plane (Fig. 2.15). This upper curved edge lies superior to the right and left bile ducts, the most superior structures in the porta hepatis. It is this taut, firm, upper curved edge of the hilar plate which is dissected free from the underside of the liver when 'lowering the hilar plate'.

The sheath of the right portal pedicle extends off the hilar plate like a sleeve in our example. It carries into the liver surrounding the portal structures, i.e. portal vein, hepatic artery and bile duct. The combined structure, consisting of a hepatic artery, bile duct and portal vein surrounded by its fibrous sheath, is referred to as a 'portal pedicle'. As the right portal pedicle enters the liver it divides into a right anterior and right posterior portal pedicle supplying the respective sections and then segmental pedicles supplying the four segments. On the left side only, the segmental structures are sheathed. There is no **sheathed** main portal pedicle because the main portal vein, proper hepatic artery and common hepatic duct are not close enough to the liver to be enclosed in a sheath.

The cystic plate is the ovoid fibrous sheet on which the gallbladder lies (Fig. 2.15). When performing a cholecystectomy this plate is normally left behind. In its posterior extent the cystic plate narrows to become a stout cord which attaches to the anterior surface of the sheath of the right portal pedicle. The latter is a point of anatomical importance for the surgeon wishing to expose the anterior surface of the right portal pedicle, since this cord must be divided to do so as we have described.[11] The other plates are the umbilical and arantian, which underlie the umbilical portion of the left portal vein and the ligamentum venosum respectively (Fig. 2.15). The other sheaths carry segmental bilo-vascular pedicles of the left liver and caudate lobe.

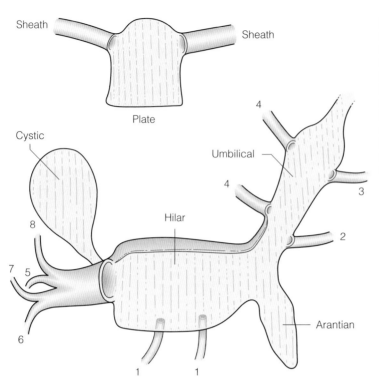

Figure 2.15 • Plate/sheath system of the liver with inset showing a schematic of a plate with two sheaths (see text). Reproduced from Strasberg SM, Linehan DC, Hawkins DC. Isolation of right main and right sectional portal pedicles for liver resection without hepatotomy or inflow occlusion. J Am Coll Surg 2008; 206:390–6. With permission of the Journal of the American College of Surgeons.

In performing a right hepatectomy, there are two methods of managing the right-sided portal vessels and bile ducts. The first is to isolate the hepatic artery, portal vein and bile duct individually and either control them or ligate them extrahepatically, and the second is to isolate the entire portal pedicle and staple the pedicle. Isolation of the right portal pedicle can be performed by making hepatotomies above the right portal pedicle in Sg4 and in the gallbladder fossa after removing the gallbladder. A finger is passed through the hepatotomy to isolate the right portal pedicle. This technique usually requires inflow occlusion. It can also be done without inflow occlusion by lowering the hilar plate and coming around the right portal pedicle directly on its surface, as we have recently described (**Fig. 2.16**).[10] It is advisable to divide caudate veins in the area below the vena caval ligament before performing pedicle isolation, since haemorrhage from these veins can be considerable if they are injured during isolation of the right portal pedicle. The advantage of pedicle isolation over isolation of individual vessels and the bile duct is that sectional resections require isolation of pedicles (Fig. 2.16).[10] Furthermore, pedicle isolation is much easier to do laparoscopically than individual structure isolation.

Liver capsule and attachments

The liver is encased in a thin fibrous capsule which covers the entire organ except for a large bare area posteriorly where the organ is in contact with the IVC and with the diaphragm to the right of the IVC. The bare area stretches superiorly to include the termination of the three hepatic veins and ends in a point, which is also where the attachment of the falciform ligament ends. The limit of the bare area, where the peritoneum passes between the body wall and the liver, is called the coronary ligament. It is one of three structures which connect the liver to the abdominal wall 'dorsally', the other two being the right and left triangular ligaments. The liver also has another bare area, best thought of as a bare crease where the hepato-duodenal ligament and the lesser omentum attach on the 'ventral' surface. It is through this crease that the portal structures enter the liver at the hilum (hilum = 'a crease on a seed'). The other ligamentous structures of interest to surgeons are the ligamentum teres, falciform ligament and the ligamentum venosum. The ligamentum teres (teres = 'round') is the obliterated left umbilical vein and runs in the free edge of the falciform ligament from the umbilicus to the termination of the umbilical portion of the left portal vein. The falciform (falciform = 'scythe shaped') is the filmy fold that runs between the anterior abdominal wall above the umbilicus and attaches to the anterior surface of the liver between the left medial and left lateral sections.

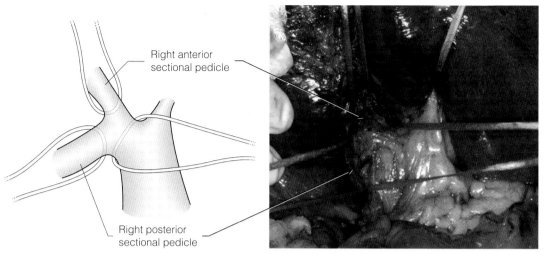

Right anterior
sectional pedicle

Right posterior
sectional pedicle

Figure 2.16 • Isolation of right portal pedicle and sectional pedicles by technique of dissection on surface of pedicles. No inflow occlusion or separate hepatotomies are used (see Ref. 10). The umbilical tape in the upper right of the photograph is around the bridge of liver tissue over the umbilical fissure. Reproduced from Strasberg SM, Linehan DC, Hawkins DC. Isolation of right main and right sectional portal pedicles for liver resection without hepatotomy or inflow occlusion. J Am Coll Surg. 2008; 206:390–6. With permission of the Journal of the American College of Surgeons.

Surface anatomy

Numerous terms for surface anatomy exist. They are of minimal surgical importance. Since the term 'lobe' has been used in different ways by various anatomists and surgeons it is best avoided except in reference to the caudate lobe. Fissure and scissure or scissura are similarly confusing terms since they apply only to clefts in casts of the liver. The ligaments of the liver are of surgical importance and are described under capsule and attachments.

Pathological conditions may distort or alter the position of normal hepatic structures. Tumours may push vessels so that they are stretched and curved over the surface of the tumour, narrowing or occluding them by direct pressure. Tumours may partially or completely occlude vessels by mural invasion, by inducing bland thrombi or by entering the lumen and producing tumour thrombi. They may cause bile ducts to dilate to a size many times normal. Atrophy of a portion of the liver will be induced by processes that occlude either the portal vein or bile duct. Since the liver will undergo hyperplasia to maintain a constant volume of liver cells, atrophy of one part of the liver is usually accompanied by growth of another. If the right portal vein is occluded by a tumour, the right liver will atrophy and the left liver will grow. When seen from below, this process will exert a counter-clockwise rotational effect on the porta hepatis, rotating the bile duct posteriorly, the hepatic artery to the right, and the portal vein to the left and anteriorly.

Gallbladder and extrahepatic bile ducts

Gallbladder

The gallbladder lies on the cystic plate. The edge of the gallbladder forms one side of the hepatocystic triangle. The other two sides are the right side of the common hepatic duct and the liver. Eponyms covering this anatomy (Calot, Moosman, etc.) are confusing and should be abandoned. The hepatocystic triangle contains the cystic artery and cystic node and a portion of the right hepatic artery, as well as fat and fibrous tissue. Clearance of this triangle along with isolation of the cystic duct and elevation of the base of the gallbladder off the lower portion of the cystic plate gives the 'critical view of safety' that we have described for identification of the cystic structures during laparoscopic cholecystectomy.[12]

A large number of curiosities of the gallbladder such as the phrygian cap have been described. The following are anomalies of importance to the biliary surgeon.

Agenesis of the gallbladder

Agenesis occurs in about 1 in 8000 individuals and can be difficult to recognise. An ultrasonographer may describe a 'shrunken' gallbladder. When agenesis is suspected it may be confirmed by axial imaging but if doubt remains, laparoscopy is definitive.

Double gallbladder

This is also a very rare anomaly but can be the cause of persistent symptoms after resection of one gallbladder. A gallbladder may also be bifid, which usually does not cause symptoms or have an hourglass constriction that may cause symptoms due to obstruction of the upper segment.

Cystic duct

This structure is normally 1–2 cm in length and 2–3 mm in diameter. It joins the common hepatic duct at an acute angle to form the common bile duct. The cystic duct normally joins the common hepatic duct approximately 4 cm above the duodenum. However, the cystic duct may enter at any level up to the right hepatic duct and down to the ampulla. The cystic duct may also join the right hepatic duct either when the right duct is in its normal position or in an aberrant location.

There are three patterns of confluence of the cystic duct and common hepatic duct (**Fig. 2.17**). In the 20% of patients in which there is a parallel union, the surgeon is prone to injure the side of the former structure when approaching the common hepatic duct by dissecting the cystic duct (Fig. 2.17). Also, when making a choledochotomy at this level the incision should be started slightly to the left side of the midplane of the bile duct in order to avoid entering a septum between the two fused cystic/common hepatic ducts. When performing cholecys-

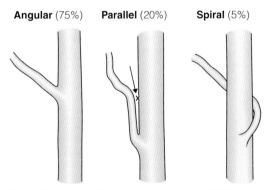

Angular (75%)   **Parallel** (20%)   **Spiral** (5%)

Figure 2.17 • The three types of cystic duct/CHD confluence. The parallel union confluence is shown in the middle. Dissection of this type of cystic duct (arrow) may lead to injury to the side of the CHD. During laparoscopic cholecystectomy this is often a cautery injury. Adapted from Warrren KW, McDonald WM, Kune GA. Bile duct strictures: new concepts in the management of an old problem. In: Irvine WT (ed.) Modern trends in surgery. London: Butterworth, 1966. With permission from Elsevier.

tectomy the cystic duct should be occluded in such a way that there is a visible section of cystic duct below the clip closest to the common bile duct.

Although a gallbladder with two cystic ducts has been described the author has not seen convincing proof that this anomaly actually exists. If it does it must be an anomaly of extreme rarity. When two 'cystic ducts' are identified, it is likely that the cystic duct is congenitally short or has been effaced by a stone and that the two structures thought to be dual cystic ducts are, in fact, the common bile duct and the common hepatic duct.

Cystic artery

The cystic artery is about 1 mm in diameter and normally arises from the right hepatic artery in the hepatocystic triangle. The cystic artery may arise from a right hepatic artery that runs anterior to the common hepatic duct. The cystic artery may also arise from the right hepatic artery on the left side of the common hepatic duct and run anterior to this duct, while the right hepatic artery runs behind it. Such cystic arteries tend to tether the gallbladder and make dissection of the hepatocytic triangle more difficult. The cystic artery may arise from an aberrant right hepatic artery coming off the superior mesenteric artery (SMA). In this case the cystic artery and not the cystic duct tends to be in the free edge of the fold leading from the hepatoduodenal ligament to the gallbladder. This should be suspected whenever the 'cystic duct' looks smaller than the 'cystic artery'.

Normally the cystic artery runs for 1–2 cm to meet the gallbladder superior to the insertion of the cystic duct. The artery ramifies into an anterior and posterior branch at the point of contact with the gallbladder and these branches continue to divide on their respective surfaces. Sometimes the cystic artery divides into branches before the gallbladder edge is reached. In such cases, the anterior branch may be mistaken to be the cystic artery proper and the posterior branch will not be discovered until later in the dissection, when it may be divided inadvertently. The artery may ramify into several branches before arriving at the gallbladder, giving the impression that there is no cystic artery. The anterior and posterior branches may arise independently from the right hepatic artery, giving rise to two distinct cystic arteries.

Multiple small cystic veins drain into intrahepatic portal vein branches by passing into the liver around or through the cystic plate. Sometimes there are cystic veins in the hepatocystic triangle that run parallel to the cystic artery to enter the main portal vein.

Small bile ducts may penetrate the cystic plate to enter the gallbladder. These 'ducts of Luschka' are very small, usually submillimetre accessory ducts. However, when divided during a cholecystectomy postoperative bilomas may occur. Bilomas and haemorrhage may also be caused by penetration of the cystic plate during dissection. In about 10% of patients there is a large peripheral bile duct immediately deep to the plate, disruption of which will cause copious bile drainage. The origin of the middle hepatic vein is also in this location, and if it is injured massive haemorrhage may ensue. There is areolar tissue between the muscularis of the gallbladder and the cystic plate. At the top of the gallbladder the layer is very thin. As one progresses downwards the areolar layer thickens. If dissection from the top of the gallbladder downward is continued on the gallbladder leaving the areolar tissue on the cystic plate, one will arrive onto the posterior surface of the cystic artery and cystic duct. Conversely, if it is continued downward on the cystic plate leaving the areolar tissue on the gallbladder one will arrive onto the surface of the right portal pedicle. If this is not anticipated, structures in the right portal pedicle may be injured. Therefore the proper plane of dissection is between the gallbladder and the areolar tissue.

Extrahepatic bile ducts

The common hepatic duct (CHD) is formed by the union of left and right ducts, and normally occurs at the right extremity of the base of Sg4 anterior and superior to the bifurcation of the portal vein. The CHD travels in the right edge of the hepatoduodenal ligament for 2–3 cm, where it joins with the cystic duct to form the common bile duct (CBD). The latter has a supraduodenal course of 3–4 cm and then passes behind the duodenum to run in or occasionally behind the pancreas to enter the second portion of the duodenum. Details of its lower section and relation to the pancreatic duct are described in the final section of this chapter. The external diameter of the CBD varies from 5 to 13 mm when distended to physiological pressures. However, the duct diameter at surgery, i.e. in fasting patients with low duct pressures, may be as small as 3 mm. Radiologically, the internal duct diameter is measured on fasting patients. Under these conditions the upper limit of normal is about 8 mm. Size should never be used as a sole criterion for identifying a bile duct and caution is required in situations in which a structure seems larger than the expected norm. Although the cystic duct may be enlarged due to passage of stones, the surgeon should take extra precautions before dividing a 'cystic duct' that is greater than 2 mm in diameter because the common bile duct can be 3 mm in diameter and aberrant ducts may be smaller.

Anomalies of extrahepatic bile ducts

As already noted there are biliary anomalies of the right and left ductal systems that can affect outcome of hepatic surgery. The same is true for biliary surgery. The most important clinical anomaly is low insertion of right hepatic ducts referred to above. Because of its low location, it may be mistaken to be the cystic duct and be injured. This is even more likely to occur when the cystic duct unites with an aberrant duct as opposed to joining the common hepatic duct. An extremely rare (if it exists at all) and even more hazardous anomaly occurs when an aberrant right hepatic duct joins the infundibulum of the gallbladder. This anomaly will in most instances not be recognised and lead to an injury of the duct. In most cases, this appearance is probably due to a Mirizzi syndrome of the type in which the anterior wall of the common hepatic duct has been destroyed, giving the appearance that the right hepatic duct enters the gallbladder. Left hepatic ducts can also join the CHD at a low level. They are less prone to be injured since the dissection during cholecystectomy is on the right side of the biliary tree.

Extrahepatic arteries

Anomalies of the hepatic arteries may be important in gallbladder surgery. Normally the right hepatic artery passes posterior to the bile duct (80%) and gives off the cystic artery in the hepatocystic triangle. However, in 20% of cases the right hepatic artery runs anterior to the bile duct. The right hepatic artery may lie very close to the gallbladder and chronic inflammation can draw the right hepatic artery directly onto the gallbladder, where it lies in an inverse U-loop and is prone to injury. In the 'classical injury' in laparoscopic cholecystectomy in which the common bile duct is mistaken for the cystic duct, an associated right hepatic artery injury is very common, since that right hepatic artery is considered to be the cystic artery.

Blood supply of bile ducts

Bile ducts receive supply only from the hepatic artery. Blood supply to the bile duct is axial.[13] Inferiorly the common bile duct receives supply from the retroduodenal arteries, branches of the gastroduodenal arcade. These arteries pass onto the bile duct at the 3 and 9 o'clock positions and run upward along the CBD. Superiorly, branches pass from the proper, right and left hepatic arteries onto the CHD at the level of the confluence of the right and left bile ducts (**Fig. 2.18**). Arteries pass onto the bile duct at the 3 and 9 o'clock positions and run downward along the CBD and anastomose with the longitudinal arteries coming up from below. Between

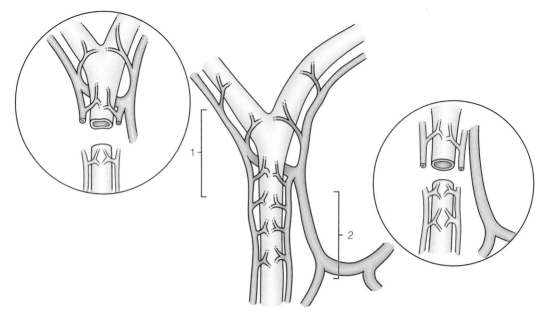

Figure 2.18 • Blood supply to bile ducts. Longitudinal 3 and 9 o'clock arteries are enlarged and hatched. **(1)** Transection 1 cm below confluence. Blood supply at lower cut margin is tenuous. **(2)** Transection 1 cm below confluence. Blood supply at upper cut margin is tenuous. © Washington University in St Louis.

the level of the duodenum and the liver edge there are few arteries that pass directly onto the bile duct. There is a watershed of arterial blood supply on the bile duct. If the CHD is transected at a high level, i.e. close to the confluence, the arterial blood supply to the inferior cut edge of the CHD will come from the retroduodenal arteries through the longitudinal vessels running along the supraduodenal bile duct to the level of transection – a distance of several centimetres. Consequently, ischaemia of the inferior cut edge of the bile duct is possible (**Fig. 2.18, 1**). Similarly, if the bile duct is transected at the level of the duodenum, the upper cut edge of the CBD may be ischaemic (**Fig. 2.18, 2**). The clinical implication is that whenever hepatico-jejunostomy is performed the bile duct should be divided 1–2 cm below the normal site of confluence of left and right ducts to ensure good blood supply to the bile duct. A corollary is that choledocho-choledochototomy is inherently risky because of the potential for one or other of the cut ends to be ischaemic depending on the level of transection.

Pancreas

The pancreas is a retroperitoneal organ lying obliquely across the upper abdomen so that the tail is superior to the head. It is formed by the fusion of ventral and dorsal anlages in utero, the ventral pancreas rotating to come behind and fuse with the dorsal pancreas. On average it is 22 cm in length. The head of the pancreas is discoid in shape and terminates inferiorly and medially in the hook-like uncinate process. The neck, body and tail are shaped like a flattened cylinder, sometimes somewhat triangular in cross-section with a flat anterior and pointed posterior surface. These divisions of the organ are somewhat arbitrary; the neck of the pancreas sits anterior to the superior mesenteric and portal veins. Normally the consistency of the gland is soft.

Pancreatic ducts

The prevailing anatomical pattern of the pancreatic duct is the result of union of the ventral duct (Wirsung) with the dorsal duct (Santorini) along with partial regression of the dorsal duct in the head. The 'genu' of the duct (genu = knee) is the bend in the duct concave inferiorly where the ventral duct joins the dorsal. In the prevailing pattern both ducts communicate with the duodenum, the dorsal duct entering at the minor papilla about 2 cm above and 5 mm anterior to the major papilla. Other ductal patterns are possible, which involve various degrees of dominance or regression of the portions of the ducts in the head of the pancreas. For instance, the ducts may not unite resulting in separate drainage from the ventral and dorsal pancreas (pancreas divisum), the dorsal duct may lose its connection to the duodenum or the dorsal duct in the head may lose its connection to the rest of the ductal system and drain only a small section of the head into the duodenum. Alternatively, the ventral duct may regress and the dorsal duct drains more or all of the pancreas through the minor ampulla. The uncinate process is served by its own duct, which joins the main pancreatic duct 1–2 cm from its entry into the duodenum.

The pancreatic duct (and pancreas) is often referred to as proximal (head) and distal (tail). These are confusing terms – as are the terms proximal and distal on the bile duct. Adding to the confusion is that 'distal' on the bile duct is near the ampulla, but that site is 'proximal' on the pancreatic duct. Instead, that part of the bile duct should be referred to as the pancreatic portion or lower bile duct while that near the bifurcation should be called the upper extrahepatic or hilar bile duct. In the case of the pancreas, the duct should be referred to as the 'pancreatic head duct', 'pancreatic body duct', etc.

The ventral duct usually joins the CBD to form a common channel several millimetres from the ampulla of Vater, usually within the wall of the duodenum. The bile duct traverses the duodenal wall obliquely and the pancreatic duct at a right angle. Each duct and the common channel have their own sphincters. The sphincters can be palpated from within the duodenum and form part of the raised 'major papilla' at whose apex the opening of the common channel can be seen. The common channel may be longer or absent, with both ducts entering the duodenum separately, the pancreatic duct more inferiorly. In performing a sphincteroplasty, it is advisable to open the common channel superiorly (10–12 o'clock position in the mobilised duodenum) to avoid the orifice of the pancreatic duct (4 o'clock). The ampulla is normally at the midpoint of the second part of the duodenum. It is rarely higher but can be as low as the midpoint of the third part of the duodenum. When the dorsal duct has its own communication with the duodenum it is found at the 'minor papilla', about 2 cm proximal and 1 cm anterior to the major papilla.

Blood supply of the pancreas

The arterial supply of the pancreas consists of two vascular systems, one supplying the head and uncinate and the other the body and tail. The neck is a watershed between these two areas of supply.[14] The head and uncinate process are supplied by the pancreatico-duodenal arcade, which consists of two to several loops of vessels that arise from the superior pancreatico-duodenal (branch of gastroduodenal) and inferior pancreatico-duodenal (branch of the SMA). The arcades run on the anterior and posterior surface of the pancreas next to the duodenum, the anterior arcade lying somewhat

closer to the duodenum. The second system arises from the splenic artery, which gives three arteries into the dorsal surface of the gland (**Fig. 2.19**). The dorsal pancreatic artery is the most medial of the three and the most important. It anastomoses with the pancreatico-duodenal arcade in the neck of the pancreas. It is the most aberrant artery in the upper abdomen and may arise from vessels that are routinely occluded during pancreatico-duodenectomy, which may account in part for fistula formation after this procedure.

Venous drainage generally follows arterial supply. The veins of the body and tail of the pancreas drain into the splenic vein, where it lies partly embedded in the posterior surface of the gland. These veins are short and fragile. The head and uncinate process veins drain into the superior mesenteric vein (SMV) and portal vein on the right lateral side of these structures. Uncinate veins often drain into a large first jejunal tributary vein, which then empties into the SMV. A nearly constant posterior superior pancreatico-duodenal vein enters the right lateral side of the portal vein at the level of the duodenum. The inferior mesenteric vein (IMV) does not normally drain the pancreas but its anatomy is important to the surgeon since it may become a draining vein of the pancreas if the termination of the splenic vein is surgically occluded during a resection of a pancreatic tumour. The IMV may drain into the SMV, the splenic vein or into the confluence of these veins. Only when it drains into the splenic vein can it decompress the splenic vein when it is occluded at the confluence with the SMV.

Lymphatics of the pancreas

For surgical purposes the lymphatic drainage of the pancreas is best considered in relation to the two main surgical procedures, resection of the pancreatic head and resection on the pancreatic body and tail. The aim of lymphatic resection during these procedures is to resect the primary lymph nodes, which receive lymph directly from pancreatic tissue (N1 nodes) as opposed to nodes that receive drainage from N1 nodes (N2 nodes). There is a ring of nodes around the pancreas that drain the adjacent sections of the gland (N1 nodes).[15] These in turn drain into nodes along the SMA, coeliac artery and aorta (axial nodes).[15] The axial nodes, which are N2 for most areas of the pancreas, are also N1 for portions of the pancreatic head, body and uncinate process that lie close to the aorta. The lymphatics of the body and tail are shown in **Figure 2.20**. The lymphatics of the head and uncinate process drain into a nodal ring for this part of the gland consisting of lymph nodes in the pancreatico-duodenal groove anteriorly and posteriorly, into subpyloric

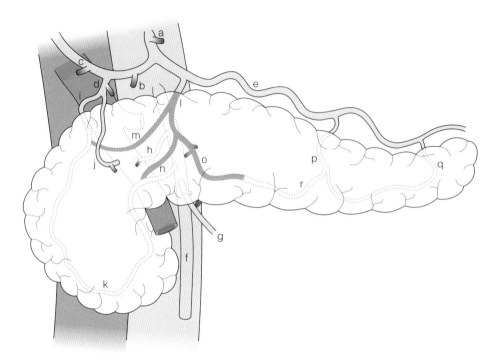

Figure 2.19 • Arterial blood supply to the pancreas. The dorsal pancreatic artery is shown shaded. Alternate origins of the artery are shown as black stumps. Key: a, coeliac artery; b, common hepatic artery; c, right hepatic artery; d, gastroduodenal artery; e, splenic artery; f, superior mesenteric artery; g, middle colic artery; h, right hepatic artery (aberrant); i, superior pancreatico-duodenal artery; j, right gastroepiploic artery; k, inferior pancreatico-duodenal artery; l, dorsal pancreatic artery (DPA); m, right anastomotic branch of DPA to superior part of pancreatico-duodenal arcade; n, right anastomotic branch of DPA to inferior part of pancreatico-duodenal arcade; o, left anastomotic branch of DPA becomes transverse pancreatic artery; p, pancreatica magna artery; q, caudal pancreatic artery; r, transverse pancreatic artery. © Washington University in St Louis.

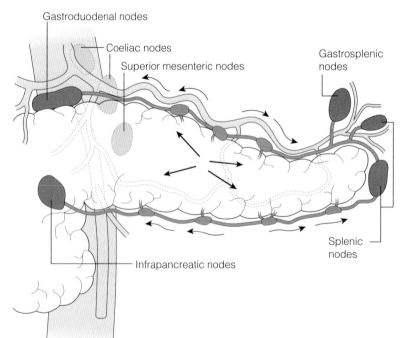

Figure 2.20 • Lymphatic drainage of the body and tail of the pancreas. The intraparenchymal lymphatics from the four quadrants empty into lymphatic vessels on the superior and inferior borders of the pancreas (arrows). Small nodes are found along these vessels. The lymph flows to the nodes of the 'ring'. These are N1 nodes, although some of the lymph may have passed through the smaller nodes as described. The nodes of the ring empty into nodes along the SMA, coeliac artery and aorta. The latter are therefore N2 nodes, but they are also N1 nodes for the more central part of the pancreas. © Washington University in St Louis.

nodes inferiorly, into nodes adjacent to the CBD and hepatic artery superiorly and into nodes along the SMA medially. These are N1, but as noted above so are some of the axial nodes. The standard node dissection for a Whipple procedure removes all of these nodal groups. This removes the N1 nodes unless there is direct lymphatic drainage to the left side of the SMA or to nodes around the coeliac artery, which does occur in a small proportion of patients.

Anatomical relations and ligaments of the pancreas

The pancreas is a deeply seated organ which, unlike the liver and most of the biliary tree, is not obvious when opening the abdomen. The anatomical relations of the pancreas are very important in pancreatic surgery. The structures emphasised in the following section are those which are commonly invaded by tumours.

Posteriorly the pancreas is related from right to left to the right kidney and perinephric fat, to the IVC and right gonadal vein, aorta, the left renal vein (slightly inferior), **retropancreatic fat**, the **left adrenal gland** and the superior pole of the left kidney. The **SMV** and **portal vein** are posterior relations of the neck of the pancreas and **splenic vein** of the body and tail. The **SMA** is a posterior relation of the junction of the neck and body of the gland lying posterior and to the right of the SMV. The SMA and SMV are both related to the uncinate process and give branches into (SMA) and receive **tributaries from** (SMV) the uncinate process. Often the uncinate veins enter a large tributary of the SMV, the first jejunal vein, which also abuts the uncinate process. These short arteries and veins are of importance surgically as they are divided when the head of the pancreas is resected; the veins tend to be fragile. The **coeliac artery** rises vertically superior to the SMA close to the superior edge of the pancreas, where it gives off the common hepatic artery and the **splenic artery**. The former runs anteriorly and to the left in approximation to the superior border of the pancreas. At the point where the artery passes in front of the portal vein it divides into the **gastroduodenal artery**, which passes anterior to the neck of the pancreas, sometimes buried within it. It terminates in the right gastroepiploic artery that rises in a fold of tissue toward the pylorus, a fold that also contains the right gastroepiploic vein and subpyloric nodes. The splenic artery snakes along the superior border of the pancreas to leave it 2–3 cm from the termination of the pancreas. The head of the pancreas is wrapped in the first three parts of the duodenum and the tail ends in relation to the splenic hilum. There is variability in the proximity of the tail of the pancreas to the spleen. In some cases the pancreas terminates 2 cm from the splenic substance and in others it abuts it. The anterior surface of the body and tail of the pancreas is covered by peritoneum, which is the posterior wall of the lesser sac, and then by the posterior wall of the stomach anterior to this. The transverse mesocolon is related to the inferior border of the pancreas, and the right and left extremities of the transverse colon are related to the head and tail of the gland. The IMV is related to the inferior border of the neck of the pancreas and may pass behind it to enter the splenic vein or turn medially to enter the SMV.

The pancreas is normally accessed surgically by entering the lesser sac either by division of the greater omentum below the gastroepiploic arcade or by releasing the greater omentum from its attachment to the transverse colon. When the lesser sac is entered the anterior surface of the neck body and tail are often visible but may be obscured by congenital filmy adhesions to the posterior wall of the stomach. To expose the head of the pancreas it is necessary to mobilise the right side of the transverse colon and hepatic flexure inferiorly and to divide the right gastroepiploic vein. The latter crosses the inferior border of the pancreas to join with the middle colic vein to form the gastrocolic trunk, which then enters the SMV. For complete exposure, e.g. for a Frey procedure, the right gastroepiploic artery is also divided and it and the subpyloric nodes are swept upwards off the pancreas. To access the SMV at the inferior border of the pancreas the peritoneum at the inferior border of the neck is divided and the dissection is continued inferiorly and laterally to open a groove between the uncinate process and the mesentery. Division of the right gastroepiploic vein at the inferior border of the pancreas greatly facilitates this manoeuvre. Normally no veins enter the SMV or portal vein from the posterior surface of the neck of the pancreas. Consequently, the neck of the pancreas can be separated from the anterior surface of the SMV/portal vein in this avascular plane. The peritoneum at the inferior border of the neck, body and tail of the pancreas is avascular, and there are few vascular connections between the back of the body and tail of the pancreas and retroperitoneal tissues. As a result the pancreas may be readily dissected free from retroperitoneum. The splenic vein is partly embedded in the back of the pancreas from the point that it reaches the gland on the left to about 1 cm from its termination at its confluence with the SMV.

> **Key points**
>
> - A prevailing pattern of hepatic, biliary and pancreatic anatomy exists but variations (anomalies) are frequent.
> - All HBP operations should be conducted with the strong suspicion that an anatomical anomaly may be present.

References

1. Terminology Committee of the IHPBA. The Brisbane 2000 Terminology of Liver Anatomy and Resections. HPB 2000; 2:333–9.

2. Healey JE, Schroy PC. Anatomy of the biliary ducts within the human liver; analysis of the prevailing pattern of branchings and the major variations of the biliary ducts. Arch Surg 1953; 66:599–616.

3. Couinaud C. Paris. Le foie. Etudes anatomiques et chirugicales. Paris: Masson & Cie, 1957.

4. Hjortsjo C-H. The topography of the intrahepatic duct systems. Acta Anat 1951; 11:599–615.

5. Botero AC, Strasberg SM. Division of the left hemiliver in man – segments, sectors, or sections. Liver Transpl Surg 1998; 4:226–31.

6. Masselot R, Leborgne J. Anatomical study of hepatic veins. Anat Clin 1978; 1:109–25.

7. Kawasaki S, Makuuchi M, Miyagawa S et al. Extended lateral segmentectomy using intra-operative ultrasound to obtain a partial liver graft. Am J Surg 1996; 171:286–8.

8. Makuuchi M, Yamamoto J, Takayama T et al. Extrahepatic division of the right hepatic vein in hepatectomy. Hepato-Gastroenterology 1991; 38:176–9.

9. Belghiti J, Guevara OA, Noun R et al. Liver hanging maneuver: a safe approach to right hepatectomy without liver mobilization. J Am Coll Surg 2001; 193:109–11.

10. Strasberg SM, Linehan DC, Hawkins DC. Isolation of right main and right sectional portal pedicles for liver resection without hepatotomy or inflow occlusion. J Am Coll Surg 2008; 206:390–6.

11. Strasberg SM, Picus DD, Drebin JA. Results of a new strategy for reconstruction of biliary injuries having an isolated right-sided component. J Gastroint Surg 2001; 5:266–74.

12. Strasberg SM, Hertl M, Soper NJ. An analysis of the problem of biliary injury during laparoscopic cholecystectomy. J Am Coll Surg 1995; 180: 101–25.

13. Northover JM, Terblanche J. A new look at the arterial supply of the bile duct in man and its surgical implications. Br J Surg 1979; 66: 379–84.

14. Michels NA. Blood supply and anatomy of the upper abdominal organs. Philadelphia: JB Lippincott, 1955.

15. O'Morchoe CC. Lymphatic system of the pancreas. Microsc Res Tech 1997; 37:456–77.

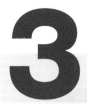

3

Laparoscopy in staging and assessment of hepatobiliary disease

Niels A. van der Gaag
Olivier R.C. Busch
Willem A. Bemelman
Dirk J. Gouma

Introduction

Accurate staging is of utmost importance in patients with hepatobiliary diseases since non-surgical palliation can be considered for advanced disease. Whenever surgical palliation is preferred, laparotomy is indicated, regardless of tumour resectability. Laparoscopy for hepato-pancreato-biliary (HPB) tumours was originally introduced as an additional diagnostic procedure for staging of patients deemed resectable by radiological imaging.[1] In particular, the procedure enabled detection of small metastatic tumour deposits on the liver surface and peritoneum which could be easily missed with standard radiological techniques. The addition of laparoscopic ultrasonography could also detect small hepatic metastases and local ingrowth in vascular structures.

However, the value of laparoscopy for HPB tumours is dependent on the specific indication and the associated end-points. In the selection of patients for curative resection, success can be defined as additional findings (such as liver cysts), a change in treatment strategy (bypass instead of resection) or the avoidance of unnecessary laparotomy (detection of metastases followed by non-surgical palliation). Studies on the value of diagnostic laparoscopy and laparoscopic ultrasonography have shown beneficial results but these have been influenced by various factors, such as the quality of the prelaparoscopy non-invasive imaging modalities and the timing of the laparoscopy in the staging process. Other fac-

tors include the expertise of the surgeon, the diligence of searching for metastases, the definition of local resectability, and whether a simple search for occult metastasis or an extended laparoscopy with exploration of the lesser sac, the porta hepatis, duodenum, transverse mesocolon and mesenteric vessels is performed. Furthermore, in selecting the most appropriate treatment, successful laparoscopy might also identify patients for chemoradiation (locally advanced disease) or chemotherapy only (metastatic disease).

Diagnostic laparoscopy and laparoscopic ultrasonography have been extensively evaluated in patients with HPB malignancies in our institution. These studies have focused mainly on diagnostic laparoscopy as a procedure to prevent unnecessary laparotomies – in our opinion, the most important end-point of success of the procedure. This chapter reports on the findings of these studies and provides an update of the current literature on HPB tumours. Some issues will be discussed for HPB tumours in general, whereas other key management points will be dealt with for each specific tumour location (pancreatic, proximal bile duct and liver).

Technical details

Diagnostic laparoscopy and subsequent therapeutic laparotomy are performed as separate procedures at our institution for logistical reasons, whereas others perform both procedures in one setting. In

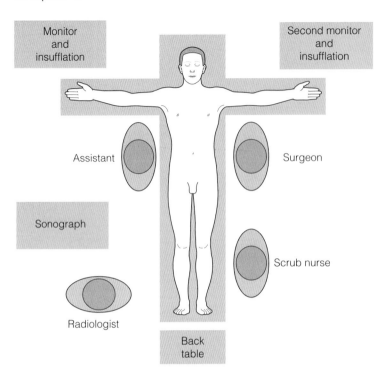

Figure 3.1 • Position in the operating theatre during laparoscopy and laparoscopic ultrasonography (LUS).

doing so, the scheduling of surgery may be difficult, but the patient can be spared a second procedure. The procedure is performed under general anaesthesia with the patient in a supine position and the surgeon standing on the left side of the patient (**Fig. 3.1**). A CO_2 pneumoperitoneum is established using a pressure of 12–15 mmHg by an open technique. A subumbilical trocar is introduced for a zero-degree camera and two other 10–11 mm trocars are placed in the left and right subcostal regions (**Fig. 3.2**). Inspection of the abdominal cavity is performed and the peritoneum is explored to identify tumour spread. The visceral peritoneum, the left lobe of the liver, the anterior aspect of the stomach, lesser and greater omentum, and the spleen are inspected. The right side of the abdominal cavity is investigated by passing the camera beneath the falciform ligament. The Treitz ligament, mesenteric root and pancreatic head are exposed by moving the omentum and the transverse colon in front of the stomach. The mesocolon and duodenal curve can be evaluated for possible ingrowth of pancreatic tumour at this point. Improved exposure may be obtained by placing the patient in a reverse Trendelenburg position and tilting the table laterally from side to side. Inspection can be performed from different angles because all trocars allow introduction of the camera, and this can be helpful in evaluating liver tumours. The lesser sac can be opened to provide a direct view of the pancreas and spleen, important for assessment of local ingrowth and evaluation of suspicious

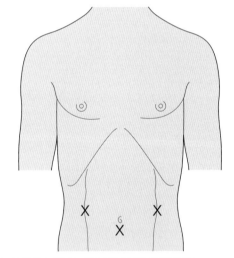

Figure 3.2 • Trocar placement for diagnostic laparoscopy and laparoscopic ultrasonography.

coeliac lymph nodes in cases of pancreatic body and tail tumours.

Peritoneal lavage can be performed prior to dissection or biopsy to prevent contamination of the lavage sample. Isotonic saline (500–1500 ml) is instilled into the subhepatic space and dispersed by abdominal agitation. The fluid is drained through the left subcostal trocar and collected for cytological evaluation. When distant metastases or tumour

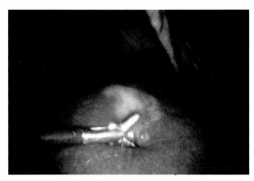

Figure 3.3 • Visual guided biopsy during laparoscopy.

ingrowth in the hepatoduodenal ligament or meso-colon are not detected or proven by frozen section, laparoscopic ultrasonography can be performed using either 10-mm-diameter rigid or flexible ultra-sound probes. Isotonic saline is instilled in the peri-toneal cavity to provide an acoustic window, and the abdominal pressure can be decreased to 7–8 mmHg to improve contact with the liver surface.[2] We use a rigid 7.5 MHz linear array laparoscopic ultrasound (LUS) probe wrapped in a sterile poly-ethylene cover sheet, filled with sterile ultrasonic gel, to examine the liver, hepatoduodenal ligament, coeliac axis, gallbladder and pancreas, as well as lymph nodes. The patient is scanned from multiple ports to evaluate the tumour from different angles. Biopsies of suspicious lesions are taken at the end of the procedure under direct laparoscopic vision or by laparoscopic ultrasound guidance using biopsy forceps (**Fig. 3.3**) or Tru-cut® (Travenol; Baxter Healthcare Corporation, Deerfield, IL, USA) and Rotex® (Ursus Konsult AB, Stockholm, Sweden) biopsy needles. In suspected liver cirrhosis, a visu-ally guided biopsy of the liver is taken for histolog-ical investigation and grading of the cirrhosis. The abdominal cavity is decompressed and the wounds are closed in a standard fashion.

Safety and complications

Diagnostic laparoscopy is a safe procedure with low morbidity, while complications have been reported in 0.15–3% of cases, and almost without mortal-ity (0.05%).[3] In a prospective series of 420 patients, three patients (1%) had major complications, including anaphylactic shock, small bowel perfo-ration and bile leakage after liver biopsy, a poten-tial risk when biopsies are taken from lesions in an inadequately drained liver segment.[4] Twelve patients (3%) had minor complications: four wound infec-tions; two wound haematomas; three patients with undefined upper abdominal pain; one aspiration pneumonia; one urinary retention; and one inci-

sional hernia. There was no mortality in this series and patients were discharged at a mean of 1.5 post-operative days.

The introduction of the first trocar is the most hazardous part of any laparoscopic procedure, due to the associated risk of vascular and bowel lesions. However, the incidence of serious vas-cular lesions is extremely low (0.001–0.005%), although mortality in patients with such a com-plication may reach 17%.[5] The incidence of lapa-roscopy-induced bowel injury is 0.13% and such injury is usually discovered during the operation.[6] Nevertheless, laparoscopy-induced bowel injury is also associated with a mortality rate of 3.6%. If the patient has undergone a previous laparot-omy, such as in colorectal cancer, the incidence of vascular and bowel injury increases. We recom-mend that the first trocar is introduced by an open procedure using the Hasson® or TrocDoc trocar, which is no more time-consuming.[7] Although there remains a risk of delayed bowel injury due to dia-thermy injury, we believe that the open procedure reduces the risk of perforating intra-abdominal organs, with the advantage of directly recognising the injury when it occurs.

 Port-site metastases are a feared complication of diagnostic laparoscopy in suspected intra-abdominal malignancies, although the expected risk is probably overestimated and cannot be used as an argument against laparoscopy.

In our series of 420 patients, port-site metastases occurred in only eight patients (2%) after a median follow-up period of 5 months. Furthermore, all patients had advanced disease at the time the port-site metastases were discovered. These data are sim-ilar to those of Shoup and colleagues, who reported a 0.8% port-site metastasis rate in a similar group of patients.[8] In patients undergoing an open proce-dure after laparoscopy the incidence of incisional site recurrence was not significantly different. Importantly, all patients in both series had perito-neal tumour spread present at the time of diagno-sis. Nevertheless, this small possibility of port-site metastases underlines the importance of careful assessment in patients with small, potentially resect-able tumours.[9] In selecting patients for resection, biopsies of the primary tumour or regional lymph nodes are never performed in our institution to establish pathology-proven diagnosis. Only vis-ible, suspicious distant metastases are biopsied to exclude definitively the possibility of resection. The dramatic consequences in these patients outweigh the potential risks of port-site metastases, which do not influence prognosis in pathology-proven metastatic disease.

Pancreatic and periampullary cancer

Pancreatic cancer still has a poor prognosis, since the majority of patients present with advanced disease. Surgical resection is the only treatment with a chance of definitive cure, but surgical exploration is applicable in only 10–20% of patients, due to distant metastases and/or locally advanced disease at time of presentation.[10] In patients with pancreatic or periampullary cancer, minimally invasive palliative techniques, such as endoscopic stenting, can relieve jaundice as an alternative to surgical bypass and have changed the approach to patients with irresectable disease. The detection of small liver and peritoneal metastases (**Fig. 3.4**) is an important motivation for performing diagnostic laparoscopy, since this might avoid open exploration.

CT and resectability

At present the best initial imaging modality for assessment of patients with suspected pancreatic cancer is high quality multislice spiral CT.[11–13]

Thin slice (2–3 mm), high-speed scanning with optimal use of contrast medium enables detection and characterisation of smaller lesions and provides detailed information on the relationship of the primary tumour with surrounding structures. CT has excellent accuracy in predicting irresectability (specificity 90–100%); however, sensitivity for assessment of irresectability remains much lower (70%). This is due to its inability to detect very small metastatic liver lesions (<1 cm) or peritoneal deposits (**Fig. 3.5**) and, to a lesser extent, in assessing accurately the presence of subtle vascular invasion.

The yield of additional laparoscopic staging is influenced greatly by the quality of the prelaparoscopic

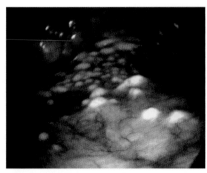

Figure 3.4 • Peritoneal metastases from pancreatic cancer.

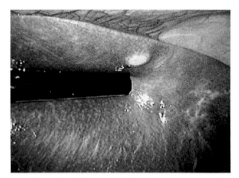

Figure 3.5 • Small liver metastases from pancreatic cancer during laparotomy.

staging process and unfortunately information on the scanning protocol and use of high-quality spiral CT is often lacking in most series. Incorrect staging with poor quality CT, for example, results in an overestimation in the yield of diagnostic laparoscopy and laparoscopic ultrasonography. Pisters and colleagues[14] stated that detection of occult metastatic disease should be less than 20% during laparoscopy, otherwise the quality of prediagnostic imaging should be considered inadequate. Table 3.1[15–21] summarises a number of studies from experienced centres in which the potential benefit of diagnostic laparoscopy in detecting metastases was undertaken after high-quality spiral CT. The results should be interpreted cautiously since many of these studies assessed the role of staging laparoscopy indirectly by examining the number of unsuspected metastases encountered at open exploration after negative preoperative imaging.[10] Moreover, the potential benefit of laparoscopy was attributed to detection of distant metastases only, irrespective of the additional value of laparoscopic ultrasound and peritoneal cytology.

Studies that correlate CT findings with operative and histopathological findings underline the importance of thin-slice CT in resectability assessment. Sensitivity and specificity were 78% and 76%, respectively, when 5-mm slices were used, compared with 91% and 90% for a slice thickness of 3 mm.[22,23] Furthermore, it has been shown that a high predicted risk for irresectability with CT is associated with significantly poorer survival. In a study of 71 consecutive patients with potentially resectable pancreatic head cancer, Phoa et al.[24] reported a median survival of 21 months for patients staged as resectable by CT compared to 9.7 months for the patients staged as unresectable. For the resected tumours, survival was relatively poor if tumours were larger than 3 cm or if CT signs of local irresectability were noted (hazard ratio 3.2). In a study by Thomson et al.,[25] laparoscopy with ultrasound identified

Table 3.1 • Peritoneal and/or liver metastases detected during laparotomy after high-quality spiral CT scan (± EUS)

Author	Year	Patients considered resectable	Resection rate (%)	Patients with metastases	Maximum % prevented
Spitz et al.[15]	1997	118	80	18	15
Friess et al.[16]	1998	159	75	16	10
Saldinger et al.[17]	2000	68	76	3	4
Schlieman et al.[18]	2003	89	45	24	27
Maire et al.[19]	2004	69	77	9	13
Morganti et al.[20]	2005	54	57	6	11
Ellsmere et al.[21]	2005	44	52	8	18

Adapted from Pisters et al.[14]

27 of 88 (31%) patients with Loyer CT grade A–D lesions as having unresectable disease and 17 of 29 (59%) with grade E lesions. The authors concluded that in patients with grade A–D lesions, laparoscopy should continue to be used, but selectively in grade E and not for grade O (no evident mass lesion) or grade F tumours (vascular occlusion).

While the most important objective in laparoscopy is to prevent unnecessary laparotomy, a number of patients do need a subsequent laparotomy for further palliation (e.g. bypass procedure for gastrointestinal obstruction). A further study assessed 233 patients with upper gastrointestinal malignancy, of whom 114 patients had a periampullary tumour.[26] Laparotomy was avoided initially in 17 patients (15%) but 5 of these patients (29%) subsequently required laparotomy for duodenal obstruction. This reduced the overall efficacy of laparoscopy in preventing unnecessary laparotomies from 15% to 11%. In a more recent study of 297 patients, the laparoscopic yield decreased to 13% (39 patients), probably due to improved radiological staging techniques.[27] This, combined with an increasingly critical view of resectability and palliation, has resulted in a decreased benefit of laparoscopic staging. Having abandoned the use of routine diagnostic and staging laparoscopy in patients with periampullary tumours in our own institution, we investigated

the implementation of this strategy in 186 consecutive patients.[28] At laparotomy, 63 patients (34%) had unresectable disease, while metastases were found in 29 patients (16%). Considering the previous accuracy of laparoscopy of 59%, the potential benefit was only 10%. The results in Table 3.2 document the decline in benefit of diagnostic laparoscopy and the evolution of radiological staging modalities in our centre. Recently, other large studies[2,25,27,29–31] (Table 3.3) have shown varying results when addressing the effectiveness of staging laparoscopy in identifying patients with unsuspected unresectable disease and in decreasing the number of unnecessary laparotomies.

 Based on these results the routine use of diagnostic laparoscopy in pancreatic cancer cannot be recommended.

At the present time, the controversy is focused on whether diagnostic laparoscopy should be used selectively for patients with questionably resectable pancreatic cancer based on preoperative imaging. To identify variables that might enhance the yield of laparoscopy by its selective use, two studies found that larger tumours (size >3 cm) on preoperative

Table 3.2 • Influence of radiological imaging and time period on the yield of diagnostic laparoscopy for periampullary cancer in the Academic Medical Center (AMC)

	Period	Prevented laparotomy (%)	Radiological staging
Introduction	1993–94	19	Ultrasonography
Late laparotomy	1993–95	15	Ultrasonography + conventional CT scan
Randomised trial	1995–98	13	5-mm sliced spiral CT scan
Implementation study	1999–2001	9.5	3-mm sliced spiral CT scan

Table 3.3 • Studies on the value of staging laparoscopy for pancreatic head or periampullary cancer and detection of unresectable disease at laparotomy (recent studies with >80 patients)

Author	Year	Patients	Study type	Unresectable found at laparoscopy (%)	Additional unresectable found at laparotomy (%)	Total unresectable patients (%)
Conlon et al.[2]	1996	108	Prosp	39	5	41
Jimenez et al.[29]	2000	125	Retro	31	6	37
Vollmer et al.[30]	2002	88	Retro	30	15	46
Van Dijkum et al.[27]	2003	297	Prosp	13	24	37
Doran et al.[31]	2004	305	Prosp	15	16	31
Thomson et al.[25]	2006	152	Retro	37	22	59

Adapted from Stefanidis et al.[10]

imaging had significantly more unsuspected metastases at exploration compared with those with smaller tumours (<3 cm).[10] Preoperative serum carbohydrate antigen (CA) 19-9 level has been shown to increase the yield of laparoscopy in three studies.[10,32] In patients with adenocarcinoma of the pancreas, low CA19-9 levels (<100 or 150 U/ml for the respective studies) predicted a low probability of metastatic disease, and the authors concluded that laparoscopy can be avoided in those patients. Patients with elevated CA19-9 have an increased probability of metastatic disease and may benefit from laparoscopy. Finally, it has been shown that the yield of laparoscopy is much higher in patients with pancreatic body and tail tumours than for periampullary tumours.[10]

 Assessment of tumour size, preoperative serum CA19-9 level and tumour location is of value in selecting patients that might benefit from staging laparoscopy.

Obviously, resectability rate and, consequently, the yield of laparoscopy following spiral CT is totally dependent of what constitutes irresectability. Spitz et al.[15] reported a series of 118 patients of whom only 2 (1%) had unresectable disease, whereas 25 patients (21%) required vascular resection and reconstruction for local ingrowth of tumour into a major vessel. At our institution, gross ingrowth of a pancreatic tumour in the portal vein or superior mesenteric vein is considered a criterion for irresectability because it is associated with a dismal prognosis. In an earlier report from our institution, the median survival was only 6 months after segmental venous resection.[33] In a large review of 1646 patients that underwent portal-superior mesenteric vein resection of varying

extent, the median survival was only 13 months and was probably skewed by a positive publication bias.[34] In our present series of patients with minimal vascular involvement, a survival of 14 months was observed and therefore only partial rather than extensive (segmental) resection and reconstruction is performed. Pancreatic resection with resection of small, synchronous liver metastases in well-selected patients with low-volume metastatic liver disease did not result in long-term survival in the overwhelming majority of patients.[35]

Extended laparoscopy

Some authors have extended staging laparoscopy in periampullary cancer to imitate open exploration so as to gain more information about the possible tumour invasion of retroperitoneal vessels.[2] In a series of 103 pancreatic cancers, examination was performed of the primary tumour, liver and porta hepatis, with division of the gastrohepatic omentum, inspection of the vena cava, caudate lobe, coeliac axis and lesser sac, as well as examination of local tumour spread to the mesocolon, duodenum, jejunum and ligament of Treitz. Although Conlon's criteria of irresectability are not accepted universally, they found that the extension of the procedure identified irresectability in 14 patients (12%). However, others have stated that this approach is time-consuming and potentially dangerous.[29] Part of the time needed for the laparoscopic procedure could be regained when the therapeutic laparotomy is performed immediately after the laparoscopy. However, extended laparoscopy may lead to troublesome bleeding when assessing local tumour extension into major vessels and biopsying for pathological examination.

Laparoscopic ultrasonography

Laparoscopic ultrasonography has been introduced as an additional procedure to increase the detection of small intrahepatic liver metastasis (**Fig. 3.6**), to identify enlarged and suspicious lymph nodes, and to evaluate local ingrowth into the vascular structures. Some authors who found a high yield for this procedure have staged all liver lesions detected by ultrasonography without verification by pathological examination. Similarly, enlarged lymph nodes have been considered a finding of irresectability without biopsy or local suspected tumour ingrowth. Such features should only have therapeutic consequences when they are proven histopathologically. Metastases detected by laparoscopic ultrasonography that were not found during preoperative imaging are often too small for successful laparoscopic ultrasonography-guided puncture to confirm the diagnosis histopathologically (**Fig. 3.7**). Interpretation of the literature on the additional value of laparoscopic ultrasonography is difficult due to differences in patient selection, criteria of success and prelaparoscopic imaging techniques. The predictive value of local tumour ingrowth into major blood vessels is high with laparoscopic ultrasonography and it may therefore be useful in patients who show equivocal findings at spiral CT scanning. Most series do not give information on the additional value of laparoscopic ultrasonography after laparoscopic evaluation did not show irresectability.

We analysed the additional value of laparoscopic ultrasonography in 223 patients with periampullary cancer in detecting metastases and/or local tumour ingrowth (**Fig. 3.8**), compared with radio-

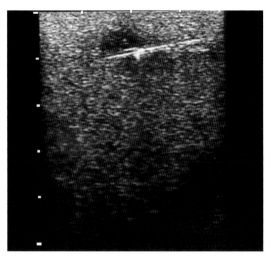

Figure 3.7 • Ultrasonographic guided biopsy of liver lesion.

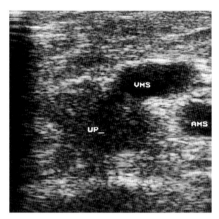

Figure 3.8 • Local ingrowth in the superior mesenteric vein (SMV) of pancreatic tumour visualised by laparoscopic ultrasonography. AMS, superior mesenteric artery; UP, tumour in uncinate process.

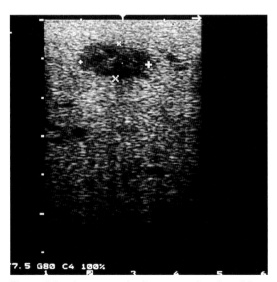

Figure 3.6 • Laparoscopic ultrasonography of small liver lesion.

logical investigations and also whether these findings could be proven by pathological examination. In 17 patients, metastases were found during laparoscopic ultrasonography, but most of these lesions had already been identified or suspected following US or CT. In only three patients (1%) could these lesions be considered a new finding, and in only two patients was this confirmed pathologically. Detection of tumour ingrowth in major vessels was suspected in 22% but it was reported as a new finding in only 5%. In none of the patients could biopsy prove local invasion but it is accepted that this is a limitation of any imaging modality. The additional value of laparoscopic ultrasonography on local ingrowth of pancreatic cancer is difficult to establish from some other studies[36–41] (Table 3.4).

Table 3.4 • Benefit of laparoscopic ultrasonography on determining vascular tumour ingrowth in patients with periampullary cancer

Author	Year	Patients	Unresectable at laparoscopy alone	Unresectable at LUS*	Benefit of LUS (overall %)
Minnard et al.[37]	1998	90	41	8	9
Catheline et al.[38]	1999	26	n/a[†]	7	27
Schachter et al.[39]	2000	67	8	16	24
Taylor et al.[40]	2001	51	n/a	11	22
Hünerbein et al.[41]	2001	77	35	3	4

*Laparoscopic ultrasound.
†n/a, not available.

Considering the improved quality of endoscopic ultrasonography currently in our centre, laparoscopic ultrasonography is not considered useful in the work-up of patients with pancreatic carcinoma.

Palliation

The evaluation of staging procedures is incomplete without considering the consequences for treatment, which should be aimed at improving outcome. Therefore, in extending the value of laparoscopy as a diagnostic tool, we investigated the consequences of laparoscopically detected and histologically proven unresectable cancer, in terms of hospital-free survival, by randomising patients for palliative treatment to endoscopic stenting or subsequent surgical bypass.[27] In this study, histologically proven metastases were detected at laparoscopy in 39 of the 297 patients (13%). The average hospital-free survival for those patients that subsequently underwent endoscopic stenting was 94 days compared to 164 days for patients that underwent surgical palliative treatment. This study confirmed a limited benefit for laparoscopy in preventing laparotomy, but more importantly demonstrated no improvement in hospital-free survival after non-surgical palliation in these patients. Patients with a high risk of irresectability suspected on CT staging or those who are unlikely to benefit from surgical palliation could be selected for this staging procedure.

On the other hand, there is evidence that the majority of patients who are treated endoscopically do not require surgical palliation.[42] Furthermore, a recent Cochrane meta-analysis of 21 randomised controlled trials actually demonstrated that endoscopic (metal) stents are the intervention of choice in patients with malignant distal obstructive jaundice due to irresectable pancreatic carcinoma.[43] Evidence on the feasibility of performing a bypass laparoscopically for malignant gastric outlet obstruction is emerging. In a prospective randomised trial, Mehta and colleagues found that laparoscopic gastrojejunostomy was as safe a means of palliation as duodenal stenting.[44] There were no complications, a shorter hospital stay (5.2 vs. 11.4 days) and an improvement in physical health at 1 month.

Patients with a high a priori risk of irresectability will benefit from diagnostic laparoscopy, either to prove irresectability and initiate endoscopic palliation, or to proceed to laparotomy for resection or surgical palliation.

Advanced disease

Patients with locally advanced disease have distinct treatment options and outcome when compared to patients with metastatic disease, most importantly in the application of radiation-based protocols for locoregional control. Since locally advanced cancer is more likely to be associated with peritoneal or liver metastases, failure to detect these metastases results in understaging of disease. Chemoradiation will not be of benefit to such patients but, moreover, might result in unnecessary treatment-related morbidity. Several authors have therefore suggested that diagnostic laparoscopy should be performed to select those patients with true locally advanced disease, thereby excluding patients with CT-occult metastatic disease from further treatment and unnecessary morbidity.[10,45,46] Liu and Traverso found that occult distant disease was detected by laparoscopy in 34% of patients shown to have locally unresectable disease by CT, and body and tail tumours were twice as likely to have unsuspected metastasis (53%) as pancreatic head tumours (28%).[47] They concluded that laparoscopic staging should be used routinely for locally extensive pancreatic cancer when therapies directed at the primary tumour are being considered. When inappropriately applied, the effect of treatment will result in falsely low survival statistics, since patients with distant metastasis are known to have a poor outlook.

Diagnostic laparoscopy is advised to identify true locally advanced disease when chemoradiation, as opposed to systemic chemotherapy, is being considered as palliative treatment.

Proximal bile duct tumours

Differentiation of bile duct cancer infiltrating the liver hilum from gallbladder cancer or even benign pathology as a cause of proximal bile duct obstruction may be difficult. Hilar cholangiocarcinomas are often small and do not form a bulky mass, which makes them very difficult to visualise on any imaging modality. Occlusion of the portal venous system is usually well seen with CT and magnetic resonance imaging (MRI), but more limited tumour ingrowth can be hard to determine. Moreover, accurate evaluation of the extent of intrahepatic tumour extension can be difficult without performing direct cholangiography (ERCP or percutaneous transhepatic cholangiography). Therefore, the surgeon dealing with malignant proximal bile duct obstruction is often faced with significant discrepancy between the findings of preoperative investigations and those visualised at the time of exploration. Tumours infiltrating the proximal bile ducts in particular tend to be unresectable and, because palliation is invariably non-surgical, these patients might benefit from laparoscopic staging to avoid unnecessary laparotomy.[48] Obviously, there is no rationale for laparoscopic staging if intrahepatic biliary bypass surgery is the preferred method of palliation in these patients.[49]

Large gallbladder cancers are recognised easily by preoperative assessment or during laparoscopy. Characteristic findings at laparoscopy include a thickened whitish-coloured wall, neovascularisation of the wall, omentum adherent to the gallbladder and infiltration of tumour into the adjacent liver. Surgical technique is critically important in situations where the preoperative profile and the intraoperative findings suggest the possibility of malignancy. Thus, if the dissection is difficult, or the risk of gallbladder rupture appears high, conversion to an open procedure may avoid the intraperitoneal spread of malignant cells.[50] Laparoscopy may also be useful in those patients in whom an early stage tumour has been diagnosed incidentally following gallbladder removal and where liver resection and lymphadenectomy is being considered. In advanced disease, histological confirmation of peritoneal or liver metastases may be required but in most cases this will be apparent prior to exploration.

Diagnostic and staging laparoscopy

Information on the additional value of diagnostic laparoscopy for malignant proximal bile duct obstruction is limited. In a pilot study from our institution, advanced disease was diagnosed in 19 (40%) of the 47 patients by laparoscopy.[4] These results were explained, in part, by a change in diagnosis after laparoscopy from a primary bile duct tumour to a locally invasive gallbladder cancer. A more recent study of 110 consecutive patients in our institution has confirmed these data.[51] Laparoscopy revealed histologically proven incurable disease in 44 (41%) patients. Of the 65 patients who underwent laparotomy, 35 patients (54%) were unresectable. Although laparotomy was avoided in 41% of cases, laparoscopy could not assess resectability correctly in 44% of patients.

These findings agree with a study from the Memorial Sloan Kettering Cancer Center[52] involving 100 patients with carcinoma of the extrahepatic biliary tree. Thirty-five patients (35%) were identified as having unresectable disease at laparoscopy. Of the 65 patients who underwent laparotomy, a further 34 tumours (52%) were unresectable, resulting in an overall accuracy of 51% for detecting unresectable disease. The yield of laparoscopy was greater for gallbladder cancer than for hilar cholangiocarcinoma, as was also found by others.[30] Similarly, Agrawal et al. performed laparoscopic staging for gallbladder cancer in the same setting with subsequent laparotomy.[53] Laparoscopy avoided further surgery in 35 patients (38%) after detection of liver and peritoneal metastases or extensive locally advanced disease (6 patients) that was missed on imaging. Finally, in a series of 401 patients with hepatobiliary cancer, the highest yield for laparoscopy was found in patients with biliary cancer, but the study emphasised that the surgeon's preoperative impression of resectability was as important as the laparoscopic staging procedure.[54]

Laparoscopy should be employed to stage proximal bile duct tumours, and in particular gallbladder cancer, due to the associated high yield and subsequent option for non-surgical palliation for irresectable disease.

Laparoscopic ultrasonography

Laparoscopic ultrasonography has not been very useful in staging the local tumour spread of proximal bile duct cancer. In our recent series of 110 proximal bile duct lesions, laparoscopic ultra-sonography staged only one patient as unresect-able.[51] These data are comparable to the findings of Vollmer and colleagues,[30] who identified 2 of 23 patients (9%) as having unresectable disease as a result of laparoscopic ultrasonography alone. The New York study confirmed that patients with unre-sectable disease most often had locally advanced tumours, but laparoscopic ultrasonography did not contribute to the assessment of resectability in these patients.[52] Furthermore, extensive biliary and vascular involvement can be determined with high accuracy (91%) by external colour Doppler ultra-sonography, as well as thin-slice contrast-enhanced multislice CT.[55]

The additional value of laparoscopic ultrasonogra-phy is therefore too low for it to be performed rou-tinely in patients with proximal bile duct tumours.

Palliation

Although the most appropriate palliation of malig-nant proximal biliary obstruction is still controver-sial, we prefer a non-surgical approach and therefore laparoscopic staging has substantial benefit.[56] In these patients laparoscopic palliation appears to have lit-tle role despite innovative descriptions of combined radiological and endoscopic techniques.

Hepatic malignancies

Diagnostic laparoscopy

For hepatic malignancy, the major imaging modal-ities include US and contrast-enhanced spiral CT. Recent developments in gradient coil design, the use of body phased array coils and the availability of novel MR contrast agents show promise, and have resulted in MRI being recognised increas-ingly as the preoperative standard in this group of patients.[57]

 FDG-PET has been shown in three meta-analyses not only to be the most sensitive means of detecting intrahepatic metastases but, in a recent review, for also identifying extrahepatic metastases in patients with potentially resectable colorectal liver metastases.[58]

Accordingly, the precise role of laparoscopy in hepatic malignancy, at least for secondary lesions, is subject to considerable change. Traditionally, lapa-roscopy is considered useful in patients with hepatic malignancy because there is usually no indication for surgical palliation if curative resection is not pos-sible. Laparoscopy can be used for examination of the abdominal cavity to rule out extrahepatic meta-static disease and can provide information on the presence of superficial liver lesions and character-ise small (<1 cm) intrahepatic lesions. Close inspec-tion of the liver is particularly relevant in patients with cirrhosis, because it is difficult to detect lesions against the nodular, inhomogeneous background of cirrhosis, and to differentiate malignant lesions from regenerative or dysplastic nodules. Evaluation of the degree of liver cirrhosis is important prior to resec-tion of hepatocellular carcinoma, and laparoscopic guided biopsies can be performed safely to assess the quality of the remaining liver. In a study looking at 58 biopsies in 22 consecutive patients with a pro-longed prothrombin time, prolonged bleeding time or thrombocytopenia, Inabnet and Deziel[59] identi-fied only one patient (5%) who required transfu-sion and laparotomy for haemostatic control. Most patients with secondary liver malignancies have pre-viously undergone a laparotomy, making the visu-alisation of intra-abdominal organs more difficult due to adhesions. The failure rate of laparoscopy in these patients is reported as 5–15% in most series. It is important, therefore, to use an open technique for introduction of the first trocar. Unfortunately, some pitfalls remain in applying laparoscopy to the evaluation of liver malignancy. The relative ease with which iatrogenic injury can be caused to the hepatic parenchyma by retraction and manipulation remains a concern.

Laparoscopic ultrasonography is attractive as a means of evaluating liver lesions and most studies reporting on the value of laparoscopy in primary and secondary liver malignancies have added this to their procedure. The gold standard for detecting secondary liver lesions is still intraoperative palpa-tion and ultrasonography, but it has been demon-strated that laparoscopic ultrasonography detects these lesions effectively.

Primary liver malignancy

Lo and colleagues[60] found that laparoscopic evalua-tion avoided exploratory laparotomy in 63% of the unresectable patients with primary liver cancer. The procedure was accurate in assessing the quality of the liver remnant and the presence of intrahepatic metastases, but it was less sensitive in determin-ing the presence of tumour thrombi in major vas-cular structures and the extent of local invasion, especially in large (>10 cm) tumours. The study of Ido et al.[61] clearly showed the value of lapa-roscopic ultrasonography in detecting and diagnosing small hepatocellular carcinomas; 134 new nodules were visualised by this technique in 64 (34%) of 186 patients in whom 28 nodules (in 23 patients) were histologically diagnosed as hepatocellular carcinoma. Of these 23 patients, 18 had been diagnosed as solitary hepatocellular carcinoma before laparoscopy. Similarly, Montorsi and colleagues[62] found new lesions of histologically proven hepatocellular carcinoma in 22% of patients. Even when preoperative staging includes a high-speed spiral CT, Foroutani et al.[63] demonstrated that laparoscopic ultrasonography was superior in detecting additional tumours. Ultrasonography confirmed all 201 tumours seen on CT and detected 21 additional tumours (9.5%) ranging in size from 0.3 to 2.7 cm in 11 patients (20%).

 These series and our recent study[4,60–62,64,65] (Table 3.5) suggest that laparoscopic staging is useful in patients with primary liver malignancies since these tumours tend to be at high risk of being unresectable. The value of laparoscopic staging is doubled due to its capacity to facilitate guided biopsies to determine the quality of the liver remnant in cirrhotic patients.

Colorectal cancer liver metastases

There has been a change in the approach to the management of colorectal cancer liver lesions over the last decade, which has influenced the yield of laparoscopy in these patients. The indications for resection for metastases have changed towards a more aggressive approach for multiple lesions (more than four) and bilobar disease. The under-

standing of liver anatomy and familiarity with intraoperative ultrasonography has led to a segment-oriented approach and has made repeated resections feasible. Furthermore, the use of local ablative techniques such as radiofrequency ablation (RFA) in combination with resection has extended the possibilities for curative surgical treatment. Currently the only absolute restrictions for curative resection include irresectable extrahepatic dissemination and failure of function of the (future) liver remnant, for which nowadays portal vein embolisation might be used to induce hypertrophy. In addition to this more aggressive surgical approach, improved imaging techniques in recent years have impacted on the value of laparoscopy with ultrasonography in patients with secondary liver malignancy. In a recent analysis of our data, we found a decreased yield of laparoscopy in such patients.[65] We failed to perform a full examination in 11 of the 51 patients (20%) due to adhesions. Five of 43 patients were staged correctly as unresectable, giving a yield of 12% in this group. In 5 of 12 patients (42%), unresectable disease was identified by laparoscopy and laparoscopic ultrasonography. This yield is considerably less compared to a previous study in which 7 of 27 patients (26%) with colorectal liver metastases were prevented from undergoing an unnecessary laparotomy. Several other series[63,64,66–68] have reported variable success rates for laparoscopy in patients with secondary liver malignancy of colorectal cancer (Table 3.5). It should be noted that some of these series considered bilobar disease as an exclusion for resection, which may have resulted

Table 3.5 • Selected studies on diagnostic laparoscopy in primary and secondary liver malignancy

Author	Year	Primary or secondary	Patients	Number unresectable detected by laparoscopy (%)
Lo et al.[60]	1998	Primary	12	8 (67)
Van Dijkum et al.[4]	1999	Primary	10	4 (25)
		Secondary	33	11 (33)
Ido et al.[61]	1999	Primary	186	64 (34)
Jarnagin et al.[64]	2000	Primary/secondary	104	26 (25)
Foroutani et al.[63]	2000	Primary	9	1 (11)
		Secondary	46	10 (22)
Montorsi et al.[62]	2001	Primary	70	14 (22)
Metcalfe et al.[66]	2003	Secondary	24	12 (50)
De Castro et al.[65]	2004	Primary	33	15 (45)
		Secondary	43	5 (12)
Thaler et al.[67]	2005	Secondary	136	34 (25)
Mann et al.[68]	2007	Secondary	200	39 (20)

in a higher yield for diagnostic laparoscopy than would have been found if modern resection criteria were used.

Nowadays, several centres favour the selective use of laparoscopy in patients with colorectal metastases. Jarnagin et al.[69] have described a clinical risk score (CRS) that predicted survival after hepatic resection and was suitable in identifying high-risk patients most likely to benefit from laparoscopy. In a study of 103 patients, occult unresectable disease was found in 12% of patients with a low score versus 42% of patients with a high score. In a recent publication, the authors reported similar findings which in their opinion underlined the indication for selective use of laparoscopy.[70] Similarly, in a series of 200 patients, Mann and colleagues[68] reported a detection rate of only 6% for patients with the lowest CRS, whereas this rate was 75% for the highest CRS scores. Metcalfe et al.[66] demonstrated a yield of 50% in a selected group of patients, whereas in the group of 49 patients selected for direct surgical exploration 46 patients (94%) were resected. Although their selection criteria for laparoscopy were not very strict, they found that the likelihood of being unresectable is in part predicted by the disease-free interval and the number of hepatic metastases.

Non-colorectal cancer liver metastases

In a limited experience of eight patients with secondary non-colorectal liver malignancy, we identified unresectable disease in three patients (38%). Only one unresectable tumour was missed by laparoscopic staging. A larger series of 30 consecutive patients with non-colorectal cancer metastases from the Memorial Sloan-Kettering Cancer Center staged 6 of the 30 patients' tumours (20%) as unresectable.[71] Laparoscopy detected 6 of the 9 patients (67%) with unresectable disease.

Laparoscopic staging is indicated for primary liver tumours due to the higher yield, while in patients with colorectal hepatic metastases, the indication for laparoscopy seems to be limited to patients with high CRS, especially with the availability of FDG-PET scans.

Laparoscopic treatment and palliation

A recent meta-analysis of eight (non-randomised) studies, comparing open and laparoscopic surgery, showed that laparoscopic resection for benign and malignant neoplasms results in reduced operative blood loss and earlier recovery with oncological clearance comparable with open surgery.[72] When performed by experienced surgeons in selected patients it may be a safe and feasible option. However, the authors emphasise the risk of the potential of significant bias from these reported studies and stress that further randomised controlled trials should be undertaken to confirm or exclude this bias and to assess long-term survival rates. Surgery is seldom required for palliation of malignant liver tumours but occasionally endocrine liver tumours need to be resected for palliation.

Radiofrequency tumour ablation has been shown to be safe and effective in reducing tumour load in patients with primary and secondary liver tumours. Since radiofrequency ablation can be performed during laparoscopy and laparoscopic guided ultrasonography it seems appropriate to perform this procedure directly after the staging laparoscopy. A recent review of relevant studies which included at least 10 patients reported rates of complete tumour ablation, local recurrence or survival after treatment.[73] Hepatic resection remains the standard of care when feasible and radiofrequency ablation cannot be considered as equivalent, but does appear to have a role in treating unresectable disease or may also be used in conjunction with resection to extend its limits.

Cytology of peritoneal lavage

The rationale for performing peritoneal lavage cytology lies in the detection of free cancer cells, which are believed to indicate early seeding of peritoneal metastases. The sixth edition of the American Joint Commission on Cancer (AJCC) Cancer Staging Manual classifies positive peritoneal cytology as M1 (stage IV) disease.[10] In gastric cancer patients it has been shown that patients with positive cytology of their peritoneal washings (**Fig. 3.9**) had a worse prognosis than those who

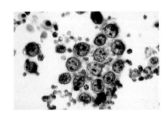

Figure 3.9 • Peritoneal washing with malignant cells from pancreatic cancer.

Table 3.6 • Peritoneal lavage during laparoscopic staging in patients with periampullary carcinoma

Author	Year	Patients	Positive cytology	Percentage
Van Dijkum et al.[75]	1998	236	7	3
Nakao et al.[77]	1999	74	22	29
Konishi et al.[78]	2002	151	36	24
Liu and Traverso[47]	2005	74	9	12*
Ferrone et al.[76]	2006	462	77	17

*Only patients with evidence of metastatic disease with CT scan of locally unresectable disease.

have not.[74] In our study of 449 patients, 362 of whom had potentially resectable HPB tumours, diagnostic laparoscopy was combined with peritoneal lavage.[75] Positive cytology was evident in only 20 patients (6%), of whom 15 (75%) had already proven metastases during laparoscopy. Of the whole group, 236 patients had pancreatic or periampullary carcinoma but in only 7 patients with pancreatic tumours (3%) was lavage positive. In most patients, metastases had already been visualised during laparoscopy and peritoneal lavage provided additional value in only 2 patients (0.9%). The sensitivity and specificity of lavage for detection of metastasis were 18% and 99% respectively. Although a positive peritoneal lavage was associated with a significant decreased median survival in our study, it was not an independent predictor for survival. Others have found that positive cytology was not associated with survival in irresectable disease; however, it was associated with poor survival in resected patients, equal to stage IV patients, and as a result should be considered as a separate procedure in high-risk patients.[76] Although a straightforward procedure, its value in HPB tumours is therefore still subject to debate, as evidenced by the wide reported range in yield of detecting cancer cells[47,75–78] (Table 3.6).

 Routine cytology of peritoneal lavage cannot be advised currently because of the low additional benefit and limited prognostic value, but might be of value in high-risk patients.

New techniques might increase the yield. A pilot study found that detection of micrometastases in peritoneal washings of pancreatic cancer patients by reverse transcriptase–polymerase chain reaction (RT–PCR), using a panel of tumour markers, was a sensitive method for detection of subclinical peritoneal tumour dissemination.[79]

Conclusions

Laparoscopic staging for HPB tumours is only appropriate when non-surgical palliation is preferred for unresectable patients, while the main objective is the avoidance of an unnecessary laparotomy. Ongoing improvements in preoperative radiological imaging have led to a more accurate prediction of resectability of HPB tumours and, as such, have decreased the yield of both laparoscopy and laparoscopic ultrasonography to a level that routine laparoscopy cannot now be advocated. Laparoscopy in the preoperative work-up is indicated only for those tumours with a high a priori chance of irresectability, such as proximal bile duct tumours including gallbladder cancer, pancreatic body and tail tumours, and primary liver tumours. For other tumour locations selective use of laparoscopy is indicated.

Selective use of laparoscopy for pancreatic or periampullary cancers is restricted to patients with a high risk of occult metastases, such as larger primary tumours (>3 cm), the presence of low-volume ascites, CT findings indicating possible carcinomatosis or small hypodense regions suggesting hepatic metastases that are inaccessible to percutaneous biopsy, or subtle clinical and laboratory findings suggesting advanced disease such as increased CA19-9 levels. In the presence of irresectable locally advanced disease, laparoscopy is indicated when chemoradiation-based palliative protocols as opposed to systemic chemotherapy are being considered for metastatic disease. Selective use of laparoscopy for secondary hepatic malignancies is indicated in the presence of a lymph-node-positive primary tumour, a disease-free interval of less than a year after colorectal cancer diagnosis, more than one hepatic lesion and a largest tumour diameter of >5 cm, which have all been shown to be predictors of survival.[80]

References

1. Warshaw AL, Tepper JE, Shipley WU. Laparoscopy in the staging and planning of therapy for pancreatic cancer. Am J Surg 1986; 151:76–80.

2. Conlon KC, Dougherty E, Klimstra DS et al. The value of minimal access surgery in the staging of patients with potentially resectable peripancreatic malignancy. Ann Surg 1996; 223:134–40.

   Early report of the potential role of extended laparoscopy in 115 patients with potentially resectable peripancreatic malignancy.

3. Boyd WP, Jr, Nord HJ. Diagnostic laparoscopy. Endoscopy 2000; 32:153–8.

4. Nieveen van Dijkum EJ, de Wit LT, van Delden OM et al. Staging laparoscopy and laparoscopic ultrasonography in more than 400 patients with upper gastrointestinal carcinoma. J Am Coll Surg 1999; 189:459–65.

5. Bateman BG, Kolp LA, Hoeger K. Complications of laparoscopy – operative and diagnostic. Fertil Steril 1996; 66:30–5.

6. van der Voort M, Heijnsdijk EA, Gouma DJ. Bowel injury as a complication of laparoscopy. Br J Surg 2004; 91:1253–8.

7. Bemelman WA, de Wit LT, Busch OR et al. Establishment of pneumoperitoneum with a modified blunt trocar. J Laparoendosc Adv Surg Tech A 2000; 10:217–8.

8. Shoup M, Brennan MF, Karpeh MS et al. Port site metastasis after diagnostic laparoscopy for upper gastrointestinal tract malignancies: an uncommon entity. Ann Surg Oncol 2002; 9:632–6.

   Report of 1965 laparoscopic procedures for cancer demonstrating that the very small risk of port-site recurrence (0.8%) cannot be used as an argument against laparoscopy in upper GI malignancy.

9. Tjalma WA. Laparoscopic surgery and port-site metastases: routine measurements to reduce the risk. Eur J Gynaecol Oncol 2003; 24:236.

10. Stefanidis D, Grove KD, Schwesinger WH et al. The current role of staging laparoscopy for adenocarcinoma of the pancreas: a review. Ann Oncol 2006; 17:189–99.

    Extensive review that underlines the role of variables enhancing the yield of laparoscopy.

11. Bipat S, Phoa SS, van Delden OM et al. Ultrasonography, computed tomography and magnetic resonance imaging for diagnosis and determining resectability of pancreatic adenocarcinoma: a meta-analysis. J Comput Assist Tomogr 2005; 29:438–45.

    Meta-analysis concluding that helical CT is preferable as an imaging modality for the diagnosis and assessment of resectability of pancreatic compared with MRI and US.

12. Bao PQ, Johnson JC, Lindsey EH et al. Endoscopic ultrasound and computed tomography predictors of pancreatic cancer resectability. J Gastrointest Surg 2008; 12:10–16.

13. Zamboni GA, Kruskal JB, Vollmer CM et al. Pancreatic adenocarcinoma: value of multidetector CT angiography in preoperative evaluation. Radiology 2007; 245:770–8.

14. Pisters PW, Lee JE, Vauthey JN et al. Laparoscopy in the staging of pancreatic cancer. Br J Surg 2001; 88:325–37.

15. Spitz FR, Abbruzzese JL, Lee JE et al. Preoperative and postoperative chemoradiation strategies in patients treated with pancreaticoduodenectomy for adenocarcinoma of the pancreas. J Clin Oncol 1997; 15:928–37.

16. Friess H, Kleeff J, Silva JC et al. The role of diagnostic laparoscopy in pancreatic and periampullary malignancies. J Am Coll Surg 1998; 186:675–82.

17. Saldinger PF, Reilly M, Reynolds K et al. Is CT angiography sufficient for prediction of resectability of periampullary neoplasms?. J Gastrointest Surg 2000; 4:233–7.

18. Schlieman MG, Ho HS, Bold RJ. Utility of tumor markers in determining resectability of pancreatic cancer. Arch Surg 2003; 138:951–5.

19. Maire F, Sauvanet A, Trivin F et al. Staging of pancreatic head adenocarcinoma with spiral CT and endoscopic ultrasonography: an indirect evaluation of the usefulness of laparoscopy. Pancreatology 2004; 4:436–40.

20. Morganti AG, Brizi MG, Macchia G et al. The prognostic effect of clinical staging in pancreatic adenocarcinoma. Ann Surg Oncol 2005; 12:145–51.

21. Ellsmere J, Mortele K, Sahani D et al. Does multidetector-row CT eliminate the role of diagnostic laparoscopy in assessing the resectability of pancreatic head adenocarcinoma? Surg Endosc 2005; 19:369–73.

22. Diehl SJ, Lehmann KJ, Sadick M et al. Pancreatic cancer: value of dual-phase helical CT in assessing resectability. Radiology 1998; 206:373–8.

23. Phoa SS, Reeders JW, Rauws EA et al. Spiral computed tomography for preoperative staging of potentially resectable carcinoma of the pancreatic head. Br J Surg 1999; 86:789–94.

24. Phoa SS, Tilleman EH, van Delden OM et al. Value of CT criteria in predicting survival in patients with potentially resectable pancreatic head carcinoma. J Surg Oncol 2005; 91:33–40.

25. Thomson BN, Parks RW, Redhead DN et al. Refining the role of laparoscopy and laparoscopic ultrasound in the staging of presumed pancreatic head and ampullary tumours. Br J Cancer 2006; 94:213–17.

26. Nieveen van Dijkum EJ, de Wit LT, van Delden OM et al. The efficacy of laparoscopic staging in patients with upper gastrointestinal tumors. Cancer 1997; 79:1315–19.

27. Nieveen van Dijkum EJ, Romijn MG, Terwee CB et al. Laparoscopic staging and subsequent palliation in patients with peripancreatic carcinoma. Ann Surg 2003; 237:66–73.
    Large study on 287 consecutive patients with peripancreatic malignancy demonstrating a detection rate for laparoscopic staging of 35% and biopsy-proven irresectable disease in 13%. The study also suggested that there was no apparent gain for non-surgical palliation.

28. Tilleman EH, Kuiken BW, Phoa SS et al. Limitation of diagnostic laparoscopy for patients with a periampullary carcinoma. Eur J Surg Oncol 2004; 30:658–62.

29. Jimenez RE, Warshaw AL, Rattner DW et al. Impact of laparoscopic staging in the treatment of pancreatic cancer. Arch Surg 2000; 135:409–14.

30. Vollmer CM, Drebin JA, Middleton WD et al. Utility of staging laparoscopy in subsets of peripancreatic and biliary malignancies. Ann Surg 2002; 235:1–7.

31. Doran HE, Bosonnet L, Connor S et al. Laparoscopy and laparoscopic ultrasound in the evaluation of pancreatic and periampullary tumours. Dig Surg 2004; 21:305–13.

32. Karachristos A, Scarmeas N, Hoffman JP. CA 19-9 levels predict results of staging laparoscopy in pancreatic cancer. J Gastrointest Surg 2005; 9:1286–92.

33. Allema JH, Reinders ME, van Gulik TM et al. Portal vein resection in patients undergoing pancreatoduodenectomy for carcinoma of the pancreatic head. Br J Surg 1994; 81:1642–6.

34. Siriwardana HP, Siriwardena AK. Systematic review of outcome of synchronous portal-superior mesenteric vein resection during pancreatectomy for cancer. Br J Surg 2006; 93:662–73.

35. Gleisner AL, Assumpcao L, Cameron JL et al. Is resection of periampullary or pancreatic adenocarcinoma with synchronous hepatic metastasis justified?. Cancer 2007; 110:2484–92.

36. Callery MP, Strasberg SM, Doherty GM et al. Staging laparoscopy with laparoscopic ultrasonography: optimizing resectability in hepatobiliary and pancreatic malignancy. J Am Coll Surg 1997; 185:33–9.

37. Minnard EA, Conlon KC, Hoos A et al. Laparoscopic ultrasound enhances standard laparoscopy in the staging of pancreatic cancer. Ann Surg 1998; 228:182–7.

38. Catheline JM, Turner R, Rizk N et al. The use of diagnostic laparoscopy supported by laparoscopic ultrasonography in the assessment of pancreatic cancer. Surg Endosc 1999; 13:239–45.

39. Schachter PP, Avni Y, Shimonov M et al. The impact of laparoscopy and laparoscopic ultrasonography on the management of pancreatic cancer. Arch Surg 2000; 135:1303–7.

40. Taylor AM, Roberts SA, Manson JM. Experience with laparoscopic ultrasonography for defining tumour resectability in carcinoma of the pancreatic head and periampullary region. Br J Surg 2001; 88:1077–83.

41. Hünerbein M, Rau B, Hohenberger P et al. Value of laparoscopic ultrasound for staging of gastrointestinal tumors. Chirurg 2001; 72:914–19.

42. Espat NJ, Brennan MF, Conlon KC. Patients with laparoscopically staged unresectable pancreatic adenocarcinoma do not require subsequent surgical biliary or gastric bypass. J Am Coll Surg 1999; 188:649–55.

43. Moss AC, Morris E, Mac MP. Palliative biliary stents for obstructing pancreatic carcinoma. Cochrane Database Syst Rev 2006; CD004200.

    Meta-analysis concluding that endoscopic metal stents are the intervention of choice at present in patients with malignant distal obstructive jaundice due to pancreatic carcinoma.

44. Mehta S, Hindmarsh A, Cheong E et al. Prospective randomized trial of laparoscopic gastrojejunostomy versus duodenal stenting for malignant gastric outflow obstruction. Surg Endosc 2006; 20:239–42.

    Only (small) randomised trial performed that favoured duodenal stenting over (laparoscopic) gastrojejunostomy for malignant gastric outflow in irresectable pancreatic cancer.

45. Shoup M, Winston C, Brennan MF et al. Is there a role for staging laparoscopy in patients with locally advanced, unresectable pancreatic adenocarcinoma? J Gastrointest Surg 2004; 8:1068–71.

    Prospective study in which the authors concluded patients considered for treatment for locally advanced disease should be staged laparoscopically before initiation of therapy.

46. Butturini G, Crippa S, Bassi C et al. The role of laparoscopy in advanced pancreatic cancer diagnosis. Dig Surg 2007; 24:33–7.

47. Liu RC, Traverso LW. Diagnostic laparoscopy improves staging of pancreatic cancer deemed locally unresectable by computed tomography. Surg Endosc 2005; 19:638–42.

48. Garner PD, Hall LD, Johnstone PA. Palliation of unresectable hilar cholangiocarcinoma. J Surg Oncol 2000; 75:95–7.

49. Jarnagin WR, Burke E, Powers C et al. Intrahepatic biliary enteric bypass provides effective palliation in selected patients with malignant obstruction at the hepatic duct confluence. Am J Surg 1998; 175:453–60.

50. Shih SP, Schulick RD, Cameron JL et al. Gallbladder cancer: the role of laparoscopy and radical resection. Ann Surg 2007; 245:893–901.

51. Tilleman EH, de Castro SM, Busch OR et al. Diagnostic laparoscopy and laparoscopic ultrasound for staging of patients with malignant proximal bile duct obstruction. J Gastrointest Surg 2002; 6:426–30.

    Authors' study of 110 patients demonstrating that laparoscopy avoided unnecessary laparotomy in 41% of patients and concluding that the procedure should be performed routinely in assessing patients with potentially resectable tumour.

52. Weber SM, DeMatteo RP, Fong Y et al. Staging laparoscopy in patients with extrahepatic biliary carcinoma. Analysis of 100 patients. Ann Surg 2002; 235:392–9.

53. Agrawal S, Sonawane RN, Behari A et al. Laparoscopic staging in gallbladder cancer. Dig Surg 2005; 22:440–5.

54. D'Angelica M , Fong Y, Weber et al. The role of staging laparoscopy in hepatobiliary malignancy: prospective analysis of 401 cases. Ann Surg Oncol 2003; 10:183–9.

    Study showing that one in five patients can be spared laparotomy by laparoscopic staging. Multivariate analysis showed that surgeon's preoperative impression of resectability is important.

55. Smits NJ, Reeders JW. Imaging and staging of biliopancreatic malignancy: role of ultrasound. Ann Oncol 1999; 10(Suppl 4):20–4.

56. Gerhards MF, den HD, Rauws EA et al. Palliative treatment in patients with unresectable hilar cholangiocarcinoma: results of endoscopic drainage in patients with type III and IV hilar cholangiocarcinoma. Eur J Surg 2001; 167:274–80.

57. Ward J. New MR techniques for the detection of liver metastases. Cancer Imaging 2006; 6:33–42.

58. Yang YY, Fleshman JW, Strasberg SM. Detection and management of extrahepatic colorectal cancer in patients with resectable liver metastases. J Gastrointest Surg 2007; 11:929–44.

    Comprehensive review emphasising the diagnostic role of FDG-PET for detection of intra- and extrahepatic metastases in patients with resectable colorectal liver metastases.

59. Inabnet WB, Deziel DJ. Laparoscopic liver biopsy in patients with coagulopathy, portal hypertension, and ascites. Am Surg 1995; 61:603–6.

60. Lo CM, Lai EC, Liu CL et al. Laparoscopy and laparoscopic ultrasonography avoid exploratory laparotomy in patients with hepatocellular carcinoma. Ann Surg 1998; 227:527–32.

61. Ido K, Nakazawa Y, Isoda N et al. The role of laparoscopic US and laparoscopic US-guided aspiration biopsy in the diagnosis of multicentric hepatocellular carcinoma. Gastrointest Endosc 1999; 50:523–6.

62. Montorsi M, Santambrogio R, Bianchi P et al. Laparoscopy with laparoscopic ultrasound for pretreatment staging of hepatocellular carcinoma: a prospective study. J Gastrointest Surg 2001; 5:312–15.

63. Foroutani A, Garland AM, Berber E et al. Laparoscopic ultrasound vs triphasic computed tomography for detecting liver tumors. Arch Surg 2000; 135:933–8.

64. Jarnagin WR, Bodniewicz J, Dougherty E et al. A prospective analysis of staging laparoscopy in patients with primary and secondary hepatobiliary malignancies. J Gastrointest Surg 2000; 4:34–43.

65. de Castro SM, Tilleman EH, Busch OR et al. Diagnostic laparoscopy for primary and second-

ary liver malignancies: impact of improved imaging and changed criteria for resection. Ann Surg Oncol 2004; 11:522–9.

Authors' study of 84 consecutive patients over a 6-year period demonstrating a greater role for laparoscopic staging of primary hepatic malignancy.

66. Metcalfe MS, Close JS, Iswariah H et al. The value of laparoscopic staging for patients with colorectal metastases. Arch Surg 2003; 138:770–2.

67. Thaler K, Kanneganti S, Khajanchee Y et al. The evolving role of staging laparoscopy in the treatment of colorectal hepatic metastasis. Arch Surg 2005; 140:727–34.

68. Mann CD, Neal CP, Metcalfe MS et al. Clinical Risk Score predicts yield of staging laparoscopy in patients with colorectal liver metastases. Br J Surg 2007; 94:855–9.

69. Jarnagin WR, Conlon K, Bodniewicz J et al. A clinical scoring system predicts the yield of diagnostic laparoscopy in patients with potentially resectable hepatic colorectal metastases. Cancer 2001; 91:1121–8.

A scoring system that would have reduced the need for laparoscopy in 57 of 1103 patients being assessed for resection.

70. Grobmyer SR, Fong Y, D'Angelica M et al. Diagnostic laparoscopy prior to planned hepatic resection for colorectal metastases. Arch Surg 2004; 139:1326–30.

71. D'Angelica M, Jarnagin W, Dematteo R et al Staging laparoscopy for potentially resectable noncolorectal, nonneuroendocrine liver metastases. Ann Surg Oncol 2002; 9:204–9.

72. Simillis C, Constantinides VA, Tekkis PP et al. Laparoscopic versus open hepatic resections for benign and malignant neoplasms – a meta-analysis. Surgery 2007; 141:203–11.

73. McKay A, Dixon E, Taylor M. Current role of radio-frequency ablation for the treatment of colorectal liver metastases. Br J Surg 2006; 93:1192–1201.

74. Boku T, Nakane Y, Minoura T et al. Prognostic significance of serosal invasion and free intraperitoneal cancer cells in gastric cancer. Br J Surg 1990; 77:436–9.

75. Nieveen van Dijkum EJ, Sturm PD, de Wit LT et al. Cytology of peritoneal lavage performed during staging laparoscopy for gastrointestinal malignancies: is it useful? Ann Surg 1998; 228:728–33.

76. Ferrone CR, Haas B, Tang L et al. The influence of positive peritoneal cytology on survival in patients with pancreatic adenocarcinoma. J Gastrointest Surg 2006; 10:1347–53.

77. Nakao A, Oshima K, Takeda S et al. Peritoneal washings cytology combined with immuno-cytochemical staining in pancreatic cancer. Hepatogastroenterology 1999; 46:2974–7.

78. Konishi M, Kinoshita T, Nakagohri T et al. Prognostic value of cytologic examination of peritoneal washings in pancreatic cancer. Arch Surg 2002; 137:475–80.

79. Dalal KM, Woo Y, Galanis C et al. Detection of micrometastases in peritoneal washings of pancreatic cancer patients by the reverse transcriptase polymerase chain reaction. J Gastrointest Surg 2007; 11:1598–1606.

80. Fong Y, Fortner J, Sun RL et al. Clinical score for predicting recurrence after hepatic resection for metastatic colorectal cancer: analysis of 1001 consecutive cases. Ann Surg 1999; 230:309–18.

4

Benign liver lesions

Rowan W. Parks
O. James Garden

Introduction

Benign liver lesions are common and may be difficult to differentiate from primary and secondary hepatic tumours. Such may be identified as an incidental finding when radiological investigation is undertaken for unrelated intraabdominal disease or when coexistent hepatic pathology is present giving rise to problems of diagnosis and management. Although these lesions may be of congenital origin, most are of unknown aetiology. They generally are asymptomatic but, since they are often slow growing, they may produce symptoms caused by mass effect. Rarely, such lesions may give rise to acute symptoms resulting from necrosis, thrombosis, haemorrhage or rupture.

Routine liver function tests are invariably within normal limits and are therefore of value in guiding the clinician towards a diagnosis of benign disease. Nonetheless, complications such as haemorrhage and necrosis may be associated with increases in serum transaminase levels. Elevation in tumour markers and the development of paraneoplastic syndromes such as erythrocytosis, hyperglycaemia and hypercalcaemia are observed rarely.

Characterisation of hepatic lesions is provided by imaging tests of the liver. Ultrasonography (US), computed tomography (CT) and magnetic resonance imaging (MRI) are the cornerstones of diagnosis and often complement one another. More recently, positron emission tomography (PET) has shown promise. Abdominal US will differentiate cystic forms from solid lesions, whereas CT and MRI using intravenous contrast and delayed imaging may detect the number and size of the lesions.

Hepatic angiography is employed rarely in modern clinical practice. Laparoscopy is used to allow direct visualisation of liver lesions and can be combined with laparoscopic US to provide high-resolution images.

None of these tests will provide definitive histological diagnosis but the role of needle biopsy or aspiration of suspected hepatic lesions remains much debated. Biopsy is contraindicated for patients with suspected haemangioma, haemangioendothelioma and cysts suspected of being echinococcal in origin. Needle biopsy or fine-needle aspiration cytology of suspected hypervascular solid tumours may result in haemorrhage, sampling error, misdiagnosis and needle-tract tumour seeding. Tissue from a haemangioma may resemble fibrosis, and focal nodular hyperplasia may resemble cirrhosis. Needle samples of hepatic adenoma may be interpreted as normal tissue and may be difficult to differentiate from hepatoma. Percutaneous biopsy should only be performed in those patients who are being considered candidates for surgical intervention and only where the results of biopsy might influence further management. Despite extensive radiological imaging in an attempt to characterise a lesion, the final diagnosis may not be made until the lesion has been resected and the pathologist can undertake definitive examination of the resected tissue.

The general surgeon should be thoroughly familiar with the gross appearance, clinical significance and natural history of these benign lesions as the treatment strategy may vary from simple observation (of focal nodular hyperplasia) to complex radical hepatic resection (of hepatocellular adenoma). Most symptomatic benign liver lesions are excised;

however, hepatic resection, if performed without the proper indications, can prove hazardous.

Classification

Although a variety of benign liver tumour has been described, by far the majority are sufficiently rare that they can easily be labelled medical curiosities. A detailed description of these various lesions is beyond the scope of the current text (Box 4.1). The majority of benign hepatic lesions encountered in clinical practice include haemangioma, liver cell adenoma, focal nodular hyperplasia, bile duct hamartoma and hepatic cysts. For completeness, a brief résumé is provided of less common and miscellaneous lesions which may give rise to diagnostic and management dilemmas.

Box 4.1 • Classification of benign tumours of the liver

Epithelial tumours

Hepatocellular:
• Nodular transformation
• Focal nodular hyperplasia
• Hepatocellular adenoma
Cholangiocellular:
• Bile duct adenoma
• Biliary cystadenoma

Mesenchymal tumours

Tumours of adipose tissue:
• Lipoma
• Myelolipoma
• Angiomyolipoma
Tumours of muscle tissue:
• Leiomyoma
Tumours of blood vessels:
• Infantile haemangioendothelioma
Haemangioma:
• Hereditary haemorrhagic telangiectasia
• Peliosis hepatis
Tumours of mesothelial tissue:
• Benign mesothelioma

Mixed mesenchymal and epithelial tumours

Mesenchymal hamartoma
Benign teratoma

Miscellaneous

Adrenal rest tumour
Pancreatic heterotopia
Inflammatory pseudotumour

From Ishak KG, Goodman ZD. Benign tumours of the liver. In: Berk JE (ed.) Bockus gastroenterology, 4th edn. Philadelphia: WB Saunders, 1985.

Haemangiomas

Haemangiomas are the most common benign hepatic tumours of mesenchymal origin. Small capillary haemangiomas are more common than the larger cavernous haemangiomas and are often multiple. Small lesions are asymptomatic and an incidental finding; however, they may give rise to diagnostic difficulty in patients undergoing investigation. Once accurate diagnosis has been made no further therapy is needed. Haemangiomas are probably of congenital origin rather than neoplastic and do not undergo malignant transformation. The incidence of cavernous haemangioma in autopsy series varies considerably but has been reported to be as high as 8%. These lesions are the second most common hepatic tumour in the USA, exceeded only by hepatic metastases.[1] With the more widespread use of sensitive imaging studies of the upper abdomen, the identification of such lesions as an incidental finding will undoubtedly be more common. Cavernous haemangiomas may reach an enormous size, and lesions weighing up to 6 kg are well documented. Giant haemangiomas are defined as greater than 4 cm in diameter.[2] Such haemangiomas are usually solitary, but multiple lesions have been described in about 10% of cases.[1] They may be associated with similar lesions in the skin and other organs. Lesions are usually evenly distributed throughout the liver and its substance but large lesions situated peripherally may form a pedicle.

Pathology

Cavernous haemangiomas are seen most frequently in patients in the third to fifth decades of life. They are more common and more likely to become clinically manifest at a younger age in women, are more common with increasing parity and may enlarge during pregnancy.[3–5] This indicates a possible role of female sex hormones in their development, although an association with the oral contraceptive pill has not been proven. The aetiology of liver haemangiomas is still unclear but they may represent benign congenital hamartomas. These lesions appear to grow by progressive ectasia rather than hyperplasia or hypertrophy. At operation, they appear as well-circumscribed, reddish-purple, hypervascular lesions, which may be multilobulated or have a smooth surface. There is a dissectible plane between the lesion and the normal liver parenchyma. When sectioned, the lesion will partially collapse due to the escape of blood, and it has a honeycombed cut surface. There may be gross evidence of thrombosis, fibrosis or calcification (**Fig. 4.1**). Microscopically, haemangiomas are composed of cystically dilated vascular spaces, lined by endothelial cells and separated by fibrous septa of varying thickness. There is usually a clear plane between haemangioma and

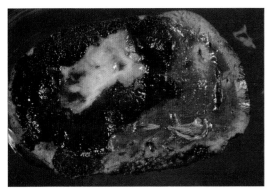

Figure 4.1 • A large haemangioma showing the characteristic honeycomb feature with a central scar.

normal liver tissue as these lesions are usually encapsulated by a rim of fibrous tissue.

Clinical presentation

Most haemangiomas are asymptomatic until they exceed 10 cm in diameter. Symptoms may include vague abdominal pain or fullness, early satiety, nausea, vomiting or fever. Rare presentations include obstructive jaundice, biliary colic, gastric outlet obstruction and spontaneous rupture. Although abdominal pain or discomfort is the most frequent indication for removing a liver haemangioma, it must be remembered that associated pathology may coexist and be the cause of the symptoms. Farges et al.[6]

reported that 42% of the patients in their series had other pathology, such as gallbladder disease, liver cysts, gastroduodenal ulcers or hiatus hernia. The difficulty of attributing symptoms to the haemangioma is evidenced by the occasional persistence of symptoms after resection.[7]

Pain related to an uncomplicated haemangioma is likely due to stretching or inflammation of Glisson's capsule. Occasionally, large lesions located in the left lobe of the liver may cause pressure effects on adjacent structures and infarction or necrosis may account for the sudden onset of pain. Intra-abdominal haemorrhage due to spontaneous or traumatic rupture of haemangioma is a very rare complication.[5] A past review of the literature included only 28 reports of spontaneous, life-threatening haemorrhage due to liver haemangiomas, a minimal figure considering the prevalence of the tumour.[8] Thrombocytopenia and hypofibrinogenaemia have also been associated with cavernous haemangiomas of the liver (Kasabach–Merritt syndrome), and this effect may be related to consumption of coagulation factors.[1]

A large haemangioma or the liver edge may be palpable on inspiration. It is difficult to differentiate the consistency of a haemangioma from normal liver through the abdominal wall unless it has calcified or undergone thrombosis or fibrosis. Occasionally, a bruit is heard over a haemangioma, but this is a non-specific finding. Liver function tests are normal in the patient presenting without complication.

Such lesions are generally hyperechoic on ultrasound examination (**Fig. 4.2**). Farges et al.[6] found

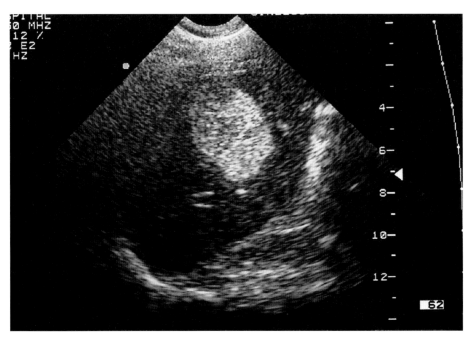

Figure 4.2 • Hyperechoic appearance of haemangioma on ultrasound examination.

the diagnosis to be established by US alone in 80% of patients with haemangiomas smaller than 6 cm. However, this investigation alone cannot differentiate a haemangioma from hepatocellular carcinoma, liver cell adenoma, focal nodular hyperplasia or a solitary metastasis. CT has proven most useful in the diagnosis of haemangiomas.[9] Prior to intravenous contrast infusion, CT shows the haemangioma to consist of a well-demarcated hypodense mass. After the intravenous injection of contrast medium, serial scans will reveal a zone of progressive enhancement peripherally that varies in thickness and often demonstrates an irregular margin (**Fig. 4.3**). The centre of the haemangioma remains hypodense and the overall lesion size does not change. Selective hepatic angiography shows a characteristic pattern consisting of normal-sized hepatic arteries without neovascularity or 'corkscrewing'. Typically there is rapid filling of the large blood-filled spaces of the haemangioma with contrast medium, producing the so-called 'cotton-wool' appearance surrounding the feeding hepatic arteries. The CT findings are often sufficiently characteristic that the role for angiography in the diagnosis of cavernous haemangiomas is limited.[9] Over the past decade MRI has emerged

as a highly accurate technique for diagnosing and characterising liver haemangioma, with a reported 90% sensitivity, 95% specificity and 93% accuracy[10,11] (**Fig. 4.4**). Haemangiomas are typically very bright (light bulb sign) on T2-weighted images and show peripheral nodular enhancement on dynamic gadolinium-enhanced T1-weighted images.[12] Single-photon emission CT (SPECT) using technetium-99m-labelled red blood cells has been shown to increase the spatial resolution of planar scintigraphy and has been shown to have a sensitivity and accuracy close to that of MRI.[13] In practice, a combination of these diagnostic modalities is preferred. Laparoscopy can also be of value for lesions situated superficially where they can be recognised on gross examination and by gentle palpation, which reveals characteristic compressibility. In addition, this technique can be effectively combined with laparoscopic contact US, which significantly adds to the diagnostic potential of laparoscopy alone.[14]

Needle biopsy of vascular liver lesions should not be performed. Diagnostic uncertainty is seldom a problem with cavernous haemangiomas, except in lesions not large enough to show cavernous characteristics, which may necessitate diagnostic removal.

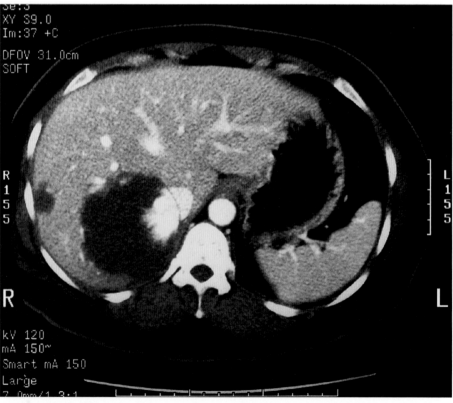

Figure 4.3 • CT scan demonstrating peripheral enhancement of a haemangioma after intravenous injection of contrast material.

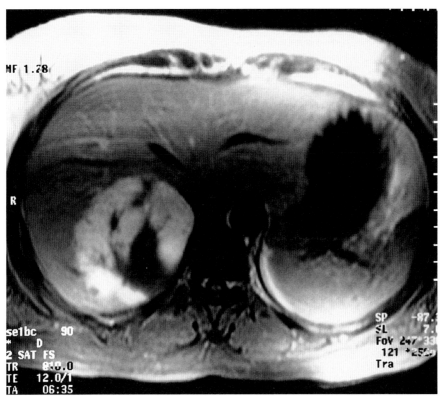

Figure 4.4 • T1-weighted MRI scan with gadolinium demonstrating the same haemangioma as in Fig. 4.3.

Management

A wide range of management strategies from observation to resection have been advocated for such lesions. Simple reassurance should be given to patients in whom small lesions (i.e. <4 cm) have been detected as an incidental finding. For larger cavernous haemangiomas, consideration should be given to weighing the risk of operation against the natural history of untreated lesions. Trastek et al.[5] followed up 34 untreated patients over a maximum period of 15 years. No patient had a lesion that bled, none reported abdominal symptoms and no patient had compromise of quality of life. A further report from the same group, when the observation period had been extended to 21 years, reported two patients with large symptomatic lesions of questionable resectability at initial presentation who remained symptomatic but with little documented growth of the haemangioma. The remainder were asymptomatic and there was no instance of rupture.[15] Two more recent longitudinal studies have supported the accepted view that asymptomatic giant haemangiomas of the liver can be managed safely by observation.[16,17]

Nichols et al.[15] reported no operative deaths and the single postoperative complication was a wound infection in 41 patients undergoing resection of such lesions. In a similar series of 69 patients, Weimann et al.[18] reported no postoperative deaths and a morbidity rate of 19%. Also in this series were 104 patients with haemangioma and 53 patients with focal nodular hyperplasia who were observed for a median of 32 months (range 7–132 months). There was no evidence of malignant transformation or tumour rupture. Therefore, safe resection is possible but there is no evidence that asymptomatic patients should undergo resection since the risk of rupture is minimal.[6,19]

When treatment is indicated, surgical excision provides the only effective therapy. Reports of the effectiveness of hepatic arterial ligation are anecdotal. Arterial ligation or embolisation may, however, be considered for the temporary control of haemorrhage in exceptional circumstances in order to allow time for transfer of a patient for definitive management in a specialist centre. The benefits of radiation therapy and corticosteroids have not been well documented and are inconsistent. It is possible that the success of non-resectional therapy may well be largely due to the naturally occurring spontaneous involution of these lesions.

The choice of excision requires consideration of the size and anatomical location of the lesion.

Haemangiomas can often be enucleated[20] to avoid loss of functional liver parenchyma, diminish blood loss and minimise postoperative bile leakage, although in some cases it may be wiser and safer to perform a formal anatomical liver resection. At enucleation, a plane between the lesion and the liver is easily found and this can be developed by blunt dissection. This can be facilitated by the use of the Cavitron ultrasonic surgical aspiration system (CUSA™) with concomitant control of the inflow vessels. Laparoscopic resection of liver haemangioma has been reported,[21] and orthotopic liver transplantation has also been used successfully to treat symptomatic patients with technically unresectable complicated giant haemangioma.[22]

 Liver haemangioma rarely causes complications and resection should only be considered for symptomatic lesions.

Liver cell adenoma

Although liver cell adenoma requires differentiation from any solid hepatic lesion, it is often considered alongside focal nodular hyperplasia.[23]

Hepatic adenomas arise in otherwise normal liver and present as a focal abnormality or mass. The true prevalence of the disease is difficult to assess but 90% develop in women in the third to fifth decades of life.[24,25] These tumours were rarely reported before 1960, but their apparent increase in incidence since then corresponded with the introduction of oral contraceptives at that time. The causal relationship between liver cell adenoma and oral contraceptives was first suggested by Baum et al.[26] in 1973. Ninety percent of patients with liver cell adenomas have used oral contraceptives and the annual incidence among oral contraceptive users has been reported to be 3–4 per 100000 if the contraceptives are taken for more than 2 years. The risk of developing a liver cell adenoma increases with the dose and duration of use of the contraceptive preparation.[24] Furthermore, pregnancy has been associated with increased symptoms and an increased risk of complications in patients with liver cell adenomas.[24,27] The introduction of low-oestrogen-containing contraceptive preparations may result in a reduction in incidence, although adenomas are also associated with non-contraceptive oestrogen use, androgenic steroid use, diabetes, glycogen storage disease, galactosaemia and iron overload. This association implicates altered carbohydrate metabolism in the formation of liver cell adenomas.[28]

Pathology

Liver cell adenomas are usually solitary, round and occasionally encapsulated. Lesions are soft and smooth surfaced, but occasionally may be pedunculated. The cut surface has a pale-yellow fleshy appearance unless haemorrhage and necrosis produce discoloration (**Fig. 4.5**). They are sharply demarcated from normal liver but without a fibrous capsule. Approximately 12–30% of these tumours are multiple, and if more than ten adenomas are present, the condition is regarded as liver adenomatosis.[29] This may be a separate pathological entity from isolated liver cell adenoma as both sexes are equally affected and oral contraceptive usage is unusual. Microscopically, there are uniform masses of benign-appearing hepatocytes without ducts or portal triads. The hepatocytes appear paler than normal because of increased glycogen or fat content. Venous lakes (peliosis hepatis) are often seen.

There is debate as to whether liver cell adenomas are precancerous. Rooks et al.[24] reported the finding of hepatocellular carcinoma 5 years after resection of a liver cell adenoma, and other authors have recognised unequivocal areas of hepatocellular carcinoma adjacent to or within liver cell adenomas.[25,30,31] Also reported is the development of hepatocellular carcinoma several years after diagnosis of biopsy-proven benign liver cell adenoma.[28,32,33] However, Tao[34] concluded on histological grounds that liver cell adenoma was not a premalignant lesion, but that liver cell dysplasia was an irreversible premalignant condition that would progress to cancer.

Clinical presentation

These lesions present frequently with abdominal pain from haemorrhage into the tumour or adjacent

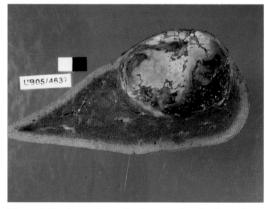

Figure 4.5 • Large liver cell adenoma showing the pale yellow fleshy appearance of its cut surface. There are areas of discoloration from haemorrhage.

liver. Some patients develop severe acute abdominal pain due to intraperitoneal rupture and haemoperitoneum, which may present as hypovolaemic shock. Up to one-third of patients sense the presence of an abdominal mass. The remainder of adenomas are discovered incidentally at autopsy, laparotomy or during radiological assessment for another problem.

Although the clinical presentation may be suggestive of liver cell adenoma, definitive preoperative diagnosis may be difficult. Liver function tests are generally normal unless tumour necrosis or haemorrhage is present. Anaemia may therefore occur. US can detect small adenomas, which characteristically display a lesion of mixed echogeneity and heterogeneous texture. CT may show evidence of recent haemorrhage or necrosis. Lesions are generally hypodense prior to infusion of contrast medium and demonstrate a wide range of densities after intravenous contrast administration. They often appear as well-demarcated, fat-containing or haemorrhagic lesions on MRI. If undertaken, selective visceral angiography shows a hypervascular tumour with irregular areas of hypovascularity secondary to haemorrhage or necrosis. Liver cell adenomas generally exhibit a peripheral blood supply. An isotope scan may be helpful in pointing towards a diagnosis of adenoma, which does not take up any isotope and therefore appears as a filling defect. Conventional radiological imaging may not be able to differentiate between liver cell adenoma and hepatocellular carcinoma; however, promising results have been reported with the use of positron emission tomography (PET) using fluorodeoxyglucose (FDG) to differentiate benign from malignant lesions.[35]

Percutaneous needle biopsy or fine-needle aspiration cytology undertaken prior to referral is often misleading. Biopsy of these vascular tumours risks precipitating haemorrhage, and even an experienced histopathologist may experience difficulty in differentiating between liver cell adenoma and a well-differentiated hepatocellular carcinoma.

Management

In the symptomatic patient, surgical intervention will be required. A minority of patients will present with intraperitoneal bleeding, the cause of which might only be identified at laparotomy. Most deaths from liver cell adenomas are secondary to haemorrhage, with intraperitoneal bleeding carrying a 20% mortality rate in one series.[24] Hepatic arterial embolisation[36] or packing might be considered to facilitate transfer of the patient to a specialist centre. Definitive control of bleeding is best achieved by formal hepatic resection. In some patients, haemorrhage may be contained within the liver or subcapsularly. If the patient remains haemodynamically stable, it may be prudent to defer elective surgical intervention to enable resolution of the haematoma, thereby enabling a more limited hepatic resection (**Fig. 4.6**).

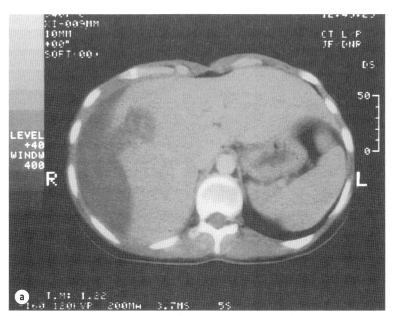

Figure 4.6 • (a) CT scan showing extensive subcapsular haematoma resulting from spontaneous haemorrhage into the liver.

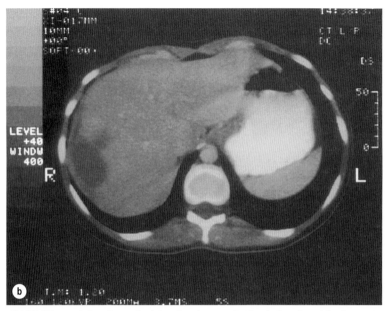

Figure 4.6 • Cont'd (b) CT scan taken 2 months later showing a reduction in the size of the haematoma. Contrast is now present within a small adenoma lying adjacent to the haematoma.

For the asymptomatic patient, surgical intervention should still be considered. Several case reports document regression of liver cell tumours following cessation of oral contraceptives,[37,38] although this is not a consistent finding, and development of hepatocellular carcinoma in the site of adenoma regression has been reported.[32] Non-operative discrimination between liver cell adenoma and hepatocellular carcinoma is difficult. Furthermore, liver cell adenomas can harbour foci of tumour and may be premalignant lesions. They more commonly produce symptoms and may result in life-threatening haemorrhage.

 Hepatic resection should be considered in all patients with a suspected liver cell adenoma; however, each case must be individually evaluated and the risk of surgery weighed against the potential for future morbidity or mortality. Orthotopic liver transplantation has been described for unresectable benign liver tumours with severe symptoms and for patients with multiple adenomas.[18,39]

Focal nodular hyperplasia

Focal nodular hyperplasia (FNH) is often difficult to differentiate from liver cell adenoma and for this reason represents a substantial proportion of benign lesions submitted to hepatic resection (Table 4.1). The incidence of FNH has

Table 4.1 • Indications for 108 hepatic resections for benign disease in the Hepatobiliary Unit, Royal Infirmary, Edinburgh (October 1988– June 2003)

Aetiology	Number of patients
Cystic disease	29
Focal nodular hyperplasia	16
Haemangioma	15
Liver cell adenoma	10
Primary sclerosing cholangitis	7
Cystadenoma	6
Hepatic pseudotumour	6
Trauma	5
Liver abscess	5
Benign bile duct stricture	3
Intrahepatic calculi	2
Bile duct injury	2
Intrahepatic leiomyoma	1
Benign schwannoma	1
TOTAL	108

been increasing, although this is more likely to be related to improvements in abdominal imaging. Many lesions are still found incidentally at laparotomy or autopsy. About 90% of cases occur in women, primarily in the second and third decades, although the condition may also afflict older women and a small number of men and children. The incidence of FNH does not appear to have increased since the introduction of oral contraceptives; however, some investigators have suggested that oral contraceptives may foster growth or increased vascularity of these lesions, and they have been implicated in the few cases that present with haemorrhage.

Pathology

FNH has many similarities to liver cell adenoma and distinguishing between the two may be difficult. FNH consists of a firm lobulated localised lesion in an otherwise normal liver. These nodules are generally several centimetres in size and occasionally can grow much larger. Lesions are well circumscribed but have no capsule. On sectioning, there is generally a central scar with fibrous radiations, which account for the nodular and sometimes umbilicated appearance. Lesions are usually similar or slightly lighter in colour than adjacent normal hepatic parenchyma (**Fig. 4.7**). FNH is multifocal in up to 20% of cases and may coexist with haemangiomas in 5–10% of patients.[1]

Microscopically, FNH looks similar to cirrhosis, with regenerating nodules and connective tissue septa. The lesions consist of many normal hepatic cells mixed with bile ducts or ductules and divided by fibrous septa. The septa contain numerous bile ducts and a moderate, predominantly lymphocytic, infiltration, and there is usually some evidence of mild cholestasis.

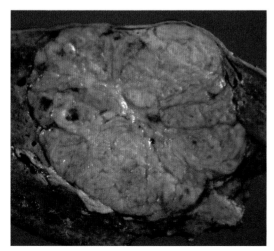

Figure 4.7 • Cut surface of focal nodular hyperplasia showing a central scar.

Clinical features

FNH is a benign process that rarely causes symptoms but the main difficulty lies in differentiating this process from other hepatic lesions. Less than 10% of patients with FNH have symptoms, the most common being mild, vague right upper quadrant abdominal pain. Acute symptoms due to haemorrhage are exceptional.

Most imaging techniques used in isolation cannot reliably establish the diagnosis of FNH. Therefore, a combination of imaging modalities is preferred.[40] The appearances on ultrasound and CT are non-specific and on occasions the lesion may not be visualised (**Fig. 4.8**). Cholescintigraphy combined with either ultrasound or CT has been shown to have an 82% sensitivity and 97% specificity for diagnosing focal nodular hyperplasia.[18] Arteriography is now used infrequently for the diagnosis of FNH. The classical appearance on arteriography is that of a sharply delineated hypervascular mass with a single central artery and centrifugal filling of the vessels (spoke-wheel pattern). Cherqui et al. reported a 70% sensitivity and 98% specificity for MRI in detecting FNH.[41]

Management

Treatment of a patient with FNH depends essentially on the certainty of the diagnosis. In asymptomatic patients with the typical features of FNH unequivocally demonstrated by one or more radiological investigations, no further treatment is required. However, a malignant tumour will be found in up to 6% of patients with an undetermined, presumed benign lesion.[42]

Many surgeons believe that patients should be submitted to open or laparoscopic biopsy because of the difficulty in establishing a diagnosis preoperatively and because of the dangers of needle biopsy. Enucleation or resection should be undertaken if it can be performed with minimal morbidity for any lesion that is increasing in size, bleeding or unequivocally symptomatic.

Recent data on the natural history of FNH have been gathered by Kerlin et al.[25] Of 41 patients studied, 11 had lesions found incidentally at autopsy. Sixteen patients had open surgical biopsies of clinically apparent lesions, with the majority of the lesions left in situ. These patients were observed for up to 15 years, during which time none of the lesions bled or increased in size. Although it could be claimed that such lesions are best managed conservatively, a balanced approach is best adopted, with surgical excision being undertaken if this can be done with minimal morbidity and mortality. Observation in selected patients may be considered if there is a significant risk of morbidity with surgical intervention.

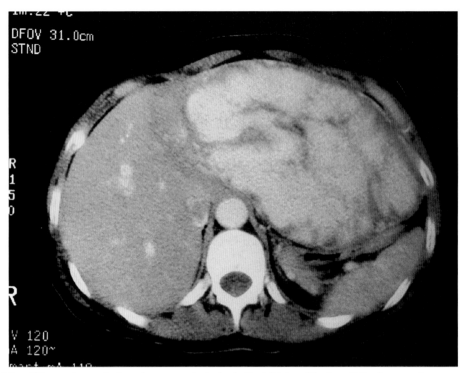

Figure 4.8 • CT scan demonstrating a large vascular lesion in the left lobe of the liver. Following resection, histopathology confirmed this to be a large area of focal nodular hyperplasia.

Nodular regenerative hyperplasia (macroregenerative nodules)

This is a benign proliferative process in which the normal hepatic architecture is entirely replaced by diffuse regenerative nodules of hepatocytes. Autopsy reports suggest the prevalence of nodular regenerative hyperplasia (NRH) is approximately 2%. It predominantly occurs in older patients, and is often associated with lymphoproliferative and rheumatological diseases or develops after organ transplantation.

The majority of patients are asymptomatic, are diagnosed incidentally and require no further treatment. The most common physical findings are splenomegaly and hepatomegaly. A small percentage of patients may develop portal hypertension due to compression of intrahepatic portal radicles by the regenerating nodules, and present with variceal bleeding or ascites. Rarely, patients may develop hepatic failure and in some instances have undergone liver transplantation. Liver function tests are usually normal or slightly elevated, and the radiological features are relatively nonspecific. The diagnosis of NRH is confirmed on the gross and histological findings of the liver.

Macroscopically, the hepatic parenchyma is entirely replaced by nodules varying in size from 0.1 to 4 cm. The histological findings of NRH are regenerating hepatocytes separated by atrophic parenchyma, curvilinear compression of the central lobule, and absence of fibrous tissue or bands of scar tissue between the nodules. NRH may be suspected when a patient presents with symptoms of portal hypertension and a liver biopsy that fails to show cirrhosis or is interpreted as being normal. Confirmation may require open or laparoscopic liver biopsy. Liver cell dysplasia is a common finding in NRH and there are a small number of case reports of hepatocellular carcinoma developing in livers with NRH, leading some authors to suggest that NRH may represent a premalignant condition in some patients.

Bile duct adenoma (bile duct hamartoma)

Surgeons should be aware of bile duct adenomas since they are common and may be mistaken at operation as liver metastases. They do not manifest clinically but are incidental findings at laparotomy or autopsy.[43] These rarely exceed 1 cm in diameter and appear as raised greyish-white areas on the liver capsule. Histologically, they are composed of a mass of mature bile ducts surrounded by fibrous stroma, which blends indistinctly into the adjacent liver. They require to be distinguished from the nests of hyperplastic bile ducts that occur in focal nodular hyperplasia and also in undifferentiated adenocarcinoma of the biliary tract type.

The only clinical significance of the bile duct adenoma is its possible confusion at laparoscopy or laparotomy with metastatic carcinoma, cholangiocarcinoma or other focal hepatic lesions. When encountered, excisional biopsy should be performed to confirm the diagnosis.

Hepatic pseudotumours

Hepatic pseudotumours may be considerable in size and can occur in any age group. These lesions are essentially overgrowths of chronic inflammatory tissue but may be mistaken for other neoplastic lesions of the liver.[44] The aetiology is not known but they may be secondary to thrombosis and infarction of a major vessel, represent a form of immune reaction, or result from resolution of an abscess. They appear as a hypodense lesion on CT, and may be either hyperechoic or hypoechoic on US. Arteriography reveals a hypervascular mass. Such pseudotumours may require resection to prevent reactivation of infection. The clinical history and presentation are likely to point towards a diagnosis of pseudotumour.

Miscellaneous benign tumours

Mesenchymal hamartomas are exceptional and probably of congenital origin. They are most commonly described in infants under 12 months; however, a few have been documented in adults.[45] Although they are entirely benign, hamartomas can compromise the liver and the individual by progressive enlargement, and therefore these lesions should be resected. Microscopically, the tumour is characterised by a myxoid background of highly cellular embryonal mesenchyme, throughout which are found random groups of hepatic cells, bile ducts and multiple cysts, which may produce a honeycomb appearance. Recurrence following excision has not been reported.

Primary myxoma in the adult is exceptional. Primary lipomas are rarely described in life but have been identified incidentally at post-mortem.[1] Other solid tumours include leiomyoma, mesothelioma and fibroma. Benign teratoma of the liver has been reported but this generally occurs in children.

Liver abscess

The incidence of pyogenic liver abscess has remained relatively constant over the past century despite earlier diagnosis and treatment of underlying causes and more aggressive antibiotic therapies. In recent years, the decrease in cases resulting from haematogenous spread from infected foci has been mirrored by an increase in cases secondary to hepatobiliary pathology. In almost half the patients reviewed in our own centre over a 5-year period, biliary sepsis was the major predisposing factor.[46] In 20% of patients, the presumed source of infection was from the portal route, but few cases were thought to have arisen from systemic infection. Hepatic abscesses secondary to ascending cholangitis are often multiple due to the distribution of the infecting organism along the biliary ductal system.[47] Early reports implicated choledocholithiasis as the main causative factor; however, more recent series document malignant biliary obstruction as a more common aetiological factor.[46,48]

Infections within organs drained by the portal vein are dependent on the underlying illness. In the early literature, portal vein pyelophlebitis secondary to appendicitis was often implicated, whereas diverticulitis, pancreatitis and diffuse peritonitis are now more frequently reported. Haematogenous spread from non-gastrointestinal sources accounts for 10–20% of liver abscesses and occurs most typically with bacterial endocarditis, other conditions associated with systemic bacteraemia such as urinary sepsis, pneumonia, osteomyelitis or following intravenous drug abuse. Abscesses may also occur from direct extension into the liver parenchyma from localised perforation of an adjacent viscus, such as the gallbladder, colon, stomach or duodenum. In a significant percentage of patients (approximately 15–35%), the aetiology of hepatic abscess remains obscure (cryptogenic abscess) despite extensive clinical and pathological investigation.

Clinical presentation

Patients present with a spectrum of symptoms and signs, the most consistent being fever associated with malaise, anorexia, weight loss and upper abdominal pain. Jaundice is a feature in approximately 50% of cases. Laboratory studies typically reflect a systemic bacterial infection. Commonly reported findings are of leucocytosis, anaemia, hyperbilirubinaemia, hypoalbuminaemia and raised levels of acute-phase proteins. US is invariably diagnostic and will often demonstrate a fluid-filled cavity. There may be a hyperechoic wall, the presence of which is dependent on the chronicity of the abscess. CT may be useful to exclude the presence of other abscesses and to identify a primary source within the abdomen (**Fig. 4.9**). Magnetic

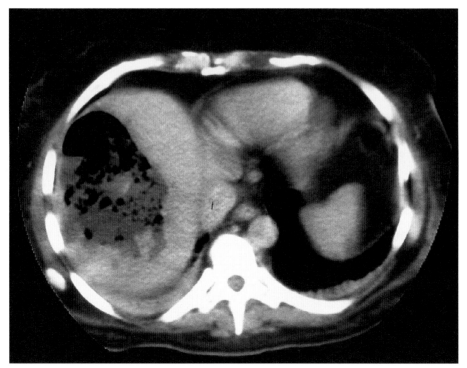

Figure 4.9 • Large liver abscess in right lobe of liver.

resonance cholangiography should be undertaken in patients with biliary symptoms, obstructive liver function tests or a dilated common bile duct, and can be combined with cross-sectional MRI to identify any hepatic parenchymal abnormality. Barium enema or colonoscopy may be indicated to exclude a colonic source of portal pyaemia.

Management

The key to successful management is drainage of the purulent collection combined with appropriate antibiotic therapy, which is determined by the results of culture of blood and aspirated pus. Although virtually all pathogenic organisms have been identified, enteric organisms predominate. Polymicrobial infection is seen frequently when hepatic abscess is secondary to infection arising from the portal venous system. Although antibiotic therapy as the sole treatment for hepatic abscess is rarely successful, prolonged systemic antibiotic administration may be the only option for patients with diffuse multiple microabscesses. In general, macroscopic hepatic collections require drainage of the purulent material. Over the past two decades, the introduction and refinement of percutaneous drainage techniques have dramatically altered the management of patients with pyogenic hepatic abscesses. Percutaneous drainage has become the first-line

therapeutic option in most centres for patients with single or multiple liver abscesses.[47,49–51] Abscess communication with the intrahepatic biliary tree does not prevent pyogenic collections being successfully treated by percutaneous techniques, although the period of drainage may be prolonged. The use of percutaneous aspiration combined with systemic antibiotics without drainage has been advocated by some groups;[52] however, in the only randomised trial comparing the two techniques, aspiration was successful in only 60% of patients whereas percutaneous catheter drainage was successful in 100% of patients.[53]

Regular irrigation of drainage catheters reduces the risk of catheter blockage due to necrotic debris. Surgical drainage is rarely employed but is usually reserved for patients who have failed percutaneous drainage and those who require surgical management of the underlying problem. Liver resection is occasionally required for patients with liver abscess.[54] The indication is usually failed non-operative management, hepatolithiasis, intrahepatic biliary stricture or gross parenchymal destruction.

Effective decompression of the biliary tree is as important as abscess drainage where obstruction of the bile duct has contributed to the development of hepatic abscess. Following successful drainage of the abscess, antibiotic administration should be continued for a prolonged period (3–6 weeks) to assist in the complete eradication of infection.

Pyogenic liver abscess still carries a significant mortality. In our experience, one-third of patients will not survive admission to hospital, although this reflects the high proportion of patients developing hepatic abscess related to underlying malignant biliary obstruction.

Amoebic abscess

This form of abscess is sufficiently common that it should be considered in the differential diagnosis of hepatic lesions. About 10% of the world's population is chronically infected with *Entamoeba histolytica*, although less than 10% of individuals are symptomatic. Liver abscess is the most common extraintestinal manifestation of amoebiasis and is reported in 3–10% of affected patients. Males are more commonly affected than females, and the highest incidence is in the 20- to 50-year-old age group.[55]

The diagnosis is likely to be straightforward in areas where amoebiasis is endemic but the liver abscess may present many years after previous intestinal infection. Some 75–90% of abscesses are in the right lobe, and involvement of the left lobe usually indicates more advanced disease. Rupture occurs in 2–17% of cases and usually occurs into the peritoneal cavity and rarely into the pleural cavity, the bronchial tree or pericardium. Signs and symptoms of amoebic infection are the same as for pyogenic abscess. On US and CT, the boundaries of the abscess are generally poorly defined (**Fig. 4.10**). Patients with amoebic liver abscess virtually always have serum antiamoebic antibodies, which can be detected by an indirect haemagglutination test or an enzyme-linked immunosorbent assay (ELISA) technique. Percutaneous aspiration produces a sterile and odourless fluid, which is described as having the appearance of 'anchovy paste'. Routine percutaneous aspiration is now regarded as superfluous in the management of amoebic liver abscess unless serology is inconclusive, a therapeutic trial with antiamoebic drugs is deemed inappropriate (as in pregnancy), or rupture is suspected to be imminent.

A preliminary diagnosis can be made on the basis of a dramatic clinical response to metronidazole, which should be commenced empirically in endemic areas.[55] If clinical symptoms do not resolve within 48–72 hours of treatment, an incorrect diagnosis or secondary bacterial infection should be suspected. Percutaneous aspiration may be beneficial for patients when medical treatment has failed. Percutaneous catheter drainage is indicated rarely as the abscess contents are viscous and bacterial superinfection may occur. Open surgical drainage is indicated in complicated cases and in those who fail to respond to conservative therapy. In a meta-analysis of 3081 patients with amoebic liver abscess the mortality rate was 4%, compared with a mortality rate of 46% in patients with pyogenic liver abscess.[56]

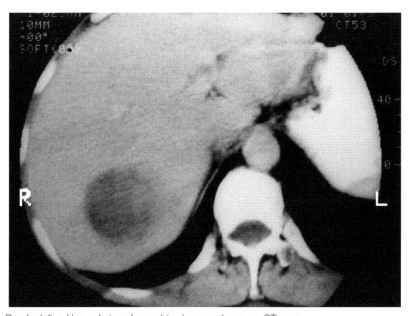

Figure 4.10 • Poorly defined boundaries of amoebic abscess shown on CT scan.

Hydatid cyst

Echinococcus infection is a zoonosis that can give rise to liver lesions. These collections are better classified as cysts rather than abscesses because the organism is almost entirely determined by the hepatic environment and little host inflammatory reaction is present. An intense fibrous reaction around the lesion is characteristic but there is no epithelial lining to the cyst. The incidence of *Echinococcus granulosus* is in decline but sporadic cases are reported in Europe, Australia, New Zealand, South America, Asia and Africa. The prevalence of human echinococciasis is directly related to contact with dogs and sheep. *Echinococcus multilocularis*, or alveolar hydatid disease, is rare, although it is a much more dangerous condition. It pursues a more invasive course than the more common form of the disease.

Hydatid cysts are most commonly unilocular and may grow as large as 20 cm. The cyst wall is about 5 mm thick and consists of an external laminated hilar membrane (ectocyst layer) and an internal enucleated germinal layer (endocyst layer), which is responsible for production of the colourless hydatid fluid, brood capsules and daughter cysts. Brood capsules are small cellular masses and together with calcareous bodies form 'hydatid sand'. About 70% of lesions are in the right lobe

and 15% in the left, with both lobes involved in approximately 15% of cases.

Clinical presentation

Many infections are probably contracted during childhood and lie latent for many years, often until complications occur. Clinical symptoms of echinococcal cystic disease are often insidious but there is usually a history of contact with dogs or sheep. Distension of the liver capsule may produce right upper quadrant pain. Jaundice is infrequent but may be due to extrinsic biliary compression or due to rupture into the biliary tree leading to obstruction by cystic debris. Secondary bacterial infection of the cyst occurs in approximately 10% of cases. Liver function tests are generally abnormal and eosinophilia is present in up to one-third of patients.

Echinococcal disease may occasionally mimic a primary liver tumour or metastatic disease. Serology may be helpful in establishing a diagnosis. Plain abdominal radiographs may reveal a calcified cyst wall. US and CT may demonstrate septa, 'hydatid sand' or daughter cysts within the main cyst cavity, which are important signs for differentiating hydatid from other benign liver cysts (**Fig. 4.11**). Percutaneous aspiration and drainage should be avoided because of the risk of dissemination or anaphylaxis.

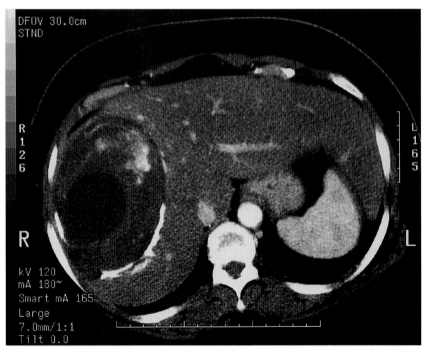

Figure 4.11 • Hydatid cyst with calcified cyst wall and a few peripheral daughter cysts.

Management

Once the diagnosis has been established, surgery is generally required as the natural history of viable hydatid cysts is one of growth and potential complications. Significant morbidity and mortality may result from rupture into the peritoneal or thoracic cavity or the development of a bronchobiliary fistula. Surgery might best be avoided in elderly frail patients with small, asymptomatic calcified cysts. Treatment with an oral anthelmintic agent, such as mebendazole or albendazole, to minimise the risks of hydatid spread at surgery or reduce the incidence of postoperative recurrence, has been advocated by some authors, although there remains considerable doubt as to its efficacy. Aspiration of the hydatid cyst with instillation of scolicidal agents, such as hypertonic saline, silver nitrate, chlorhexidine, cetrimide, hydrogen peroxide, formalin or alcohol, has generally been abandoned because of the risk of anaphylaxis or the risk of developing sclerosing cholangitis if a bile duct communication is present. These have been generally replaced by peroperative cover with an anthelmintic agent.

The main principle of surgical treatment is to eradicate the parasite, prevent intraoperative spillage of cyst contents and obliterate the residual cavity.[57] At open operation, the operating field is generally packed off with swabs. After decompression, the cyst and contents are shelled out by peeling the endocyst off the host ectocyst layer. The fibrous host wall of the residual cavity should be carefully examined for any bile leakage from biliary–cyst communications, which are then sutured. The residual cyst cavity can be marsupialised, packed with omentum or plicated.[58] Pericystectomy is advocated by some but should preserve those portions of the cyst wall that come into contact with major blood vessels. For smaller, peripheral lesions, formal hepatic resection may be considered, particularly if a diagnostic dilemma remains. The mortality for surgery of hydatid disease should be low and confined to complicated disease. In a series of 505 patients, Milicevic reported a mortality rate of 1.5% and a morbidity rate of 30%.[58]

Simple cysts of the liver

Non-parasitic cystic disease of the liver can result from a congenital malformation of the intrahepatic bile ducts. These cysts may be single, multiple or diffuse (polycystic liver disease). These contain serous fluid and do not communicate with the intrahepatic biliary tree. Small cysts are surrounded by normal liver tissue, although as these enlarge, there is displacement and atrophy of adjacent hepatic tissue. A large cyst may occupy an entire lobe of the liver and result in compensatory hypertrophy of the residual liver. Such cysts have no septa and are unilocular. Microscopically, they are lined by a single layer of cuboidal or columnar epithelial cells, which resemble those of biliary epithelium. Simple cysts have a prevalence of about 3.6%. The female to male ratio is 4:1 in asymptomatic cases, but rises to 10:1 in symptomatic or complicated simple cysts.[59] Huge cysts almost exclusively affect women over the age of 50 years.

Clinical presentation

The vast majority of simple cysts are asymptomatic and are discovered incidentally. Large cysts may cause abdominal pain or discomfort, and a mass may be palpable in the right hypochondrium. Other symptoms may include anorexia, early satiety or vomiting. Rare complications include acute onset of pain from intracystic haemorrhage, rupture, torsion or infection. Jaundice is uncommon, but may be caused by external compression of the biliary tree. Likewise, portal hypertension has been reported as a consequence of portal vein compression.

Diagnosis can be made on the basis of abdominal US, which demonstrates a circular anechoic area that has a well-defined boundary with the liver. No wall is evident and there is posterior acoustic enhancement. Intracystic haemorrhage may cause internal acoustic shadowing; however, the presence of cyst wall nodules or solid intracystic components must be considered neoplastic. US examination of the kidneys is useful to exclude the presence of polycystic disease. Further diagnostic investigation is rarely required, although where intervention is contemplated, CT or MRI will provide more accurate anatomical localisation and exclude the presence of other cysts. Cysts appear as well-rounded, water-dense lesions without septa on CT (**Fig. 4.12**). Intravenous contrast enhancement will confirm the avascularity of these lesions. Scintigraphy and angiography are not required to make a diagnosis. Where complications such as haemorrhage occur, the simple cyst may appear relatively thick-walled and may contain cystic debris. In such instances, serological tests should be undertaken to exclude parasitic infection. It should be borne in mind that calcification is rarely present in simple cysts but may be present with hydatid cysts.

Management

Asymptomatic simple cysts require no treatment; however, symptomatic or complicated simple cysts may require intervention. Percutaneous aspiration risks introducing infection and does not provide definitive therapy. However, Gigot and colleagues have advocated this technique as a diagnostic test for

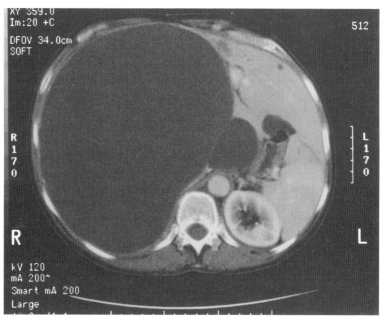

Figure 4.12 • CT scan demonstrating a large benign cyst occupying the entire right lobe of the liver. At least two further cysts are seen in the caudate and left lobes of the liver. Note the normal left kidney. This patient underwent successful laparoscopic deroofing of the cyst.

patients with questionable symptoms.[60] Aspiration followed by percutaneous instillation of sclerosant agents has shown promising results in reducing symptomatic and radiological cyst recurrence.[61] Open deroofing of simple liver cysts has, in the past, been the established conventional treatment. Total cystectomy is not required and may be hazardous since there is no plane of dissection between the cyst and the liver. In recent years, laparoscopic deroofing of such solitary cysts has been advocated. This technique was first described in 1991,[62] and is associated with higher patient acceptability and shorter postoperative stay compared with open surgical techniques. In a recent comprehensive review of 21 papers on the laparoscopic management of hepatic cysts, Klingler et al. reported 61 laparoscopic deroofing procedures with an overall morbidity rate of 10%.[63]

Even at open surgery, deroofing of large centrally placed cysts may not prevent reconstitution of the cyst with recurrence of symptoms. In such patients, we would now advocate more radical resection, which does not generally involve substantial sacrifice of functioning hepatic parenchyma.

Polycystic liver disease (PCLD)

Adult polycystic kidney disease is frequently associated with multiple liver cysts, which are macroscopically and microscopically similar to simple cysts of the liver. However, in this condition the liver cysts are multiple when present and may extensively replace both lobes of the liver (**Fig. 4.13**). In addition to the macroscopic cysts, there are usually numerous microscopic cysts and clusters of multiple bile ductules, designated as von Meyenburg complexes. The condition is an autosomal dominant disorder and carries a much more sinister prognosis because of the risk of chronic renal failure. There is an increased prevalence associated with increasing age and the female sex.[64]

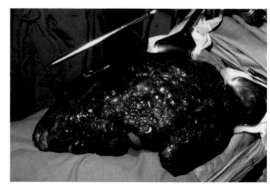

Figure 4.13 • Massive polycystic liver delivered from abdomen and pelvis before resection and deroofoing.

Clinical presentation

In most patients with adult polycystic kidney disease, the liver cysts are clinically silent. The commonest symptoms are related to increase in liver size, and include abdominal and pelvic discomfort and respiratory compromise. An abdominal mass will be present in three-quarters of patients. There are rarely signs of cholestasis, liver failure or portal hypertension, and liver function tests are usually normal. Both US and CT will demonstrate multiple fluid-filled cysts with well-defined margins in the liver and the kidneys (**Fig. 4.14**). Liver cysts increase in size slowly and complications are uncommon. Rupture and bacterial infection are reported to be more common with immunosuppression following kidney transplantation.[65]

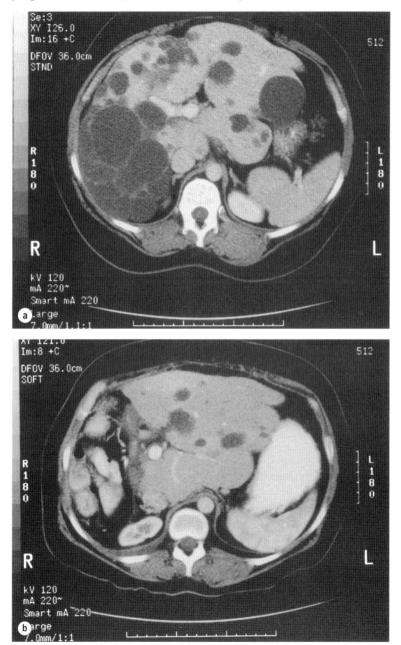

Figure 4.14 • **(a)** Contrast-enhanced CT scan demonstrating the presence of multiple cysts within the liver and kidneys. Note the predominance of large cysts within the right lobe of the liver. **(b)** CT scan taken 1 month following right hepatectomy and deroofing of the residual cyst in the same patient.

Management

Asymptomatic patients require no treatment. Percutaneous aspiration of cysts and instillation of sclerosant rarely produce satisfactory long-term relief of symptoms. Surgical deroofing or fenestration according to the technique described by Lin et al.[66] is the most widely used treatment modality for symptomatic patients but must be extensive and radical to achieve satisfactory results. Some have suggested that laparoscopic deroofing may provide good relief of symptoms.[67] However, in our own series this technique was associated with a high recurrence rate.[59] Recent evidence suggests that a more aggressive open surgical approach involving resection of the liver may provide longer-lasting relief of symptoms[68,69] but it should be appreciated that hepatic resection is difficult in such patients and is associated with significant morbidity. Nonetheless, extensive resection and cyst deroofing may allow the abdomen to better accommodate the enlarged residual liver. Surgical intervention is often associated with transient but massive ascites in the postoperative period.[70] Liver transplantation may be indicated in selected patients with hepatic failure.[71]

Cystadenoma

Cystadenoma of the liver is rare, but it has a strong tendency to recur and has a malignant potential. It is usually solitary and mainly affects women over 40 years of age. Cystadenomas are often multiloculated and may measure up to 20 cm in diameter. Histologically, the locules are mostly lined by a single layer of cuboidal or columnar cells; however, in areas the epithelium may form papillary projections. The presenting features are similar to other mass-forming hepatic pathologies, namely abdominal discomfort, anorexia, nausea and abdominal swelling. A large hepatic mass may be palpable. Liver function tests are usually normal. Diagnosis is based on US, MRI or CT (**Fig. 4.15**). US characteristics are of a large, anechoic, fluid-filled area with irregular margins. Internal echoes may be seen due to septa or papillary projections from the cyst wall. CT provides more accurate localisation, but may be less sensitive than US for demonstrating the thin septations. Cystadenomas grow very slowly and complications include biliary obstruction, intracystic haemorrhage, bacterial infection, rupture, recurrence after

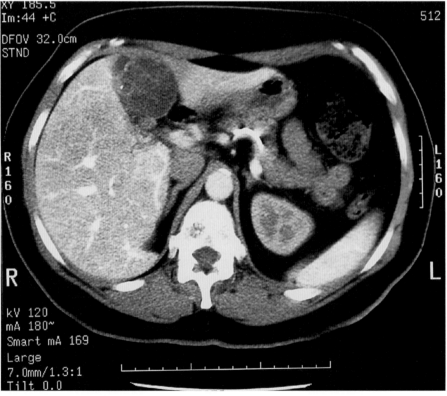

Figure 4.15 • CT scan demonstrating septa within a cystadenoma in segment 4 of the liver.

partial excision and transformation into cystade-nocarcinoma. This may be suspected radiologically by the presence of large projections into the cyst lobules and septal calcification.[72] Cystadenoma of the liver, even if asymptomatic, must be treated by complete excision.

References

1. Ishak KG, Rabin L. Benign tumors of the liver. Med Clin North Am 1975; 59:995–1013.

2. Adam YG, Huvos AG, Fortner JG. Giant heman-giomas of the liver. Ann Surg 1970; 172:239–45.

3. Schwartz SI, Husser WC. Cavernous hemangioma of the liver: a single institution report of 16 resections. Ann Surg 1987; 205:456–65.

4. Sewell JH, Weiss K. Spontaneous rupture of hemangioma of the liver. Arch Surg 1961; 83:105–9.

5. Trastek VF, van Heerden JA, Sheedy PF et al. Cavernous hemangiomas of the liver: resect or observe? Am J Surg 1983; 145:49–53.

6. Farges O, Daradkeh S, Bismuth H. Cavernous hemangiomas of the liver: are there any indications for resection? World J Surg 1995; 19:19–24.

7. Bornman PC, Terblanche J, Blumgart RL et al. Giant hemangiomas: diagnostic and therapeutic dilemmas. Surgery 1987; 101:445–9.

8. Yamamoto T, Kawarada Y, Yano T et al. Spontaneous rupture of haemangioma of the liver: treatment with transcatheter hepatic arterial embolisation. Am J Gastroenterol 1991; 86:1645–9.

9. Johnson CM, Sheedy PF, Stanson AW et al. Computed tomography and angiography of cavernous hemangiomas of the liver. Radiology 1985; 138:115–21.

10. Birnbaum BA, Weinreb JC, Mengibow AJ et al. Definitive diagnosis of hepatic hemangiomas: MR imaging versus Tc-99m labelled red blood cell SPECT. Radiology 1990; 176:95–102.

11. Choi BI, Shin YM, Chung JW et al. MR findings of hepatic cavernous hemangioma after intraarterial infusion of iodized oil. Abdom Imaging 1994; 16:507–11.

12. Mahfouz AE, Hamm B, Taupitz M et al. Hypervascular liver lesions: differentiation of focal nodular hyperplasia from malignant tumours with dynamic gadolinium-enhanced MR imaging. Radiology 1993; 186:133–42.

13. Krause T, Hauenstein K, Studier-Fischer B et al. Improved evaluation of technetium-99m-red blood cell SPECT in haemangioma of the liver. J Nucl Med 1993; 34:375–80.

14. Yamagata M, Kanematsu T, Matsumata T et al. Management of haemangioma of the liver: compa-rison of results between surgery and observation. Br J Surg 1991; 78:1223–5.

15. Nichols FC, van Heerden JA, Weiland LH. Benign liver tumors. Surg Clin North Am 1989; 69:297–314.

16. Pietrabissa A, Giulianotti P, Campatelli A et al. Management and follow-up of 78 giant haem-angiomas of the liver. Br J Surg 1996; 83:915–18.

17. Terkivatan T, Vrijland WW, Den Hoed PT et al. Size of lesion is not a criterion for resection during management of giant liver haemangioma. Br J Surg 2002; 89:1240–4.

18. Weimann A, Ringe B, Klempnauer J et al. Benign liver tumours: differential diagnosis and indications for surgery. World J Surg 1997; 21:983–91.

19. Foster JH, Adson MA, Schwartz SI et al. Symposium: benign liver tumours. Contemp Surg 1982; 21:67–102.

20. Baer HU, Dennison AR, Mouton W et al. Enucleation of giant hemangiomas of the liver. Ann Surg 1992; 216:673–6.

21. Cunningham JD, Katz LB, Brower ST et al. Laparoscopic resection of two liver hemangiomata. Surg Laparosc Endosc 1995; 5:277–80.

22. Longeville JH, de-la-Hall P, Dolan P et al. Treatment of a giant haemangioma of the liver with Kasabach–Merritt syndrome by orthotopic liver transplant, a case report. HPB Surg 1997; 10:159–62.

23. Nagorney DM. Benign hepatic tumors: focal nodular hyperplasia and hepatocellular adenoma. World J Surg 1995; 19:13–18.

24. Rooks JB, Ory HW, Ishak KG et al. Epidemiology of hepatocellular adenoma: the role of oral contraceptive use. J Am Med Assoc 1979; 242:644–8.

25. Kerlin P, Davis GL, McGill DB et al. Hepatic adenoma and focal nodular hyperplasia: clinical, pathologic and radiologic features. Gastroenterology 1983; 84:994–1002.

26. Baum JK, Bookstein JJ, Holtz F et al. Possible association between benign hepatomas and oral contraceptives. Lancet 1973; 2:926–9.

27. Kent DR, Nissen ED, Nissen SE et al. Effect of pregnancy on liver tumour associated with oral contraceptives. Obstet Gynecol 1978; 51:148–51.

28. Leese T, Farges O, Bismuth H. Liver cell adenomas: a 12 year surgical experience in a specialist hepatobiliary unit. Ann Surg 1988; 208:558–64.

29. Chiche L, Dao T, Salame E et al. Liver adenomatosis: reappraisal, diagnosis, and surgical management: eight new cases and review of the literature. Ann Surg 2000; 231:74–81.

30. Ferrell LD. Hepatocellular carcinoma arising in a focus of multilobular adenoma. Am J Surg Pathol 1993, 17:525–9.

31. Scott FR, El-Rafaie A, More L et al. Hepatocellular carcinoma arising in an adenoma: value of Qbend 10 immunostaining in diagnosis of liver cell carcinoma. Histopathology 1996; 28:472–4.

32. Gordon SC, Reddy KR, Livingstone AS et al. Resolution of a contraceptive steroid-induced hepatic adenoma with subsequent evolution into hepatocellular carcinoma. Ann Intern Med 1986; 105:547–9.

33. Gyorffy EJ, Bredfeldt JE, Black WC. Transformation of hepatic cell adenoma to hepatocellular carcinoma due to oral contraceptive use. Ann Intern Med 1989; 110:489–90.

34. Tao LC. Oral contraceptive-associated liver cell adenoma and hepatocellular carcinoma: cytomorphology and mechanism of malignant transformation. Cancer 1991; 68:341–7.

35. Delbeke D, Martin WH, Sandler MP et al. Evaluation of benign vs malignant hepatic lesions with positron emission tomography. Arch Surg 1998; 133:510–16.

36. Stoot JHMB, van der Linden E, Terpstra OT, Schaapherder AFM. Life-saving therapy for haemorrhaging liver adenomas using selective arterial embolisation. Br J Surg 2007; 94:1249–53.

37. Buhler H, Pirovino M, Akobiantz A et al. Regression of liver cell adenoma. A follow-up study of three consecutive cases after discontinuation of oral contraceptive use. Gastroenterology 1982; 82:775–82.

38. Aseni P, Sansalone CV, Sammartino C et al. Rapid disappearance of hepatic adenoma after contraceptive withdrawal. J Clin Gastroenterol 2001; 33:234–6.

39. Tepetes K, Selby R, Webb M et al. Orthoptic liver transplantation for benign hepatic neoplasms. Arch Surg 1995; 130:153–6.

40. Welch TJ, Sheedy PJ, Johnson CM et al. Focal nodular hyperplasia and hepatic adenoma: comparison of angiography, CT, US, and scintigraphy. Radiology 1985; 156:593–5.

41. Cherqui D, Rahmouni A, Charlotte F et al. Management of focal nodular hyperplasia and hepatocellular adenoma in young women: a series of 41 patients with clinical, radiological, pathological correlations. Hepatology 1995; 22:1674–81.

42. Belghiti J, Pateron D, Panis Y et al. Resection of presumed benign liver tumours. Br J Surg 1993; 80:380–3.

43. Allaire GS, Rabin L, Ishak KG. Bile duct adenoma: a study of 152 cases. Am J Surg Pathol 1988; 12:708–15.

44. Shek TWH, Ng IOL, Chan KW. Inflammatory pseudotumor of the liver: report of four cases and review of the literature. Am J Surg Pathol 1993; 17:231–8.

45. Grases PJ, Matos-Villalobos M, Arcia-Romero F et al. Mesenchymal hamartoma of the liver. Gastroenterology 1979; 76:1466–9.

46. Rintoul R, O'Riordain MG, Laurenson IF et al. The changing management of pyogenic liver abscess. Br J Surg 1996; 83:215–18.

47. Chou FF, Sheen-Chen SM, Chen YS et al. Single and multiple pyogenic liver abscesses: clinical course, etiology and results of treatment. World J Surg 1997; 21:384–9.

48. Huang CJ, Pitt HA, Lipsett PA et al. Pyogenic hepatic abscess: changing trends over 42 years. Ann Surg 1996; 223:600–9.

49. Branum GD, Tyson GS, Branum MA et al. Hepatic abscess: changes in etiology, diagnosis and management. Ann Surg 1990; 212:655–62.

50. Chu KM, Fan ST, Lai EC et al. Pyogenic liver abscess: an audit of experience over the past decade. Arch Surg 1996; 131:148–52.

51. Pearce NW, Knight R, Irving H. Non-operative management of pyogenic liver abscess. HPB 2003; 5:91–5.

52. Giorgio A, Tarantino L, Mariniello N et al. Pyogenic liver abscesses: 13 years of experience in percutaneous needle aspiration with US guidance. Radiology 1995; 195:122–4.

53. Rajak CL, Gupta S, Jain S et al. Percutaneous treatment of liver abscess: needle aspiration versus catheter drainage. Am J Roentgenol 1998; 170:1035–9.

54. Strong RW, Fawcett J, Lynch SV et al. Hepatectomy for pyogenic liver abscess. HPB 2003; 5:86–90.

55. Akgun Y, Tacyildiz IH, Celik Y. Amebic liver abscess: changing trends over 20 years. World J Surg 1999; 23:102–6.

56. Pitt HA. Surgical management of hepatic abscesses. World J Surg 1990; 14:498–504.

57. Agaoglu N, Turkyilmaz S, Arslan MK. Surgical treatment of hydatid cysts of the liver. Br J Surg 2003; 90:1536–41.

58. Milicevic M. Hydatid disease. In: Blumgart LH (ed.) Surgery of the liver and biliary tract, 3rd edn. London:WB Saunders, 2000; pp. 1167–204.

59. Martin IJ, McKinley AJ, Currie EJ et al. Tailoring the management of nonparasitic liver cysts. Ann Surg 1998; 228:167–72.

60. Gigot JF, Legrand M, Hubens G et al. Laparoscopic treatment of nonparasitic liver cysts: adequate selection of patients and surgical technique. World J Surg 1996; 20:556–61.

61. Montorsi M, Torzilli G, Fumagalli U et al. Percutaneous alcohol sclerotherapy of simple hepatic cysts. Results from a multicentre survey in Italy. HPB Surg 1994; 8:89–94.

62. Paterson-Brown S, Garden OJ. Laser assisted laparoscopic excision of liver cyst. Br J Surg 1991; 78:1047.

63. Klingler PJ, Gadenstatter M, Schmid T et al. Treatment of hepatic cysts in the laparoscopic era. Br J Surg 1997; 84:438–44.

64. Milutinovic J, Failkow PJ, Rudd TG et al. Liver cysts in patients with autosomal dominant polycystic kidney disease. Am J Med 1980; 68:741–4.

65. Bourgeois N, Kinnaert P, Vereerstraeten P et al. Infection of hepatic cysts following kidney transplantation in polycystic disease. World J Surg 1983; 7:629–31.

66. Lin TY, Chen CC, Wang SM. Treatment of nonparasitic disease of the liver: a new approach to therapy of the polycystic liver. Ann Surg 1968; 168:921–7.

67. Morino M, De Giuli M, Festa V et al. Laparoscopic management of symptomatic non-parasitic cysts of the liver: indications and results. Ann Surg 1994; 219:157–64.

68. Henne-Bruns D, Klomp HJ, Kremer B. Nonparasitic liver cysts and polycystic liver disease: results of surgical treatment. Hepatogastroenterology 1993; 40:1–5.

69. Que F, Nagorney DM, Gross JB Jr et al. Liver resection and cyst fenestration in the treatment of severe polycystic liver disease. Gastroenterology 1995; 108:487–94.

70. Farges O, Bismuth H. Fenestration in the management of polycystic liver disease. World J Surg 1995; 19:25–30.

71. Starzl TE, Reyes J, Tzakis A et al. Liver transplantation for polycystic liver disease. Arch Surg 1990; 125:575–7.

72. Korobkin M, Stephens DH, Lee JKT et al. Biliary cystadenoma and cystadenocarcinoma: CT and sonographic findings. Am J Roentgenol 1989; 153:507–11.

5

Primary malignant tumours of the liver

Olivier Farges
Jacques Belghiti

With the exception of hepatocellular carcinoma (HCC), which is one of the most common malignancies, primary tumours of the liver are relatively rare in adults. HCC arises from hepatocytes and cirrhosis is its main aetiological factor. This tumour is the subject of considerable interest due to its rising incidence and the development of innovative treatments. Intrahepatic cholangiocarcinoma (ICCA) arises from the peripheral intrahepatic biliary radicles and other rarer primary tumours arise from mesodermal cells, and include angiosarcoma, epithelioid haemangio-endothelioma and sarcoma.

Hepatocellular carcinoma

HCC accounts for 90% of all primary liver malignancy and its incidence continues to increase. It is the fifth most common neoplasm, accounting for more than 5% of all cancers, and also the third most common cause of cancer-related death. The World Health Organisation has estimated that primary liver cancer caused 619 000 deaths worldwide, as much as colon or rectum cancer.[1] HCC usually occurs in male patients, and cirrhosis precedes its development in most cases. Due to better medical management of cirrhosis, survival of cirrhotic patients has steadily increased in recent years resulting in a greater risk of developing HCC. Cohort studies have reported that in patients with HCC, the death rate due to cancer is 50–60% while hepatic failure and gastrointestinal bleeding are responsible for approximately 30% and 10% of the deaths respectively. HCC may now be identified at an early stage, particularly through the screening of high-risk patients.

Control of HCC nodules may be achieved successfully by surgical resection and by percutaneous treatment but their precise role will depend on the morphological features of the tumour and the functional status of the non-tumourous liver. Such treatments share a high incidence of tumour recurrence due to the persistence of the underlying cirrhosis, which represents a preneoplastic condition. Liver transplantation may seem a logical alternative treatment but has its own limitations, including tumour recurrence, the limited availability of grafts, and its cost. The most exciting areas of progress are the control of hepatitis B virus (HBV) or hepatitis C virus (HCV), the prevention of carcinogenesis in patients with chronic liver disease, and the development of medical therapies.

Incidence of HCC

The world age-adjusted incidence of HCC in men is 14.9 per 100 000,[2] but has geographical variation. Most cases occur in Africa and South-East Asia, with China alone accounting for more than 50% of the world cases. The incidence may be as high as 99 per 100 000 in Mongolian men. Other high-rate areas include Senegal, Gambia, South Korea, Hong Kong and Japan. North and South America, Northern Europe and Oceania are areas with low rates (less than 5 cases per 100 000). Southern European countries have intermediate rates.[3] HBV and HCV are the main risk factors, although their respective contributions differ in different areas of the world. Together they account for more than three-quarters of all cases (Table 5.1). HCC usually develops 20–40 years after the

Table 5.1 • Age and prevalence of HBV and HCV among patients with HCC in different geographical areas[6]

Area	Age (years)	HBV (%)	HCV (%)	Combined (%)
Africa	47	47	18	65
USA	63	16	48	64
South America	55	43	21	64
Western Europe	65	18	44	62
Eastern Europe	60	51	15	66
South-western Asia	52	42	27	69
Japan	65	15	75	91
China, Korea	52	70	18	88
World		53	25	78

viral contamination but cofactors may account for variations in the tumour evolution.

The age-adjusted incidence in women is two to four times less than in men and the difference is most pronounced in medium-risk south European populations and premenopausal women. Reasons for this higher rate in men include differences in exposure to risk factors, higher body mass index, higher levels of androgenic hormones and lower production or reduced response to estradiol.

The rising incidence of HCC was first documented in the USA, where this doubled between the late 1970s and the early 1990s,[4] reaching 3 cases per 100 000. Comparable increases have also been registered in Canada, Australia, Japan and various European countries. The recent epidemic of HCV infection probably accounts for a large part of this increase. It has been estimated that HCV began to infect large numbers of young adults in North America and South and Central Europe in the 1960s and 1970s as a result of intravenous drug use. The virus moved into national blood supplies and circulated until a screening test was developed in 1990, after which time rates of new infection decreased dramatically. The increase in the incidence of HCV-related HCC is, however, anticipated to persist until at least 2010 because of the delay between HCV contamination and HCC development. Alternative explanations for the increased incidence of HCC include ageing of the population, increased detection, improved survival of cirrhotic patients but also the recent epidemic of obesity and type II diabetes.

Risk factors of HCC

The main risk factor for HCC is liver cirrhosis. Once present, male gender, age (as a marker of the duration of exposure to a given aetiological agent), stage of cirrhosis and diabetes are additional independent risk factors. In contrast, coffee consumption greater than 2 cups/day could reduce the risk in both patients with and without chronic liver disease as evidenced by a recent meta-analysis.[5]

Cirrhosis vs. no underlying liver disease

Up to 90% of all HCC arises in patients with cirrhosis or extensive fibrosis. It is not clear whether this association is an effect of the regenerative process or of the underlying cause of cirrhosis. The risk of tumour development varies with the type of cirrhosis; the highest risk is reported for chronic viral hepatitis (78% of HCC worldwide[6]) whereas lower risks are associated with other forms of cirrhosis such as primary biliary cirrhosis. Multiple risk factors are increasingly identified in individual patients. The largest population at risk of chronic liver diseases and therefore HCC are patients with insulin resistance (worldwide prevalence 10%), high alcohol consumption (10%), HBV infection (5%), HCV infection (3%) and genetic haemochromatosis (0.5%).

HCC developing in the absence of cirrhosis is found in 10–20% of patients. The term 'absence of cirrhosis' appears more appropriate than 'normal liver' as these patients frequently have some degree of mild fibrosis, necroinflammation, steatosis or liver cell dysplasia. Variations in these proportions may be related to the definition of the underlying liver, method of recruitment (i.e. medical or surgical), type of material studied (liver biopsy, autopsy or surgical resection specimen) and geographical area. HCC in the absence of cirrhosis may be related to some of the same aetiologies as those responsible for HCC in cirrhotic livers. Alternatively, others are specific, such as hormonal exposure or glycogenosis.

HBV infection

It is estimated that 40 million people are currently affected worldwide by HBV, particularly in developing countries; HBV infection should, however, begin to decline as a result of increased utilisation of HBV immunisation. Areas of high prevalence for chronic HBV infection (Asia and Africa) also have the highest incidence of HCC. Conversely, vaccination campaigns against HBV in high endemic areas such as Taiwan have resulted in a decrease in hepatitis B surface antigen (HBsAg) prevalence among children from 10% to 1%, and have been associated with a 60% decrease in the incidence of HCC.[7] There is evidence that HBV-DNA sequences integrate into the genome of malignant hepatocytes and can be detected in the liver tissues of patients with HCC despite the absence of classical HBV serological markers. HBV-specific protein may also interact with liver genes. HBV is therefore a direct risk factor for HCC and can occur in patients without cirrhosis. The risk of HBV-associated HCC increases with the severity of the underlying hepatitis, age at infection and duration of infection, as well as level of viral replication.[8]

An Asian patient with HBV-related cirrhosis has a 17% cumulative risk of developing HCC over a 5-year period. In the West, this cumulative risk is 10%. This may be explained by the earlier acquisition of HBV in Asia through vertical transmission (rather than horizontal transmission in the West through sexual or parenteral routes), longer duration of disease, or additional exposure to environmental factors.

Ongoing HBV replication or hepatitis B e antigen (HBeAg) infection accelerates the progression to cirrhosis and also to HCC. A study conducted in Taiwanese men reported that the risk of HCC increased 10-fold when HBsAg was present and 60-fold when HBeAg was present.[9] Similarly, HBV-DNA levels greater than 10^4 or 10^6 copies/mL are associated with a 2.3 and 6.1 hazard risk respectively, compared to patients with lower levels of replication.[10] Additional cofactors increasing the risk of HCC are male gender (3–6 times higher risk), an age >40 years, concurrent HCV infection (twofold increased risk), HDV coinfection (threefold), heavy alcohol consumption (two- to threefold) and, in endemic regions, aflatoxin ingestion. Diabetes (two- to threefold) and central obesity are two additional emerging risk factors that are associated with HCC development independent of HBV infection.

Vaccination against HBV is the most effective means of decreasing the incidence of HBV-related HCC.

HCV infection

The expansion of HCV infection probably accounts for a significant proportion of the increased incidence of HCC observed over the past 10 years.[4] In Western countries, up to 70% of HCC patients have anti-HCV antibodies in their serum and the mean

time for developing HCC following HCV infection is approximately 30 years. Hence, it is estimated that the incidence of HCC will continue to increase during the next decade.[11]

In HCV-positive patients with initially compensated viral cirrhosis, HCC is both the most frequent and first complication.[12] The annual incidence of HCC is 0–2% in patients with chronic hepatitis and 1–4% in those with compensated cirrhosis, although rates as high as 7%/year have been reported in Japan.[13] In patients with cirrhosis, additional independent risk factors increasing the risk of HCC are age >55 years (two- to fourfold), male gender (two- to threefold), porphyria cutanea tarda (twofold), steatosis (threefold), diabetes (twofold), alcohol intake greater than 60–80 g/day (two- to fourfold) and HBV coinfection (two- to sixfold). Obesity is also a likely cofactor. In contrast, the viral genotype or viral concentration has no impact on the risk of HCC.

The mechanism of HCV-related HCC is still not very clear. The great majority of patients with HCV-related HCC have cirrhosis, suggesting that it is the presence of cirrhosis that is crucial for the development of this tumour. HCV-associated HCC has been reported in non-cirrhotic patients, although considerably less frequently than for HBV, indicating that it could also have a mutagenic effect. The core and NS3 proteins of HCV are likely oncogenic candidates.

Because anti-HCV vaccination is not available, prevention of HCV infection and of progression of chronic HCV infection to cirrhosis through antiviral treatment is the only means to reduce the incidence of HCV-related HCC.

During the past 15 years, improvements in antiviral treatments have included extension of therapy to 48 weeks, the combination of interferon with ribavirin, and the use of pegylated interferon. These have resulted in improvement in the sustained virological response (SVR) rate in randomised trials from less than 10% with a 24-week course of interferon monotherapy to as high as 50–60% with the combination of pegylated interferon and ribavirin over 48 weeks. SVR is associated with a significantly decreased risk of developing HCC.[14] Long-term follow-up of these patients should nevertheless be maintained since HCC may develop years after sustained response.

In human immunodeficiency virus (HIV)-positive patients, the prevalence of HCV infection in Europe and the USA is 35%, and even higher rates have been reported in drug users.[15] Because newer therapies are decreasing mortality from HIV infection, both conditions are observed with increasing frequency. Cirrhosis and HCC occur 15–20 years earlier than in patients infected by HCV alone. Conversely, HCV coinfection increases the risk of progression to AIDS.

Other viral infections

Infection with the hepatitis delta virus (HDV) is found in patients who are also infected with HBV (see above). Hepatitis A virus (HAV) and hepatitis E virus (HEV) infection cause neither chronic hepatitis nor HCC.

Alcohol

Heavy (>50–70 g/day) and prolonged alcohol ingestion increases the risk of HCC 13-fold. Its relative role should, however, probably be reassessed in view of the high incidence (75%) of HCV infection in HCC patients presumed to have 'alcoholic' cirrhosis. It is likely that the same occurs to some extent for the metabolic syndrome. It is estimated that alcohol accounts for 10% (Asia) to 20% (Europe and North America) of HCC. However, alcohol is such an important and frequent cofactor in the development of HCV- or HBV-related HCC[16] that it is, at least to some extent, involved in most HCC. Data available from cohort studies of European or US patients with alcohol-related cirrhosis suggest an annual incidence of HCC of 1.7% (as compared with 2.2% and 3.7% in patients of the same geographical area with HBV- or HCV-associated cirrhosis).

Non-alcoholic fatty liver disease (NAFLD)

NAFLD has recently been recognised as being one of the most common causes of liver disease in the USA[17] (and other Western countries). Histological changes in the liver range from simple steatosis to more severe forms of non-alcoholic steatohepatitis (NASH), including cirrhosis. It is closely associated with type II diabetes and obesity, as part of the metabolic syndrome, the prevalence of which has increased as an epidemic. It has been estimated that 90% of obese people (body mass index >30 kg/m^2) have some form of NAFLD, including 60% with simple steatosis or steatosis with only mild inflammation, 25–30% have NASH which is largely characterised by hepatocellular injury and some degree of fibrosis, and 3–5% have cirrhosis.[18] Similarly, it is estimated that 70% of persons with type II diabetes have some fatty liver.

 NAFLD (and the metabolic syndrome) accounts for a substantial portion of what was considered in the past as cryptogenic cirrhosis and carries an inherent risk of the development of HCC.

There is an increased prevalence of obesity and diabetes[19] in patients with HCC and no identifiable cause for chronic liver disease. Obesity increases mortality from liver cancer two- to fivefold,[20] far more than for any other cancer, and this influence persists after adjustment for alcohol use. Diabetes is also a risk factor for liver cancer, although its independent influence is more difficult to assess as cirrhotic patients have an increased prevalence of diabetes; a recent cohort study performed in patients without acute or chronic liver disease has, however, found a twofold risk of HCC in diabetics.[21]

HCC has been reported in patients with previously diagnosed NAFLD but prospective longitudinal studies are lacking that could more precisely estimate the link and incidence. There are difficulties since once cirrhosis is established, histological features of NAFLD may have disappeared. The impression is that the majority of cryptogenic cirrhosis is attributable to NAFLD and that obesity-related cryptogenic cirrhosis carries a risk of HCC similar to HCV-related cirrhosis.[22] In addition, there is evidence that, as for alcohol, it may favour the development of HCC in HCV patients.[19]

One area of uncertainty is whether metabolic syndrome favours the development of HCC in the absence of cirrhosis. Most human studies suggest that silent progression of NASH to cirrhosis is a prerequisite to the development of HCC. There are, however, animal models of fatty liver in which HCC develops without cirrhosis,[23] as well as case reports or small clinical series in which NASH-associated HCC occurs on a background of only mild fibrosis.[24]

Hereditary haemochromatosis

Hereditary haemochromatosis is a genetically mediated disorder characterised by excessive gastrointestinal absorption of iron and is a long-known risk factor for HCC. The risk for the development of HCC in haemochromatosis is estimated to be increased 100- to 200-fold[25] with a pooled prevalence of approximately 10% overall and almost twice as much in the subgroup of patients with cirrhosis.[26] More recent population-based studies have reported a 20-fold increase in standardised incidence ratio[27] and this risk was increased in the subgroup of patients with cirrhosis. Whether the risk of HCC in patients with haemochromatosis is greater than in patients with cirrhosis of other origins is controversial. The annual incidence, once cirrhosis has occurred, is estimated to be 5%. Other risk factors besides cirrhosis include male gender (29-fold in male and sevenfold in female) and diabetes. The fact that HCC may develop in patients with hereditary haemochromatosis in the absence of cirrhosis has several implications. Haemochromatosis should be ruled out when an HCC is discovered in an otherwise normal liver. Conversely, it has been estimated that early detection of the C282Y homozygote mutation in male patients would decrease the overall incidence of HCC by 10%.[28]

Interestingly, pathological conditions other than haemochromatosis that are associated with iron overload, such as homozygous β-thalassaemia or the so-called African overload syndrome, are also associated with an increased risk of HCC. Similarly, there is also evidence of a link between iron deposits within the liver and HCC in patients with and without cirrhosis.

Cirrhosis of other aetiologies

Primary biliary cirrhosis (PBC) has normally been considered as a low risk factor for HCC, not only because of its rare incidence but also because it predominantly affects women (with a sex ratio of 9:1) who are relatively spared from HCC otherwise. A recent study[29] reported an annual incidence of 0.3% in patients with early PBC and 1.5% in those with advanced PBC. All patients had stage III or IV PBC by the time HCC developed.[29] The risk is five to seven times greater in men than in women. Interestingly, previous history of blood transfusion has recently been repeatedly identified as an additional independent risk factor which is not related to HBV or HCV coinfection.[29,30] In contrast, HCC development in patients with secondary biliary cirrhosis is exceptional if it even exists.

Autoimmune hepatitis has a low risk of HCC development. Potential reasons are the female predominance and the delayed development of cirrhosis through corticosteroid therapy. HCV infection needs to be ruled out as it may induce autoantibodies. A recent literature review identified only 35 cases.[31]

Aflatoxin

Aflatoxin B1 has also long been associated with the development of HCC because areas with a large consumption of this toxin coincide with areas of high incidence of HCC (Asia and sub-Saharan Africa). Aflatoxin is ingested in food as a result of contamination of imperfectly stored staple crops by *Aspergillus flavus*. It is thought to induce HCC through mutation of the tumour suppressor gene p53. Although some studies suggest that it is an independent risk factor,[32] others suggest that it could be a co-carcinogen only in patients with HBV infection. HCC in this setting frequently develops in a non-cirrhotic liver.

Metabolic liver disease and HCC

An increased risk of HCC is recognised in some other forms of metabolic liver disease such as α_1-antitrypsin deficiency, porphyria cutanea tarda, tyrosinaemia and hypercitrullinaemia. Glycogenosis type IV, hereditary fructose intolerance and Wilson disease may also develop HCC but with a lower risk. There is evidence that iron and copper overload in haemochromatosis and Wilson disease generate, respectively, oxygen/ nitrogen species and unsaturated aldehydes that cause mutations in the p53 tumour suppressor gene.

Adenoma, contraceptives and androgens

Adenoma complicating type I glycogenosis and related to anabolic steroids or androgens may transform into HCC within non-cirrhotic livers. Fanconi disease may also be complicated by HCC, especially if it has been treated by steroids. The risk of transformation of adenomas secondary to contraceptives and estrogen treatments is real,[33] but probably less than 10%. It is, however, the main rationale for removing all adenomas. The risk of malignant transformation of polyadenomatosis is not increased despite the higher number of tumours.[34]

Transformation of adenoma apparently only occurs in tumours larger than 5 cm, is more frequent in male patients and the risk of transformation has recently been linked to some molecular characteristics and in particular β-cathenin mutation.[35] Recreational anabolic steroid use is known to potentially result in the development of adenoma and malignant transformation to HCC has been reported.[36]

Pathology of HCC and of nodular lesions in chronic liver disease

It is widely believed that a cirrhotic liver may contain preneoplastic nodules that are in an intermediate stage between non-neoplastic regenerating nodules and overtly malignant HCC. These preneoplastic or dysplastic nodules (DNs) are further divided into low and high grade depending on the degree of cytological or architectural atypia on histological examination. DNs are defined as a nodular region of less than 2 cm in diameter with dysplasia but without definite histological criteria of malignancy.[37] Encapsulation, necrosis and haemorrhage are not seen. Low-grade DNs are around 1 cm in diameter and slightly yellowish, and have a very low probability of becoming malignant. High-grade DNs are less common with slightly larger nodules (up to 2 cm) and characterised by increased cell density with an irregular thin-trabecular pattern and occasionally unpaired arteries. These are often difficult to differentiate from highly differentiated HCC. They may contain distinct foci of well-differentiated HCC and are therefore considered as precancerous lesions and become malignant in a third of cases.[38] It must, however, be appreciated that lesions smaller than 2 cm may also represent HCC, some of which have already disseminated. Tumour invasion into the portal vein and intrahepatic metastases are found in 25% and 10% respectively of such lesions. These features help in identifying the malignant nature of these early HCCs but molecular analysis will probably become the optimum tool in the future.[39] Nodules larger than 2 cm are seldom regenerative or dysplastic nodules and usually correspond to HCC.[40]

HCCs can be subdivided according to their gross morphology, degree of differentiation, vascularity, presence of a surrounding capsule and presence of vascular invasion. All of these criteria have practical implications.

On gross morphology, HCCs can be solitary or multinodular, consisting of either a collection of discrete lesions in different segments developing synchronously (multicentric HCC) or as one dominant mass and a number of 'daughter' nodules (intrahepatic metastases) located in the adjacent segments. Diffuse HCCs are relatively rare at presentation and consist of poorly defined, widely infiltrative masses that present particular diagnostic challenges on imaging. A third type is the infiltrating HCC, which typically is less differentiated with ill-defined margins.

Microscopically, HCCs exhibit variable degrees of differentiation that are usually stratified into four different histological grades, known as Edmondson grades 1–4, which correspond to well-differentiated, moderately differentiated, poorly differentiated and undifferentiated types. The degree of differentiation decreases normally as the tumour increases in diameter. Very well-differentiated HCC can resemble normal hepatocytes and the trabecular structure may reproduce a near normal lobar architecture so that histological diagnosis by biopsy or following resection may be difficult. Immunostaining with specific markers may prove useful.[40]

Vascularisation is a key parameter in differentiating HCC from regenerating nodules. Progression from macroregenerative nodule to low-grade DN, high-grade DN and frank HCC is characterised by loss of visualisation of portal tracts and development of new non-triadal arterial vessels which become the dominant blood supply in overt HCC lesions. This arterial neoangiogenesis is the landmark of HCC diagnosis and the rationale for chemoembolisation and antiangiogenic treatment.

Tumour nodules may be surrounded by a distinct fibrous capsule. This capsule, present in 80% of resected HCCs, has a variable thickness, which may not be complete, and is frequently infiltrated by tumour cells. Capsular microscopic invasion by tumour cells is present in almost one-third of tumours smaller than 2 cm in diameter, as compared with two-thirds of those with a larger diameter.[41]

HCC has a great tendency to spread locally and to invade blood vessels. The rate of portal invasion is higher in the expansive type, in poorly differentiated HCC and in large tumours. Characteristically, microscopic vascular invasion involves 20% of tumours of 2 cm in diameter, 30–60% of cases in nodules 2–5 cm and up to 60–90% in nodules above 5 cm in size. The presence of portal invasion is the most important predictive factor associated with recurrence. The tumour thrombus has its own arterial supply, mainly from the site of the original venous invasion. Once HCC invades the portal vein, tumour thrombi grow rapidly in both directions, and in particular towards the main portal vein. As a consequence, tumour fragments spread throughout the liver as the thrombus crosses segmental branches. Once the tumour thrombus has extended into the main portal vein, there is a high risk of complete thrombosis and increased portal hypertension. This accounts for the frequent presentation with fatal rupture of oesophageal varices, or liver decompensation including ascites (**Fig. 5.1**), jaundice and encephalopathy. Invasion of hepatic veins is possible, although less frequent. The thrombus eventually extends into the suprahepatic vena cava or the right atrium and is associated with a high risk of lung metastases. Rarely, HCC may invade the biliary tract and give rise to jaundice or haemobilia. Mechanisms of HCC-induced biliary obstruction include:

- intraductal tumour extension;
- obstruction by a fragment of necrotic tumour debris;
- haemorrhage of the tumour resulting in haemobilia;
- metastatic lymph node compression of major bile ducts in the porta hepatis.

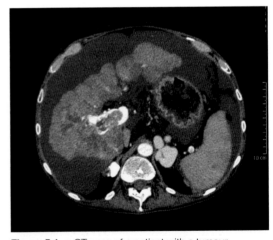

Figure 5.1 • CT scan of a patient with a tumour thrombus originating from an HCC located in the right liver. The thrombus extends in the main portal vein. Ascites is present.

The rate of invasion of the portal vein, hepatic vein and bile duct at the time of diagnosis is 15%, 5% and 3% respectively.[41] However, it is estimated that during the natural history of HCC, approximately 1 in 3 patients will develop portal vein thrombosis.

When present, metastases are most frequently found in the lung. Other locations, in decreasing order of frequency, are: adrenal glands, bones, lymph nodes, meninges, pancreas, brain and kidney. Large tumour size, bilobar disease and poor differentiation are risk factors for metastatic disease.

Clinical presentation

There are basically three circumstances of diagnosis: (1) incidental finding during routine screening; (2) incidental finding during work-up of impaired liver function tests or of another pathological condition; and (3) presence of liver- or cancer-related symptoms, the severity of which depend on the stage of the tumour and the functional status of the non-tumourous liver. In developed countries, a growing number of tumours are discovered incidentally at an asymptomatic stage. As tumours increase in size, they may cause abdominal pain, malaise, weight loss, asthenia, anorexia and fever. These symptoms may be acute as a result of tumour extension or complication.

Spontaneous rupture occurs in 5–15% of patients[42] and is observed particularly in patients with superficial or protruding tumours. The diagnosis should be suspected in patients with known HCC or cirrhosis presenting with acute epigastric pain as well as in Asian or African men who develop an acute abdomen (**Fig. 5.2**). Minor rupture manifests as abdominal pain or haemorrhagic ascites, and hypovolaemic

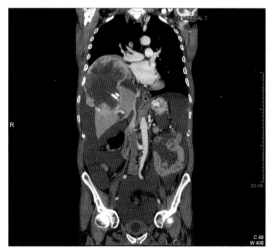

Figure 5.2 • CT scan of a patient with a ruptured HCC. Note that the rupture is limited at the upper part of the liver. This patient had haemorrhagic ascites.

shock is only present in about half of the patients. Portal vein invasion may manifest as upper gastrointestinal bleeding or acute ascites and invasion of hepatic veins or inferior vena cava may result in pulmonary embolism or sudden death.

Clinical symptoms resulting from biliary invasion or haemobilia are present in 2% of the patients. Possible paraneoplastic syndromes associated with HCC include polyglobulia, hypercalcaemia and hypoglycaemia. Finally, in patients with underlying liver disease, a sudden onset or worsening of ascites or liver decompensation may be the first evidence of HCC formation.

Clinical examination may only reveal large or superficial tumours. There may be clinical signs of cirrhosis, in particular ascites, a collateral circulation, umbilical hernia, hepatomegaly and splenomegaly.

Liver function tests and tumour markers

Liver function test impairment is non-specific and reflects the underlying liver pathology or the presence of a space-occupying lesion. Because most HCCs develop within a cirrhotic liver and since HCCs on normal livers are usually large, normal liver function tests are exceptional. Jaundice is most frequently the result of liver decompensation.

Serum α-fetoprotein (AFP) is the most widely recognised serum marker of HCC. It is secreted during fetal life but the residual levels are very low in the adult (0–20 ng/mL). It may increase in HCC patients and serum levels greater than 400 ng/mL can be considered as an indicator of an HCC with 95% confidence. These levels may exceed 10 000 ng/mL in 5–10% of HCCs.[41] Very high levels usually correlate with poor differentiation, tumour aggressiveness and vascular invasion. However, an AFP >20 ng/mL has a sensitivity of 60% (a surveillance programme using this cut-off value would miss 40% of tumours) and drops to 22% for values greater than 200 ng/mL. Only 10% of small tumours are associated with raised levels whereas 30% of patients with chronic active hepatitis without an HCC have a moderately increased AFP. This usually correlates with the degree of histological activity and raised levels of transaminase, and it may therefore fluctuate. Tumours other than HCC can also be associated with increased AFP levels but these are rare (non-seminal germinal tumours, hepatoid gastric tumours, neuroendocrine tumours). Alternative serum markers for HCC, such as des-γ-carboxy prothrombin, PIVKA-II (>40 mAU/mL) and AFP-L3 (>15%) have not come into common practice except in Japan, where they are covered under the national health insurance.

Morphological studies

The aims of imaging in the context of HCC are:

- to screen high-risk patients;
- to identify small lesions;
- to differentiate HCC from other space-occupying lesions;
- to select the appropriate treatment.

The number of lesions, their size and extent, and the presence of daughter nodules, vascular invasion, extrahepatic spread and underlying liver disease are critical in choosing the most appropriate treatment. These aims may be achieved by ultrasonography (US), contrast-enhanced US, computed tomography (CT), magnetic resonance imaging (MRI), angiography or a combination of these.

Ultrasound and contrast-enhanced ultrasound

US is the first-line investigation because of its low cost, high availability and high sensitivity in identifying a focal liver mass. In experienced hands, US may identify 85–95% of lesions of 3–5 cm diameter and 60–80% of lesions of 1 cm. Differences in accuracy worldwide may be explained by steatosis rate, spontaneous heterogeneity of the liver disease and in the ultrasonographer. Typically, small HCCs are hypoechoic and homogeneous and cannot be differentiated from regenerating or dysplastic nodules. With increasing size, they may become hypo- or hyperechoic but most importantly heterogeneous. A hypoechoic peripheral rim corresponds to the capsule. The infiltrating type is usually very difficult to identify in a grossly heterogeneous cirrhotic liver. Besides echoity, the accuracy of US depends on the dimension and location of the tumour, as well as operator experience. A 1-cm-diameter tumour can be visualised if it is deeply located, whereas the same lesion located on the surface can be missed. Similarly, tumours located in the upper liver segments or on the edge of the left lateral segment may be missed. Tumours detected at an advanced stage despite surveillance are located frequently at one of these two sites. Obesity may also prevent accurate exploration of the liver (thickened abdominal wall or steatotic liver). Doppler US may demonstrate a feeding artery and/or draining veins. US is also accurate in identifying vascular or biliary invasion and indirect evidence of cirrhosis such as segmental atrophy, splenomegaly, ascites or collateral veins. Tumour thrombosis, as opposed to cruoric thrombosis, is associated with enlargement of the vascular lumen, and an arterial signal may be detected by duplex Doppler.

To improve the accuracy of US, contrast agents (stabilised microbubbles) are being used increasingly. They are administered intravenously via bolus injection followed by saline flush. Enhancement patterns are typically described during arterial phase (10–20 s postinjection), portal venous (30–80 s) and late phase (120–360 s). Whereas US microbubbles are confined to the vascular spaces, contrast agents for CT and MRI are rapidly cleared from the blood into the extracellular space. Although contrast-enhanced US has proved very useful to characterise nodules, sensitivity is not increased. Contrast-enhanced US is subject to the same limitations as other US modes: if the baseline scan is unsatisfactory, the contrast-enhanced US study will be unsatisfactory as well.

Computed tomography

CT is more accurate than US in identifying HCCs and their lobar or segmental distribution, particularly with the development of helical and multislice spiral scanners.[43] Spiral CT is undertaken without contrast and during arterial (25–50 s), portal (60–65 s) and equilibrium (130–180 s) phases after contrast administration. In addition, it is useful for identifying features of underlying cirrhosis, accurately measuring liver and tumour volumes, and assessing extrahepatic tumour spread. HCCs are usually hypodense and spontaneous hyperdensity is usually associated with iron overload or fatty infiltration, which is seen in 2–20% of the patients. Specific features are early uptake of contrast and a mosaic shape pattern. During the portal phase, the density diminishes sharply and results in a washout (tumour is hypodense compared to adjacent parenchyma) during the late phase (**Fig. 5.3**). HCCs may show variable vascularity depending on tumour grade and some are poorly vascularised. The capsule, when present, is best seen at the portal or late phase as an enhanced thickening at the periphery (delayed vascular enhancement is characteristic of fibrosis). Vascular invasion of segmental branches may also be identified. Intratumoural arterioportal fistula may occur and present as an early enhancement of portal branches or as a triangular area distal to the tumour with contrast enhancement different from the adjacent parenchyma. Nonetheless, such fistulas are seen frequently in cirrhotic patients without HCC as infracentimetric hypervascular subcapsular lesions.

Magnetic resonance imaging

MRI tends to be more accurate than other imaging techniques in differentiating HCC from other liver tumours, especially those >2 cm. As for CT, the technique of MRI should be accurate with T1- and

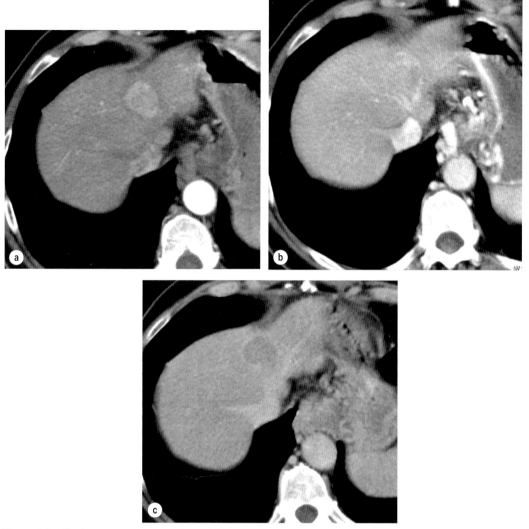

Figure 5.3 • Typical vascular kinetics of an HCC. There is early uptake of contrast at the arterial phase **(a)** that becomes isodense at the portal phase **(b)**, with washout at the late phase **(c)**.

T2-weighted images and with early, intermediate and late phase following contrast injection of gadolinium. The characteristics of an HCC are the mosaic shape structure and the presence of a capsule. Tumours are hypointense on T1-weighted images and hyperintense on T2-weighted images, but these characteristics are present in only 54% of patients; 16% of HCCs demonstrate hypointensity on both T1 and T2 images. Hyperintensity on T1-weighted images is also possible, and associated with fatty, copper or glycogen infiltration of the tumour. The kinetics of vascular enhancement following injection of contrast is the same as during CT with early uptake and late washout.

Arteriography

Although the diagnostic usefulness of angiography has been reduced, it is still widely used as part of arterial chemoembolisation. Arteriography shows early vascular uptake (blush) and if used, lipiodol injection is retained selectively for a prolonged period by the tumour. On subsequent CT, the retained radiodense Lipiodol reveals the tumour as a high-density area. Uptake within the liver is not specific for HCC, since all hypervascular liver tumours, including focal nodular hyperplasia, adenoma, angioma and metastases, will retain Lipiodol. False-negative results may be observed with avascular, necrotic or fibrotic HCC.

Accuracy of imaging techniques

CT and MRI with contrast enhancement have the highest diagnostic accuracy (>80%) and the techniques can be combined. Comparison with the pathological analysis of explanted livers of transplant candidates, however, shows that both techniques lose accuracy in assessing extension of the disease. For any technique, additional intrahepatic tumours, especially those less than 1 cm, are not diagnosed preoperatively in 30% of cases. MRI angiography with 2-mm sections is currently considered the most accurate technique, with a sensitivity of 100% for nodules more than 20 mm, 89% for nodules 10–20 mm and 34% for nodules <10 mm.[44]

Diagnosis of HCC

Although the differential diagnosis of HCC includes a number of non-neoplastic conditions and malignant tumours, the key challenge is the differentiation of HCC from other nodules within the cirrhotic liver.

The first attempt to standardise the diagnostic criteria was performed in 2000 by the European Association for the Study of Liver Disease (EASLD).[45] The advocated strategy was based on the size of the nodules:

- For nodules less than 1 cm on US, it was considered that other imaging techniques would be unlikely to confirm reliably the diagnosis. Since the accuracy of liver biopsy for such small lesions and the probability that they are HCC is low, it was felt reasonable to repeat US at 3-month intervals until the lesion exceeded 1 cm in size. However, early HCC may take more than a year to reach this size and this recall policy should be strict.
- Nodules larger than 2 cm have a much higher probability of being HCC and confirmation of the diagnosis is mandatory. In cirrhotic patients, a diagnosis of HCC was assumed if two coincident imaging techniques (US, spiral CT, MRI or angiography) demonstrated arterial hypervascularisation of the lesion or if the hypervascular mass was associated with a serum AFP >400 ng/mL.
- For 1–2 cm nodules biopsy was recommended, although it was acknowledged that a negative biopsy did not exclude the diagnosis. A recall policy was advocated for such nodules.

Subsequent to these recommendations, several studies identified delayed contrast washout as a characteristic of HCC in addition to intense early arterial uptake.[46] This feature was introduced in the refined version of the diagnostic criteria in 2005 by the AASLD.[47]

According to these new guidelines:
- the presence of early uptake and delayed washout on a single dynamic imaging study (triphasic CT, MRI with gadolinium or contrast-enhanced US) was considered characteristic of HCC for nodules >2cm;
- for nodules 1–2 cm, both characteristics had to be present on two (and not a single) dynamic imaging techniques to retain the diagnosis of HCC.

The latter proposal has recently been validated prospectively[48] with specificity and positive predictive values of 100%. However, the sensitivity was 33%, underlying the need for biopsy and recall policies when these criteria are not present.

Requirement for and reliability of histological study

Pathological confirmation of HCC can be obtained by cytology, histology or a combination of these with increasing accuracy. Routine biopsy is not indicated in cirrhotic patients, as indicated previously. Liver biopsy is limited by the potential for haemorrhage and pain, and may occasionally be responsible for neoplastic seeding and vascular spread. The reported incidence of needle tract seeding is 1–5%.[49] Tumour involvement is generally limited to subcutaneous tissues and this has a slow progression. It is possible to perform local excision without apparent impact on survival. Even if the false positive rate is low, the risk of needle tract seeding is balanced by the risk of pursuing an aggressive treatment such as resection or transplantation in a patient without malignancy. In the future, tumour biopsy may provide molecular profiling to help plan screening or treatment. It is currently inaccurate in assessing the tumour grade.[50]

There is a 30–40% false-negative rate of fine-needle biopsy and a negative result should therefore never rule out malignancy.[51]

Natural history of HCC and staging systems

Traditionally, the natural history of HCC is considered to be particularly grim, with life expectancy measurable in weeks. However, in a recent analysis of the results of the control group of randomised controlled trials (RCTs),[51] the median survival in patients with non-surgical advanced, symptomatic HCC is 6 months. Similarly, the prognosis of untreated patients who are not all end-stage at the time of presentation is better than anticipated, with 2- and 3-year survival rates of 40–56% and 13–28% respectively. In asymptomatic patients without tumoural invasion, the 3-year survival may be as high as 50%.[51] These observations have important implications for HCC diagnosed at an early stage, particularly in patients with preserved liver function.

The aim of staging systems is to predict outcome. This can either be used to anticipate prognosis and, more recently, for selection of treatment. Survival of HCC patients is mainly influenced by the morphological spread of tumour, the presence and severity of cancer-related symptoms, and the severity and evolution of the underlying cirrhosis. The most recent systems attempt to integrate all three groups of parameters.

- Although staging was assessed initially by the TNM classification, the pathological particularity of HCC has led to the successive implementation of modifications in Eastern (Liver Cancer Study Group of Japan) and Western (American Joint Committee on Cancer, International Union Against Cancer) countries. These take into account tumour number, vascular invasion and tumour size (Table 5.2). A limitation is that they are based on pathological findings and can only be applied accurately (retrospectively) in operated patients.
- Cancer-related symptoms have a detrimental impact on outcome that is assessed by the WHO performance status or the Karnofsky index. The presence of pain is a poor indicator of outcome.
- Liver damage induced by underlying liver disease has traditionally been assessed by the Child–Pugh score. This was, however, designed to assess the functional reserve of cirrhotic patients undergoing portocaval shunt surgery and is not entirely appropriate for HCC patients in whom therapeutic options may include liver transplantation and liver resection.

Several groups have attempted to combine them within integrated staging systems. There are currently six such systems designated as the CLIP (from Italy), GRETCH (from France), BCLC (from Spain), CUPI (from China), JSS and JIS (from Japan) scores. It is beyond the scope of this chapter to detail all of them (Table 5.3).[52] It should be appreciated that these scores have been computed retrospectively by multivariate analysis of a specific patient population and not all have been externally validated. Furthermore, the sample population in question was either an unse-

Table 5.2 • Comparison of the tumour (T) staging in the Liver Cancer Study Group of Japan (LCSGJ) and American Joint Committee on Cancer (AJCC) staging systems

	LCSGJ
T1	Tumour <2 cm, unique *and* without vascular invasion
T2	Tumour <2 cm, multiple *or* with vascular invasion
	Tumour >2 cm single *and* without vascular invasion
T3	Tumour <2 cm, multiple *and* with vascular invasion
	Tumour >2 cm, multiple *or* with vascular invasion
T4	Tumour >2 cm, multiple *and* with vascular invasion
	AJCC
T1	Single tumour without vascular invasion
T2	Tumour <5 cm, multiple *or* with vascular invasion
T3A	Multiple tumours, any >5 cm
	or tumour(s) involving major branch of portal or hepatic vein(s)
T3B	Any tumour N1
T4	Any tumour M1

AJCC/UICC and LCSGJ TNM classification of HCC.

lected group (GRETCH, CLIP, CUPI) or a population of HCC patients who were candidates for potentially curative treatments (BCLC). These systems apply to all patients with HCC but surgical staging systems (LCSGJ or UICC) are more accurate for patients undergoing surgery. It should be appreciated that some of these are true staging systems whereas others are used for treatment selection.

Screening for HCC

Screening is used routinely in countries where effective therapeutic interventions are available. HCC fulfils most of the criteria required for a surveillance or screening programme to be justified. HCC is common in highly endemic areas (and its incidence is growing in others) and it is associated with a high mortality. Furthermore, the survival is extremely poor by the time patients present with symptoms related to the tumour, and the population at risk is clearly defined (in particular – but not exclusively – patients with HCV- and HBV-related cirrhosis, especially when they are male and over 60 years). Acceptable screening tests of low morbidity and

Table 5.3 • Main variables retained in prognostic models

	GRETCH		CLIP		CUPI	
Tumour morphology			Multinodular extension <50%	1	TNM I and II	−3
			Multinodular extension >50%	2	TNM III	−1
					TNM IV	0
	Portal thrombosis	1	Portal thrombosis	1		
Tumour biology	AFP >35 ng/mL	2	AFP >400 ng/mL	1	AFP >500 ng/mL	3
Liver function	Bilirubin >50 μmol/L	3	Child–Pugh A	0	Bilirubin <34 μmol/mL	0
	Alk. phosph. >2N*	2	Child–Pugh B	1	Bilirubin 34–51 μmol/mL	3
			Child–Pugh C	2	Bilirubin >51 μmol/mL	4
					Alk. phosph. >200 IU/L	3
General status	Karnofsky index <80	3			Asymptomatic	−4
Score range		0–11		0–6		−7 to 12

The numbers refer to the score given to each variable. A total score is obtained by adding each individual score. In the CLIP score, the median survivals according to the score in the initial[30] and prospective validations[32] were: score 0: 36–42 months; score 1: 22–32 months; score 2: 8–16 months; score 3: 4–7 months, score 4 or above: 1–3 months.
*2N = twice normal.

high efficacy exist that allow the tumour to be recognised in the latent/early stage. Finally, effective treatments exist in selected patients.

The two most common tests used for screening of HCC are US and serum AFP measurements, although many clinicians consider the latter investigation to be of little value for screening. However, the regular increase of AFP in patients who have a normal AFP at baseline should prompt the performance of a CT or MRI scan if US is negative.

No clear evidence is available to determine the optimal interval for periodic screening. Tumour doubling times vary widely with an average of 200 days. It has been estimated that the time taken for an undetectable lesion to grow to 2 cm is about 4–12 months, and that it takes 5 months for the most rapidly growing HCC to reach 3 cm. Because treatments are most effective on tumours <3 cm, screening programmes are usually performed at 6-month intervals. However, feasibility of treatment and survival is not different for patients who have semi-annual and annual surveillance,[53] although the latter is the most cost-effective strategy. Nevertheless, conventional practice involves a 6-month interval or less (3–4 months according to the Japanese guidelines[54]) in very-high-risk patients.

There are limitations to screening programmes. Of patients presenting with HCC, 20–50% have previously undiagnosed cirrhosis and therefore escape surveillance. Access to medical care and compliance is a limitation in highly endemic areas, with 50% of patients with alcoholic cirrhosis defaulting from surveillance over 5 years. US is highly operator dependent, and the cost and invasiveness of CT and MRI make them unsuitable for screening. However, these latter modalities are particularly suited in patients with irregular background liver parenchyma or obesity.

Surveillance of at-risk patients is being used increasingly at 6-month intervals with US and AFP estimation to detect HCC at an early stage.

High-risk groups consist of those with established cirrhosis due to HBV, HCV and haemochromatosis. Male patients with alcohol-related cirrhosis abstaining from alcohol or likely to comply with treatment should also be considered.

Ultrasound is recommended as a screening tool whereas CT and MRI are most useful in confirming the diagnosis. Liver biopsy is recommended in selected cases only.

The impact of screening programmes on patient management and survival is still controversial,[55] but it is accepted that these increase the chance of successful treatment and improve survival. In the only prospective randomised controlled study involving more than

17 000 HBV patients from Shanghai, surgical resection could be performed in 70% of the screened patients compared with none of the non-screened patients,[56] with 1-year survival of 88% in the former and zero in the latter group. The variation between the studies might be related to improvements in US and medical treatment and to the causative agent of the HCC. For example, most HCCs in China are related to early HBV infection and therefore occur in relatively young patients with less severe underlying liver disease.

Physicians should take into account the presence of comorbid disease, severity of liver disease and available treatment options when deciding whether or not to screen a cirrhotic patient. Screening of Child C patients is inappropriate if they are not potential liver transplant candidates. Resection is usually contraindicated in Child B patients and there is no evidence yet that treatment, apart from transplantation, will improve survival.

Treatment options

Only transplantation for HCC treats the underlying liver disease, therefore recurrence is invariable with all other treatments in the cirrhotic patient. In patients without cirrhosis, liver resection is the ideal treatment but this group accounts for only a small proportion of HCCs. In cirrhotic patients management is more challenging and should take into account patient age, tumour extent and liver function. Using appropriate selection criteria, liver transplantation, liver resection, percutaneous treatment and chemoembolisation have, in decreasing order, the greatest efficacy but, in increasing order, the greatest feasibility and should be considered in this order.

HCC in normal livers

The indication for treatment is least controversial in patients with no or minimal coexisting fibrosis. However, risk factors such as HBV infection, genetic haemochromatosis, alcohol ingestion and steatosis require consideration. HCCs are usually large and solitary, arising in relatively young patients. Since the non-tumourous liver has a high regenerating capacity, surgical resection, through major hepatectomies, is associated with relatively low mortality, morbidity and transfusion rates less than 1%, 15% and 30% respectively.[57] Five-year survival is greater than 50%.[58] Percutaneous ablation is not undertaken due to the large tumour size. Transplantation is associated with perioperative mortality of 10%, a need for long-term immunosuppression, and has long-term results no different from those of resection.[59] Transplantation has been performed with poor results in the past in patients with tumours judged unresectable but is currently hardly ever used. Early detection of recurrence is important since it can often be managed by repeat resection. A small group of patients may benefit from

transplantation if their recurrence is confined to the liver and if repeat resection is not possible.

Liver resection of HCC in cirrhotic patients

Resection of HCC has three limitations in cirrhotic patients:

- The tumour is multifocal in 20–60% of cirrhotic livers at the time of diagnosis and liver resection can only be considered normally in patients with unifocal tumours.
- Cirrhosis is an important risk factor for the development of postoperative complications, and the rising prevalence of the dysmetabolic syndrome further increases the perioperative risk through obesity, diabetes and dyslipidaemia.
- There is ongoing risk of recurrence in the cirrhotic liver.

In-hospital death was observed in 10% of patients in the 1990s but has decreased since then as a result of improved patient selection, operative technique and perioperative management. Although some very large series report no mortality,[60] the average mortality rates in national surveys or registries are 4–6% and are therefore higher than in non-cirrhotic patients or after resection of other malignancies.

Cirrhosis is associated with poor functional reserve of the liver and impaired ability to regenerate and this correlates with the fibrosis grade,[61] although it is only in patients with extensive fibrosis or cirrhosis that this impairment has clinical impact. Typically, following a major liver resection, the prothrombin time (peak on postoperative day 1) and serum bilirubin (peak on postoperative day 5) increase. Recovery of both tests is delayed or absent in cirrhotic patients. Death when it occurs is usually delayed and results from superimposed infection.

 The predominant risk factors for postoperative liver failure are the patient's Child grade and the extent of resection. Any resection is contraindicated in patients who are grade C at the time of surgery, and only limited resection is possible in patients who are grade B. However, even in grade A cirrhotic patients with normal serum bilirubin and prothrombin time and no ascites, the risk of liver surgery is increased. Additional risk factors for liver decompensation in Child A patients include indocyanine green (ICG) retention rate at 15 minutes >20%,[62] serum transaminase level greater than twice the normal upper range[63] or hepatic venous pressure gradient (an invasive measurement of portal hypertension) >10 mmHg.[64]

Transjugular measurement is not used routinely but indirect evidence of portal hypertension includes previous history of variceal bleeding or ascites, presence of oesophageal varices, platelet count lower than $100 \times 10^9/L$ or a radiologically visible porto-systemic shunt. The three risk factors of ICG test, cytolysis and portal hypertension probably overlap but when any of these factors are present, resection should be considered with extreme caution.

There has been considerable interest during the past 5 years in the optimal management of the remnant liver. This includes more selective use of inflow occlusion[65] and avoiding excessive mobilisation of the liver.[66,67]

 When major hepatectomy is contemplated, preoperative portal vein embolisation (PVE) of the lobe to be resected should be performed to increase the volume of the remnant liver.

When right hepatectomy is contemplated, the right portal vein is percutaneously injected, under ultrasonographic guidance, with glue or ethanol. This induces atrophy of the right liver within 2–6 weeks and hypertrophy of the left future remnant liver as assessed by CT volumetry.[68] A prospective controlled trial has shown that preoperative PVE caused approximately a 50% reduction in risk of postoperative complications and in-hospital stay.[69] Hypertrophy of the left liver following right PVE does not occur if portal flow is diverted from the left portal vein through portosystemic shunts. PVE can be preceded by selective arterial embolisation to improve tumour control and enhance hypertrophy of the future remnant liver.[70] If the increase in this remnant liver is less than 10%, resection is contraindicated. PVE can therefore be viewed not only as a way to increase the volume of the future remnant liver but also as a way of testing the ability of the liver to regenerate.

There is increasing evidence that both anatomical resections (as opposed to tumourectomies) and wide (as opposed to limited) margins may improve long-term survival without increasing the perioperative risk.

 The concept of anatomical resections is to remove both the tumour and the adjacent segments that have the same portal tributaries. Several retrospective studies have reported an approximately 20% improvement in overall and disease-free survival compared to limited resections.[71,72] The impact of the margin width has been evaluated in a prospective controlled trial.[73] A 2-cm margin was associated with a 75% 5-year survival as compared to 49% for 1-cm margins.

The largest series from the Liver Cancer Study Group in Japan has reported 1-, 3-, 5- and 10-year survival rates of 87%, 66%, 48% and 21% respectively in 11 631 cirrhotic patients treated by hepatic resection between 1992 and 2003.[41] Comparable results have been reported by other groups world-wide, with no differences between Western and Asian studies.[74] Using multivariate analysis stratified by associated liver disease, independent prognostic predictors are age, degree of liver damage, AFP level, maximal tumour dimension, number of tumours, intrahepatic extent of tumours, extrahepatic metastasis, portal vein invasion, hepatic vein invasion, surgical curability and free surgical margins.[75] Survival rates as high as 68% at 5 years may be achieved in Child grade A patients with well-encapsulated tumours of 2 cm diameter or less.

Recurrence following resection of HCC

Tumour recurrence is the major cause of death following resection of HCC, although it is much more frequent in the cirrhotic patient. The frequency of tumour recurrence in cirrhotic patients is estimated at 40% within the first year, 60% at 3 years and around 80% at 5 years. However, it is invariable if follow-up is extended beyond 10 years as the precursor condition (cirrhosis) persists after surgery.[76]

It is frequently difficult to differentiate true recurrence from de novo tumours. The former tend to occur within the first 2 years and their main risk factors are vascular invasion, poor histological differentiation, presence of satellites and number of nodules. De novo recurrent tumours occur later and the main risk factors are the same as those of a primary HCC. Molecular analysis suggests that their respective proportions are 60–70% and 30–40%. Recurrence within the liver is multifocal in 50% of the patients and is associated with distant metastasis in 15%, especially in the lungs, adrenal gland or bones.[77] Extrahepatic recurrence without simultaneous intrahepatic recurrence is infrequent in cirrhotic livers.

In addition to these parameters, there is increasing evidence that the technique of resection influences long-term outcome. Intraoperative blood transfusions are associated with an increased risk of recurrence. Anatomical resection and a tumour-free margin of 2 cm are associated with improved survival.

 Strategies to prevent recurrence have been disappointing. A review of published RCTs has, in 2002,[78] concluded that preoperative chemoembolisation, adjuvant chemoembolisation and systemic chemotherapy had not shown convincing evidence of their effectiveness.

Biological treatments such as adoptive immunotherapy by activated lymphocytes with interleukin-2 and antibody to CD3 or immunotherapy with interferon have shown promising results, along with adjuvant treatment with retinoic acid and ^{131}I-labelled Lipiodol.

An update follow-up of the only randomised trial of adjuvant ^{131}I-labelled Lipiodol has shown that the improved overall and disease-free survivals in the treatment group persisted until the seventh post-operative year.[79] This study was characterised by a very high proportion of HBV-related HCC (88%) and another trial is under way in France. Two studies from Asia evaluating the use of interferon reported decreased early recurrence and improved long-term survival in patients with HBV-related cirrhosis, either for the entire group[80] or for patients with advanced disease stage III/IVa.[81] In contrast, a third study[82] from Europe in patients with HCV-related HCC (without or with HBV coinfection) experienced poor compliance and demonstrated interferon had no impact on overall or disease-free survival. The single significant difference was a reduced incidence of late recurrence in purely HCV-positive patients. No study has confirmed the potential efficacy of retinoic acid.

For the present, the best way to improve survival is to monitor resected patients regularly as some may benefit from the treatment of recurrence if it is confined to the liver.[83] These treatments may rely on re-resection, transarterial chemoembolisation, percutaneous treatment or liver transplantation. Treatment of recurrence has been suggested to be one of the main reasons for the improved survival following resection observed over the past 10 years.[84] The risk and outcome of a repeat resection appears comparable to that of a first hepatectomy.[85]

Liver transplantation

HCC is the only tumour for which transplantation plays a significant role, and this is the most attractive therapeutic option because it removes both detectable and undetectable tumour nodules together with all the preneoplastic lesions that are present in the cirrhotic liver. In addition, it simultaneously treats the underlying cirrhosis and prevents the development of postoperative or distant complications associated with portal hypertension and liver failure.

Liver transplantation was performed initially in patients in whom partial liver resection could not be considered and HCC accounted for almost 40% of indications in Europe in the 1980s. Results were disappointing, even after ruling out extra-hepatic disease or hilar lymph node metastases with a high rate of early recurrence.[86] Furthermore, the use of immunosuppressive treatments accelerated markedly the course of recurrence. Outcome was clearly poorer than for other transplant indications, although a 30% 5-year survival was considered a fair result for malignancy. Donor shortages resulted in high mortality rates for patients on liver transplantation waiting lists and all these factors led to the consensus that transplantation should not be proposed for cirrhotic patients with large or multifocal HCCs.

Conversely, the outcome in patients transplanted with an incidental HCC was extremely favourable, with a small incidence of tumour recurrence and survival comparable to patients transplanted without malignancy.

Several groups in the 1990s found that limited tumour involvement – defined by the presence of a single tumour less than 5 cm or the presence of two or three tumours less than 3 cm in patients with no vascular invasion and no extrahepatic disease (the so-called Milan criteria) – was associated with a much better outcome.[87] With the adoption of these criteria by the United Network for Organ Sharing (UNOS), the 5-year survival has increased in the USA from 25% in the period 1987–91 to 61% in the period 1997–2001.[88] These good results have been reproduced by others worldwide with 5-year survival currently ranging between 60% and 75%.[87,89–91]

However, because of these strict oncological limitations, less than 5–10% of HCC patients are potential transplant candidates, and HCC currently accounts for only 10% of all liver transplantations.

Besides these carcinological considerations, there are various limitations to liver transplantation. Firstly, it is not readily available in high endemic areas of HCC. When available, the average time from listing to transplantation has increased to 10–12 months in Europe and the USA and it is not uncommon for patients to be excluded from the waiting list due to disease progression. The cumulative drop-out from the waiting list has been estimated to be 7–15% at 6 months and 25% at 12 months.[89] In Barcelona, although the 2-year survival has been reported to be 84% after transplantation, on an intention-to-treat basis this figure drops to 54% from the time of listing.[90] Similarly, the UCSF group reported a 73% 5-year survival after transplantation but a 73% 2-year survival from the time of listing.[89] The final limitation to transplantation is that not all patients with an HCC fulfilling the criteria are potential transplant candidates. Age above 60–65 years is a contraindication in many centres due to donor shortage, although outcome in selected older patients is not very different from that of younger patients. This is a major limitation to transplantation for HCV-related HCC in the Western world, as more than 50% of these patients are 60 years or more. Transplantation is contraindicated in patients with HBV-DNA replication or persistent alcohol consumption, as cirrhosis is likely to recur within the graft.

Since the turn of the millennium, liver transplantation for HCC has entered a third period aimed at increasing the proportion of patients who could benefit from transplantation. This has been attempted by a careful and progressive expansion of the Milan criteria, an improvement in the availability by changing the allocation systems of cadaver grafts prioritising HCC patients and developing living-related liver transplantation and controlling for tumour progression while patients are on the waiting list.

 There is consensus that expansion of the Milan criteria would be acceptable if associated with a 10–20% 5-year recurrence rate and greater than 50% 5-year survival rate.

There are four main factors affecting recurrence after transplantation for HCC. Macroscopic vascular invasion is correlated with circulating tumoural cells with a potential for re-colonisation of the graft.[92] The nodule size correlates with vascular invasion, although it is not clear that a tumour size threshold identifies risk of recurrence. The total number of nodules in multifocal tumour is an adverse factor as very small nodules are frequently unrecognised with current imaging techniques. Poorly differentiated tumours were found to have post-transplantation recurrence rates about twice as high as that of patients with well-differentiated tumours.[91] Up to now, attempts to expand the criteria have relied mainly on the number and size of nodules since percutaneous biopsy and imaging studies are still somewhat inaccurate in assessing tumour differentiation and vascular invasion. Among the proposed expansion criteria,[89] the UCSF criteria (single tumour nodule up to 6.5 cm, or three or fewer tumours, the largest of which is <4.5 cm with the sum of the tumour diameters <8 cm) is the most widely used, but most patients are also within the Milan criteria. Interestingly, the 5-year survival of patients within the UCSF but outside the Milan criteria is 48%. Obviously, the relatively low accuracy of imaging techniques in staging tumours is an important limiting factor for the expansion of the criteria. The number of small nodules is underestimated in 70% of patients, and macroscopic vascular invasion and satellite nodules are present in 5% and 40% of patients fulfilling the Milan criteria. Predicting tumour biology through molecular profiling rather than tumour morphology is the aim of current research in this field.[93]

Until the accuracy of imaging studies is improved, one way to identify patients as having favourable histology is to resect the tumour prior to listing the patient for transplantation. Similarly, a high (>300 ng/mL) or rapidly increasing AFP level is often associated with macroscopic vascular invasion and is often considered by many centres as a contraindication to transplantation.

Living-donor liver transplantation (LDLT) is an alternative source of grafts but has its own drawbacks, including the inherent risk for the donor, the risk of small-for-size grafts and the fact that only 25–30% of transplant candidates have a potential donor. However, it has the advantage of being performed rapidly, so avoiding drop-out on the waiting lists. Some centres recommend extended use of transplantation for malignancy, even in those patients with a high risk of recurrence. This issue is highly controversial and the overall number of LDLT cases in Western countries has decreased and the trend favours cadaveric transplantation through changes in the allocation of cadaver grafts. In the USA, the adoption of the Model of End-stage Liver Disease (MELD) organ allocation policy in 2002 has given priority to candidates with HCC within the Milan criteria. Waiting times have shortened, obviating the need for LDLT. Similar policies have been applied in other countries such as France and the UK.

Limiting tumour progression during the waiting period has relied on transarterial chemoembolisation (TACE), percutaneous ablation or partial liver resection. There is some evidence that these treatments may reduce the drop-out rates on the waiting lists but it is not clear if the outcome is the same for patients within or beyond the Milan criteria. The impact of these treatments on downstaging and post-transplantation survival is similarly uncertain.

No RCT has compared liver resection and transplantation and interpretation of retrospective studies is difficult because there is generally a greater proportion of Child B and C patients and of small and multiple tumours in transplantation groups. Liver transplantation is the best option for patients with HCC and decompensated liver disease but, given the graft shortage, the optimal treatment strategy for patients with preserved liver function and small cancers is not well established. For selected patients, this has led to the concept of bridge or salvage transplantation,[94] where liver resection is performed first and the patient is listed either immediately for transplantation if there is risk of early recurrence or secondarily should recurrence occur and if this falls within the Milan criteria.

Transarterial chemoembolisation (TACE) of HCC

Arterial embolisation is the most widely used initial treatment in patients with unresectable HCC. Its rationale is that HCC, in contrast to the liver parenchyma, receives almost 100% of its blood supply from the artery (whereas 70% of the liver parenchyma blood supply comes from the portal vein).

When the artery is obstructed, the tumour experiences an ischaemic insult that results in extensive necrosis. Several agents may be used to achieve this, including gelfoam, starch microspheres and metallic coils. Injection of iodised oil has been combined to improve the efficacy of embolisation of the tumour arterial supply. Iodised oil (Lipiodol), which is hyperdense on CT scan, is cleared from the normal hepatic parenchyma but retained in malignant tumours for periods ranging from several weeks to over a year. This accumulation, which is not associated with significant adverse effects, may be used for targeting cytotoxic drugs by increasing their concentration in the tumour cells. Cytotoxic drugs employed in chemoembolisation include 5-fluorouracil (5-FU), doxorubicin, mitomycin C, epirubicin or cisplatin and iodine-131. Contraindications for TACE include liver decompensation, biliary obstruction, bilioenteric anastomosis, impaired kidney function and portal vein thrombosis, as simultaneous arterial embolisation may lead to liver necrosis. However, the latter contraindication is relative provided the patient has compensated liver disease and the embolisation is performed selectively on a limited tumour volume.

In patients with good liver function, arterial embolisation is usually well tolerated. In contrast, a pre-embolisation abnormal serum bilirubin or prothrombin time is associated with a risk of liver decompensation, either as a result of embolisation or if the dosage of chemotherapy is not decreased. The mortality associated with this procedure ranges between 0% and 2% in Child A patients,[95] but is 8% and 37% in Child grade B and C patients respectively.[96] Overall, more than 75% of the patients develop a postembolisation syndrome characterised by fever, abdominal pain, nausea and raised serum transaminase level. These symptoms, which are not prevented by antibiotics or anti-inflammatory drugs, are self-limiting and last for less than 1 week. A more severe form requiring prolonged hospitalisation is observed in 15%. The postembolisation syndrome, which was attributed to tumour necrosis, in fact seems to be related to injury of the non-tumourous liver, with a higher rate of fever and cytolysis in patients with minor fibrotic changes.[97] This tends to become less severe if the procedure is repeated. More severe complications occur in less than 5% of patients and include, in decreasing order of frequency: cholecystitis or gallbladder infarction, gastric or duodenal wall necrosis, and acute pancreatitis. These are probably related to the inadvertent migration of embolisation material in the cystic, pyloric or gastroduodenal artery, and they have become less frequent with the use of supraselective embolisation. Ulcer prophylaxis should nevertheless be routine, and an ultrasound scan should be performed if pain or fever persists. Hepatic abscess

formation is rare, occurring in 0.3%, but is associated with high mortality, close to 50%.[98] The main risk factors are a previous history of bilioenteric anastomosis (the rationale for excluding such patients from embolisation), large tumours, biliary lithiasis and portal thrombosis. An early CT scan may show the presence of gas in the tumour, which is more frequently due to the inadvertent injection of air during the procedure than an anaerobic superinfection.

The efficacy of TACE is assessed by dynamic CT (usually at 1 month) as the disappearance of the arterial vascular supply to the tumour, which is frequently associated with a dense and massive uptake of Lipiodol by the tumour and a decrease in its diameter. These features do not necessarily evolve in parallel. A decrease in tumour size may, for example, be associated with persistent vascularisation (i.e. residual tumour), whereas compact Lipiodol uptake without residual vascularisation may indicate complete tumour necrosis despite no significant decrease in size.

One of the largest recent studies is a prospective Japanese nationwide survey[99] reporting median and 1-, 3-, 5- and 7-year survivals of 34 months, 82%, 47%, 26% and 16% respectively, with a TACE-related mortality of 0.5%. Independent predictors of survival were, by decreasing order of influence, the degree of liver damage, portal vein invasion, maximum tumour size and number of lesions, and AFP levels.

The clinical efficacy of TACE has been compared in seven RCTs, including a total of 516 patients who were further included into a meta-analysis. Initial trials failed to demonstrate significant improved survival despite an antitumour effect.[95,100] These were, however, criticised for having included patients with advanced tumour stage and poor hepatic function. More recently, two excellent trials focusing on patients with unresectable HCC, but applying stricter selection criteria by excluding patients with diffuse neoplasm and severe liver failure, have shown significant survival advantage with an active retreatment schedule.[101,102] These results have been confirmed by meta-analysis.[103]

Variables associated with improved survival following TACE, besides treatment response, are a hypervascular HCC at baseline,[104] a compact uptake of Lipiodol within the tumour,[105] and the repetition of the procedures.

TACE is therefore a validated treatment option in selected patients with irresectable HCC.

Although this treatment has been used routinely for more than 25 years and the technique of the procedure has evolved significantly to become more selective, standardisation of the end-points that should be reached during the procedure is still lacking, and there is no good evidence for the best chemotherapeutic agent or the optimum retreatment strategy. TACE used to be repeated at fixed intervals (2–3 months), until an arbitrarily planned number of courses was reached, technical difficulties were encountered, arteries became obstructed as a result of chemotherapy-induced endothelial injury or the patient died. Discontinuation is, however, reasonable if there is either progression despite two procedures or, conversely, if there is evidence of complete tumour necrosis. Patients are thereafter submitted to regular follow-up and treatment is repeated in case of local or de novo recurrence. With the development of more hyperselective embolisations, greater attention is paid to accessory arteries that may contribute to tumour vascularity, such as the diaphragmatic or mammary arteries, that should also be embolised to achieve adequate control.

Percutaneous local ablative therapy

Locoregional therapies are those percutaneous treatment modalities that allow the injection of a damaging agent directly into the tumour or the application of an energy source.

- Damaging agents include chemicals such as ethanol or acetic acid. Percutaneous ethanol injection (PEI) was introduced in the 1980s and causes dehydration and necrosis of cells as well as thrombosis of small blood vessels.
- Energy sources either aim at increasing temperature by radiofrequency microwave or interstitial laser photocoagulation or, alternatively, at decreasing temperature (cryoablation). Radiofrequency (RF) was introduced in 1993 and has emerged as the most effective of these techniques. It exploits the conversion of electromagnetic energy into heat via a needle electrode (15–18G) with an insulated shaft and a non-insulated tip, positioned into the tumour while the patient is made into an electric circuit by placing grounding pads on his or her thighs. The RF emitted from the tip causes ionic agitation and frictional heat, which leads to cell death from coagulation necrosis. The objective is to maintain a 55–100°C temperature throughout the entire target volume for a sufficient period of time. Monitoring the impedance is important because excessive heating results in tissue charring, increased tissue impedance and decreased energy absorption.

These methods have common advantages and limitations. On the one hand, they are minimally invasive, preserve the uninvolved liver parenchyma, have no systemic side-effects, and avoid the mortality and morbidity of major hepatic surgery. On the other hand, only tumours less than 5 cm are likely to be treated successfully but the smaller the diameter, the greater the probability of complete local control. The presence of multiple tumours (more than three) is also a limitation because of the need for repeated punctures. In addition, multiple tumours are either the result of multifocal carcinogenesis or vascular extension, and a focal treatment is therefore unlikely to be very effective. Obviously, a common requirement is also the need to clearly visualise the tumour by US. Hence, isoechoic HCC or tumours located in the upper part of segments 4, 7 and 8 may occasionally be unsuitable for treatment, although intraoperative RF may overcome this limitation. Finally, whichever technique is used, the needle should not enter the tumour directly but pass through the hepatic parenchyma so as to prevent intraperitoneal bleeding or seeding of tumour cells. This may prove impossible for some superficial or protruding tumours.

Common contraindications include gross ascites which favours intraperitoneal bleeding, coagulopathy that cannot be corrected, and obstructive jaundice due to the risk of abscess formation or bile peritonitis. Additional contraindications specific to radiofrequency are the proximity of the tumour to the colon, duodenum and stomach, which may be perforated by the heating process, with the biliary confluence, the presence of a biliodigestive anastomosis and a pacemaker. Whereas PEI is a short and very cheap procedure performed under light sedation, RF is more costly, prolonged (20–90 minutes) and painful, and therefore generally performed under general anaesthesia.

 All RCTs[106] comparing the various techniques of ablation have suggested that the actuarial probability of local recurrence was significantly lower in the RF arm compared with either PEI arm or percutaneous acetic acid injection arms and that RF required fewer treatment sessions to achieve comparable antitumoural effects.

Diffusion of ethanol within the tumour may be limited by fibrotic septa and, whereas the capsule may prevent diffusion of ethanol beyond the tumour, RF may produce a safety margin. There is evidence that this margin decreases the recurrence rate provided it encompasses the potential satellite nodules. The incidence of these nodules increases with poorer differentiation of the tumour, but for tumours less than 3 cm remains confined to a distance of 10 mm of its border. Whether this improved local control translates into improved survival remains controversial.

Percutaneous ablative therapies have initially been performed in patients who were unsuitable for resective surgery and both the EASLD[45] and AASLD[47] have recommended this strategy. RF has, however, now demonstrated its effectiveness to a point where it is considered by some centres as the first-line treatment for single nodules less than 2–3 cm.

Evidence supporting this new attitude come in particular from the progressive increase in the diameter of necrosis achieved through improvements in the design of the electrodes (J-hooked needles, cooled electrodes) or combining RF with TACE, or simultaneous occlusion of the arterial supply. Furthermore, experienced radiologists have the ability to overcome the so-called high-risk locations (defined as less than 5 mm distance between the tumour and a large vessel that may produce a cooling effect) or an extrahepatic organ.[107] The results of two RCTs comparing ablation and resection in patients with early HCC[108,109] demonstrated no difference but a large multicentre phase 2 trial reported a 97% sustained complete response and a 68% actuarial 5-year survival in patients with HCC of 2 cm or less.[110]

The technique of RF and accuracy of monitoring are important. The current approach is to perform RF with a targeted safety margin of 1 cm to encompass potential satellite nodules. Treatment response is assessed by CT or MRI no earlier than 1 month after the procedure. RF may result in a rim of fibrotic tissue (hypervascular at the late phase of MRI or CT scan) at the periphery of the tumour and should not be mistaken for residual tumour tissue. Follow-up thereafter relies on imaging studies at 3-month intervals to ensure that there is no recurrence of contrast enhancement.

In a recent literature review of the side-effects of RF, the mortality was 0.5% and the morbidity was 9%.[111] The most frequent complications are pleural effusion and segmental intrahepatic dilatation, which have no or limited impact. Severe complications include, in particular, abscess formation, perforation of adjacent organs and intraperitoneal bleeding. Perforation of adjacent organs can be overcome by performing the RF under laparoscopy and separating these adjacent organs from the tumour. Tumour seeding seems a more frequent occurrence than after PEI because of the larger needle diameter. Risk factors include subcapsular location and poor histological differentiation of the tumour. Coagulating the needle tract while removing the needle may reduce this risk.

Palliative treatments

Systemic and regional chemotherapy

Systemic chemotherapy has had very limited value in the past as a primary treatment modality for HCC, as only a very small number of patients obtained meaningful palliation using conventional drugs. Several RCTs have assessed the role of systemic chemotherapy by the intravenous route – using either single agents (doxorubicin, cisplatin, mitomycin C, 5-FU) or combined agents – on tumour progression and survival. These trials have described an overall partial response rate of less than 20%, with a negligible complete response rate.[103] Therefore, there is no rationale for using chemotherapy in unresectable HCC outside of clinical trials.

A recent trial using molecularly targeted agents has, however, for the first time demonstrated an improved overall survival in this disease and sets the new standards for the first-line treatment of advanced HCC. These new agents target angiogenesis and epidermal growth factor (EGF) receptor pathways.

Sorafemib (Nexavar®) exerts an antiangiogenic effect by targeting the tyrosine kinases vascular endothelial growth factor (VEGF) receptors 2 and 3, and the platelet-derived growth factor receptor β. In the SHARP phase 3 trial presented at the 2007 ASCO meeting, the median overall survival in Child–Pugh A cirrhotic patients with histologically proven and advanced HCC was 10.7 months in the treated group (400 mg twice daily orally) versus 7.9 months in the placebo double-blinded controlled arm of the study ($P = 0.00058$) and the median times to tumour progression were 24 weeks and 12 weeks respectively ($P = 0.000007$).[112] Side-effects included diarrhoea (39%), hand–foot syndrome (21%), anorexia (14%) and alopecia (14%). Interestingly, despite these unique results, the response rate, as assessed by the RECIST criteria (that take into account the size of the tumour) was only 2%. This observation has contributed to a changing trend in the evaluation of the response of HCC to various treatments.

Other agents with comparable action pathways have been evaluated in phase 2 trials and include bevacizumab and sunitinib. Anti-EGF receptor agents such as tarceva and cetuximab also show promising results in phase 2 studies. Contraindications to these treatments include coronary artery disease, cardiac failure, systemic hypertension and Child B or C cirrhosis.

External and internal radiation therapy

External beam radiation therapy has been of limited value in treating HCC because the tumour is relatively radioresistant whereas the normal liver parenchyma is very radiosensitive. Maximum tolerance of the normal liver to irradiation is generally accepted to be between 2500 and 3000 Gy. Above these values, the risk of radiation hepatitis increases quickly and is associated with a mortality rate close to 50%. In addition, it is difficult to protect the surrounding organs such as the colon, duodenum and kidney.

Greater interest has therefore been placed on injecting radioisotopes such as iodine-131-iodised oil and ^{90}Y-labelled microspheres directly into the hepatic artery, which offers the advantage of increased delivery within the tumour and decreased systemic toxicity. The former agent has an efficacy comparable to that of chemoembolisation in patients with HCC not complicated by portal thrombosis.[113] In contrast its superiority has been demonstrated in patients with portal thrombosis, being associated with a 6-month survival rate of 48% as compared with 0% in a control group receiving only medical support.[114] The use of ^{90}Y microspheres is more recent and has been shown in a phase 2 trial to be safe and effective, in particular in patients with portal vein thrombosis.[115] The planned phase 3 trial has been delayed with the positive results of the SHARP study that targeted the same population.

Hormone therapy

Antiandrogenic and antioestrogenic treatment has been used in palliation of HCC. Results with antiandrogens have been disappointing.[103] There has been more interest regarding the use of antioestrogenic treatment with tamoxifen. Results of controlled studies are controversial but, overall, this treatment has no impact on 1-year survival[103] and is therefore no longer used.

Somatostatin analogues

There has been hope that somatostatin analogues could be effective in HCC since 40% of these tumours express somatostatin receptors. A small randomised trial suggested longer survival in those treated with short-acting octreotide than in an untreated control group (median survival 13 vs. 4 months, 12-month survival 56% vs. 13%).[116] These results have not been reproduced by trials using long-acting octreotide, even after stratifying for the CLIP score.[117]

Defining a treatment strategy

Uncomplicated HCC associated with chronic liver disease

Treatment algorithms have to take account of variations in different geographical areas including the availability of treatments, presence or absence of screening policies, and aetiology and severity of the underlying liver disease.

- Liver transplantation, when available, is considered first and attention is therefore paid to the extent of liver disease, patient age and presence or absence of associated conditions.
- If transplantation is not available or not indicated, resection should be considered. Limiting factors are the number of nodules (ideally there should be only one) and the severity of underlying liver disease (patients should have normal prothrombin time and serum bilirubin and neither cytolysis, portal hypertension or impaired ICG tests). If a right hepatectomy is considered it should be preceded by PVE (with or without TACE).
- If resection is not considered due to the severity of the underlying liver disease and the nodule is single (or if there are less than three nodules), RF is the treatment of choice provided the tumour is less than 3–5 cm. For single tumours 2 cm or less, RF is a first-line treatment in some centres, as an alternative to resection.
- If neither resection nor RF is considered, TACE is performed provided there is no ascites or liver failure (and in particular that serum bilirubin is less than 50 μmol/L) and that the tumour burden is not too extensive.
- Remaining patients are currently considered for antiangiogenic treatments provided there is neither liver failure nor vascular disease.

According to this algorithm, it may be considered that the proportion of patients who are candidates for transplantation is 5–10%, for resection 10–15%, for RF 15–20% and for TACE 20–30%.

Treatment of complicated HCC

HCC with portal vein invasion is a contraindication for liver transplantation, ablative treatments and traditionally arterial chemoembolisation unless it is performed highly selectively, with reduced doses and partial arterial occlusion as the end-point. Embolisation with radioactive microspheres may be considered. TACE or US-guided injection of chemotherapy or alcohol within the thrombus is exceptionally effective. If thrombus does not extend into the main portal vein, surgical resection can be considered in the small proportion of young patients with good general condition, preserved liver function and limited tumour extension provided the tumour is also removed. Antiangiogenic therapy is otherwise indicated.

Ruptured HCC should not always be considered as a contraindication to treatment. Without treatment, the mortality of this complication is almost 100%. The primary aim of treatment is to stop bleeding since ascites and impaired coagulation usually impair haemostasis. Several methods of haemostasis have been advocated, including TACE, hepatic artery ligation, local control through suture plication, or packing and resection of the tumour.[118] It is very difficult to compare the results of treatments since some patients experienced tumour rupture as a terminal presentation with multiple tumours, portal thrombosis and liver insufficiency. Initial haemostasis by TACE may allow subsequent hepatectomy after evaluation of tumour extent and functional liver reserve. Although rupture of HCC may be associated with peritoneal seeding of tumour cells, this should not be regarded as a contraindication to radical treatment. Data available from the literature indicate that the 1-year survival of patients undergoing second-stage hepatectomy is 40%, and long-term survival has been reported.

Fibrolamellar carcinoma (FLC)

FLC is a rare variant of HCC,[55] with several pathological and clinical features distinct from HCC. It is most frequently observed in the Western hemisphere, where it accounts for approximately 1% of all HCCs.[119] These tumours occur at a younger age than HCC (20–35 years) and there is no apparent relationship with gender. FLC rarely occurs on a background of chronic liver disease. As a consequence:

- The tumour is usually large at the time of diagnosis (8–10 cm), and the common presenting symptoms are a palpable mass, abdominal pain, weight loss, malaise and anorexia.
- The prognosis is better than that of HCC overall and comparable to that of HCC within 'normal' liver. Five-year survival following resection is 50–75%.[120] Prolonged survival has been reported in patients with advanced tumour stage.[121]
- Resection is preferred to transplantation, since long-term results are comparable.

FLC usually presents as a large solitary hypervascular heterogeneous liver mass with a central hypodense region due to central necrosis or fibrosis. On MRI, the central scar of FLC tumours has low attenuation on T2 images, whereas the central scar of focal nodular hyperplasia has high attenuation. They have well-defined margins, calcification is present in 68% and abdominal lymphadenopathy in up to 60% of patients. Histology demonstrates deeply eosinophilic, polygonal neoplastic cells surrounded by a dense, layered fibrous stroma.

AFP levels are raised in less than 10% of patients.[120] Lymph node invasion within the hepatic pedicle is high and if resection is considered, simultaneous lymphadenectomy of the hepatic pedicle is recommended. There is a significant risk of recurrence, not only within the liver but also as lymph node or distant metastases with a recurrence-free survival of 20%.[120] Close long-term follow-up is mandatory since recurrence and death beyond 5 years are common. Repeat surgery is a reasonable option in this younger patient population due to the relatively indolent course of the disease and the relative inefficacy of non-surgical treatments.

Intrahepatic cholangiocarcinoma (ICCA)

ICCA, also known as peripheral cholangiocarcinoma, is a rare (but the second most common) tumour accounting for 5–10% of all primary malignant liver tumours. It arises from the peripheral intrahepatic biliary radicles, which differentiates them from hilar (Klatskin tumours) and common bile duct cholangiocarcinoma. It has a poor overall prognosis.

ICCA has only recently been identified as a separate entity. Many cases were probably misclassified in the past as metastatic adenocarcinoma of unknown origin. The diagnosis is currently ascertained through immunostaining that shows that they are CK7+ and CK20− (colorectal metastases are CK7− and CK20+). In the UK, it is only since 2001 that ICCA has been provided a specific code in the International Classification of Diseases (C22.1).

Furthermore, cholangiocarcinomas are still frequently analysed in the literature as a group, irrespective of their anatomical origin. There is, however, evidence that not only their clinical presentation but also their epidemiology, molecular biology and natural history are distinct.

Incidence

Recent reports, from different areas of the world, suggest that the incidence of ICCA is increasing, particularly in the USA, UK, France, Italy, Japan and Australia.[122] In contrast, it appears to have decreased in other countries.[123] In the USA, the incidence is 3 per million,[124] 10 times less than HCC. There is evidence that this increase is real, not as a consequence of improved detection or classification and related to an as yet unidentified environmental factor.

Risk factors

The traditional risk factors for cholangiocarcinoma include chronic biliary inflammation such as primary sclerosing cholangitis, chronic choledocholithiasis, hepatolithiasis, parasitic biliary infestation, and chronic typhoid carrier state or abnormal bile such as bile duct adenoma, biliary papillomatosis, Caroli's disease and choledochal cyst. These apply to all cholangiocarcinomas but most cases (with the exception of some geographical area of Asia and in particular in north-eastern Thailand, where *Opisthorcis viverrini* infection is particularly high) cannot be linked to ICCA. The results of case–control studies[125–127] have suggested that chronic non-alcoholic liver disease, HBV infection, HCV infection, obesity and smoking are observed with increased frequency in ICCA compared to controls, whereas diabetes, thyrotoxicosis, chronic pancreatitis, non-specific liver cirrhosis and alcohol are found with higher rates in both intra- and extrahepatic cholangiocarcinoma compared to controls. Interestingly, HBV and HCV nucleic acids have been detected in ICCA, and biliary dysplasia (the precursor lesion of ICCA) has been observed with increasing frequency in patients with HCV or alcohol-related cirrhosis.[128] Besides epidemiological studies, there is therefore other evidence for a link between ICCA and chronic liver disease. However, in contrast to HCC, most ICCAs develop without a background of liver disease. In surgical series, 75% of patients have normal livers, 16% have chronic hepatitis/liver fibrosis and 9% have cirrhosis.[41]

Classification

The Liver Cancer Study Group of Japan proposed a gross classification of ICCA into three types on the basis of the macroscopic finding of the cut surface of the tumour: mass forming, which is by far the commonest type (75% in Asian series) and presents as a tumour; periductal infiltrating, which spreads along the bile ducts; and intraductal growth type.[129] However, tumours may have mixed components and in particular a combination of mass forming and periductal infiltrating, which has a worse prognosis. The intraductal growth type of ICCA appears, on the contrary, to have a more favourable prognosis after resection.[130]

For patients with the **mass-forming** type, a staging system has been devised based on the analysis of survival following resection. Stage I disease is defined as a solitary tumour without vascular invasion, stage II disease as a solitary lesion with vascular invasion, stage IIIA disease as multiple tumours with or without vascular invasion, stage IIIB disease with regional lymph node metastasis, and stage IV disease with distant metastases. Estimated 3-year survival rates are 74% for stage I, 48% for stage II, 18% for stage IIIA and 7% for stage IIIB.[131] Multiple tumours and lymph node invasion are present in 50% and 40% of patients undergoing resection respectively.[131] Both are correlated with tumour size[132] and therefore have a major impact on survival.

A final consideration is the potential association of ICCA and HCC, also known as hepatocholangiocarcinoma. This entity includes the presence of two distinct tumours each having one of the two phenotypes or the presence, within the same tumour, of both biliary and hepatocyte differentiation. When this is the case, the prognosis is that of the biliary component, which is worse than that of the HCC component.

Pathology and progression analysis

Two distinct conditions preceding invasive cholangiocarcinoma have been identified. The first is a flat or micropapillary growth of atypical biliary epithelium, which has been called biliary dysplasia or biliary intraepithelial neoplasia. The second is an intraductal papillary neoplasm of the bile duct with malignant potential, which is histologically characterised by the prominent papillary growth of atypical biliary epithelium with distinct fibrovascular cores and frequent mucin over-production. These preneoplastic conditions are observed with varying frequency depending on the cause of biliary inflammation. They have mainly been analysed in hepatolithiasis and are observed more frequently in large bile ducts as hilar tumours than in small septal–interlobular bile ducts such as with ICCA.[132,133] The dysplasia–carcinoma sequence therefore appears more obvious for hilar lesions than peripheral lesions. This suggests that an alternative source of ICCA could be the canals of Hering or hepatic progenitor cells, which are a target cell population for carcinogenesis in chronic liver disease.[134]

Clinical presentation and laboratory tests

Owing to its intrahepatic location, the tumour rarely produces early symptoms and is generally discovered at an advanced stage, declaring itself with abdominal pain and weight loss. The serum alkaline phosphatase level is usually elevated but jaundice is infrequent and occurs late due to extrinsic compression of the hepatic confluence. Serum markers such as carcinoembryonic antigen (CEA) and carbohydrate antigen (CA) 19-9 may be elevated. CEA exceeds 20 ng/mL in 15% and CA19-9 is greater than 300 U/mL in 40% of cases. AFP exceeds 200 ng/mL in only 6% of patients.[41]

Imaging studies

The main characteristic of mass-forming ICCA is that it is a fibrous tumour and therefore displays no enhancement at the arterial phase and delayed enhancement at the late phase. This may be seen both on CT and MRI. On MRI, they are hypointense on T1-weighted images and moderately to markedly hyperintense on T2-weighted images (**Fig. 5.4**). They are typically large, non-encapsulated, heterogeneous, associated with narrowing of portal adjacent veins and a retraction of the liver capsule.[135] As the tumour grows, satellite nodules frequently develop in the vicinity, or in the contralateral lobe (**Fig. 5.5**). When superficial, these satellite nodules may not be visible on imaging, which is a rationale for staging laparoscopy. There is a greater propensity for lymph node invasion of the hepatic pedicle and for peritoneal metastases. In contrast to HCC, it does not invade the lumen of the portal veins but may encase them, producing segmental liver atrophy. Localised dilatation of intrahepatic bile ducts is also possible.

Diagnosis

The main differential diagnoses of ICCA are other fibrous tumours and in particular metastases from colorectal cancer. Both tumours may easily be confused on imaging studies. In cases of uncertainty a colonoscopy can be performed or a percutaneous liver biopsy provided it is coupled with immunostaining with CK7 (positive in ICCA) and CK20 (positive in colon metastases).

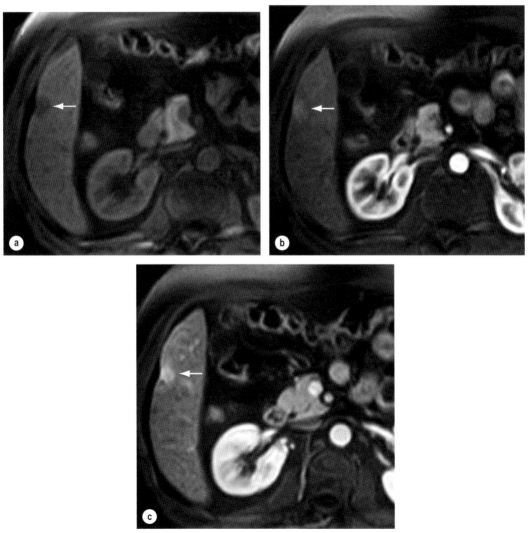

Figure 5.4 • Vascular kinetics of a small cholangiocarcinoma on MRI (arrowed). Note that the lesion is spontaneously hypointense **(a)**, that the uptake of vascular contrast is more pronounced at the late phase **(c)** than at the arterial phase **(b)** and that there is a retraction of the capsule.

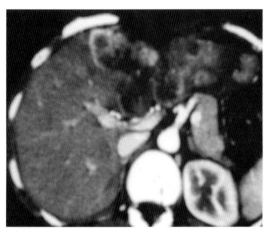

Figure 5.5 • CT scan of a patient with an intrahepatic/peripheral cholangiocarcinoma. Note the presence of typical satellite nodules at the periphery of the tumour.

Treatment

Surgical resection is the only effective treatment[136] but surgical series are still limited by inclusion of small numbers of patients. They are generally diagnosed at an advanced stage and in some series only 30% of these patients have resectable tumours.[137] Owing to the usually large tumour size at diagnosis and their frequent central location, most can only be removed by major hepatectomies. There is a significant risk (30%) that, even despite adequate preoperative imaging work-up, a laparotomy discovers contraindications to a curative resection. Staging laparotomy has been advocated[138] but also has high false-negative rates and, as a consequence, patients should be warned preoperatively about this possibility. The extensive nature of resection results in significant postoperative mortality rates of 3–7% and the 5-year survival rates are less than 40%. Survival is influenced by the presence of satellite nodules or positive lymph nodes. Few patients with one or the other feature survive for more than 3 years. Intraductal ICCAs have a better long-term prognosis, and the mass-forming has a better prognosis than the infiltrating type.[139] The difference in the proportion of each subtype may account for the difference in survival, which seems better in Asian than in Western series. The worse prognosis of the infiltrating type is due to spread along Glisson's capsule and the high incidence of lymph node involvement.

Intrahepatic recurrences are the most common cause of death. These recurrences are usually not accessible to any form of treatment, in contrast to hepatocellular carcinoma. Liver transplantation is usually not considered as an effective therapy for ICCA since the 5-year survival is less than 30%.

Systemic chemotherapy traditionally has little effect in this disease and there is no consensus that it should be used in the adjuvant setting. It is frequently performed in the palliative setting. Demonstration of the efficacy of new regimens, including gemcitabine–oxaliplatin and/or antiangiogenic treatments is awaited.[140]

Epithelioid haemangioendothelioma (EHE)

EHEs are neoplasms of vascular origin that arise predominantly from soft tissues, bones and visceral organs, in particular the lung and the liver. Primary hepatic EHE develops from the endothelial cells lining the sinusoids and progresses along the sinusoids and vascular pedicles. It is extremely rare with an incidence of less than 1 per million population. It does not arise on a background of liver disease and there is no identified causative factor. Mean age at presentation is 42 years with a female to male ratio of 3:2.[141] Half present as right upper quadrant pain, a quarter incidentally and the remainder with severe symptoms such as ascites, jaundice, weakness and weight loss. Liver failure as a result of massive infiltration has been described.

These tumours are usually discovered at an advanced stage; almost 90% are multifocal and then usually involve both lobes. Approximately one-third of the patients have extrahepatic spread to regional lymph nodes, peritoneum, lung and spleen.

Although the diagnosis is obvious when appropriate immunohistochemical staining is performed on tumour samples, it is frequently misdiagnosed on other investigations. Laboratory parameters are non-specific and tumour markers are normal. On imaging studies, the lesions are frequently confused with cholangiocarcinoma, metastatic carcinoma, sclerosing angioma or inflammatory pseudotumours. They are usually hypoechoic or heterogeneous on US, hypodense on CT with peripheral and/or central enhancement, hypointense on T1-weighted MRI, and hyperintense on T2-weighted images with similar contrast enhancement as that seen on CT. Multiplicity of lesions (especially if coalescent), their subcapsular location with liver capsule retraction and the presence of calcification (10–30%) or central necrotic and haemorrhagic areas should raise the suspicion of the diagnosis, especially in young patients. Histology shows a tumour composed of epithelioid and dendritic cells in variable proportions with a propensity for invasion of hepatic and portal veins, with an overall ill-defined growth pattern and infiltrative margins. These features are difficult to identify or differentiate from other tumours on a percutaneous biopsy sample due to the epithelioid shape of the tumour cells and the dense fibrotic stroma. In contrast, immunostaining for factor VIII-related antigens is highly specific, demonstrating endothelial differentiation. Most tumours also stain positive for CD34 and CD31 endothelial markers. Epithelial markers including cytokeratins are negative.

The natural history of this tumour is highly variable. Although exceptional, prolonged survival of more than 10 years (and up to 27 years) has been reported without treatment,[142] and both partial and complete spontaneous tumour regression has even been described.[143] On the other hand, some patients die within 2 weeks of diagnosis and 20% are dead within 1 year. Overall, only 20–40% survive more than 5 years.[141] Because of the rarity of this tumour and its highly variable course, there is no widely accepted therapeutic strategy.

Partial hepatectomy is rarely feasible due to the invariable multifocal involvement of the liver. Palliative resection is not advocated as some have raised concerns that liver regeneration could promote a flare of residual tumours. Conversely, extrahepatic spread at the time of liver resection does not correlate with survival. Reports of favourable outcome with an estimated 5-year survival of 75%[141] probably represent a highly selected subgroup.

The place of liver transplantation has recently been clarified by a multi-institutional analysis.[144] In 59 patients reported to the European Liver Transplant Registry, impressive 5- and 10-year survival rates of 83% and 74% respectively were reported. Invasion of lymph nodes and presence of restricted extrahepatic involvement had limited impact on survival and should therefore not be considered formal contraindications to transplantation. The current shortage of liver grafts and the prolonged waiting time may dictate that liver transplantation is only indicated in very selected patients. Experience with locoregional or systemic chemotherapy is small and these are usually considered of limited value, especially as first-line therapies. Neoadjuvant combination therapies using anti-VEGF antibodies, however, deserve investigation.

Angiosarcoma

Angiosarcomas of the liver are rare tumours with a dismal prognosis. A recent European survey estimated its incidence as being 0.1 per million/year, being less than 1% of primary liver tumours. The 1-, 3- and 5-year survival rates were 20%, 8% and 5% respectively.[145] Despite its rarity, it has received attention because of its frequent association with environmental carcinogens. There is clear association with prior exposure to thorium dioxide (Thorotrast), arsenicals and vinyl chloride.[146] Association with androgenic anabolic steroids, estrogens, oral contraceptives, phenelzine and cupric acid has also been reported. Overall, up to 50% of angiosarcomas are associated with previous exposure to a chemical carcinogenic agent.

These environmental risk factors may account for the male predominance (gender ratio of 3:1) and the age at the time of diagnosis (50–70 years). Patients usually experience non-specific symptoms such as abdominal pain, weakness, fatigue, anorexia and weight loss, but acute abdomen related to tumour rupture is a classical presentation. Biological abnormalities may include haemolytic anaemia and thrombocytopenia, which are related to microangiopathic haemolysis and intravascular coagulation respectively.

Morphologically, angiosarcoma may present as a large solitary mass or as multinodular lesions. On CT, they are usually hypodense and remain so after contrast injection except for occasional focal areas of central or peripheral ring-shaped enhancement. At delayed imaging, the lesion continues to enhance compared with that of the early-phase images. On MRI, the lesions tend to be hyperintense on T2-weighted images and heterogeneous on T1-weighted images, with focal hyperintensity on a background of hypointensity. Enhancement on the arterial and portal phases is heterogeneous.[147] Although the progressive enhancement could mimic that of angioma, angiosarcomas clearly differ in that they are usually multiple and more heterogeneous, and enhancement is of lower intensity compared to the aorta, whereas it is the same for angioma. Additional radiological features allowing differentiation from HCC or neuroendocrine liver metastases (both of which may also be multiple with early enhancement) include continuing progressive enhancement on delayed phase and the presence of splenic metastases.

The tumour develops from endothelial cells lining the hepatic sinusoids, and grows along these and the blood vessels. Disruption of hepatic plates may result in the development of cavities filled with tumour debris or haematoma, which favours the invasion of hepatic and portal veins. These tumours have ill-defined borders and typically involve the entire liver.

Angiosarcomas are rapidly growing and median survival is 6 months. Most patients have metastases at presentation, most notably in the lung and spleen. The latter may be involved in up to half of patients[147] and it is difficult to determine whether the liver or spleen is the primary lesion. Death results from liver failure or intraperitoneal bleeding due to tumour rupture. Bleeding is a risk because of the vascularity of the tumour, the associated thrombocytopenia or liver failure. Prolonged survival beyond 7 years has been reported[148] and it is therefore considered reasonable to attempt resection and to administer chemotherapy. However, a recent report recorded only four patients surviving for more than a year after resection. Transplantation has not been associated with survival beyond 3 years due to tumour recurrence, and is therefore not indicated. Radiation therapy may have some value in this particular tumour.

Other sarcomas, including leiomyosarcoma, should be resected if feasible.[149,150]

Primary hepatic lymphoma

Although malignant lymphoma frequently involves the liver, primary hepatic lymphomas are rare.[151] Gross examination reveals a single large tumour mass or multiple small masses with a diffuse hepatic involvement in about 10% of cases. Most primary hepatic lymphomas are classified as diffuse large-cell lymphomas of B-cell lineage. Some cases of primary hepatic lymphomas have been reported in association with AIDS or with chronic liver disease.

Since primary lymphoma of the liver may not necessarily represent disseminated disease, resection should be considered, when possible, in addition to chemotherapy.

Key points

- The incidence of HCC is rising.
- Its development is closely linked to the presence of an underlying liver disease. Viral infection or coinfection, alcohol ingestion and excessive weight are frequently implicated in its development.
- The annual incidence of HCC, once cirrhosis has developed, is 2–7%.
- Surveillance of cirrhotic patients is recommended to detect HCC at an early stage provided treatment is feasible.
- US is recommended as a screening tool while CT and MRI are most useful to confirm the diagnosis. Liver biopsy is recommended in selected cases.
- Liver transplantation is the treatment of choice in cirrhotic patients with limited tumour involvement.
- Liver resection is the treatment of choice in patients with normal livers and is indicated in cirrhotic patients with preserved liver function, no severe portal hypertension and no associated active hepatitis.
- Percutaneous treatments are effective in patients with small tumours.
- Selective chemoembolisation is effective in selected patients with preserved liver function.

References

1. World Health Organisation. The World Health Report 2003: shaping the future. Geneva: World Health Organisation, 2003. Available at: http://www.who.int/whr/2003/en/whr03_en.pdf/

2. Ferlay J, Bray F, Pisani P et al. GLOBOCAN 2000/ Cancer incidence, mortality and prevalence worldwide, version 1.0. IARC Cancer Base No. 5. Lyon: IARC, 2001.

3. Parkin DM. Cancer incidence in five continents. IARC scientific publications, Vol. VIII (No. 155). Lyon: IARC Press, 2002.

4. El Serag HB, Andrew C. The increasing incidence of hepatocellular carcinoma in the United States. N Engl J Med 1999; 340:745–50.

5. Larsson SC, Wolk A. Coffee consumption and risk of liver cancer: a meta-analysis. Gastroenterology 2007; 132:1740–5.

6. Perz JF, Armstrong GL, Farrington LA et al. The contributions of hepatitis B virus and hepatitis C virus infections to cirrhosis and primary liver cancer worldwide. J Hepatol 2006; 45:529–38.

7. Chang MH, Chen CJ, Lai MS et al. Universal hepatitis B vaccination in Taiwan and the incidence of hepatocellular carcinoma in children. Taiwan Childhood Hepatoma Study Group. N Engl J Med 1997; 336:1855–9.

   Vaccination significantly reduces the risk of HCC.

8. Fatovich G, Bortolotti F, Donato F. Natural history of chronic hepatitis B: special emphasis on disease progression and prognostic factors. J Hepatol 2008; 48:335–52.

9. Yang HI, Lu SN, Liaw YF et al. Hepatitis B e antigen and the risk of hepatocellular carcinoma. N Engl J Med 2002; 347:168–74.

10. Chen CJ, Yang HI, Su J et al. REVEAL-HBV Study Group. Risk of hepatocellular carcinoma across a biological gradient of serum hepatitis B virus DNA level. JAMA 2006; 295:65–73.

11. Salomon JA, Weinstein MC, Hammitt JK et al. Empirically calibrated model of hepatitis C virus infection in the United States. Am J Epidemiol 2002; 156:761–73.

12. Benvegnù L, Gios M, Boccato S et al. Natural history of compensated viral cirrhosis: a prospective study on the incidence and hierarchy of major complications. Gut 2004; 53:744–9.

13. Fattovich G, Stroffolini T, Zagni I et al. Hepatocellular carcinoma in cirrhosis: incidence and risk factors. Gastroenterology 2004; 127:S35–50.

14. Braks RE, Ganne-Carrie N, Fontaine H et al. Effect of sustained virological response on long-term clinical outcome in 113 patients with compensated hepatitis C-related cirrhosis treated by interferon alpha and ibavirin. World J Gastroenterol 2007; 13: 5648–53.

15. Verucchi G, Calza L, Manfredi R et al. Human immunodeficiency virus and hepatitis C virus co-infection: epidemiology, natural history, therapeutic options and clinical management. Infection 2004; 32:33–46.

16. Yamauchi M, Nakahara M, Maezawa Y et al. Prevalence of hepatocellular carcinoma in patients with alcoholic cirrhosis and prior exposure to hepatitis C. Am J Gastroenterol 1993; 88:39–43.

17. Marrero JA, Fontana RJ, Su GL et al. NAFLD may be a common underlying liver disease in patients with hepatocellular carcinoma in the United States. Hepatology 2002; 36:1349–54.

18. Neuschwander-Tetri BA, Caldwell SH. Nonalcoholic steatohepatitis: summary of an AASLD Single Topic Conference. Hepatology 2003; 37:1202–19.

19. Regimbeau JM, Colombat M, Mognol P et al. Obesity and diabetes as a risk factor for hepatocellular carcinoma. Liver Transpl 2004; 10(2, Suppl 1): S69–73.

20. Calle EE, Rodriguez C, Walker-Thurmond K et al. Overweight, obesity, and mortality from cancer in a prospectively studied cohort of U.S. adults. N Engl J Med 2003; 348:1625–38.

21. El Serag HB, Tran T, Everhart JE. Diabetes increases the risk of chronic liver disease and hepatocellular carcinoma. Gastroenterology 2004; 126:460–8.

22. Caldwell SH, Crespo DM, Kang HS et al. Obesity and hepatocellular carcinoma. Gastroenterology 2004; 127:S97–103.

23. Soga M, Kishimoto Y, Kawamura Y et al. Spontaneous development of hepatocellular carcinomas in the FLS mice with hereditary fatty liver. Cancer Lett 2003; 196:43–8.

24. Hashizume H, Sato K, Takagi H et al. Primary liver cancers with nonalcoholic steatohepatitis. Eur J Gastroenterol Hepatol 2007; 19:827–34.

25. Hsing AW, McLaughlin JK, Olsen JH et al. Cancer risk following primary hemochromatosis: a population-based cohort study in Denmark. Int J Cancer 1995; 60:160–2.

26. Adams PC. Hepatocellular carcinoma in hereditary hemochromatosis. Can J Gastorenterol 1993; 7:37–41.

27. Elmberg M, Hultcrantz R, Ekbom A et al. Cancer risk in patients with hereditary hemochromatosis and in their first-degree relatives. Gastroenterology 2003; 125:1733–41.

28. Haddow JE, Palomaki GE, McClain M et al. Hereditary haemochromatosis and hepatocellular carcinoma in males: a strategy for estimating the potential for primary prevention. J Med Screen 2003; 10:11–13.

29. Shibuya A, Tanaka K, Miyakawa H et al. Hepatocellular carcinoma and survival in patients with primary biliary cirrhosis. Hepatology 2002; 35:1172–8.

30. Suzuki A, Lymp J, Donlinger J et al. Clinical predictors for hepatocellular carcinoma in patients with primary biliary cirrhosis. Clin Gastroenterol Hepatol 2007; 5:259–64.

31. Nishiyama R, Kanai T, Abe J et al. Hepatocellular carcinoma associated with autoimmune hepatitis. J Hepatobiliary Pancreat Surg 2004; 11:215–19.

32. Chen CJ, Wang LY, Lu SN et al. Elevated aflatoxin exposure and increased risk of hepatocellular carcinoma. Hepatology 1996; 24:38–42.

33. Leese T, Farges O, Bismuth H. Liver cell adenomas. A 12-year surgical experience from a specialist hepatobiliary unit. Ann Surg 1988; 208:558–64.

34. Chiche L, Dao T, Salame E et al. Liver adenomatosis: reappraisal, diagnosis, and surgical management: eight new cases and review of the literature. Ann Surg 2000; 231:74–81.

35. Bioulac-Sage P, Rebouissou S, Thomas C et al. Hepatocellular adenoma subtype classification using molecular markers and immunohistochemistry. Hepatology 2007; 46:740–8.

36. Gorayski P, Thompson CH, Subhash HS et al. Hepatocellular carcinoma associated with recreational anabolic steroid use. Br J Sports Med 2008; 42:74–5.

37. Borzio M, Fargion S, Borzio F et al. Impact of large regenerative, low grade and high grade dysplastic nodules in hepatocellular carcinoma development. J Hepatol 2003; 39:208–14.

38. Takayama T, Makuuchi M, Hirohashi S et al. Malignant transformation of adenomatous hyperplasia to hepatocellular carcinoma. Lancet 1990; 336:1150–3.

39. Nam SW, Park JY, Ramasamy A et al. Molecular changes from dysplastic nodule to hepatocellular carcinoma through gene expression profiling. Hepatology 2005; 42:809–18.

40. Coston WM, Loera S, Lau SK et al. Distinction of hepatocellular carcinoma from benign hepatic

mimickers using Glypican-3 and CD34 immuno-histochemistry. Am J Surg Pathol 2008; 32: 433–44.

41. Ikai I, Arii S, Okasaki M et al. Report of the 17th nationwide follow-up survey of primary liver cancer in Japan. Hepatol Res 2007; 37:676–91.

42. Yeh CN, Lee WC, Jeng LB et al. Spontaneous tumour rupture and prognosis in patients with hepatocellular carcinoma. Br J Surg 2002; 89:1125–9.

43. Murakami T, Kim T, Takahashi S et al. Hepatocellular carcinoma: multidetector row helical CT. Abdom Imaging 2002; 27:139–46.

44. Burrel M, Llovet JM, Ayuso C et al. MRI angiography is superior to helical CT for detection of HCC prior to liver transplantation: an explant correlation. Hepatology 2003; 38:1034–42.

45. Bruix J, Sherman M, Llovet JM et al. Clinical management of hepatocellular carcinoma. Conclusions of the Barcelona 2000 EASL conference. J Hepatol 2001; 35:421–30.

    EASL consensus statement on HCC management.

46. Bolondi L, Gaiani S, Celli N et al. Characterization of small nodules in cirrhosis by assessment of vascularity: the problem of hypovascular hepatocellular carcinoma. Hepatology 2005; 42:27–34.

47. Bruix J, Sherman M. Management of hepatocellular carcinoma. Hepatology 2005; 42:1208–36.

48. Forner A, Vilana R, Ayuso C et al. Diagnosis of hepatic nodules 20 mm or smaller in cirrhosis: prospective validation of the noninvasive diagnostic criteria for hepatocellular carcinoma. Hepatology 2008; 47:97–104.

49. Stigliano R, Marelli L, Yu D et al. Seeding following percutaneous diagnostic and therapeutic approaches for hepatocellular carcinoma. What is the risk and the outcome? Seeding risk for percutaneous approach of HCC. Cancer Treat Rev 2007; 33:437–47.

50. Pawlik TM, Gleisner AL, Anders RA et al. Preoperative assessment of hepatocellular carcinoma tumour grade using needle biopsy: implications for transplant eligibility. Ann Surg 2007; 245: 435–42.

51. Llovet JM, Bustamante J, Castells A et al. Natural history of untreated nonsurgical hepatocellular carcinoma: rationale for the design and evaluation of therapeutic trials. Hepatology 1999; 29:62–7.

52. Wildi S, Pestalozzi BC, McCormack L et al. Critical evaluation of the different staging systems for hepatocellular carcinoma. Br J Surg 2004; 91:400–8.

53. Trevisani F, De Notariis S, Rapaccini G et al. Semiannual and annual surveillance of cirrhotic patients for hepatocellular carcinoma: effects on cancer stage and patient survival (Italian experience). Am J Gastroenterol 2002; 97:734–44.

54. Makuuchi M, Kokudo N, Arii S et al. Development of evidence-based clinical guidelines for the diagnosis and treatment of hepatocellular carcinoma in Japan. Hepatol Res 2008; 38:37–51.

55. Yuen MF, Lai CL. Screening for hepatocellular carcinoma: survival benefit and cost-effectiveness. Ann Oncol 2003; 14:1463–7.

56. Yang B, Zhang B, Xu Y et al. Prospective study of early detection for primary liver cancer. J Cancer Res Clin Oncol 1997; 123:357–60.

    Randomised controlled trial in which a significantly greater number of patients underwent liver resection as a result of screening.

57. Belghiti J, Hiramatsu K, Benoist S et al. Seven hundred forty-seven hepatectomies in the 1990s: an update to evaluate the actual risk of liver resection. J Am Coll Surg 2000; 191:38–46.

58. Chang CH, Chau GY, Lui WY et al. Long-term results of hepatic resection for hepatocellular carcinoma originating from the noncirrhotic liver. Arch Surg 2004; 139:320–5.

59. Iwatsuki S, Starzl TE, Sheahan DG et al. Hepatic resection versus transplantation for hepatocellular carcinoma. Ann Surg 1991; 214:221–9.

60. Imamura H, Seyama Y, Kokudo N et al. One thousand fifty-six hepatectomies without mortality in 8 years. Arch Surg 2003; 138:1198–206; discussion 1206.

61. Farges O, Malassagne B, Flejou JF et al. Risk of major liver resection in patients with underlying chronic liver disease: a reappraisal. Ann Surg 1999; 229:210–15.

62. Makuuchi M, Kosuge T, Takayama T et al. Surgery for small liver cancers. Semin Surg Oncol 1993; 9:298–304.

63. Noun R, Jagot P, Farges O et al. High preoperative serum alanine transferase levels: effect on the risk of liver resection in Child grade A cirrhotic patients. World J Surg 1997; 21:390–4.

64. Bruix J, Castells A, Bosch J et al. Surgical resection of hepatocellular carcinoma in cirrhotic patients: prognostic value of preoperative portal pressure. Gastroenterology 1996; 111:1018–22.

65. Belghiti J, Noun R, Malafosse R et al. Continuous versus intermittent portal triad clamping for liver resection. Ann Surg 1999; 229:369–75.

66. Belghiti J, Guevara OA, Noun R et al. Liver hanging maneuver: a safe approach to right hepatectomy without liver mobilization. J Am Coll Surg 2001; 193:109–11.

67. Liu CL, Fan ST, Cheung ST et al. Anterior approach versus conventional approach right hepatic resection for large hepatocellular carcinoma: a prospective randomized controlled study. Ann Surg 2006; 244:194–203.

    Survival advantage for author approach.

68. Abdalla EK, Hicks ME, Vauthey JN. Portal vein embolization: rationale, technique and future prospects. Br J Surg 2001; 88:165–75.

69. Farges O, Belghiti J, Kianmanesh R et al. Portal vein embolization before right hepatectomy: prospective clinical trial. Ann Surg 2003; 237:208–17.

PVE resulted in a 50% reduction in risk of post-operative complications and hospital stay.

70. Ogata S, Belghiti J, Farges O et al. Sequential arterial and portal vein embolizations before right hepatectomy in patients with cirrhosis and hepatocellular carcinoma. Br J Surg 2006; 93:1091–8.

71. Hasegawa K, Kokudo N, Imamura H et al. Prognostic impact of anatomic resection for hepatocellular carcinoma. Ann Surg 2005; 242:252–9.

72. Wakai T, Shirai Y, Sakata J et al. Anatomic resection independently improves long-term survival in patients with T1–T2 hepatocellular carcinoma. Ann Surg Oncol 2007; 14:1356–65.

73. Shi M, Guo RP, Lin XJ et al. Partial hepatectomy with wide versus narrow resection margin for solitary hepatocellular carcinoma: a prospective randomized trial. Ann Surg 2007; 245:36–43.

A 2 cm resection margin was associated with significantly improved survival.

74. Pawlik T, Esnoala NF, Vauthey JN. Surgical treatment of hepatocellular carcinoma: similar long term results despite geographic variations. Liver Transpl 2004; 10:S74–80.

75. Ikai I, Arii S, Kojiro M et al. Reevaluation of prognostic factors for survival after liver resection in patients with hepatocellular carcinoma in a Japanese nationwide survey. Cancer 2004; 101:796–802.

76. Belghiti J, Panis Y, Farges O et al. Intrahepatic recurrence after resection of hepatocellular carcinoma complicating cirrhosis. Ann Surg 1991; 214:114–17.

77. Chen MF, Hwang TL, Jeng LB et al. Postoperative recurrence of hepatocellular carcinoma. Arch Surg 1994; 129:738–42.

78. Schwartz JD, Schwartz M, Mandeli J et al. Neoadjuvant and adjuvant therapy for resectable hepatocellular carcinoma: review of the randomised clinical trials. Lancet Oncol 2002; 3:593–603.

79. Lau WY, Lai EC, Leung TW et al. Adjuvant intra-arterial iodine-131-labeled lipiodol for resectable hepatocellular carcinoma: a prospective randomized trial-update on 5-year and 10-year survival. Ann Surg 2008; 247:43–8.

A significant survival benefit for patients receiving adjuvant treatment.

80. Sun HC, Tang ZY, Wang L et al. Postoperative interferon alpha treatment postponed recurrence and improved overall survival in patients after curative resection of HBV-related hepatocellular carcinoma: a randomized clinical trial. J Cancer Res Clin Oncol 2006; 132:458–65.

81. Lo CM, Liu CL, Chan SC et al. A randomized, controlled trial of postoperative adjuvant interferon therapy after resection of hepatocellular carcinoma. Ann Surg 2007; 245:831–42.

82. Mazzaferro V, Romito R, Schiavo M et al. HCC Italian Task Force. Prevention of hepatocellular carcinoma recurrence with alpha-interferon after liver resection in HCV cirrhosis. Hepatology 2006; 44:1543–54.

83. Poon RTP, Fan ST, Lo CM et al. Intrahepatic recurrence after curative resection of hepatocellular carcinoma. Long-term results of treatment and prognostic factors. Ann Surg 1999; 229:216–22.

84. Taura K, Ikai I, Hatano E et al. Implication of frequent local ablation therapy for intrahepatic recurrence in prolonged survival of patients with hepatocellular carcinoma undergoing hepatic resection: an analysis of 610 patients over 16 years old. Ann Surg 2006; 244:265–73.

85. Farges O, Regimbeau JM, Belghiti J. Aggressive management of recurrence following surgical resection of hepatocellular carcinoma. Hepatogastroenterology 1998; 45:S1275–80.

86. Ringe B, Pichlmayr R, Wittekind C et al. Surgical treatment of hepatocellular carcinoma: experience with liver resection and transplantation in 198 patients. World J Surg 1991; 15:270–85.

87. Mazzaferro V, Regalia E, Doci R et al. Liver transplantation for the treatment of small hepatocellular carcinomas in patients with cirrhosis. N Engl J Med 1996; 334:693–9.

88. Yoo HY, Patt CH, Geschwind JF et al. The outcome of liver transplantation in patients with hepatocellular carcinoma in the United States between 1988 and 2001: 5-year survival has improved significantly with time. J Clin Oncol 2003; 21:4329–35.

89. Yao FY, Ferrell L, Bass NM et al. Liver transplantation for hepatocellular carcinoma: comparison of the proposed UCSF criteria with the Milan criteria and the Pittsburgh modified TNM criteria. Liver Transpl 2002; 8:765–74.

90. Llovet JM, Fuster J, Bruix J. Intention-to-treat analysis of surgical treatment for early hepatocellular carcinoma: resection versus transplantation. Hepatology 1999; 30:1434–40.

91. Jonas S, Bechstein WO, Steinmuller T et al. Vascular invasion and histopathological grading determine outcome after liver transplantation for hepatocellular carcinoma. Hepatology 2001; 33:1081–6.

92. Kar S, Carr BI. Detection of liver cells in peripheral blood of patients with advanced stage hepatocellular carcinoma. Hepatology 1995; 21:403–7.

93. Lee JS, Chu IS, Heo J et al. Classification and prediction of survival in hepatocellular carcinoma by gene expression profiling. Hepatology 2004; 40:667–76.

94. Belghiti J, Cortes A, Abdalla EK et al. Resection prior to liver transplantation for hepatocellular carcinoma. Ann Surg 2003; 238:885–92.

95. Groupe d'étude et de traitement du carcinome hépatocellulaire. A comparison of lipiodol chemoembolisation and conservative treatment for unresectable hepatocellular carcinoma. N Engl J Med 1995; 332:1256–61.

96. Bismuth H, Morino M, Sherlock D et al. Primary treatment of hepatocellular carcinoma

by arterial chemoembolisation. Am J Surg 1992; 163:387–94.

97. Paye F, Farges O, Dahmane M et al. Cytolysis following chemoembolisation for hepatocellular carcinoma. Br J Surg 1999; 86:176–80.

98. Ong GY, Changchien CS, Lee CM et al. Liver abscess complicating transcatheter arterial embolization: a rare but serious complication. A retrospective study after 3878 procedures. Eur J Gastroenterol Hepatol 2004; 16:737–42.

99. Takayasu K, Arii S, Ikai I et al. Liver Cancer Study Group of Japan. Prospective cohort study of transarterial chemoembolization for unresectable hepatocellular carcinoma in 8510 patients. Gastroenterology 2006; 131:461–9.

100. Bruix J, Llovet JM, Castells A et al. Transarterial embolization versus symptomatic treatment in patients with advanced hepatocellular carcinoma: results of a randomized controlled trial in a single institution. Hepatology 1998; 127:1578–83.

101. Lo CM, Ngan H, Tso WK et al. Randomized controlled trial of transarterial lipiodol chemoembolization for unresectable hepatocellular carcinoma. Hepatology 2002; 35:1164–71.

102. Llovet JM, Real MI, Montana X et al. Arterial embolisation or chemoembolisation versus symptomatic treatment in patients with unresectable hepatocellular carcinoma: a randomised controlled trial. Lancet 2002; 359:1734–9.

103. Llovet JM, Bruix J. Systematic review of randomized trials for unresectable hepatocellular carcinoma: chemoembolization improves survival. Hepatology 2003; 37:429–42.
   Review of evidence demonstrating survival advantage with chemoembolization.

104. Katyal S, Oliver JH, Peterson MS et al. Prognostic significance of arterial phase CT for prediction of response to transcatheter arterial chemoembolization in unresectable hepatocellular carcinoma: a retrospective analysis. Am J Roentgenol 2000; 175:1665–72.

105. Lee HS, Kim KM, Yoon JH et al. Therapeutic efficacy of transcatheter arterial chemoembolization as compared with hepatic resection in hepatocellular carcinoma patients with compensated liver function in a hepatitis B virus-endemic area: a prospective cohort study. J Clin Oncol 2002; 20:4459–65.

106. Lopez P, Villanueva A, Llovet JM. Updated systematic review of randomized controlled trials in hepatocellular carcinoma, 2002-2005. Aliment Pharmacol Ther 2006; 23:1535–47.
   Review demonstrating significant reduction in local recurrence with RF compared to other ablative techniques.

107. Teratani T, Yoshida H, Shiina S et al. Radiofrequency ablation for hepatocellular carcinoma in so-called high-risk locations. Hepatology 2006; 43:1101–8.

108. Chen MS, Li JQ, Zheng Y et al. A prospective randomized trial comparing percutaneous local ablative therapy and partial hepatectomy for small hepatocellular carcinoma. Ann Surg 2006; 243:321–8.

109. Lu MD, Kuang M, Liang LJ et al. Surgical resection versus percutaneous thermal ablation for early-stage hepatocellular carcinoma: a randomized clinical trial. Zhonghua Yi Xue Za Zhi 2006; 86:801–5.

110. Livraghi T, Meloni F, Di Stasi M et al. Sustained complete response and complications rates after radiofrequency ablation of very early hepatocellular carcinoma in cirrhosis: is resection still the treatment of choice? Hepatology 2008; 47:82–9.

111. Mulier S, Mulier P, Ni Y et al. Complication of radiofrequency coagulation of liver tumours. Br J Surg 2002; 89:1206–22.

112. Llovet J, Ricci S, Mazzaferro V et al. Sorafenib in advanced hepatocellular carcinoma (HCC). N Engl J Med 2008; 359:378–98.
   Randomized trial showing beneficial effect on survival with sorafenib.

113. Raoul JL, Guyader D, Bretagne JF et al. Prospective randomized trial of chemoembolization versus intra-arterial injection of ^{131}I-labeled-iodized oil in the treatment of hepatocellular carcinoma. Hepatology 1997; 26:1156–61.

114. Raoul JL, Guyader D, Bretagne JF et al. Randomised controlled trial for hepatocellular carcinoma with portal vein thrombosis versus medical support. J Nucl Med 1994; 35:1782–7.

115. Kulik LM, Carr BI, Mulcahy MF et al. Safety and efficacy of ^{90}Y radiotherapy for hepatocellular carcinoma with and without portal vein thrombosis. Hepatology 2008; 47:71–81.

116. Kouroumalis E, Skordilis P, Thermos K et al. Treatment of hepatocellular carcinoma with octreotide: a randomised controlled study. Gut 1998; 42:442–7.

117. Becker G, Allgaier HP, Olschewski M et al. HECTOR Study Group. Long-acting octreotide versus placebo for treatment of advanced HCC: a randomized controlled double-blind study. Hepatology 2007; 45:9–15.

118. Leung KL, Lau WY, Lai PBS et al. Spontaneous rupture of hepatocellular carcinoma. Arch Surg 1999; 134:1103–7.

119. El-Serag HB, Davila JA. Is fibrolamellar carcinoma different from hepatocellular carcinoma? A US population-based study. Hepatology 2004; 39:798–803.

120. Stipa F, Yoon SS, Liau KH et al. Outcome of patients with fibrolamellar hepatocellular carcinoma. Cancer 2006; 106:1331–8.

121. Craig JR, Peters RL, Edmondson HA et al. Fibrolamellar carcinoma of the liver: a tumour of adolescents and young adults with distinctive clinicopathologic features. Cancer 1980; 46:372–9.

122. Khan SA, Taylor-Robinson SD, Toledano MB et al. Changing international trends in mortality

rates for liver, biliary and pancreatic tumours. J Hepatol 2002; 37:806–13.

123. Jepsen P, Vilstrup H, Tarone RE et al. Incidence rates of intra- and extrahepatic cholangiocarcinomas in Denmark from 1978 through 2002. J Natl Cancer Inst 2007;99:895-7.

124. Patel T. Increasing incidence and mortality of primary intrahepatic cholangiocarcinoma in the United States. Hepatology 2001; 33:1353–7.

125. Welzel TM, Graubard BI, El-Serag HB et al. Risk factors for intrahepatic and extrahepatic cholangiocarcinoma in the United States: a population-based case–control study. Clin Gastroenterol Hepatol 2007; 5:1221–8.

126. Shaib YH, El-Serag HB, Nooka AK et al. Risk factors for intrahepatic and extrahepatic cholangiocarcinoma: a hospital-based case–control study. Am J Gastroenterol 2007; 102:1016–21.

127. Yamamoto S, Kubo S, Hai S et al. Hepatitis C virus infection as a likely etiology of intrahepatic cholangiocarcinoma. Cancer Sci 2004; 95:592–5.

128. Torbenson M, Yeh MM, Abraham SC. Bile duct dysplasia in the setting of chronic hepatitis C and alcohol cirrhosis. Am J Surg Pathol 2007; 31: 1410–13.

129. Yamasaki S. Intrahepatic cholangiocarcinoma: macroscopic type and stage classification. J Hepatobiliary Pancreat Surg 2003; 10:288–91.

130. Suh KS, Roh HR, Koh YT et al. Clinicopathologic features of the intraductal growth type of peripheral cholangiocarcinoma. Hepatology 2000; 31:12–17.

131. Okabayashi T, Yamamoto J, Kosuge T et al. A new staging system for mass-forming intrahepatic cholangiocarcinoma: analysis of preoperative and postoperative variables. Cancer 2001; 92:2374–83.

132. Aishima S, Kuroda Y, Nishihara Y et al. Proposal of progression model for intrahepatic cholangiocarcinoma: clinicopathologic differences between hilar type and peripheral type. Am J Surg Pathol 2007; 31:1059–67.

133. Zen Y, Sasaki M, Fujii T et al. Different expression patterns of mucin core proteins and cytokeratins during intrahepatic cholangiocarcinogenesis from biliary intraepithelial neoplasia and intraductal papillary neoplasm of the bile duct – an immunohistochemical study of 110 cases of hepatolithiasis. J Hepatol 2006; 44:350–8.

134. Roskams T. Liver stem cells and their implication in hepatocellular and cholangiocarcinoma. Oncogene 2006; 25:3818–22.

135. Lim JH. Cholangiocarcinoma: morphologic classification according to growth pattern and imaging findings. Am J Roentgenol 2003; 181:819–27.

136. Khan SA, Davidson BR, Goldin R et al. Guidelines for the diagnosis and treatment of cholangiocarcinoma: consensus document. Gut 2002; 51(Suppl 6):VI1–9.

137. Nagorney DM, Donohue JH, Farnell MB et al. Outcomes after curative resections of cholangiocarcinoma. Arch Surg 1993; 128:871–7.

138. Goere D, Wagholikar GD, Pessaux P et al. Utility of staging laparoscopy in subsets of biliary cancers: laparoscopy is a powerful diagnostic tool in patients with intrahepatic and gallbladder carcinoma. Surg Endosc 2006; 20:721–5.

139. Tajima Y, Kuroki T, Fukuda K et al. An intraductal papillary component is associated with prolonged survival after hepatic resection for intrahepatic cholangiocarcinoma. Br J Surg 2004; 91:99–104.

140. Paule B, Herelle MO, Rage E et al. Cetuximab plus gemcitabine–oxaliplatin (GEMOX) in patients with refractory advanced intrahepatic cholangiocarcinomas. Oncology 2007; 72(1–2):105–10.

141. Mehrabi A, Kashfi A, Fonouni H et al. Primary malignant hepatic epithelioid hemangioendothelioma: a comprehensive review of the literature with emphasis on the surgical therapy. Cancer 2006; 107:2108–21.

142. Makhlouf HR, Ishak KG, Goodman ZD. Epithelioid hemangioendothelioma of the liver: a clinicopathologic study of 137 cases. Cancer 1999; 85:562–82.

143. Otrock ZK, Al-Kutoubi A, Kattar MM et al. Spontaneous complete regression of hepatic epithelioid haemangioendothelioma. Lancet Oncol 2006; 7:439–41.

144. Lerut JP, Orlando G, Adam R et al. European Liver Transplant Registry. The place of liver transplantation in the treatment of hepatic epitheloid hemangioendothelioma: report of the European liver transplant registry. Ann Surg 2007; 246:949–57; discussion 957.

145. Gatta G, Ciccolallo L, Kunkler I et al. EUROCARE Working Group. Survival from rare cancer in adults: a population-based study. Lancet Oncol 2006; 7:132–40.

146. Weinman MD, Chopra S. Tumours of the liver, other than primary hepatocellular carcinoma. Gastroenterol Clin North Am 1987; 16:627–50.

147. Koyama T, Fletcher JG, Johnson CD et al. Primary hepatic angiosarcoma: findings at CT and MR imaging. Radiology 2002; 222:667–73.

148. Locker GY, Doroshow JH, Zwelling LA et al. The clinical features of hepatic angiosarcoma: a report of four cases and a review of the English literature. Medicine 1979; 58:48–64.

149. Poggio JL, Nagorney DM, Nascimento AG et al. Surgical treatment of adult primary hepatic sarcoma. Br J Surg 2000; 87:1500–5.

150. Weitz J, Klimstra DS, Cymes K et al. Management of primary liver sarcomas. Cancer 2007; 109: 1391–6.

151. Aozasa K, Mishima K, Ohsawa M. Primary malignant lymphoma of the liver. Leuk Lymphoma 1993; 10:353–7.

6

Colorectal liver metastases

Derek A. O'Reilly
Graeme J. Poston

Introduction

Colorectal cancer is the commonest gastrointestinal malignancy and the second commonest cause of cancer death in Western society. It is estimated to cause 57 100 deaths per annum in the USA and 17 000 deaths per annum in the UK.[1] The liver is usually the first site of metastatic disease and may be the only site in 30–40% of patients with advanced disease.[2] At the time of initial diagnosis of colorectal cancer, 20–25% of patients will have clinically detectable liver metastases. A further 40–50% will develop liver metastases, usually within the first 3 years of follow-up after successful resection of the primary tumour.[3]

Without treatment, the median survival for colorectal liver metastases (CRLMs) is just 6–8 months, varying with the extent of disease at presentation. The prognosis is best for those whose metastases are isolated to a single lobe of the liver or are limited in number.[3] However, even for the best prognostic groups, very few survive 5 years. Surgery is the only treatment that offers the prospect of cure for CRLMs. Until recently, only 10–20% of patients were considered suitable for attempted curative resection; the remaining patients were offered palliative and symptomatic treatment.

This review focuses on a variety of recent strategies that have been designed to increase the pool of patients for whom curative treatment may be possible. These include improved preoperative staging techniques, new standards for surgical resection, novel surgical strategies, the application of modern systemic chemotherapy in a neoadjuvant setting, an emerging role for ablative therapies and an emphasis on the collaborative, multidisciplinary management of this disease.

Preoperative staging: the key to selection of candidates for curative treatment

Individual imaging techniques used in preoperative staging have different strengths and weaknesses, but consensus is now emerging on the optimal choice of technique and the sequence with which it should be employed.[4,5]

Computed tomography (CT)

Recent advances in CT technology, such as helical CT and multidetector row helical CT, have improved the performance of CT in terms of speed of acquisition, resolution and ability to image the liver during various phases of contrast enhancement with greater precision. Intravenous iodinated contrast media should be used routinely. This helps characterise liver lesions based on their enhancement patterns during the various phases of contrast circulation in the liver.[6] During the portal venous phase, normal liver parenchyma usually enhances intensely while liver metastases (with their dominant arterial supply) appear as relatively hypodense, hypovascular lesions. In small-sized liver metastases, arterial dominant phase imaging may be useful to detect faint peripheral rim enhancement. Delayed images should be obtained 4–5 minutes after contrast injection. This is helpful in differentiating metastases from benign liver lesions, particularly a haemangioma.[7] CT has become the imaging modality of choice for evaluating suspected liver metastases. However, limitations include the need for a high radiation dose and low sensitivity for the detection and characterisation of lesions smaller than 1 cm (**Figs. 6.1–6.5**).

Magnetic resonance imaging (MRI)

MRI is also a highly effective imaging modality for detecting and characterising liver lesions as it provides high lesion-to-liver contrast without using ionising radiation. Typically, CRLMs show low signal intensity on T1-weighted images and moderately high signal intensity on T2-weighted images with fat suppression. Gadolinium, the most commonly used MRI contrast agent, behaves similarly to the iodinated contrast agents used in CT. Liver-specific contrast media such as superparamagnetic iron oxide (SPIO) may further improve the contrast between liver and metastases, as this is taken up predominantly by Kupffer cells of the reticulo-endothelial system.[7] Because metastases do not have these cells, there is no SPIO uptake and they appear as high-signal-intensity lesions. Mangafodipir trisodium (Mn DPDP, Teslascan) is another MR contrast agent with comparable ability to detect and characterise CRLMs.[7] Limitations of MRI include a low sensitivity for detecting extrahepatic disease in the peritoneum and chest. It is particularly useful in problem-solving: evaluating indeterminate lesions detected on CT, in patients with fatty infiltration of the liver and in distinguishing small metastases from small cysts.[5,7] It can be used safely in patients with allergies to iodinated contrast agents (**Figs. 6.2 and 6.5**).

Positron emission tomography (PET)

PET has emerged as an important diagnostic tool in the evaluation of CRLMs. A greater metabolic activity in malignant tissue is accompanied by a greater glucose uptake relative to that of surrounding normal tissues, identified with [^{18}F]fluoro-2-D-glucose (FDG-PET). This modality is highly sensitive; however, any focal area of hypermetabolism can give a false-positive result. Other disadvantages include high cost, poor lesion localisation and limited sensitivity for lesions smaller than 1 cm. PET-CT combines the advantages of CT with the functional ability of PET, by the fusion of PET images with CT images acquired at the same time, helping to accurately localise the area of increased metabolic activity.[8] It should be considered in patients at high risk of disseminated disease at presentation or of recurrence (**Figs. 6.6 and 6.7**).

Staging laparoscopy

Staging laparoscopy is an excellent technique to detect occult metastatic disease in patients with gastrointestinal malignancies, but the yield can vary depending on the extent and quality of preoperative imaging and on the histological type of cancer. Although highly sensitive for the detection of peritoneal or surface liver metastases, laparoscopy is less sensitive in detecting locally advanced disease or nodal spread.[9]

The utility of laparoscopy for CRLMs has changed over time due to improving radiology and changing

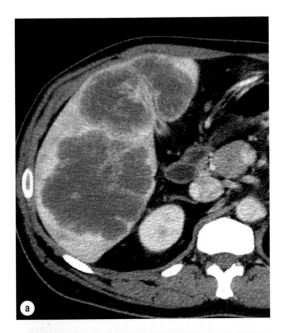

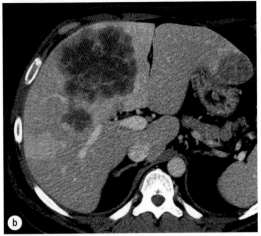

Figure 6.1 • (a,b) Large hepatic metastases. Contrast-enhanced CT shows multiple low-attenuation hepatic metastases and bilateral tumour infiltration.

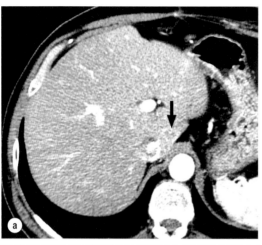

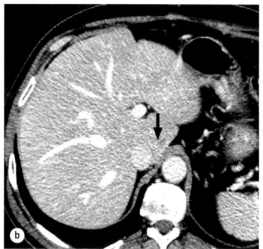

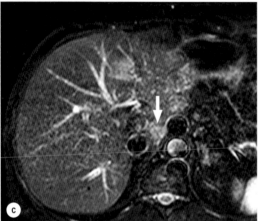

Figure 6.2 • Tiny liver metastases from colon carcinoma. **(a)** Contrast-enhanced arterial-dominant phase shows the metastasis as an area of intense ring enhancement (arrow). **(b)** Contrast-enhanced portal venous phase shows the tumour as an ill-defined area of low density (arrow). **(c)** Axial T2-weighted fast spin-echo (FSE) MRI image shows the metastases that have moderately high signal intensity compared with the liver.

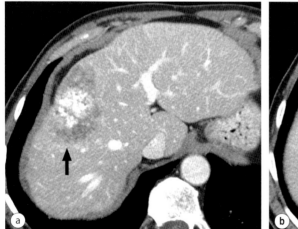

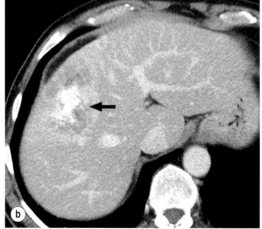

Figure 6.3 • Calcified liver metastases of colon carcinoma. Contrast-enhanced portal phase **(a)** and delayed phase **(b)** exhibit a hypodense mass (arrow) with internal calcium deposits (arrowhead).

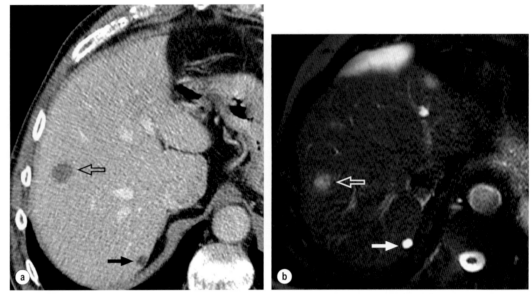

Figure 6.4 • Colorectal metastases with coincidental multiple liver cyst. **(a)** Axial CT in portal phase in a patient who has known colon carcinoma shows a hypodense metastasis in segment VIII (open arrow) and a second lesion (arrow) 'too small to characterise'. **(b)** Axial T2-weighted fast spin-echo shows a metastasis (open arrow) that has moderately high signal intensity compared with the liver and much lower signal intensity than the bright fluid-like signal intensity of the cysts (arrows).

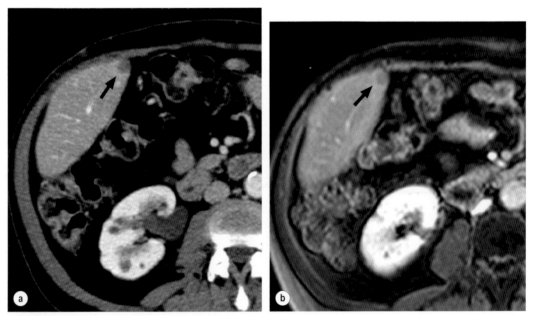

Figure 6.5 • Focal hepatic steatosis in a patient with liver metastases from colorectal cancer. **(a,b)** Axial CT images show diffuse fatty infiltration of liver and hypodense lesion (arrow) suspicious for metastasis in segment V.

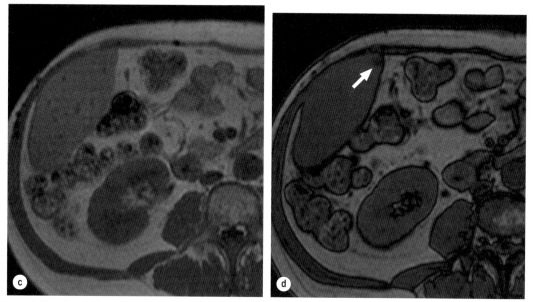

Figure 6.5 • Cont'd (c,d) Axial in-phase **(c)** and out-of-phase **(d)** images show greater signal drop of lesion in **(d)** (arrow), consistent with hypersteatosis (more fatty) compared with diffusely fatty infiltrated liver.

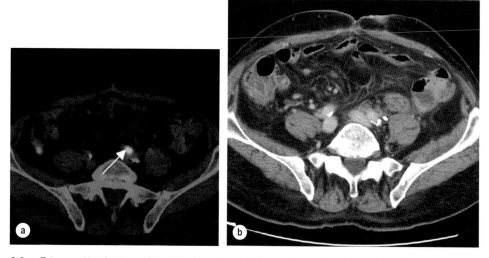

Figure 6.6 • False-positive finding of PET-CT. **(a)** Postsurgical fibrosis in a patient with colorectal carcinoma resection. Transverse FDG-PET-CT images show avid focus (arrow) with FDG uptake in the retroperitoneal space that was considered metastatic. **(b)** Activity seen on PET-CT coincides with fibrous changes after surgery on CT without evidence of metastasic foci. At histopathological examination the lesion was benign (granulomatous reaction).

indications for operation. Overall, the yield of laparoscopy for metastatic colorectal cancer to the liver ranges from 6% to 36% and is 10% in the largest series.[10-14] The overall accuracy ranges from 38% to 75%.

New studies have addressed factors that enhance our understanding of selection criteria to increase the yield of staging laparoscopy to reduce the number of patients undergoing laparoscopy who will not benefit from the procedure. The Clinical Risk Score (CRS) has been applied in this setting.[15] CRS ranges from 0 to 5 based on the presence of the following characteristics: node-positive primary tumour, prehepatectomy carcinoembryonic antigen (CEA)

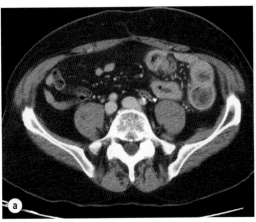
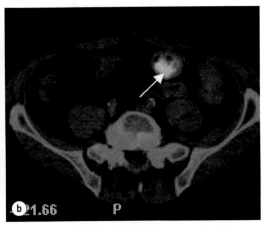

Figure 6.7 • Locoregional recurrence after resection. **(a)** CT at the level of the iliac crests shows postsurgical changes after right colectomy without evidence of tumour recurrence. **(b)** PET-CT shows highly metabolic area adjacent to ileocolic anastomosis (arrow) consistent with tumour recurrence.

greater than 200 ng/mL, more than one liver tumour, liver tumour size greater than 5 cm, and disease-free interval of less than 1 year. In the Memorial Sloan Kettering Cancer Center study, only 4% of patients' tumours were unresectable at scores of 0–1 but none were found at laparoscopy. At scores of 2–3, 21% of lesions were unresectable and only one-half were found at laparoscopy (yield of 11%). The highest yield was at scores of 4–5, where the yield of laparoscopy was 24%.[14] This study provides a very useful basis for determining which patients are most likely to benefit from staging laparoscopy.

The optimum means of assessing liver involvement and resectability in advanced colorectal cancer is based generally on local expertise and availability of imaging modalities. The evidence points towards contrast-enhanced multi-sliced CT being the most widely available and used, with MRI and PET-CT employed when further analysis is required. There is some evidence that biopsy of resectable lesions may compromise long-term survival after hepatectomy.

Surgery: the old and the new standards for resection

Criteria for resection

If CRLMs are resectable, patients can look forward to a 5-year survival of 40% and 10-year survival of 24%, with age being no barrier to resection if fit (**Figs. 6.8 and 6.9**). In the past, the decision to resect CRLMs was relatively straightforward; on the basis of old studies that established certain adverse clinicopathological factors, liver resection was attempted only in patients who had one to three unilobar metastases, preferably presenting at least 12 months after resection of the primary tumour, whose disease was resectable with at least a 1-cm margin of healthy liver tissue and who had no hilar lymphadenopathy or extrahepatic disease.

More recently, experience has demonstrated that patients with the above traditional adverse factors can experience long-term survival following liver resection.[16,17] Thus, a shift has occurred in the criteria used for assessing resectability, from morphological criteria to new ones based on whether a macroscopically and microscopically complete (R0) resection of the liver can be achieved. Instead of resectability being defined by what is removed, resectability should now be determined by what will remain.

The American Hepato-Pancreato-Biliary Association (AHPBA) 2006 consensus conference on hepatic colorectal metastases concluded that CRLMs should be determined as resectable if (i) the disease can be completely resected, (ii) two adjacent liver segments can be spared with adequate vascular inflow and outflow and biliary drainage, and (iii) the volume of the liver remaining after resection, i.e. the 'future liver remnant' (FLR), will be adequate.[5] Clearly, the FLR limit for safe resection varies from patient to patient but in those with an otherwise normal liver, the safe FLR volume is 20%.[18] A recent pan-European consensus statement concluded that resection should be performed whatever the margin and is only contraindicated when all the metastases cannot be cleared. Additional criteria for unresectability are invasion of one branch of the liver pedicle, and contact with the contralateral branch,

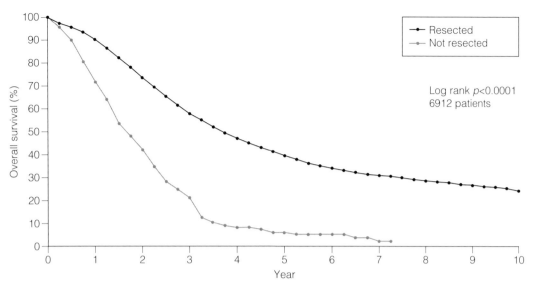

Figure 6.8 • LiverMetSurvey (with permission). Ten-year survival following hepatectomy for colorectal liver metastases comparing those who were resected (*n* = 6519) to those patients who only underwent exploratory laparotomy (*n* = 393).

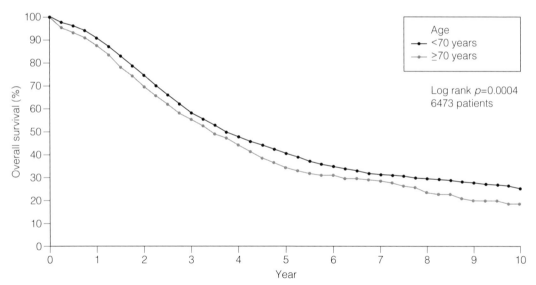

Figure 6.9 • LiverMetSurvey (with permission). Ten-year survival following hepatectomy for colorectal liver metastases comparing those <70 years of age (*n* = 5189) to those patients >70 years of age (*n* = 1284).

contact with the inferior vena cava, invasion of all three hepatic veins, the presence of coeliac lymph nodes and the presence of non-resectable extrahepatic disease[19] (**Figs. 6.10–6.13**).

The 'one centimetre rule'

These new standards clearly challenge the '1 cm rule', which required that liver resection only be attempted if a margin of at least 1 cm could be achieved. Some studies, in fact, show that the width of the surgical margin has no effect on survival, so long as the margin is microscopically clear.[20] However, in a study of 1019 patients, uniformly resected using the clamp-crushing technique, patients with a >1 cm margin had a statistically significant improvement in long-term outcome when compared with patients with lesser margins.[21] It was emphasised that even in patients with subcentimetre resections, the long-term survival is still favourable and inability

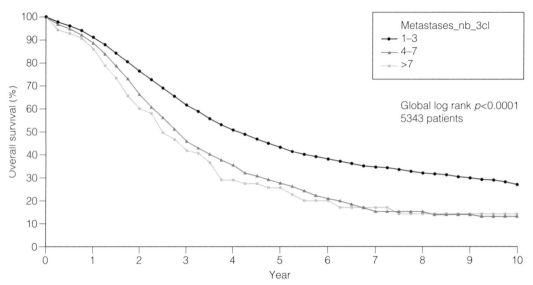

Figure 6.10 • LiverMetSurvey (with permission). Ten-year survival following hepatectomy for colorectal liver metastases comparing those who were resected with one to three metastases (*n* = 4225) to those patients who were resected with four to seven (*n* = 858) and eight or more metastases (*n* = 260).

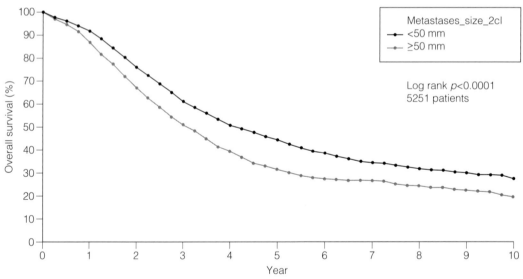

Figure 6.11 • LiverMetSurvey (with permission). Ten-year survival following hepatectomy for colorectal liver metastases comparing those who were resected with metastases <50 mm diameter (*n* = 3808) to those patients who were resected with metastases >50 mm diameter (*n* = 1443).

to obtain >1 cm margin should not preclude hepatic resection. Differing parenchymal transaction techniques potentially confound the effect of margin width and it should also be recognised that several millimetres worth of resection margin may be removed during the course of liver transection, if an ultrasonic aspirating dissector (CUSA) is used so that a margin that appeared adequate during surgery may then be reported as inadequate by the pathologist.[1] It is also possible to destroy a field of liver parenchyma adjacent to the resection margin with argon beam coagulation or ablative therapy to a depth of several millimetres.

Without resection very few patients with colorectal liver metastases are alive 5 years after their detection.

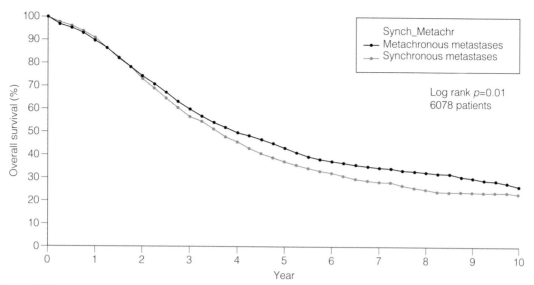

Figure 6.12 • LiverMetSurvey (with permission). Ten-year survival following hepatectomy for colorectal liver metastases comparing those who were resected with synchronous metastases (*n* = 2965) to those patients who were resected with metachronous metastases (*n* = 3113).

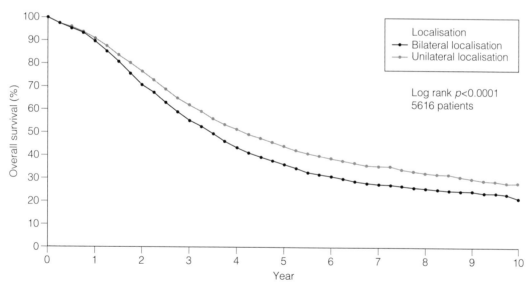

Figure 6.13 • LiverMetSurvey (with permission). Ten-year survival following hepatectomy for colorectal liver metastases comparing those who were resected with unilateral metastases (*n* = 3385) to those patients who were resected with bilateral metastases (*n* = 2231).

New surgical strategies to improve resectability

Portal vein embolisation

New surgical strategies have been increasingly employed in patients with unresectable CRLMs to improve resectability. Portal vein embolisation (PVE) induces atrophy of the liver to be resected and hypertrophy of the liver that will remain (i.e. increases the future liver remnant) with the aim of avoiding post-resection hepatic insufficiency, liver failure and death (**Fig. 6.14**). A meta-analysis of 1088 patients confirms that this technique increases significantly the FLR, making more patients suitable for liver resection.[22] The overall morbidity rate was 2.2% without mortality. Following PVE,

930 (85%) of patients underwent attempted major hepatectomy, which proved not feasible in 158 (17%) patients; 131 patients did not undergo laparotomy after PVE due to inadequate hypertrophy of the FLR or due to disease progression. Before and after PVE, all patients underwent volumetric assessment of liver volumes, which serves as a surrogate marker of remnant liver function. Although there is no consensus on what constitutes a safe volume of remnant liver, minimum values of 20–25% for patients with normal livers, 30% following chemotherapy and 40% in the presence of chronic liver disease have been suggested.[5,23,24] PVE appears to be safe, even when combined with neoadjuvant chemotherapy[25] (**Figs. 6.14 and 6.15**).

Two-stage hepatectomy

Similarly, two-stage hepatectomy involves delayed rehepatectomy after hypertrophy of the residual liver and may be used for large bilateral lesions in which a one-stage resection of all the involved segments would lead to liver failure.[26] The first stage involves the lesser resection of metastases from the FLR followed by a period of liver regeneration and, typically, PVE (or ligation during surgery) and chemotherapy. The second stage is performed 2–3 months later and consists of the major hepatectomy. One- and 3-year survival rates were 70.0% and 54.4% respectively in 25 of 33 patients in whom a two-stage hepatectomy could be completed.[27] There was no operative mortality; postoperative morbidity was 15.1% and 56.0% after first- and second-stage hepatectomy respectively (**Fig. 6.16**).

Repeat hepatectomy

Repeat hepatectomy for patients with colorectal cancer metastases is safe and provides survival benefit equal to that of a first liver resection. A meta-analysis of 21 studies, comprising 3741 patients, showed that there was no difference in

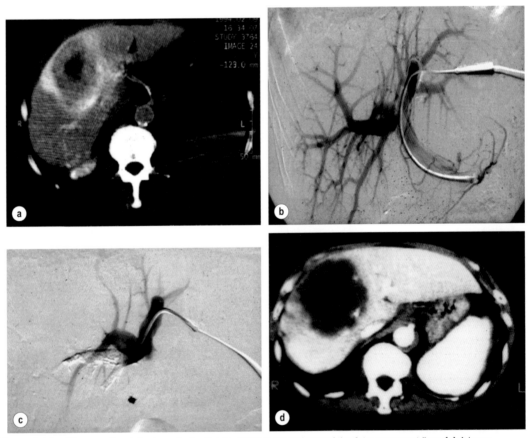

Figure 6.14 • The use of portal vein embolisation to increase the volume of the future remnant liver. **(a)** A large metastasis involving segments 4, 5 and 8 with a small left lateral segment. **(b,c)** Percutaneous catheterisation of the left portal vein, subsequently embolising the anterior and posterior divisions of the right portal vein. **(d)** The hyperplastic left lateral segment (FRL) 4 weeks later, prior to subsequently successful extended right hepatectomy.

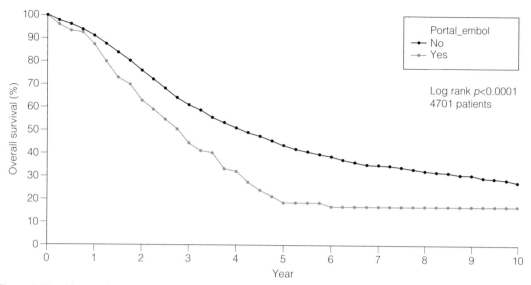

Figure 6.15 • LiverMetSurvey (with permission). Ten-year survival following hepatectomy for colorectal liver metastases comparing those who were initially resectable at detection (*n* = 4320) to those patients who were brought to resection using portal vein embolisation (*n* = 381).

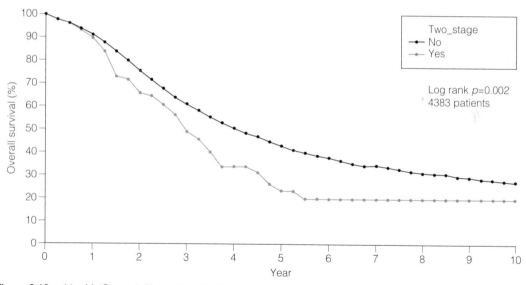

Figure 6.16 • LiverMetSurvey (with permission). Ten-year survival following hepatectomy for colorectal liver metastases comparing those who were initially resectable at detection (*n* = 4160) to those patients who underwent a two-stage liver resection to eradicate all disease detected at presentation (*n* = 223).

perioperative morbidity, mortality or long-term survival between patients undergoing a first or a repeat hepatectomy[28] (**Fig. 6.17**).

Extreme liver surgery

Resection of tumours involving the hepatic vascular inflow have been described, utilising a variety of techniques, including portal vein resection and reconstruction, hepatic artery resection and reconstruction (or arterialisation of the portal vein as an alternative).[29] Resection of tumours with involvement of the inferior vena cava (IVC) or the three major hepatic veins has also been performed, using techniques such as total hepatic vascular exclusion, in situ hypothermic perfusion and ex vivo (bench) hepatic resection.[30–32] These techniques are at the frontier of what is currently feasible and are associated with significant morbidity and mortality. Nonetheless, this aggressive surgical

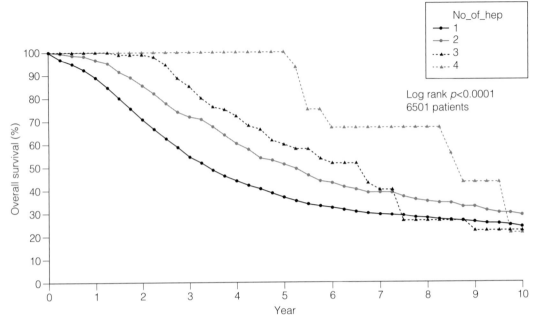

Figure 6.17 • LiverMetSurvey (with permission). Ten-year survival following hepatectomy for colorectal liver metastases comparing those who underwent one (*n* = 5657) or repeated liver resections on two (*n* = 721), three (*n* = 105) or four (*n* = 18) occasions.

approach may offer hope for patients with hepatic tumours involving the IVC, who would otherwise have a poor prognosis.

Extrahepatic colorectal disease

Extrahepatic colorectal metastases may be resected with curative intent, such as direct diaphragmatic invasion, adrenal metastases and lung metastases that are few in number and readily resectable. Reported long-term survival after pneumonectomy for colorectal metastases mirrors very closely that seen after hepatectomy (overall median survival at 5 years after thoracotomy of 41%), with similar low operative morbidity and mortality[33,34] (**Fig. 6.18**).

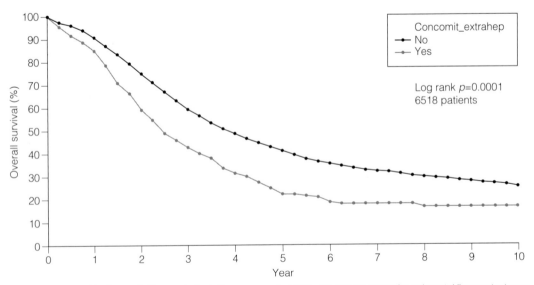

Figure 6.18 • LiverMetSurvey (with permission). Ten-year survival following hepatectomy for colorectal liver metastases comparing those who were resected with metastases confined to the liver (*n* = 5884) to those patients who were resected with both resectable liver and extrahepatic metastases (*n* = 634).

Using these advanced techniques, more than 20% of patients with colorectal liver metastases can be brought to surgical resection with curative intent.

New technologies for liver resection: better than the old?

Transection techniques

Technological innovations in liver surgery have mainly focused on minimising blood loss during transection of the hepatic parenchyma, because excessive blood loss and the associated need for blood transfusion are associated with increased postoperative morbidity and mortality, as well as reduced long-term survival.[35] Inflow occlusion (Pringle manoeuvre) and low central venous pressure (CVP) anaesthesia minimise blood loss but may cause liver damage by ischaemia and reperfusion injury. Consequently, there has been a growing interest in new devices that facilitate a more bloodless liver transection, obviating the need for inflow occlusion associated with the traditional clamp-crushing technique.

The most popular of these techniques include the ultrasonic aspirating dissector (CUSA) using ultrasonic energy, the Hydojet using a pressurised jet of water and the dissecting sealer (TissueLink) using radiofrequency energy. Most evidence with these techniques is retrospective but a recent randomised controlled trial compared all four of the aforementioned techniques in CRLMs.[36] The clamp-crushing technique was the most efficient in terms of resection time, blood loss and blood transfusion requirement compared with the other techniques. It was also the most cost efficient, with a cost saving potential of between 600 and 2400 euros per case. The degree of postoperative reperfusion injury (transaminase level) and complication rate were not significantly different among the groups. A randomised clinical trial of radiofrequency-assisted versus clamp-crushing transection in 50 patients showed a higher rate of postoperative complications: abscess in six, biliary fistula in three and biliary stenosis in one patient in the radiofrequency group, compared with none in the clamp-crushing group.[37]

Fibrin sealants

Fibrin sealants have also become popular as a means of improving perioperative haemostasis and reducing biliary leakage after liver surgery. However, a randomised study of 300 patients showed no differences in transfusion requirement, overall drainage, incidence of biliary fistula or postoperative morbidity between those receiving fibrin glue application and controls.[38] Application of fibrin sealant may be difficult to justify; its discontinuation from use would result in considerable cost savings. Pressure on healthcare costs is likely to focus scrutiny on expensive transection and sealant devices, especially where simpler techniques with comparable or better efficacy are available.

Laparoscopic liver surgery: less is more?

Laparoscopic surgery for hepatic neoplasms aims to provide curative resection while minimising complications. A meta-analysis of series published between 1998 and 2005 has been performed,[39] including eight non-randomised studies, reporting on 409 resections of hepatic neoplasms, of which 165 (40.3%) were laparoscopic and 244 (59.7%) were open. Operative blood loss and duration of hospital stay were reduced significantly after laparoscopic surgery. These findings remained consistent when considering studies matched for the presence of malignancy and segment resection. There was no difference in postoperative adverse events and extent of oncological clearance. The largest single-centre experience subsequently published reported on 300 minimally invasive procedures compared to 100 contemporaneous, cohort-matched open resections.[40] The majority of the resections in the minimally invasive group were for benign pathology but included 60 resections for 'metastatic tumours'. Resections comprised 110 segmentectomies, 63 bisegmentectomies, 47 left hepatectomies, 64 right hepatectomies, eight extended right hepatectomies and eight caudate lobe resections. Laparoscopic resections compared favourably with standard open techniques: operative times (99 vs. 182 min), blood loss (102 vs. 325 ml), transfusion requirement (2 of 300 vs. 8 of 100), length of stay (1.9 vs. 5.4 days), overall operative complications (9.3% vs. 22%) and local malignancy recurrence (2% vs. 3%).

Laparoscopic resection has the potential to reduce operative blood loss and earlier recovery with oncological clearance comparable with open surgery. Because of the potential of significant bias arising from case series, randomised controlled trials are recommended, to eliminate bias and to compare long-term survival rates.

Morbidity, mortality and survival after liver resection for CRLMs

The utility of surgical resection of CRLMs is clearly established. A large number of substantial prospective and retrospective studies consistently show 5-year survival rates following liver resection of 30–50%, depending on selection criteria. A major systematic review of surgical resection for CRLMs was undertaken to assess the published evidence for its efficacy and safety and to identify prognostic factors.[41] Thirty independent studies met all the eligibility criteria for the review and data on 30-day mortality and morbidity only were included from a further nine studies. The best available evidence came from prospective case series, but only two studies reported outcomes for all patients undergoing surgery. The remainder reported outcomes for selected groups of patients: those undergoing hepatic resection or those undergoing curative resection.

Death within 30 days of hepatic resection was reported by 24 studies, ranging from 0% to 6.6% of patients (median 2.8%). A further nine studies reported perioperative mortality within an undefined time period (1.3–4.6%, median 3.6%) and two studies reported 60-day mortality (3.4–5.5%). Mortality was not reported by four studies. Cause of death was reported by 15 studies for a total of 103 patients. The commonest specified causes of fatal complications were, in descending order of frequency: hepatic failure, postoperative haemorrhage, generalised sepsis, cardiac failure, multiorgan failure, pulmonary embolism, bile leak and anastomotic leak.[41]

Perioperative complications, including indicators of morbidity such as length of hospital stay, were reported by 29 studies. Commonest causes of both fatal and non-fatal morbidity, again in descending order of frequency, were: wound infection (5.4%), generalised sepsis (4.6%), pleural effusion (4.3%), bile leak (4.0%), perihepatic abscess (3.0%), hepatic failure (2.8%), arrhythmia (2.8%), postoperative haemorrhage (2.7%), cardiac failure (2.4%) and pneumonia (1.9%).

Two studies reported overall survival at 5 years for all patients undergoing surgery (resection and laparotomy only), median 23% (15–31%). Studies in which it was unclear whether resections were R0 or R1/2, or only presented data for both types of resection combined, had a median 5-year survival of 32% (9–63%). Sixteen studies presented 5-year survival for patients undergoing R0 resection, either for the whole study population or for subgroups of patients. Median 5-year survival for these studies was 30% (range 15–67%). Eleven studies reporting 5-year survival for nonradical resections had a median 5-year survival of 7.2% (range 0–30%), and six studies reporting patients who did not undergo resection had a median 5-year survival of 0% (range 0–6%). Disease-free survival was reported by fewer studies. Median disease-free survival was a median 14.3 months for radically resected patients and a

median of 17.2 months for patients with unspecified resections.

Twenty-two percent of all patients experienced recurrence in the liver only, although this is likely to be underestimated as two studies did not specify the proportion of liver-only recurrences. Liver plus extrahepatic recurrences and extrahepatic-only recurrences were experienced by 16% and 24% of patients respectively. In addition, one study reported recurrences in 235 (62.5%) radically resected patients, although sites of recurrence were not specified.

This systematic review was undertaken because ascertaining the benefits of surgical resection of colorectal hepatic metastases is difficult in the absence of randomised trials. However, it is clear that there is a biologically distinct group of patients with liver metastases who may become long-term disease-free survivors following hepatic resection. Such survival is rare in apparently comparable patients who do not have surgical treatment.

The value of these new treatment strategies is reenforced by LiverMetSurvey, a prospective international registry of surgically treated patients with CRLMs.[42] This collects, on a multi-institutional basis, data concerning the demography, treatment (chemotherapy, surgery, combined ablation) and outcome, and analyses prospectively the results of surgically treated patients. Ultimately, it aims to define guidelines of optimal treatment and strategy, and will be particularly useful in those clinical situations that remain controversial with regards to the benefit of surgery or to its combination with other therapies.

Classification of CRLMs

Staging systems and terminology

As the definition of resectability has changed, so too has the classification of CRLMs. The 2003 French guidelines on the management of CRLMs recommended four categories that could be defined: (i) easily resectable liver metastases, (ii) resectable liver metastases involving five to six liver segments and/or contralateral major vascular structures, (iii) liver metastases that are initially unresectable but may become resectable after chemotherapy and (iv) definitely unresectable.[43] It was recommended that patients with tumours in the second class should only undergo resection by experienced liver surgeons working within a recognised major liver unit but that tumours in the first class should be within the ability of most hepatobiliary surgeons. Since these guidelines were produced, progress in surgical and medical oncology has increased the proportion of patients deemed resectable from the outset and the proportion that become resectable after pre-operative chemotherapy.

The present American Joint Committee on Cancer (AJCC) stage IV does not distinguish between patients who are currently incurable, with a prognosis of less than 6 months, from those who are potentially curable. A recent proposal distinguished between a stage IV-R for patients with resectable disease and a stage IV-U for patients with unresectable disease.[44,45] Furthermore, stage IV-R could be further divided into IV-Ra (resectable liver only), IV-Rb (resectable extrahepatic only) and IV-Rc (resectable hepatic and extrahepatic). Stage IV-U could be similarly subdivided, after assessment by an experienced site-specific surgical oncologist.

Alternatively, the European Colorectal Metastases Treatment group has proposed a staging system based upon the French classification:[19]

- IVa – easily resectable with curative intent at detection (French classification 1)
- IVb – technically difficult/borderline resectable at detection (French classification 2)
- IVc – potentially resectable after neo-therapeutic chemotherapy
- IVd – little or no hope of being rendered resectable with curative intent after conventional chemotherapy
- Va – resectable extrahepatic disease
- Vb – unresectable extrahepatic disease.

Such systems require prospective validation but would allow clinicians to stratify patients according to prognosis, guide therapeutic decisions, and allow comparison of results of radical and non-radical treatments.

'Downstaging' of colorectal liver metastases

Studies of modern chemotherapy for unresectable CRLMs

In the past, 5-fluorouracil (5-FU) with folinic acid (leucovorin) was the only chemotherapy available for patients with unresectable CRLMs, but this rarely provided sufficient intrahepatic tumoricidal effect to render disease resectable. Modern chemotherapeutic regimens combining 5-FU, folinic acid and oxaliplatin and/or irinotecan are associated with much higher response rates and can allow 10–30% of patients with initially unresectable disease to be treated successfully with liver surgery (Table 6.1).[26,46–50]

The largest study reported so far[26] was a consecutive series of 1104 patients who were initially considered unresectable and treated with chemotherapy (5-FU and folinic acid combined with oxaliplatin (70%), irinotecan (7%), or both (4%)); 138 (12.5%) had a good response to chemotherapy, enabling potentially curative liver surgery to be performed in 93% of cases. Recurrence was frequent but treated in 52 patients by repeat hepatectomy (71 procedures) and by extrahepatic resection in 42 patients (77 procedures). Survival was 33% and 23% at 5 and 10 years respectively, although this was significantly lower than that of patients resected primarily within the same period at the same institution (48% and 30% at 5 and 10 years respectively). Subsequent trials have confirmed the ability of modern chemotherapy to render patients resectable (Table 6.1). The best combination or sequence of systemic therapies is not yet clear but is the subject of current clinical studies (**Fig. 6.19**).

Table 6.1 • Summary of studies evaluating modern neoadjuvant chemotherapy in patients with initially unresectable colorectal liver metastases

Reference	Number of patients	Chemotherapy	Number of curative (R0) resections	Survival
Adam (2004)[26]*	1104	5-FU/LV/OX and/or IR	129 (11.7%)	5-year: 33% 10-year: 23%
Pozzo (2004)[46]	40	5-FU/LV/IR	13 (32.5%)	MDFS: 14.3 months
Tournigand (2004)[49]	109 111	5-FU/LV/IR 5-FU/LV/OX	8 (7%) 14 (13%)	MOS: 47 months MOS: not reached
Alberts (2005)[47]	42	5-FU/LV/OX	14 (33.3%)	3-year: 67%
Ho (2005)[50]	40	5-FU/LV/IR	4 (10%)	MOS: 33 months
Masi (2006)[48]	74	5-FU/LV/OX/IR	12 (16.2%)	4-year: 37%

Abbreviations: 5-FU, 5-fluorouracil; IR, irinotecan; LV, leucovorin; MDFS, median disease-free survival; MOS, median overall survival; OX, oxaliplatin.

*This updates previous studies from the Hopital Paul Brousse group.

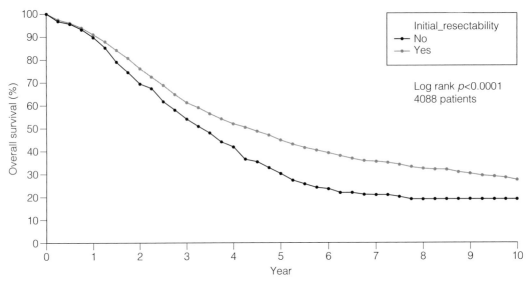

Figure 6.19 • LiverMetSurvey (with permission). Ten-year survival following hepatectomy for colorectal liver metastases comparing those who were initially resectable at detection to those patients who were considered initially unresectable but were brought to resection using systemic chemotherapy.

Patient selection and timing of surgery

Cross-study comparison is hampered by variation in the definition of what constitutes 'unresectability'. Recently, a shift has occurred in the criteria used for assessing resectability, from morphological criteria to new ones based on whether a macroscopically and microscopically complete (R0) resection of the liver can be achieved while leaving an adequate future liver remnant (FLR).[1,5,51] Although the FLR limit for safe resection varies in those patients with an otherwise normal liver, the safe FLR volume is at least 20%. An additional benefit of neoadjuvant chemotherapy on patient selection is that response to chemotherapy may well be a surrogate marker for the success of liver surgery.[52,53] Few patients who experience progression on chemotherapy and yet maintain resectable disease are alive 5 years after hepatectomy.

To optimise the timing of resection, repeat imaging should be obtained during chemotherapy. Resection should take place as soon as neoadjuvant chemotherapy renders the lesions resectable, rather than continued to best response. This strategy avoids unnecessary hepatic injury associated with prolonged chemotherapy and reduces the difficulty of interpretation of imaging caused by the absence of visible tumour and by chemotherapy-induced steatosis. This concept has been reinforced by a recent study, which demonstrated that for most patients, a complete radiological response does not mean a cure. In 55 (83%) of 66 CRLMs that had a complete

radiological response to chemotherapy, persistent macroscopic or microscopic residual disease was found in those who underwent surgery, or recurred in situ within 1 year in those who did not.[54]

Chemotherapy-associated steatohepatitis

The consequences of intra-arterial hepatic chemotherapy and systemic chemotherapy with 5-FU are well recognised, but increasing use of neoadjuvant treatment means that 'chemotherapy-associated steatohepatitis (CASH)' has become more common. The term 'blue liver syndrome' has also been used to describe the vascular alterations that result in bluish discoloration, oedema and a spongiform consistency similar to that seen with early cirrhosis.[55] Objective evidence is derived from a recent study that compared 45 patients who received systemic chemotherapy less than 2 months prior to major liver resection with 22 patients who did not receive any chemotherapy in the 6 months prior to resection.[56] There were no postoperative deaths in either group but postoperative complications were significantly more common in the chemotherapy group, occurring in 17 of 45 patients (37.8%) compared to 3 of 22 patients (13.6%) in the no-chemotherapy group ($p = 0.03$). Liver failure occurred in five patients in the chemotherapy group but did not occur in the no-chemotherapy group. Moreover, postoperative morbidity was correlated with the number of cycles of chemotherapy administered before surgery. Pathological examination of the

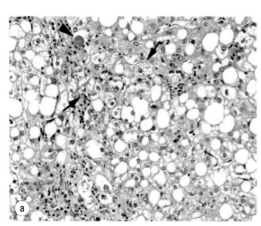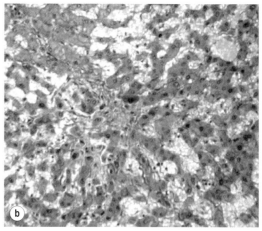

Figure 6.20 • Effects of preoperative chemotherapy on the subsequently operated liver. **(a)** Steatohepatitis which is seen following excessive pretreatment with irinotecan. The features of ballooned hepatocytes (arrowhead) and Mallory bodies (arrows) are shown. **(b)** Sinusoidal congestion and thrombosis seen after excessive pretreatment with oxaliplatin.

non-tumourous liver parenchyma showed that systemic chemotherapy was associated with microvascular changes, such as sinusoidal dilatation, atrophy of hepatocytes and hepatocyte necrosis.

Other studies have shown that postoperative complications and mortality are significantly more common after chemotherapy. In a recent study that included 248 patients who received preoperative chemotherapy, oxaliplatin was associated with sinusoidal dilatation and irinotecan with steatohepatitis (**Fig. 6.20**). Moreover, patients with steatohepatitis had increased 90-day mortality.[57] Sinusoidal injury has been significantly associated with higher morbidity and longer hospital stay in patients with CRLMs who underwent major hepatectomy after oxaliplatin-based chemotherapy.[58] This sinusoidal injury resulted in a poorer liver functional reserve preoperatively, as measured by the indocyanine green method. This factor, along with abnormal preoperative aspartate transaminase (AST), female gender and the administration of six or more cycles of oxaliplatin, were independent risk factors for sinusoidal injury.

Clearly the advent of neoadjuvant chemotherapy will present challenges as well as benefits. Greater knowledge of the pathogenesis of CASH is required. Currently, it is prudent to require a larger FLR of at least 30% after resection, in patients who have received extensive preoperative systemic chemotherapy.[5] It is apparent that liver damage is a product of life-saving chemotherapy. Newer agents, such as bevacizumab, may affect wound healing and liver regeneration. Therefore research is needed to elucidate the pathogenesis of CASH and find new therapies that will modulate these new toxicities. A crucial unanswered question is how long new therapies should be withheld before surgery is safe.

Adjuvant and 'perioperative' chemotherapy

That adjuvant chemotherapy improves the cure rate in early stage colorectal cancer indicates that it eradicates residual microscopic disease in some patients. As these are the source of ultimately fatal recurrences in patients who experience disease relapse after liver surgery, the logic of extrapolating the experience of adjuvant therapy after early stage colorectal cancer to the resected CRLM setting appears sound. In a study evaluating chemotherapy with 5-FU, folinic acid and oxaliplatin (FOLFOX) 3 months before and 3 months after the operation (**Fig. 6.21**), patients with initially resectable liver metastases from colorectal cancer chemotherapy had improved outcome and progression-free survival compared with patients who were treated with surgery alone.[59]

Hepatic arterial infusion

Hepatic arterial infusion chemotherapy (HAC) maximises hepatic drug exposure by delivering drugs via the hepatic artery and by using agents with high first-pass hepatic extraction rates. The principle is based on the understanding that metastases derive their blood supply largely from the hepatic artery whereas the normal liver is mainly supplied by the portal vein. Trials of a multimodality approach that combine systemic chemotherapy with hepatic arterial infusion chemotherapy show high response rates and the possibility of conversion to resectability of CRLMs that have progressed on prior systemic regimens.[60] Further studies of this approach are warranted.

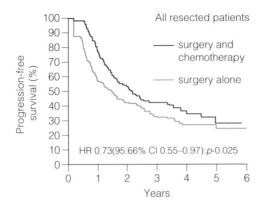

Figure 6.21 • The 33% improvement in 3-year disease-free survival demonstrated following perioperative chemotherapy using oxaliplatin compared to surgery alone for colorectal liver metastases in the EPOC trial (EORTC 40983).[57]

Number of patients at risk

Surgery	152	85	59	39	24	10
PeriOpCT	151	118	76	45	23	6

Downstaging or downsizing: neoadjuvant versus neotherapeutic chemotherapy

Recent advances have highlighted the deficiencies of our nomenclature on advanced colorectal cancer. There is clearly a difference between true neoadjuvant chemotherapy, having determined that the patient is resectable with curative intent at the outset and the administration of chemotherapy to patients with unresectable CRLMs, with the intention of rendering this disease resectable. A better term might be 'neotherapeutic chemotherapy' or 'induction chemotherapy', to differentiate this latter intention from that of true neoadjuvant chemotherapy.[44,45]

Monoclonal antibodies

Trials evaluating novel biological agents, such as the monoclonal antibodies (mAb) directed against vascular endothelial growth factor (VEGF), e.g. bevacizumab, and epidermal growth factor receptor (EGFR), e.g. cetuximab, matuzumab, panitumumab and nimotuzumab, hold out hope that even more patients with initially unresectable CRLMs may respond to treatment with combinations of biological agents and systemic treatments.

The epidermal growth factor receptor

The EGFR is a transmembrane glycoprotein that consists of an extracellular ligand-binding domain, a transmembrane domain and an intracellular domain with tyrosine kinase activity for signal transduction. Activation signals multiple biological processes including apoptosis, differentiation, cellular proliferation and regulation of survival. It enhances several processes responsible for tumour growth and progression, including proliferation, angiogenesis, invasion and metastasis, and inhibition of apoptosis. High expression of EGFR has been observed in several cancers and is expressed in 75–90% of colorectal cancers, especially in regions of deepest invasion and in advanced disease.[61]

Cetuximab is a recombinant, human/mouse chimeric immunoglobulin G1 mAb that binds specifically to the extracellular domain of the human EGFR and is the most advanced anti-EGFR mAb in clinical development. It has been approved for treatment of patients with metastatic colorectal cancer with tumours expressing EGFR and refractory to irinotecan in the USA and Europe based on the results of the BOND study, where the combination of cetuximab and irinotecan had a greater response rate, time to progression and overall survival, compared with cetuximab monotherapy.[62] Response was greatest in patients who developed an acne-like skin rash, which has led to the hypothesis that this rash may be a surrogate marker of treatment efficacy with cetuximab.[63] Efficacy has also been demonstrated in a number of trials that combined cetuximab with oxaliplatin- and irinotecan-based regimens in first-line therapy in patients with metastatic colorectal cancer,[61] and is being investigated currently in the pre- and postoperative setting in patients with resectable CRLMs (New EPOC trial).

Adam and colleagues have reported the outcome of 25 patients who underwent resection for CRLMs after stabilisation or response using cetuximab with irinotecan- or oxaliplatin-containing regimens. Patients were treated with cetuximab as second-line or higher-line chemotherapy after the failure of first-line chemotherapy.[64] Among 133 patients treated for unresectable or marginally resectable disease, nine (7%) subsequently underwent successful resection. Thus, the addition of cetuximab allowed 7% of patients with disease refractory to first-line therapy to undergo resection, thereby increasing the number of patients able to undergo resection from the previously reported 14% resectability rate achieved by the same institution after first-line, oxaliplatin-based chemotherapy without biological therapy for unresectable disease.[26] This improvement in resectability is consistent with the

10–16% additional response rate achieved with cetuximab, and with a previous analysis reporting an almost linear correlation between response and resectability for metastases confined to the liver.[65]

Vascular endothelial growth factor

VEGF is one of the most important regulators of the dynamic balance between proangiogenic and antiangiogenic factors that are crucial to the facilitation of tumour growth and metastasis. It stimulates proliferation and migration of endothelial cells and enhances microvascular permeability. VEGF is upregulated in a variety of human cancers and there is increasing evidence that anti-VEGF agents have a direct antiangiogenic effect and an additive or synergistic antitumour effect because of an improvement on delivery of chemotherapy by altering tumour vasculature.[61]

Bevacizumab has been approved for use as first-line treatment of metastatic colorectal cancer in combination with any fluorouracil-containing regimen, and is currently being studied in second-line and adjuvant settings.

There are concerns, however, that the anti-VEGF effects of bevacizumab may have a negative effect on liver regeneration and wound healing in a neo-adjuvant setting and an unresolved question is how long new therapies, such as bevacizumab, should be withheld before surgery is safe.

What role for ablative therapies?

Ablative therapy takes numerous forms. Cryotherapy, laser hyperthermia and ethanol injection are decreasing in popularity due to high complication rates or lack of efficacy. Radiofrequency ablation (RFA) has significant advantages over older ablative techniques and is increasingly used. Clarification of whether ablation is equal to surgery for resectable CRLMs or whether it offers additional survival benefit over modern systemic chemotherapy in the treatment of non-resectable disease awaits the outcome of clinical trials. Technological advances are focused on faster and more powerful delivery systems, using electrolytic and microwave destruction systems.

Cryotherapy

Cryotherapy, involving circulation of liquid nitrogen through metallic probes inserted into the tumour, results in rapid freezing of tissue to produce tumour necrosis. This technique has largely been abandoned because of its high complication rate and mortality rate of about 7%. Specific complications include major haemorrhage from cracking of the liver parenchyma and capsule during thawing and cryoshock, a syndrome of severe coagulopathy, disseminated intravascular coagulopathy and multiple organ failure.[66]

Radiofrequency ablation (RFA)

RFA has largely superseded cryotherapy, because of its superior safety profile. However, a major limitation is the increased risk of local recurrence and diminished survival with lesions greater than 2 cm.[67] RFA produces localised tumour destruction by means of alternating current passing through the RFA needle to create local tissue temperatures of 70–100°C, resulting in cell death through protein denaturation and microvascular injury.[68]

Much of the current interest in RFA derives from its low morbidity and mortality. A recent meta-analysis of 95 published series reported a complication rate of 8.9%, with intra-abdominal bleeding, sepsis and biliary tree injury being the commonest complications,[67] and mortality rates range from 0% to 0.5%. RFA has a high rate of local recurrence, ranging from 1.8% to 12% with a surgical approach, to as high as 40% with percutaneous placement. Undoubtedly, this relates to the type of lesions being treated by RFA. Ablative therapies are often used for the treatment of metastases that are often too close to major vascular structures to be considered resectable with a clear margin. Just as a surgical margin would be likely to be compromised, blood flow will conduct away heat, leading to incomplete ablation and recurrence.

The efficacy of RFA in unresectable CRLMs has been established by several large cohort studies with median survivals of 29–36 months being achieved.[69] There are currently no prospective randomised controlled trials to show an advantage for RFA over chemotherapy alone in unresectable CRLMs, but this deficiency is being addressed by a trial of chemotherapy plus local ablation versus chemotherapy alone (the CLOCC trial). A significant improvement in the chemotherapy plus RFA group would provide strong evidence of its value. While surgical resection remains the current standard of care, RFA may have a future role in combination with surgery as part of the effort to expand the definition of resectability.

Microwave ablation

Microwave ablation has been designed to overcome the limitations of previous ablative techniques. Under imaging guidance, the tumour is localised and a thin microwave antenna is placed directly into it. Electromagnetic microwaves agitate water molecules in the surrounding tissue, produce friction and heat, inducing tumour cell death by coagulation necrosis. The main advantages of microwave technology, when compared with existing techniques such as RFA and cryotherapy, include consistently higher intratumoural temperatures, larger tumour ablation volumes and faster ablation times.[70] In particular, low-frequency systems allow tumours of up to 8 cm to be successfully treated.

Selective internal radiation treatment (SIRT)

SIRT is the delivery of radiation treatment via intrahepatic arterial administration of yttrium-90 (Y-90) microspheres. Y-90 is a high-energy, beta-particle-emitting isotope. Resin microspheres measure 20–40 µm, remain in the liver permanently and have been approved for use in CRLMs. Selectivity is due to the preferential supply of tumour from the hepatic artery. Because of the half-life of Y-90 (2.67 days), 94% of the radiation dose is delivered during the 11 days following treatment.[71]

The first randomised phase 3 trial in 74 patients with CRLMs compared SIRT plus hepatic intra-arterial chemotherapy (HAC) with floxuridine versus HAC alone. In the combination treatment arm, a significantly increased complete and partial response rate, prolonged time to disease progression and a trend towards improved survival were observed.[72]

Complications of SIRT include a transient abdominal pain, fever, lethargy and nausea in up to one-third of patients. Gastroduodenal ulcers have been reported and are avoided by a meticulous administration technique that avoids reflux of Y-90 microspheres into the gastrointestinal vasculature. Because of the short range of beta particles, distant organs, such as gonads, are not subjected to beta radiation. SIRT-associated hepatic injury differs from the veno-occlusive injury associated with external beam irradiation and manifests as a cholangiopathy, because of the deposition of the microspheres in the region of the portal triad and away from the central vein.[71]

Further clinical studies are required, in neoadjuvant and salvage settings, to clarify the role of SIRT in optimal multimodality treatment strategies.

Multidisciplinary team approach

The current management of CRLMs is complex and this is likely to become increasingly so in the future. Because most patients with colorectal liver metastases present to general surgeons and oncologists without a specialist interest in their management, a computer program (OncoSurge) has been created that identifies individual patient resectability and recommends optimal treatment strategies.[73,74] The RAND Corporation/University of California Los Angeles Appropriateness Method (RAM) was used to assess strategies of resection, local ablation and chemotherapy. After a comprehensive literature review, an expert panel rated appropriateness of each treatment option for a total of 1872 ratings decisions in 252 cases. A decision model was constructed, consensus measured and results validated using 48 virtual cases and 34 real cases with known outcomes. Consensus was achieved with overall agreement rates of 93.4–99.1%.

The OncoSurge decision model allows a clinician to derive a choice of treatment strategies for an individual patient with colorectal liver metastases and compares this choice with the expert's view. Thus, the OncoSurge strategy combines the best available scientific evidence with the collective judgement of worldwide experts to yield a statement regarding the appropriateness of performing liver resection and/or local destruction, with or without chemotherapy for each patient. The computer program can be accessed at www.evidis.com/oncosurge.

Multidisciplinary teams are becoming increasingly common but are not yet ubiquitous. It should be stressed that in order to exploit every opportunity to achieve cure, the management of CRLMs should be undertaken in a multidisciplinary setting, with a medical and surgical oncologist involved in the care of every patient.[75]

Conclusions

The key recent advance in the management of CRLMs has been the availability of new, more effective chemotherapy, with the ability to convert inoperable liver disease to resectability. In tandem, surgery for patients with colorectal liver metastases has been applied in a wider range of clinical circumstances. Furthermore, the practice of re-resecting subsequent metastases has become more established as a viable life-prolonging and, in some cases, life-saving procedure. With this combined modality approach, the key contemporary developments in surgery and chemotherapy for CRLMs are brought together into an integrated framework to create a significantly expanded population of patients who can be treated with curative intent. By bringing surgical and medical paradigms together, significant advances can now be made.

Key points

- Surgery is the only treatment that offers the prospect of cure for CRLMs. The criteria now used for assessing resectability are based on whether a macroscopically and microscopically complete (R0) resection of the liver can be achieved, and whether the volume of the liver remaining after resection will be adequate.
- New surgical strategies to improve resectability include portal vein embolisation, two-stage hepatectomies, re-resection and serial liver resections, and resection of extrahepatic colorectal metastases with curative intent.
- Novel chemotherapeutic regimens combining 5-FU, folinic acid and oxaliplatin (FOLFOX) and/or irinotecan (FOLFIRI) can allow 10–30% of patients with initially unresectable disease to be successfully treated with liver surgery. Trials evaluating novel biological agents, such as bevacizumab and cetuximab, hold out hope that even more patients with initially unresectable CRLMs may respond to treatment with combinations of systemic treatments in the future.
- Increasing use of neoadjuvant treatment means that chemotherapy-associated steatohepatitis (CASH) has become more common and is associated with increased postoperative morbidity.
- The management of CRLMs should be undertaken in a multidisciplinary setting, with a medical and surgical oncologist involved in the care of every patient.

References

1. Poston GJ. Surgical strategies for colorectal liver metastases. Surg Oncol 2004; 13:125–36.

2. Weiss L, Grundmann E, Torhorst J et al. Hematogenous metastatic patterns in colonic carcinoma: an analysis of 1541 necropsies. J Pathol 1986; 150:195–203.

3. Stangl R, Altendorf-Hofmann A, Charnley RM et al. Factors influencing the natural history of colorectal liver metastases. Lancet 1994; 343:1405–10.

4. McLoughlin JM, Jensen EH, Malafa M. Resection of colorectal liver metastases. Cancer Control 2006; 13:32–41.

5. Abdalla EK, Adam R, Bilchik AJ et al. Improving respectability of hepatic colorectal metastases: expert consensus statement. Ann Surg Oncol 2006; 13:1271–80.

6. Saini S. Imaging of hepatobiliary tract. N Engl J Med 1997; 336:1889–94.

7. Martinez L, Puig I, Valls C. Colorectal liver metastases: radiological diagnosis and staging. Eur J Surg Oncol 2007; 33:S5–17.

8. Israel O, Mor M, Gaitini D et al. Combined structural and functional evaluation of cancer patients with a hybrid camera based PET/CT system using ^{18}F-FDG. J Nucl Med 2002; 43:1129–36.

9. D'Angelica M, Hiotis SP, Kim HJ et al. Laparoscopic staging for liver, biliary, pancreas, and gastric cancer. Curr Prob Surg 2007; 44:228–69.

10. de Castro SMM, Tilleman EHBM, Busch ORC et al. Diagnostic laparoscopy for primary and secondary liver malignancies: impact of improved imaging and changed criteria for resection. Ann Surg Oncol 2004; 11:522–9.

11. Rahusen FD, Cuesta MA, Borgstein PJ et al. Selection of patients for resection of colorectal metastases to the liver using diagnostic laparoscopy and laparoscopic ultrasonography. Ann Surg 1999; 230:31–7.

12. Koea J, Rodgers M, Thompson P et al. Laparoscopy in the management of colorectal cancer metastatic to the liver. Aust NZ J Surg 2004; 74:1056–9.

13. Metcalfe MS, Close JS, Iswariah H et al. The value of laparoscopic staging for patients with colorectal metastases. Arch Surg 2003; 138:770–2.

14. Grobmyer SR, Fong YM, D'Angelica M et al. Diagnostic laparoscopy prior to planned hepatic resection for colorectal metastases. Arch Surg 2004; 139:1326–30.

15. Fong Y, Fortner J, Sun RL et al. Clinical score for predicting recurrence after hepatic resection for metastatic colorectal cancer: analysis of 1001 consecutive cases. Ann Surg 1999; 230:309–18.

16. Elias D, Liberale G, Vernerey D et al. Hepatic and extrahepatic colorectal metastases: when resectable, their localization does not matter, but their total number has a prognostic effect. Ann Surg Oncol 2005; 12:900–9.

17. Minagawa M, Makuuchi M, Torzilli G et al. Extension of the frontiers of surgical indications in the treatment of liver metastases from colorectal cancer: long-term results. Ann Surg 2000; 231:487–99.

18. Vauthey JN, Pawlik TM, Abdalla EK et al. Is extended hepatectomy for hepatobiliary malignancy justified? Ann Surg 2004; 239:722–32.

19. Van Cutsem, Nordlinger B, Adam R et al. Towards a pan-European consensus on the treatment of patients with colorectal liver metastases. Eur J Cancer 2006; 42:2212–21.

20. Pawlik TM, Scoggins CR, Zorzi D et al. Effect of surgical margin status on survival and site of recurrence after hepatic resection for colorectal metastases. Ann Surg 2005; 241:715–24.

21. Are C, Gonen M, Zazzali K et al. The impact of margins on outcome after hepatic resection for colorectal metastases. Ann Surg 2007; 246:295–300.

22. Abulkhir A, Limongellin P, Healey AJ et al. Preoperative portal vein embolisation for major liver resection: a meta-analysis. Ann Surg 2008; 247:49–57.

23. Chun YS, Vauthey JN. Extending the frontiers of resectability in advanced colorectal cancer. Eur J Surg Oncol 2007; 33:S52–8.

24. Ribero D, Abdalla EK, Madoff DC et al. Portal vein embolisation before major hepatectomy and its effects on regeneration, resectability and outcome. Br J Surg 2007; 94:1386–94.

25. Covey AM, Brown KT, Jarnagin WR et al. Combined portal vein embolisation and neoadjuvant chemotherapy as a treatment strategy for resectable hepatic colorectal metastases. Ann Surg 2008; 247:451–5.

26. Adam R, Delvart V, Pascal G et al. Rescue surgery for unresectable colorectal liver metastases downstaged by chemotherapy: a model to predict longterm survival. Ann Surg 2004; 240:644–57.

27. Jaeck D, Oussoultzoglou E, Rosso E et al. A twostage hepatectomy procedure combined with portal vein embolization to achieve curative resection for initially unresectable multiple and bilobar colorectal liver metastases. Ann Surg 2004; 240:1037–51.

28. Antoniou A, Lovegrove RE, Tilney HS et al. Meta-analysis of clinical outcome after first and second liver resection for colorectal metastases. Surgery 2007; 141:9–18.

29. Kondo S, Hirano S, Ambo Y et al. Arterioportal shunting as an alternative to microvascular reconstruction after hepatic artery resection. Br J Surg 2004; 91:248–51.

30. Lodge JP, Ammori BJ, Prasad KR et al. Ex vivo and in situ resection of inferior vena cava with hepatectomy for colorectal metastases. Ann Surg 2000; 231:471–9.

31. Hemming AW, Reed AI, Langham MR Jr et al. Combined resection of the liver and inferior vena cava for hepatic malignancy. Ann Surg 2004; 239:712–21.

32. Azoulay D, Andreani P, Maggi U et al. Combined liver resection and reconstruction of the supra-renal vena cava: the Paul Brousse experience. Ann Surg 2006; 244:80–88.

33. Shiono S, Ishii G, Nagai K et al. Predictive factors for local recurrence of resected colorectal lung metastases. Ann Thorac Surg 2005; 80:1040–5.

34. Yedibela S, Klein P, Feuchter K et al. Surgical management of pulmonary metastases from colorectal cancer in 153 patients. Ann Surg Oncol 2006; 13:1538–44.

35. Kooby DA, Stockman J, Ben-Porat L et al. Influence of transfusions on perioperative and long-term outcome in patients following hepatic resection for colorectal metastases. Ann Surg 2003; 237:860–70.

36. Lesurtel M, Selzner M, Petrowsky H et al. How should transection of the liver be performed? A prospective randomized study in 100 consecutive patients: comparing four different transection strategies. Ann Surg 2005; 242:814–22.

A prospective randomised study providing evidence of efficiency and cost-effectiveness for the clamp-crushing technique.

37. Lupo L, Gallerani A, Panzera P et al. Randomised clinical trial of radiofrequency-assisted versus clamp-crushing liver resection. Br J Surg 2007; 94:287–91.

38. Figueras J, Llado L, Miro M et al. Application of fibrin glue sealant after hepatectomy does not seem justified: results of a randomized study in 300 patients. Ann Surg 2007; 245:536–42.

39. Simillis C, Constantinides VA, Tekkis PP et al. Laparoscopic versus open hepatic resections for benign and malignant neoplasms – a meta-analysis. Surgery 2007; 141:203–11.

40. Koffron AJ, Auffenberg G, Kung R et al. Evaluation of 300 minimally invasive liver resections at a single institution: less is more. Ann Surg 2007; 246:385–94.

41. Simmonds PC, Primrose JN, Colquitt JL et al. Surgical resection of hepatic metastases from colorectal cancer: a systematic review of published studies. Br J Cancer 2006; 94:982–99.

A systematic review of all prospective published single-centre series of liver resection for colorectal liver metastases.

42. http://www.livermetsurvey.org. Accessed 5 April 2008.

43. Chiche L. Recommendations for clinical practice: therapeutic management of hepatic metastases from colorectal cancers. Gastroenterol Clin Biol 2003; special issue II.

44. Poston G, Adam R, Vauthey JN. Downstaging or downsizing: time for a new staging system in advanced colorectal cancer? J Clin Oncol 2006; 24:2702–6.

45. O'Reilly DA, Poston GJ. Classification of colorectal liver metastases. Adv Gastrointest Cancers 2007; 5:6–9.

46. Pozzo C, Basso M, Cassano A et al. Neoadjuvant treatment of unresectable liver disease with irinotecan and 5-fluorouracil plus folinic acid in colorectal cancer patients. Ann Oncol 2004; 15:933–9.

47. Alberts SR, Horvarth WL, Sternfeld WC et al. Oxaliplatin, fluorouracil, and leucovorin for patients with unresectable liver-only metastases from colorectal cancer: a North Central Cancer Treatment Group phase II study. J Clin Oncol 2005; 23:9243–9.

48. Masi G, Cupini S, Marcucci L et al. Treatment with 5-fluorouracil/folinic acid, oxaliplatin and irinotecan enables surgical resection of metastases in patients with initially unresectable metastatic colorectal cancer. Ann Surg Oncol 2006; 13:58–65.

49. Tournigand C, Andre T, Achille E et al. FOLFIRI followed by FOLFOX6 or the reverse sequence in advanced colorectal cancer: a randomized GERCOR study. J Clin Oncol 2004; 22:229–37.

50. Ho WM, May B, Mok T et al. Liver resection after irinotecan, 5-fluorouracil, and folionic acid for patients with unresectable colorectal liver metastases: a multicentre phase II study by the Cancer Therapeutic Research Group. Med Oncol 2005; 22:303–12.

51. O'Reilly DA, Poston GJ. Colorectal liver metastases: current and future perspectives. Future Oncol 2006; 2:525–31.

52. Adam R, Pascal G, Castaing D. Tumor progression while on chemotherapy: a contraindication to liver resection for multiple colorectal metastases? Ann Surg 2004; 240:1052–64.

53. Allen PJ, Kemeny N, Jarnagin W et al. Importance of response to neoadjuvant chemotherapy in the treatment of multiple colorectal metastases to the liver. J Gastrointest Surg 2003; 7:108–15.

54. Benoist S, Broquet A, Penna C et al. Complete response of colorectal liver metastases after chemotherapy: Does it mean cure? J Clin Oncol 2006; 24:3939–45.

55. Bilchik AJ, Poston G, Curley SA et al. Neoadjuvant chemotherapy for metastatic colon cancer: a cautionary note. J Clin Oncol 2005; 23:9073–8.

56. Karoui M, Penna C, Amin-Hashem M. Influence of preoperative chemotherapy on the risk of major hepatectomy for colorectal liver metastases. Ann Surg 2006; 243:1–7.

57. Vauthey JN, Pawlik TM, Ribero D et al. Chemotherapy regimen predicts steatohepatitis and an increase in 90-day mortality after surgery for hepatic colorectal metastases. J Clin Oncol 2006; 24:2065–72.

58. Nakano H, Oussoultzoglou E, Rosso E et al. Sinusoidal injury increases morbidity after major hepatectomy in patients with colorectal liver metastases receiving preoperative chemotherapy. Ann Surg 2008; 247:118–24.

59. Nordlinger B, Sorbye H, Glimelius B et al. Perioperative chemotherapy with FOLFOX4 and surgery versus surgery alone for resectable liver metastases from colorectal cancer (EORTC Intergroup trial 40983): a randomised controlled trial. Lancet 2008; 371:1007–16.

The first prospective randomised phase III trial designed to demonstrate the survival benefit of perioperative chemotherapy with liver resection for colorectal liver metastasis.

60. Zelek L, Bugat R, Cherqui D et al. Multimodal therapy with intravenous biweekly leucovorin, 5-fluorouracil and irinotecan combined with hepatic arterial infusion pirarubicin in non-resectable hepatic metastases from colorectal cancer (a European Association for Research in Oncology trial). Ann Oncol 2003; 14:1537–42.

61. Capdevila J, Saura C, Macarulla T et al. Monoclonal antibodies in the treatment of advanced colorectal cancer. Eur J Surg Oncol 2007; 33:S24–34.

62. Cunningham D, Humblet Y, Siena S et al. Cetuximab monotherapy and cetuximab plus irinotecan in irinotecan-refractory metastatic colorectal cancer. N Engl J Med 2004; 351:337–45.

63. Bianchini D, Jayanth A, Chua YJ et al. Epidermal growth factor receptor inhibitor-related skin toxicity: mechanisms, treatment, and its potential role as a predictive marker. Clin Colorectal Cancer 2008; 7:33–43.

64. Adam R, Aloia T, Levi F et al. Hepatic resection after rescue cetuximab treatment for colorectal liver metastases previously refractory to conventional systemic therapy. J Clin Oncol 2007; 25:4593–602.

65. Folprecht G, Grothey A, Alberts S et al. Neoadjuvant treatment of unresectable colorectal liver metastases: correlation between tumour response and resection rates. Ann Oncol 2005; 16:1311–19.

66. Garrean S, Hering J, Helton WS et al. A primer on transarterial, chemical and thermal ablative therapies for hepatic tumours. Am J Surg 2007; 194:79–88.

67. Mulier S, Ni Y, Jamart J et al. Local recurrence after hepatic radiofrequency coagulation – Multivariate meta-analysis and review of contributing factors. Ann Surg 2005; 242:158–71.

68. Mulier S, Mulier P, Ni Y et al. Complications of radiofrequency coagulation of liver tumours. Br J Surg 2002; 89:1206–22.

69. Feliberti EC, Wagman LD. Radiofrequency ablation of liver metastases from colorectal cancer. Cancer Control 2006; 13:48–51.

70. Simon CJ, Dupuy DE, Mayo-Smith WW. Microwave ablation: principles and applications. Radiographics 2005; 25:S69–84.

71. Gulec SA, Fong Y. Yttrium 90 microsphere selective internal radiation treatment of hepatic colorectal metastases. Arch Surg 2007; 142:675–82.

72. Gray B, Van Hazel G, Hope M et al. Randomised trial of SIR-Spheres plus chemotherapy vs chemotherapy alone for treating patients with liver metastases from primary large bowel cancer. Ann Oncol 2001; 12:1711–20.

73. Poston GJ, Adam R, Alberts S et al. OncoSurge: a strategy for improving resectability with curative intent in metastatic colorectal cancer. J Clin Oncol 2005; 23:7125–34.

74. O'Reilly DA, Chaudhari M, Ballal M et al. The Oncosurge strategy for the management of colorectal liver metastases – an external validation study. Eur J Surg Oncol 2008; 34:538–40.

75. Garden OJ, Rees M, Poston GJ et al. Guidelines for resection of colorectal cancer liver metastases. Gut 2006; 55:1–8.

7

Non-colorectal hepatic metastases

Lynn Mikula
Steven Gallinger
Carol-Anne Moulton

Introduction

Colorectal cancer (CRC) is the most common source of secondary liver tumours, although almost any solid malignancy can metastasise to the liver. Tumour cells from gastrointestinal tract malignancies reach the liver directly via the portal circulation. Liver metastases may occur either in apparent isolation, as is sometimes seen in CRC, or in association with widespread systemic disease, as in pancreatic and gastric adenocarcinoma. In contrast, metastases from non-gastrointestinal tumours reach the liver via the systemic circulation and are generally indicative of disseminated disease.

The development of liver metastases was often considered a preterminal event and treatment was limited to palliation, but the success of hepatectomy in improving outcomes in metastatic CRC has generated enthusiasm for surgical approaches to liver metastases from non-colorectal primary tumours. Liver resection has become the standard of care for CRC liver metastases and many centres are adopting an increasingly aggressive approach with reported 5-year survival rates approaching 50%.[1,2] The complementary use of portal vein embolisation, radiofrequency ablation and staged resection strategies has increased the proportion of patients eligible for resection. At the same time, advances in surgical technique and knowledge of liver anatomy have

reduced significantly the morbidity and mortality associated with liver resection to less than 5% and 20% respectively.[2,3]

Liver metastases of non-colorectal origin constitute a diverse group of tumours but the majority arise from gastrointestinal sites. Primary tumours leading to liver metastases can be broadly divided into neuroendocrine and non-neuroendocrine malignancies, but these have markedly different natural histories. Neuroendocrine tumours (NETs) are often indolent, and hepatectomy for NET liver metastases can result in 5-year survival rates in excess of 75%.[4] While hepatectomy is an increasingly accepted management strategy for NETs, it is performed infrequently for non-neuroendocrine tumours with less favourable results.

The evidence regarding hepatectomy for non-colorectal metastases consists largely of retrospective reviews reporting several decades of experience.[5–8] Many studies do not distinguish between metastases of NET and non-NET origin. Even when that distinction is made, the non-NET metastases are usually considered as a single group despite comprising a heterogeneous set of pathologies. Reports focusing on a single tumour type are usually based on small case series. The available comparison group consists of those patients who, by virtue of already having worse disease, were not considered candidates for hepatectomy.

Due to the paucity of prospective, controlled data, the appropriate indications for hepatectomy for non-CRC metastases are unclear. Two factors are associated frequently with improved outcomes: a long disease-free interval between the treatment of the primary and the development of the liver metastases, and the ability to technically resect all liver metastases leaving no residual disease (R0 resection).[5] Both these factors are surrogates for tumour biology. Patients with less aggressive tumours are most likely to derive significant survival benefit from hepatectomy. Unfortunately, no single measure of tumour biology yet exists.

Pathophysiology and molecular basis of liver metastases

Achieving cure in cancer requires the complete eradication of all tumour cells. Thus, for most solid tumours, complete surgical excision is the cornerstone of treatment. In the presence of metastases there is an apparent contradiction in using a local therapy – surgery – to treat what is considered disseminated disease.

The rationale behind a surgical approach to metastatic disease is based on the concept of site-specific metastasis. First proposed by Paget in 1889, this 'seed and soil' hypothesis argues that solid tumours have a distinct pattern of distant organ involvement created by the target organ microenvironment. Ewing proposed a 'mechanical' theory in which the metastatic pattern is determined by the venous drainage of the primary tumour.[9] Neither theory takes into account the complexity of the metastatic process, which requires that a cancer cell gains specific invasion and metastatic potential before it can disseminate. The clonal selection model of the metastatic process suggests that heterogeneity develops within a population of cancer cells through mutational events, allowing a subpopulation to acquire randomly the necessary traits to disseminate successfully.[10] Alternatively, it has been argued that within cancers of the same pathological type, i.e. breast cancer, some tumours are a priori more likely to develop metastases than others. This is supported by gene expression data where specific molecular signatures have been found to predict accurately prognosis in breast cancer,[11] ovarian cancer[12] and melanoma.[13] Similarly, in CRC the genotype of microsatellite instability correlates with a decreased likelihood of metastatic spread.[14]

A recent refinement to Paget's hypothesis, based on molecular genetic research, suggests that the primary tumour is itself capable of preparing the soil by creating a 'premetastatic niche'.[15] Every cancer has a type-specific pattern of cytokine expression which appears to direct both malignant and non-malignant cells to specific distant organs. The influx and clustering of bone-marrow-derived haematopoietic cells is one of the earliest events in the development of a metastatic deposit. This is closely followed by local inflammation and the release of matrix metalloproteinases. These local events appear to mediate remodelling of the extracellular matrix, creating a more permissive microenvironment for the eventual deposition and growth of malignant cells.[16] Thus, the primary tumour both chooses and alters the sites to which it metastasises. For reasons not yet understood, many solid tumours metastasise preferentially to the liver.

If the site-specific hypothesis of metastatic spread is correct, complete surgical excision of liver metastases can remove the only site of disease and offers a chance for cure. Nonetheless, residual micrometastatic disease may exist within the liver, and hepatic recurrences are a common cause of treatment failure following hepatectomy. Even in the presence of micrometastases, the removal of all macroscopic disease may have immunological benefits. The immune-suppressing effects of cancers are well accepted: malignant cells can induce both specific and general immune suppression, facilitating tumour growth.[17] The degree of immune suppression correlates with the tumour burden[18] and if all gross metastatic disease can be removed, host defences may attack more effectively micrometastatic deposits. The use of neoadjuvant and/or post-liver resection chemotherapy may improve cure rates by controlling micrometastases.[19,20]

Clinical approach to non-colorectal liver metastases

Routine clinical, radiological and serological assessments for liver metastases should be guided by the propensity for liver metastases of each specific tumour type and the ability of potential treatments to alter the outcome of the metastatic disease. In imaging the liver, the choice of transabdominal ultrasound, contrast-enhanced ultrasound, contrast-enhanced triphasic computed tomography (CT), magnetic resonance imaging (MRI) and positron emission tomography (PET) will be dictated by tumour type as well as local availability and expertise.

Some cancers can be assessed for recurrence using more targeted techniques and biochemical markers (i.e. CA-125 for ovarian cancer, chromogranin A for NET). Nuclear imaging can detect NETs expressing somatostatin receptors with 80–90% sensitivity. PET scanning using a new somatostatin analogue, [68Ga]DOTA-TOC, has been found to be even more sensitive and specific for NETs.[21] Occasionally, the original presentation of an NET will be a liver metastasis from an unidentified primary, and the investigative focus is the localisation of the primary tumour.

When a patient is under consideration for hepatic metastasectomy, the most critical component of the clinical assessment is an accurate determination of the extent of metastatic spread, including a thorough assessment for extra-abdominal disease. The anatomic areas targeted for investigation (brain, lung, bone) will be determined by the known metastatic pattern of the primary tumour.

Certain tumours, such as gastric, breast and ovarian cancer, have a predilection for intraperitoneal spread. Carcinomatosis can be difficult to assess on preoperative imaging but is easily visualised during laparoscopy. Routine laparoscopy with laparoscopic ultrasound for patients with potentially resectable non-colorectal liver metastases has been found to result in a change in management in 20% of cases[22] and may be used in preoperative staging.

Treatment strategies

Several treatment modalities exist and the therapeutic approach must be tailored to the tumour type, the performance status of the patient and the extent of disease, made in the setting of a multidisciplinary conference. Ablative strategies and systemic or locally delivered chemotherapy can be used as adjuncts to resection. Radiofrequency ablation (RFA) has been reported to be safe and successful at achieving local control in patients with liver metastases from breast cancer,[23] ovarian cancer[24] and NETs,[25] but its major limitation is the difficulty of achieving complete necrosis in tumours larger than 3 cm.

Transarterial embolisation (TAE) takes advantage of the differential blood supply of liver metastases, which depend mainly on the hepatic arteries, and the normal parenchyma, which rely more heavily on the portal vein. Transarterial chemoembolisation (TACE) involves the local delivery of a drug prior to occluding the artery and allows prolonged exposure of the tumour to the agent without increasing systemic toxicity. Both TAE and TACE have been well described for the treatment of unresectable hepatocellular carcinoma[26] and the symptomatic relief of NETs.[27]

Neuroendocrine tumours

Gastrointestinal NETs are a diverse group of tumours that originate throughout the gastrointestinal tract and can be classified into carcinoid and pancreatic histological subtypes. Carcinoid tumours arise most commonly in the midgut and may secrete serotonin and other bioactive amines. Pancreatic NETs can be non-functional or can produce hormonally active substances (e.g. insulin, glucagon, gastrin, vasoactive intestinal peptide).

Most NETs of gastrointestinal origin demonstrate indolent growth. Nonetheless, the majority will have disseminated disease at the time of diagnosis and 5-year survival is 50–80%.[28,29] Systemic chemotherapy regimens are associated with a response of limited duration, significant toxicity and no impact on overall survival. Somatostatin analogues such as octreotide can achieve symptomatic relief in 70–80% of patients, but an antiproliferative effect is seen in less than 10% of cases.[30] As a result, efforts to improve both palliative and curative therapies have focused on cytoreductive surgery.

NETs metastasise preferentially to the liver, and in many patients the liver remains the only site of metastatic disease for a prolonged period of time. The majority of patients have multifocal, bilobar disease, and more than half will have involvement of >50% of the liver[31] (**Fig. 7.1a,b**). Liver resection may be performed with curative intent, for symptom control, or prolongation of survival in the palliative setting.

Liver resection with curative intent is reserved for procedures that aim to leave no residual disease (R0 resection) in both primary and secondary sites, and studies have demonstrated 5-year survival rates of up to 85%.[27,32] Optimal cytoreduction aims to reduce tumour volume by at least 90%.[4] Although there are no data from randomised trials, large series using historical controls or contemporary cases matched for stage have demonstrated that liver resection with optimal cytoreduction results in improved survival.[31,33,34]

A recently published review demonstrated that hepatic resection for metastatic NETs resulted in almost double 5-year survival rates over the unresected group, from 30–40% to 47–82%.[35] In addition, cytoreduction offers the most effective and durable palliation from symptoms.[33,36] As a result, surgical debulking has been advocated for both functional and non-functional tumours.[4,35] An aggressive approach, sometimes combining liver resection with other ablative strategies, is warranted (**Fig. 7.2a,b**).

Most series of hepatic resection for metastatic NETs include an occasional case with an unknown primary, despite thorough imaging and endoscopy. Although survival data are sparse, centres with expertise in the field advocate an aggressive resectional approach for these patients as well[31] (Fig. 7.2b).

RFA used in isolation can achieve symptomatic relief and local control in 60–80% of NET patients with liver metastases, but the duration of response is variable.[4] TAE and TACE have also been shown to achieve reasonable palliation for very bulky or symptomatic unresectable tumours.[4] The duration

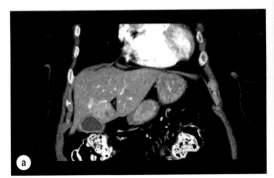
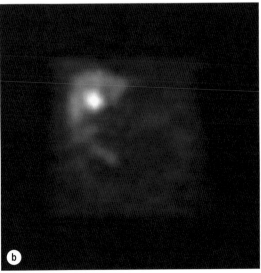

Figure 7.1 • (a) A 67-year-old female with a node-positive distal jejunal carcinoid tumour, and synchronous solitary liver metastasis in segment 4B. **(b)** Octreotide scan of the same patient. Transaxial SPECT demonstrates abnormal activity in segment 4B corresponding to known metastasis on CT.

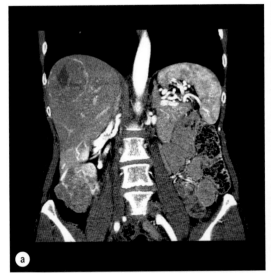
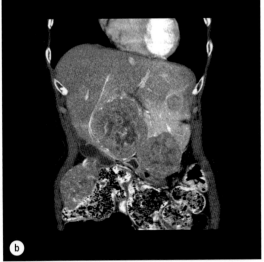

Figure 7.2 • (a) A 59-year-old female with an incidental finding of multiple NET metastases. There was no evidence of primary tumour on octreotide scan and endoscopy. Note multiple hypervascular, large metastases with central necrosis. **(b)** Same patient as in **(a)**. A debulking operation to remove 90% of tumour burden would be possible by performing an extended right hepatic lobectomy with wedge resections from segment 2.

of response is short: tumours develop collaterals quickly and repeat embolisation is necessary to maintain symptomatic control.[35] Involvement of greater than 50% of the liver is generally cited as a contraindication to TAE due to the risk of liver failure. Other complications of TAE include carcinoid crisis or other symptoms related to acute hormone release and tumour lysis syndrome.[4]

In general, aggressive multimodality therapy with embolic, ablative and systemic strategies is recommended to debulk or downstage metastatic NET.[35] The duration of response following hepatectomy is related to the completeness of resection[31] and can be predicted by the normalisation of tumour markers such as 5-hydroxyindoleacetic acid (5-HIAA) and chromogranin A. Chromogranin A is more sensitive than 5-HIAA in identifying disease progression and high levels have been shown to predict poor outcomes. A reduction in chromogranin A levels of >80% predicts a good outcome following cytoreductive hepatectomy, even when complete resection has not been achieved.[37]

Liver transplantation has been advocated as an option for patients with extensive, unresectable liver metastases with no extrahepatic disease. The largest single-centre series reported retrospective data with a 5-year survival of 80% following orthotopic liver transplantation for metastatic NETs,[38] although other results have been less favourable.[39,40] Nonetheless, liver transplantation does appear to confer long-term survival in carefully selected patients.[41]

Gastrointestinal stromal tumours

Gastrointestinal stromal tumours (GISTs) represent a group of mesenchymal malignancies that originate from the interstitial cells of Cajal of the gastrointestinal tract. Up to 90% of GISTs harbour a mutated c-kit proto-oncogene, which results in the constitutive activation of the receptor tyrosine kinase and unregulated cell growth. Exon 11 mutations account for approximately 70% of mutations in GIST.[42] Less than 5% of GISTs have wild type c-Kit, and many of these harbour mutations in the platelet-derived growth factor receptor α (PDGFRA) kinase.[43]

Primary GISTs arise in the stomach (60%), small intestine (25%), and colon and rectum (10%), with the remainder found in various other sites (gallbladder, appendix, omentum or mesentery). Surgery is the treatment of choice for resectable primary GISTs. Commonly the primary tumour is classified into four prognostic categories, ranging from very low risk to high risk, according to size of the lesion and the number of mitotic figures identified.[44]

Imatinib mesylate is a selective tyrosine kinase inhibitor and has become first-line therapy for unresectable GISTs.[45] Response to imatinib is greatest in tumours that harbour the c-Kit exon 11 mutation, but is also seen to a lesser extent in GISTs that express other isoforms of c-Kit and PDGFRA.[43] The use of imatinib in the adjuvant setting is less well defined and is currently being assessed in three randomised trials (EORTC 62024, SCANDIA and ACOSOG Z9001) and one completed phase II trial (ACOSOG A9000). The ACOSOG Z9001 trial, which examined the use of adjuvant imatinib in resected, c-Kit-positive tumours >3 cm in size, was recently stopped to accrual due to the finding of significantly higher recurrence-free survival (RFS) in the imatinib group (97% at 1 year versus 83%, hazard ratio 0.325 (95% CI 0.2–0.53), although follow-up is immature[46]).

The treatment of unresectable primary and metastatic GISTs has been revolutionised by imatinib. Between 40% and 60% of resected patients with primaries in the intermediate- to high-risk categories recur, most commonly with one of two metastatic patterns: local recurrence with peritoneal disease or intraparenchymal liver metastases.[47] Liver metastases are frequently multiple, large and bilobar, making curative resection an unlikely option.[44] Most patients with metastatic GISTs will receive imatinib as first-line treatment, with a clinical response demonstrated in 80%. This response is durable with a median survival in excess of 24 months.[48] Eventually, though, many patients develop imatinib resistance and disease progression.[49] Second-line agents (e.g. sunitinib and nilotinib) are being tested in patients that are resistant to imatinib.[50]

 The efficacy and low side-effect profile of imatinib prompted initial enthusiasm for the combined use of surgery and imatinib in the management of metastatic GISTs.[51] Surgical resection was proposed for patients with a long disease-free interval or those who developed imatinib resistance.[44] However, longer-term follow-up has provided no clear evidence that resection of metastatic GISTs improves survival. Surgery for disease that does not respond to imatinib is associated with uniformly poor results and is not recommended.[52]

A subset of GIST patients develop a pattern of disease progression where isolated nodular foci progress within a pre-existing tumour mass in a patient already on imatinib. Such cases of partial progression have the same median survival as patients who meet standard criteria for disease progression.[53] There is currently no rationale for resection in this group. The benefit of surgical resection in the group of patients with disease that is stable or responding to imatinib is not clear.[52,54] Randomised trials evaluating adjuvant surgery following response to imatinib in metastatic GISTs are currently underway.

In general, GIST metastatic to the liver is rarely amenable to resection. As such, imatinib is accepted as the first-line treatment for metastatic disease. Disease progression is managed by dose escalation followed by second-line agents such as sunitinib. In the event of tumour rupture or haemorrhage, surgery or hepatic artery embolisation may be performed in an emergency setting.[51]

Breast cancer

The surgical management of breast cancer hepatic metastases is controversial. The widely held concept that liver metastases in breast cancer reflect diffuse systemic disease has led to a nihilistic view of the role of liver resection in this setting. However, an aggressive surgical approach has been adopted recently by a number of groups, with seemingly favourable results in highly selected patients.[55–57] Unfortunately, the data are mostly retrospective and are based on heterogeneous indications, making it difficult to provide strong evidence-based guidelines.

Although breast cancer is common, isolated liver lesions in metastatic breast cancer patients are rare (1–5% of patients).[58] Sakamoto et al.[57] reported only 34 patients with resectable liver metastases among 11 000 breast cancer patients treated over an 18-year period. Selection criteria for such metastases are inconsistent in surgical series. For example, Sakamoto et al.[57] and Adam et al.[56] offered liver resection for patients with treated extrahepatic disease, while others considered liver resection only when disease was limited to the liver.[59,60] Patients with positive portal nodes have had hepatic resections,[55,57] as have patients with synchronous hepatic metastases.[56,57,60] In short, there are no clear selection criteria for resection.

Response to chemotherapy appears to be an important predictor of survival following liver resection for metastatic breast cancer. In the largest series, patients whose disease remained stable or progressed during prehepatectomy chemotherapy were 3.5 times more likely to die than responders.[56] Preoperative chemotherapy has been recommended in all cases, with hepatectomy reserved for those who show objective response.[60]

Despite the heterogeneous selection criteria, 5-year survival rates fall into two groups. Several reports describe 5-year overall survival of approximately 25%;[55,57,59] however, others have 5-year survival between 45% and 60%.[60,61] These disparate results cannot be explained by differences in study design or treatment factors. Outcomes following hepatic resection may therefore merely reflect differences in tumour biology. Furthermore, 5-year disease-free survival rates are much lower than overall survival rates, suggesting that liver resection may function as a cytoreductive rather than curative procedure in these highly selected patients.[55,56] A prospective, multicentre trial would help establish evidence-based guidelines concerning the role of hepatic resection.

Ovarian cancer

Epithelial ovarian cancer is a chemosensitive disease, and platinum-based therapies result in a significant diminution of tumour volume in the majority of patients. Unfortunately, most develop chemoresistance after 24–36 months and median survival for advanced (stage III–IV) disease is 3.5 years.[62] Nonetheless, many centres have become very aggressive with surgical debulking. Optimal cytoreduction (residual disease <1 cm) results in improved survival in advanced stage ovarian cancer.[63] Intraperitoneal (i.p.) chemotherapy has been demonstrated to further improve survival compared to intravenous therapy, and this is the current aim of treatment in many large centers. To be eligible for i.p. chemotherapy patients must undergo maximal debulking.[63] Successful cytoreduction is thus a crucial step in the management of advanced ovarian cancer.

Although the liver is rarely the only site of metastatic disease in ovarian cancer, hepatectomy can be an important component of a primary cytoreduction strategy. Ovarian cancer can involve the liver through the development of peritoneal lesions on the surface of the liver (stage III – **Fig. 7.3**) or intraparenchymal metastases (stage IV – **Fig. 7.4**). Survival is improved for patients with stage IV disease who have undergone adequate debulking surgery including hepatectomy.[64,65]

Percutaneous RFA has also been found to be effective in achieving local control in these cases and is a useful adjunct to an aggressive surgical approach.[24]

Hepatectomy has also been associated with favourable outcomes in the setting of recurrent disease. In one retrospective review of 24 patients with recurrent ovarian and fallopian tube cancer who underwent hepatectomy, the median survival was 62 months. In this study the median time between treatment of the primary cancer and the

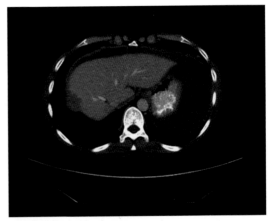

Figure 7.3 • Stage III ovarian cancer with hepatic involvement. Note direct invasion of liver capsule by peritoneal tumour plaque.

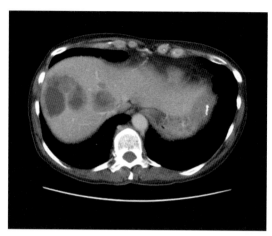

Figure 7.4 • Stage IV ovarian cancer with intraparenchymal liver metastases.

development of recurrent disease was more than 5 years, suggesting that this represented a subset of patients with very favourable biology.[66]

Renal cell carcinoma

Metastases develop in 50% of patients with renal cell carcinoma (RCC) and liver involvement is present in approximately 20% of those with metastatic disease. The presence of liver metastases usually signifies widespread systemic disease, and overall 1-year survival is less than 10% in this setting.[67] Fewer than 5% of patients have metastases restricted to the liver.[67] Until recently there has been no effective systemic chemotherapy for the treatment of metastatic RCC. Sunitinib and surafenib, oral small-molecule tyrosine kinase inhibitors, have now been shown to be more effective in inducing measurable responses compared to placebo in metastatic RCC.[68]

The available data on hepatic resection for RCC metastases are mostly limited to case reports. The largest published series describes 31 patients with metastatic RCC who underwent liver resection. In this cohort, Thelen et al.[69] reported a 5-year survival rate of 39%, a median survival of 48 months and a median time to recurrence of 27 months. Most (25/31) patients had metachronous metastases and three had positive portal nodes (of eight cases that were sampled). The major prognostic factor in multivariate analysis was margin status of the liver resection.[69]

Alves et al.[70] described 14 liver resections for metastatic, mainly metachronous, lesions with no evidence of extrahepatic disease at the time of liver resection, with a 2-year survival of 56%. The interval between resection of the primary tumour and hepatectomy was the most significant prognostic feature. Although these data appear favourable,

the authors also summarised results for 46 RCC patients who underwent liver resection for metastases reported in 12 additional smaller series, with a 5-year survival of only 13%.[70]

These limited data indicate variable results for hepatic resection in metastatic RCC. Use of the new tyrosine kinase inhibitors as either neoadjuvant or post-liver resection therapy may improve these results. An evidence-based approach to combining surgery with sunitinib or surafenib will hopefully be forthcoming with prospectively collected data.

Melanoma

The prognosis for patients with metastatic melanoma is poor, and there are no systemic treatment options that offer survival advantage. Historically, the median survival for American Joint Committee on Cancer (AJCC) stage IV melanoma with liver metastases is 2–7 months.[71] Palliative radiotherapy and systemic chemotherapy have not been shown to prolong survival. Although biological agents such as interferon-α and interleukin-2 have yielded promising response rates, these are rarely durable and are associated with significant toxicity.[72] However, numerous retrospective studies have demonstrated a survival advantage following resection of highly selected patients with metastases to the lung, soft tissues or gastrointestinal tract.[73,74]

The available evidence for hepatectomy for metastatic melanoma consists largely of subset analyses from larger series of patients with non-colorectal liver metastases. One report retrospectively reviewed the experiences of two of the largest melanoma databases in the world.[75] In this series, only 2% of the 1750 patients (n = 34) identified with hepatic metastases underwent an exploratory laparotomy with intent to resect; the selection criteria used to define this group are not stated. Of the 34 patients undergoing exploratory laparotomy, 24 (71%) underwent hepatic resection and 18 of these were considered complete. The remaining six were considered palliative or debulking procedures. Of those who underwent hepatic resection, the 5-year overall survival was 29%, with a median survival of 28 months and a median interval of 12 months to disease recurrence. The unresected group had a 5-year overall survival of 4% and a median survival of 6 months.[75] The ability to achieve a macroscopically complete resection is an important predictor of survival following hepatectomy for metastatic melanoma.[72,75]

The biological behaviour of metastatic melanoma depends in part on the site of origin of the primary tumour.[76] Cutaneous melanoma is more common than ocular melanoma.[77] While both metastasise to the liver, they appear to do so with distinct patterns of disease. Ocular melanoma metastasises to the liver more frequently, but is more likely to be associated with isolated liver metastases than cutaneous melanoma.[76,77] Survival following hepatectomy appears to be more favourable in the highly selected but rare group of patients with melanoma of ocular origin. Pawlik et al. reported 5-year survival of 21% for ocular primaries, with no 5-year survivors when the initial site of disease was cutaneous. However, 75% of resected patients in this study developed recurrent disease, and the rate of recurrence was similar between the ocular and cutaneous groups.[77]

It is impossible from the available studies to estimate the impact that liver resection has on the survival of patients with melanoma. It seems reasonable to adopt a resectional approach in highly selected patients, i.e. patients with a long disease-free interval from primary to metastases, and patients that can be rendered disease-free following surgery. This will occasionally lead to long-term survival, but for the most part patients with metastatic melanoma have a poor prognosis.

Non-colorectal gastrointestinal adenocarcinoma

Liver metastases from non-colorectal gastrointestinal (GI) adenocarcinomas can arise from the oesophagus, stomach, pancreas, gallbladder, ampulla, small bowel and distal bile duct. Hepatic resection is rarely performed for these indications and the available literature is scant.

Metastatic oesophageal cancer is usually broadly disseminated and is associated with a 5-year survival of 3–5% when multiple sites of disease are present and 7–8% when disease is limited to the liver.[78] Two case reports in the English-language literature describe hepatectomy for isolated, synchronous liver metastases.[79,80] In both cases hepatectomy was performed simultaneously with oesophagectomy and was followed by hepatic arterial chemotherapy. Both patients developed multiple liver metastases at 6[79] and 7[80] months postoperatively. These recurrences responded partially to systemic chemotherapy, and patients were alive with disease at 14[79] and 18[80] months following hepatectomy. Thus, although rarely feasible, hepatectomy followed by hepatic arterial chemotherapy may provide a limited survival benefit in chemosensitive oesophageal cancer with isolated liver metastases.

Gastric adenocarcinoma is the second most common cause of cancer-related death worldwide, and

the liver is a major site of spread. Hepatectomy for gastric cancer metastases is therefore the best described of the non-colorectal GI primaries. A recent Japanese retrospective review of 42 patients is the largest reported series. In 20 cases, the liver metastases were synchronous and the median disease-free interval was 11 months. Cases of direct liver invasion by the primary tumour were excluded. The authors reported a 5-year survival of 42%, a median survival of 34 months and eight 5-year survivors. Independent predictors of good survival from a multivariate analysis were solitary liver metastasis and the absence of serosal invasion of the primary tumour.[81]

The available evidence for hepatectomy in the management of metastases from non-colorectal, non-neuroendocrine GI primaries is extremely limited, and few meaningful statements can be made as to the utility of this treatment strategy. Nonetheless, most authors agree that these tumours are associated with poor outcomes following hepatectomy.[82–84]

Testicular cancer

Metastasectomy is well established in the management of disseminated non-seminomatous germ cell testicular carcinoma that does not completely respond to chemotherapy. Although it can be difficult to differentiate active residual tumour from post-treatment fibrosis or necrosis, the probability of achieving cure by surgical resection is high. Furthermore, residual teratoma has the potential for sarcomatous transformation. For these reasons, lymphadenectomy and visceral resection are recommended whenever there is radiographic evidence of residual disease.[85]

Two studies have specifically addressed the role of hepatectomy for metastatic testicular carcinoma. One single-institution review of 57 liver resections performed over a 22-year period reported that 60% of patients were alive and disease-free at last follow-up. The greatest benefit was seen in patients with either no residual or residual teratoma in the specimen. Patients with carcinoma in the specimen and persistent elevation of serum tumour markers had the worst prognosis.[86] A second published report found that 62% of patients were alive without disease after a mean follow-up of 66 months following hepatectomy for testicular germ cell tumours.[87] Negative prognostic indicators included viable tumour in the resected specimen, metastases greater than 3 cm in diameter and pure embryonal carcinoma in the primary lesion.

Urothelial cancer

The data for metastasectomy in the management of disseminated urothelial cancer are sparse, and no studies specifically address the role of hepatectomy. Five-year survival of 33% has been reported following resection of lung, brain or lymph node metastases in combination with chemotherapy.[88] Metastasectomy has also been employed successfully for palliation.[85] A handful of single-institution reviews of hepatectomy for non-colorectal metastases have included one or two bladder cancer patients,[7,83] but no study was powered to explore survival differences between individual tumour types and they do not comment specifically on outcomes for urothelial cancers.

Lung cancer

The management of metastatic lung cancer is largely restricted to radiation and chemotherapy. Surgery has been advocated in rare instances, such as for patients with isolated brain and adrenal metastases.[89] Liver involvement is managed surgically only under exceptional circumstances. Liver resection for metastatic lung cancer has been described only in the context of broader reviews of non-colorectal liver metastases, and individual survival figures were not provided in these studies.[7,83,84]

Adrenocortical tumours

Malignant phaeochromocytoma with liver metastases is rare, and literature on the management of this disease is anecdotal. Case reports have described the use of TAE for symptomatic relief.[90,91] In their series of non-colorectal liver metastases, Weitz et al. report three 5-year survivors following hepatic resection for metastatic adrenocortical tumours, including one 11-year survivor.[8]

Endometrial cancer

Metastatic endometrial cancer is usually multifocal in nature and not generally managed operatively. One report described hepatic trisegmentectomy followed by chemotherapy for two cases of metastatic endometrial cancer. One patient survived for 33 months with no recurrence of liver disease, although brain metastases developed 12 months following liver resection. The second case had a pulmonary recurrence 8 months after combined lung and liver resection.[92] Other isolated reports of long-term survivors exist in the context of larger studies of non-colorectal liver metastases.[8]

Conclusion

The recent success of an aggressive surgical approach to the management of CRC liver metastases has, in part, provided the impetus for stimulating the use of liver resection for non-colorectal cancer hepatic metastatic disease. Extrapolating surgical strategies from one malignancy to another is reasonable in some cases; however, fundamental biological differences between various neoplasms require thoughtful consideration of differences in the natural history and non-surgical treatment modalities that are available for each tumour site. Unfortunately, strong evidence-based data are lacking and it therefore behoves the treating surgeon to have a good working knowledge of the biology and management of various malignancies. In many cases, this is augmented by the availability of multidisciplinary tumour boards and a critical mass of subspecialists to assist in decision-making.

It is worth emphasising that in most cases liver resection should be performed with curative intent. Exceptions include liver metastases from NETs, epithelial ovarian cancer and testicular malignancies, where 'debulking' is considered useful as a palliative manoeuvre to improve overall survival. The case for resection of breast cancer metastases is evolving, with some liver surgeons advocating resection as one of various 'cytoreductive' therapies for this disease, perhaps no different than the use of multiple different chemotherapeutic and biological therapies which prolong survival in breast cancer. There is no evidence that non-curative intent surgery is helpful for patients with liver metastases from gastrointestinal tract primaries, lung and other cancers.

The presence of extrahepatic disease is almost always a contraindication to liver resection, except within the context of a prospective trial. The critical variables that usually predict cure after liver resection of secondary cancer of almost all types include prolonged disease-free interval from resection of the primary tumour, negative resection margins and performance status.

Future efforts should be directed toward the conduct of randomised trials designed to test the role of liver surgery for the common non-colorectal malignancies, and the discovery of genetic and proteomic signatures as better prognostic and predictive markers.

References

1. Shah SA, Bromberg R, Coates A et al. Survival after liver resection for metastatic colorectal carcinoma in a large population. J Am Coll Surg 2007; 205:676–83.

2. Fong Y, Fortner J, Sun RL et al. Clinical score for predicting recurrence after hepatic resection for metastatic colorectal cancer: analysis of 1001 consecutive cases. Ann Surg 1999; 230:309–18; discussion 318–21.

3. Abad A, Massuti B, Anton A et al. Colorectal cancer metastasis resectability after treatment with the combination of oxaliplatin, irinotecan and 5-fluorouracil. Final results of a phase II study. Acta Oncol 2007; 22:1–7.

4. Madoff DC, Gupta S, Ahrar K et al. Update on the management of neuroendocrine hepatic metastases. J Vasc Interv Radiol 2006; 17:1235–49; quiz 1250.

5. Adam R, Chiche L, Aloia T et al. Hepatic resection for noncolorectal nonendocrine liver metastases: analysis of 1,452 patients and development of a prognostic model. Ann Surg 2006; 244: 524–35.

6. O'Rourke TR, Tekkis P, Yeung S et al. Long-term results of liver resection for non-colorectal, non-neuroendocrine metastases. Ann Surg Oncol 2008; 15:207–18.

7. Lendoire JMM, Andriani O, Grondona J et al. Liver resection for non-colorectal, non-neuroendocrine metastases: analysis of a multicenter study from Argentina. HPB 2007; 9:435–9.

8. Weitz J, Blumgart LH, Fong Y et al. Partial hepatectomy for metastases from noncolorectal, nonneuroendocrine carcinoma. Ann Surg 2005; 241:269–76.

9. Ribatti D, Mangialardi G, Vacca A. Stephen Paget and the 'seed and soil' theory of metastatic dissemination. Clin Exp Med 2006; 6:145–9.

10. Fidler IJ. The pathogenesis of cancer metastasis: the 'seed and soil' hypothesis revisited. Nat Rev Cancer 2003; 3:453–8.

11. van't Veer LJ, Dai H, van de Vijver MJ et al. Gene expression profiling predicts clinical outcome of breast cancer. Nature 2002; 415(31):530–6.

12. Spentzos D, Levine DA, Ramoni MF et al. Gene expression signature with independent prognostic significance in epithelial ovarian cancer. J Clin Oncol 2004; 22(1):4700–10.

13. Winnepenninckx V, Lazar V, Michiels S et al. Gene expression profiling of primary cutaneous melanoma and clinical outcome. J Natl Cancer Inst 2006; 98(5):472–82.

14. Gryfe R, Kim H, Hsieh ET et al. Tumor microsatellite instability and clinical outcome in young patients with colorectal cancer. N Engl J Med 2000; 342(13):69–77.

15. Kaplan RN, Rafii S, Lyden D. Preparing the "soil": the premetastatic niche. Cancer Res 2006; 66(1):11089–93.

16. Kaplan RN, Riba RD, Zacharoulis S et al. VEGFR1-positive haematopoietic bone marrow progenitors initiate the pre-metastatic niche. Nature 2005; 438(8):820–7.

17. Wojtowicz-Praga S. Reversal of tumor-induced immunosuppression by TGF-beta inhibitors. Invest New Drugs 2003; 21(1):21–32.

18. Morton DL, Holmes EC, Golub SH. Immunologic aspects of lung cancer. Chest 1977; 71:640–3.

19. Tabernero J, Van Cutsem E, Diaz-Rubio E et al. Phase II trial of cetuximab in combination with fluorouracil, leucovorin, and oxaliplatin in the first-line treatment of metastatic colorectal cancer. J Clin Oncol 2007; 25(20):5225–32.

20. Znajda TL, Hayashi S, Horton PJ et al. Postchemotherapy characteristics of hepatic colorectal metastases: remnants of uncertain malignant potential. J Gastrointest Surg 2006; 10:483–9.

21. Gabriel M, Decristoforo C, Kendler D et al. ^{68}Ga-DOTA-Tyr3-octreotide PET in neuroendocrine tumors: comparison with somatostatin receptor scintigraphy and CT. J Nucl Med 2007; 48:508–18.

22. D'Angelica M, Jarnagin W, Dematteo R et al. Staging laparoscopy for potentially resectable non-colorectal, nonneuroendocrine liver metastases. Ann Surg Oncol 2002; 9:204–9.

23. Sofocleous CT, Nascimento RG, Gonen M et al. Radiofrequency ablation in the management of liver metastases from breast cancer. AJR 2007; 189:883–9.

24. Gervais DA, Arellano RS, Mueller PR. Percutaneous radiofrequency ablation of ovarian cancer metastasis to the liver: indications, outcomes, and role in patient management. AJR 2006; 187:746–50.

25. Gillams A, Cassoni A, Conway G et al. Radiofrequency ablation of neuroendocrine liver metastases: the Middlesex experience. Abdom Imaging 2005; 30:435–41.

26. Ribero D, Curley SA, Imamura H et al. Selection for resection of hepatocellular carcinoma and surgical strategy: indications for resection, evaluation of liver function, portal vein embolization, and resection. Ann Surg Oncol 2008; 15:986–92.

27. Yao KA, Talamonti MS, Nemcek A et al. Indications and results of liver resection and hepatic chemoembolization for metastatic gastrointestinal neuroendocrine tumors. Surgery 2001; 130:677–82; discussion 682–5.

28. Rothenstein JC, Pond SP, Dale GR et al. Neuroendocrine tumors of the gastrointestinal tract: a decade of experience at the Princess Margaret Hospital. Am J Clin Oncol 2007; 30:1–7.

29. Modlin IM, Lye KD, Kidd M. A 5-decade analysis of 13,715 carcinoid tumors. Cancer 2003; 97(15):934–59.

30. Faiss S, Pape UF, Bohmig M et al. Prospective, randomized, multicenter trial on the antiproliferative effect of lanreotide, interferon alfa, and their combination for therapy of metastatic neuroendocrine gastroenteropancreatic tumors – the International Lanreotide and Interferon Alfa Study Group. J Clin Oncol 2003; 21(15):2689–96.

Symptomatic relief but limited response to treatment.

31. Touzios JG, Kiely JM, Pitt SC et al. Neuroendocrine hepatic metastases: does aggressive management improve survival? Ann Surg 2005; 241(5):776–83; discussion 783–5.

32. McEntee GP, Nagorney DM, Kvols LK et al. Cytoreductive hepatic surgery for neuroendocrine tumors. Surgery 1990; 108:1091–6.

33. Chamberlain RS, Canes D, Brown KT et al. Hepatic neuroendocrine metastases: does intervention alter outcomes? J Am Coll Surg 2000; 190:432–45.

34. Musunuru S, Chen H, Rajpal S et al. Metastatic neuroendocrine hepatic tumors: resection improves survival. Arch Surg 2006; 141:1000–4; discussion 10005.

35. Hodul P, Malafa M, Choi J et al. The role of cytoreductive hepatic surgery as an adjunct to the management of metastatic neuroendocrine carcinomas. Cancer Control 2006; 13:61–71.

36. Osborne DA, Zervos EE, Strosberg J et al. Improved outcome with cytoreduction versus embolization for symptomatic hepatic metastases of carcinoid and neuroendocrine tumors. Ann Surg Oncol 2006; 13:572–81.

37. Jensen EH, Kvols L, McLoughlin JM et al. Biomarkers predict outcomes following cytoreductive surgery for hepatic metastases from functional carcinoid tumors. Ann Surg Oncol 2007; 14:780–5.

38. Rosenau J, Bahr MJ, von Wasielewski R et al. Ki67, E-cadherin, and p53 as prognostic indicators of long-term outcome after liver transplantation for metastatic neuroendocrine tumors. Transplantation 2002; 73(15):386–94.

39. Florman S, Toure B, Kim L et al. Liver transplantation for neuroendocrine tumors. J Gastrointest Surg 2004; 8:208–12.

40. Marin C, Robles R, Fernandez JA et al. Role of liver transplantation in the management of unresectable neuroendocrine liver metastases. Transpl Proc 2007; 39:2302–3.

41. van Vilsteren FG, Baskin-Bey ES, Nagorney DM et al. Liver transplantation for gastroenteropancreatic neuroendocrine cancers: defining selection criteria to improve survival. Liver Transpl 2006; 12:448–56.

42. Corless CL, Fletcher JA, Heinrich MC. Biology of gastrointestinal stromal tumors. J Clin Oncol 2004; 22:3813–25.

43. Heinrich MC, Corless CL, Duensing A et al. PDGFRA activating mutations in gastrointestinal stromal tumors. Science 2003; 299:708–10.

44. D'Amato G, Steinert DM, McAuliffe JC et al. Update on the biology and therapy of gastrointestinal stromal tumors. Cancer Control 2005; 12:44–56.

45. Dagher R, Cohen M, Williams G et al. Approval summary: imatinib mesylate in the treatment of metastatic and/or unresectable malignant gastrointestinal stromal tumors. Clin Cancer Res 2002; 8:3034–8.

46. DeMatteo R, Owzar K, Maki R et al. and the American College of Surgeons Oncology Group (ACOSOG) Intergroup Adjuvant GIST Study Team. Adjuvant imatinib mesylate increases recurrence free survival (RFS) in patients with completely resected localized primary gastrointestinal stromal tumor (GIST): North American Intergroup Phase III trial ACOSOG Z9001. ASCO Annual Meeting, 2007.

47. DeMatteo RP, Lewis JJ, Leung D et al. Two hundred gastrointestinal stromal tumors: recurrence patterns and prognostic factors for survival. Ann Surg 2000; 231:51–8.

48. Benjamin R, Rankin C, Fletcher C et al. for the Sarcoma Intergroup. Phase III dose-randomized study of imatinib mesylate (STI571) for GIST: Intergroup S0033 early results. Proc Am Soc Clin Oncol 2003; 22.

49. Gorre ME, Mohammed M, Ellwood K et al. Clinical resistance to STI-571 cancer therapy caused by BCR-ABL gene mutation or amplification. Science (New York) 2001; 293:876–80.

50. von Mehren M. Beyond imatinib: second generation c-KIT inhibitors for the management of gastrointestinal stromal tumors. Clin Colorectal Cancer 2006; 6(Suppl 1):S30–4.

51. Barnes G, Bulusu VR, Hardwick RH et al. A review of the surgical management of metastatic gastrointestinal stromal tumours (GISTs) on imatinib mesylate (Glivec). Int J Surg 2005; 3:206–12.

52. DeMatteo RP, Maki RG, Singer S et al. Results of tyrosine kinase inhibitor therapy followed by surgical resection for metastatic gastrointestinal stromal tumor. Ann Surg 2007; 245:347–52.

Patients with responsive disease may benefit from surgery.

53. Desai J, Shankar S, Heinrich MC et al. Clonal evolution of resistance to imatinib in patients with metastatic gastrointestinal stromal tumors. Clin Cancer Res 2007; 13(15):5398–405.

54. Gronchi A, Fiore M, Miselli F et al. Surgery of residual disease following molecular-targeted therapy with imatinib mesylate in advanced/metastatic GIST. Ann Surg 2007; 245:341–6.

55. Elias D, Maisonnette F, Druet-Cabanac M et al. An attempt to clarify indications for hepatectomy for liver metastases from breast cancer. Am J Surg 2003; 185:158–64.

56. Adam R, Aloia T, Krissat J et al. Is liver resection justified for patients with hepatic metastases from breast cancer? Ann Surg 2006; 244:897–907; discussion 908.

57. Sakamoto Y, Yamamoto J, Yoshimoto M et al. Hepatic resection for metastatic breast cancer: prognostic analysis of 34 patients. World J Surg 2005; 29:524–7.

58. Martinez SR, Young SE, Giuliano AE et al. The utility of estrogen receptor, progesterone receptor, and Her-2/neu status to predict survival in patients undergoing hepatic resection for breast cancer metastases. Am J Surg 2006; 191:281–3.

59. Selzner M, Morse MA, Vredenburgh JJ et al. Liver metastases from breast cancer: long-term survival after curative resection. Surgery 2000; 127:383–9.

60. Vlastos G, Smith DL, Singletary SE et al. Long-term survival after an aggressive surgical approach in patients with breast cancer hepatic metastases. Ann Surg Oncol 2004; 11:869–74.

61. Carlini M, Lonardo MT, Carboni F et al. Liver metastases from breast cancer. Results of surgical resection. Hepatogastroenterology 2002; 49:1597–601.

62. Chi DS, McCaughty K, Diaz JP et al. Guidelines and selection criteria for secondary cytoreductive surgery in patients with recurrent, platinum-sensitive epithelial ovarian carcinoma. Cancer 2006;106(1):1933–9.

63. Armstrong DK, Bundy B, Wenzel L et al. Intraperitoneal cisplatin and paclitaxel in ovarian cancer. N Engl J Med 2006; 354(5):34–43.

64. Bristow RE, Montz FJ, Lagasse LD et al. Survival impact of surgical cytoreduction in stage IV epithelial ovarian cancer. Gynecol Oncol 1999; 72:278–87.

65. Naik R, Nordin A, Cross PA et al. Optimal cytoreductive surgery is an independent prognostic indicator in stage IV epithelial ovarian cancer with hepatic metastases. Gynecol Oncol 2000; 78:171–5.

66. Yoon SS, Jarnagin WR, Fong Y et al. Resection of recurrent ovarian or fallopian tube carcinoma involving the liver. Gynecol Oncol 2003; 91:383–8.

67. Dekernion JB, Ramming KP, Smith RB. The natural history of metastatic renal cell carcinoma: a computer analysis. J Urol 1978; 120:148–52.

68. Goodman VL, Rock EP, Dagher R et al. Approval summary: sunitinib for the treatment of imatinib refractory or intolerant gastrointestinal stromal tumors and advanced renal cell carcinoma. Clin Cancer Res 2007;13(1):1367–73.

69. Thelen A, Jonas S, Benckert C et al. Liver resection for metastases from renal cell carcinoma. World J Surg 2007; 31:802–7.

70. Alves A, Adam R, Majno P et al. Hepatic resection for metastatic renal tumors: is it worthwhile? Ann Surg Oncol 2003; 10:705–10.

71. Balch CM, Soong SJ, Gershenwald JE et al. Prognostic factors analysis of 17,600 melanoma patients: validation of the American Joint Committee on Cancer melanoma staging system. J Clin Oncol 2001; 19(15):3622–34.

72. Wood TF, DiFronzo LA, Rose DM et al. Does complete resection of melanoma metastatic to solid intra-abdominal organs improve survival? Ann Surg Oncol 2001; 8:658–62.

73. Hodgson R, Fink MA, Jones RM. The role of abdominal resectional surgery in metastatic melanoma. Aust NZ J Surg 2007; 77:855–9.

74. Tafra L, Dale PS, Wanek LA et al. Resection and adjuvant immunotherapy for melanoma metastatic to the lung and thorax. J Thorac Cardiovasc Surg 1995; 110:119–28; discussion 129.

75. Rose DM, Essner R, Hughes TM et al. Surgical resection for metastatic melanoma to the liver: the John Wayne Cancer Institute and Sydney Melanoma Unit experience. Arch Surg 2001; 136:950–5.

76. Albert DM, Ryan LM, Borden EC. Metastatic ocular and cutaneous melanoma: a comparison of patient characteristics and prognosis. Arch Ophthalmol 1996; 114:107–8.

77. Pawlik TM, Zorzi D, Abdalla EK et al. Hepatic resection for metastatic melanoma: distinct patterns of recurrence and prognosis for ocular versus cutaneous disease. Ann Surg Oncol 2006; 13:712–20.

78. Daly JM, Karnell LH, Menck HR. National Cancer Data Base report on esophageal carcinoma. Cancer 1996; 78(15):1820–8.

79. Yamamoto T, Tachibana M, Kinugasa S et al. Esophagectomy and hepatic arterial chemotherapy following hepatic resection for esophageal cancer with liver metastasis. J Gastroenterol 2001; 36:560–3.

80. Hanazaki K, Kuroda T, Wakabayashi M et al. Hepatic metastasis from esophageal cancer treated by surgical resection and hepatic arterial infusion chemotherapy. Hepatogastroenterology 1998; 45:201–5.

81. Koga R, Yamamoto J, Ohyama S et al. Liver resection for metastatic gastric cancer: experience with 42 patients including eight long-term survivors. Jpn J Clin Oncol 2007; 37:836–42.

82. Hemming AW, Sielaff TD, Gallinger S et al. Hepatic resection of noncolorectal nonneuroendocrine metastases. Liver Transpl 2000; 6:97–101.

83. Ercolani G, Grazi GL, Ravaioli M et al. The role of liver resections for noncolorectal, nonneuroendocrine metastases: experience with 142 observed cases. Ann Surg Oncol 2005; 12:459–66.

84. Earle SA, Perez EA, Gutierrez JC et al. Hepatectomy enables prolonged survival in select patients with isolated noncolorectal liver metastasis. J Am Coll Surg 2006; 203:436–46.

85. Rasco DW, Assikis V, Marshall F. Integrating metastasectomy in the management of advanced urological malignancies – where are we in 2005? J Urol 2006; 176:1921–6.

86. Hahn TL, Jacobson L, Einhorn LH et al. Hepatic resection of metastatic testicular carcinoma: a further update. Ann Surg Oncol 1999; 6:640–4.

87. Rivoire M, Elias D, De Cian F et al. Multimodality treatment of patients with liver metastases from germ cell tumors: the role of surgery. Cancer 2001; 92(1):578–87.

88. Siefker-Radtke AO, Walsh GL, Pisters LL et al. Is there a role for surgery in the management of metastatic urothelial cancer? The M. D. Anderson experience. J Urol 2004; 171:145–8.

89. Shen KR, Meyers BF, Larner JM et al. Special treatment issues in lung cancer: ACCP evidence-based clinical practice guidelines (2nd edition). Chest 2007; 132:290S–305S.

90. Takahashi K, Ashizawa N, Minami T et al. Malignant pheochromocytoma with multiple hepatic metastases treated by chemotherapy and transcatheter arterial embolization. Intern Med 1999; 38:349–54.

91. Watanabe D, Tanabe A, Naruse M et al. Transcatheter arterial embolization for the treatment of liver metastases in a patient with malignant pheochromocytoma. Endocr J 2006; 53(1):59–66.

92. Chi DS, Fong Y, Venkatraman ES et al. Hepatic resection for metastatic gynecologic carcinomas. Gynecol Oncol 1997; 66:45–51.

8

Portal hypertension

John A.C. Buckels
Geoffrey H. Haydon
Simon P. Olliff

Introduction

The management of portal hypertension has evolved from a surgical discipline into one with the majority of patients successfully treated by medical and radiological therapies. Surgery still has a distinct role for a limited number of patients, chiefly those with extrahepatic portal hypertension and those suitable for liver transplantation (which can cure both the complications and the underlying liver disease). As patients with gastrointestinal (GI) bleeding will often be referred for a surgical opinion, it is important that the surgeon has a good understanding of the pathophysiology of variceal bleeding as well as the treatment options.

Portal hypertension itself does not require treatment, but intervention is indicated when the risk of bleeding from varices is present or when complications such as actual variceal haemorrhage or the formation of ascites occurs. The management of many patients commences with a herald variceal bleed which requires effective therapy before a plan can be made for longer-term treatment. A significant choice of options is now available, many of which are evidence-based. These include: pharmacotherapy to both prevent and treat variceal bleeding; endoscopic options of injection therapy or variceal ligation; radiologically placed transjugular intrahepatic portosystemic shunts (TIPS); and surgical options (surgical shunts and liver replacement). The selection of these options need to be tailored to the individual patients, taking into account their general fitness, including severity of any underlying liver disease and the local medical facilities and expertise available.

This chapter will briefly outline the causes, pathophysiology and natural history of portal hypertension, but will concentrate on the evaluation and the management of both asymptomatic and acutely bleeding patients with varices bleeds together with longer-term strategies. In addition, specific recommendations will be made for the management of ascites and for patients with hepatic venous outflow obstruction due to Budd–Chiari syndrome.

Aetiology and pathophysiology of portal hypertension

Traditionally, portal hypertension has been classified as prehepatic, intrahepatic or posthepatic, with the intrahepatic causes subdivided into presinusoidal, sinusoidal and postsinusoidal (Table 8.1). Prehepatic causes are usually due to portal vein thrombosis, which is discussed later in this chapter. The main cause of portal hypertension in the West is cirrhosis. This is a sinusoidal obstruction to portal flow with varying causes. Viral hepatitis and alcoholic liver disease are the most common causes, but others include primary biliary cirrhosis, primary sclerosing cholangitis and haemochromatosis. Presinusoidal obstruction due to hepatic fibrosis occurs in schistosomiasis. Worldwide, this is one of the commonest causes of portal hypertension and as it is usually associated with normal liver function has a better prognosis. The main causes of postsinusoidal portal hypertension are hepatic

Table 8.1 • Causes of portal hypertension

Presinusoidal	Sinusoidal	Postsinusoidal
Extrahepatic	**Cirrhotic**	Budd–Chiari syndrome
Portal vein thrombosis	Postviral (B,C)	Veno-occlusive disease
Splenic vein thrombosis	Alcoholic	Caval web
Increased splenic flow	Cryptogenic	Constrictive pericarditis
(tropical splenomegaly,	Primary biliary cirrhosis	
myelofibrosis)	Primary sclerosing cholangitis	
Intrahepatic	Chronic active hepatitis	
Schistosomiasis	Haemochromotosis	
Congenital hepatic fibrosis	Wilson's disease	
Sarcoidosis	**Non-cirrhotic**	
	Acute alcoholic hepatitis	
	Cytotoxic drugs	

venous thrombosis (Budd–Chiari syndrome) and veno-occlusive disease.

Experimental studies have demonstrated that the initial factor in the pathophysiology of portal hypertension is the increase in vascular resistance to portal blood flow. In cirrhosis, this increase in resistance occurs in the hepatic microcirculation (sinusoidal portal hypertension), and is a consequence of both a 'passive' and an 'active' component. The 'passive' component is the mechanical consequence of the hepatic architectural disorder resulting from histological cirrhosis, and the 'active' component the active contraction of portal/septal myofibroblasts, activated stellate cells and portal venules. The increase in intrahepatic tone is probably a consequence of an imbalance between an increase in the endogenous vasoconstrictor substances, such as endothelin, noradrenaline, the leukotrienes and angiotensin II, and a relative decrease in the endogenous vasodilator nitric oxide.[1] Vasodilatory drugs (for example, calcium channel blockers) may restore the equilibrium in intrahepatic tone, although they are not used for this indication in clinical practice.

The other major pathophysiological factor contributing to portal hypertension is an increase in portal venous blood flow through the portal circulation resulting from splanchnic arteriolar vasodilatation caused by an excessive release of endogenous arteriolar vasodilators (endothelial, neural and humoral). This can be corrected by means of splanchnic vasoconstrictors such as terlipressin and non-selective beta-blockers. Many drugs which lower portal pressure both reduce intrahepatic vascular resistance and decrease portal venous inflow.

An important but rare form, segmental or left upper quadrant portal hypertension, occurs in patients with splenic vein thrombosis. This should be suspected in patients with bleeding varices but normal liver function, particularly if there is a history of either acute or chronic pancreatitis.

The natural history of portal hypertension

The prevalence of oesophageal varices in patients with cirrhosis and portal hypertension is high. When cirrhosis is diagnosed, varices are present in 40% of compensated and 60% of decompensated cirrhotics.[2] After the initial diagnosis of cirrhosis, varices develop with an incidence of 5% per year; subsequently, they may progress from small to large at an incidence of 10–15% per year.[3] Rapid progression of hepatic decompensation is associated with a rapid increase in size, whilst improvement in liver function, particularly when associated with removal of the injurious agent (e.g. abstinence from alcohol), may result in decrease in size or disappearance of the varices.[4,5]

The overall incidence of variceal bleeding following diagnosis is of the order of 25% in unselected patients. The most important predictive factors of variceal bleeding are: severity of liver dysfunction; size of varices and intravariceal wall pressure (which although difficult to measure may correlate at endoscopy with the presence of red spots or red weals).[6] Traditionally, liver dysfunction has been classified using the Child–Pugh score[7] (Table 8.2), but a more recent scoring system, the MELD (Model for End-stage Liver Disease), may be a better prognostic indicator (Box 8.1).[8] Variceal size may be the best single predictor of variceal bleeding and

Table 8.2 • Child–Pugh classification

	Number of points		
	1	**2**	**3**
Bilirubin (μmol l⁻¹)*	<34	34–51	>51
Albumin (g l⁻¹)	>35	28–35	<28
Prothrombin time prolonged by (s)	<3	3–10	>10
Ascites	None	Slight to moderate	Moderate to severe
Encephalopathy	None	Slight to moderate	Moderate to severe

Grade A 5–6 points; Grade B 7–9 points; Grade C 10–15 points.
*In primary biliary cirrhosis, the point scoring for bilirubin level is adjusted as follows: 1 = <68, 2 = 68–170, 3 = >170.

generally it is used to decide whether a patient should be given prophylactic therapy or not. Whether a patient dies from a variceal bleed depends on the severity of the accompanying liver failure; those with a high Child–Pugh or MELD score have been reported to have as high a risk of mortality as 30–50% within 6 weeks of the index bleed.[9] However, a more accurate figure may be a mortality of 20% at 6 weeks; immediate mortality from uncontrolled bleeding is as low as 5–8%. Indeed, in 40–50% of patients who bleed and develop hypotension, variceal bleeding stops spontaneously, probably as a result of reflex splanchnic vasoconstriction with associated reduction in portal pressure and blood flow; this beneficial response is nullified by over-transfusing the patient.

The incidence of re-bleeding ranges between 30% and 40% within the first 6 weeks; this risk peaks in the first 5 days following the index bleed. Bleeding gastric varices, active bleeding at emergency endoscopy, low serum albumin levels, renal failure and a hepatic venous pressure gradient >20 mmHg have all been reported as significant indicators of an early risk of re-bleeding.[10-12] Patients surviving a first episode of variceal bleeding have a very high risk of re-bleeding (63%) and death (33%), and this is the basis for treating all patients to prevent further bleeding.[9]

Presentation

Portal hypertension may present acutely with variceal bleeding or be discovered during the investigation of a patient with liver disease. Varices are usually easily diagnosed at endoscopy and patients will then be investigated systematically. A classification of the grading of varices is given in Table 8.3. Presentation of patients with liver disease is variable and ranges from non-specific tiredness to advanced encephalopthy with decompensation. External features of advanced liver disease such as spider naevi, palmar erythema and ascites are easy to detect, although these signs will be lacking in many patients. Splenomegaly is probably the most useful physical sign, although some patients will have the classic sign of dilated umbilical vein collaterals (caput medusae).

Imaging

Doppler ultrasonagraphy is a useful and easily obtained initial imaging modality for patients

Box 8.1 • Model for End-stage Liver Disease (MELD)

MELD is calculated for patients over the age of 12 based on the following variables:

- Serum creatinine (mg/dL)
- Total bilirubin (mg/dL)
- INR (international normalised ratio).

The formula incorporates these variables as:

MELD = 3.78[Ln serum bilirubin (mg/dL)] + 11.2[Ln INR] + 9.57[Ln serum creatinine (mg/dL)] + 6.43

The following rules must be observed when using this formula:

- 1 is the minimum acceptable value for any of the three variables.
- The maximum acceptable value for serum creatinine is 4.
- The maximum value for the MELD score is 40. All values higher than 40 are given a score of 40.
- If the patient has been dialysed twice within the last 7 days, then the value for serum creatinine used should be 4.0.

In being considered for liver transplantation, patients with a diagnosis of liver cancer are assigned a MELD score based on how advanced the cancer is, using the TNM staging system.

Table 8.3 • Classification of oesophageal and gastric varices

Classification of varices		
Oesophageal varices	Grade 0 (or absent)	
	Grade 1 (or small)	Varices that collapse on insufflation of oesophagus with air
	Grade 2 (or medium)	Varices which do not collapse on air insufflation
	Grade 3 (or large)	Varices that are large enough to occlude the lumen
Gastric varices	GOV1	Gastro-oesophageal varices extending <5 cm from the oesophagus across gastro-oesophageal junction
	GOV2	Gastro-oesophageal varices extending into the fundus across gastro-oesophageal junction
	IGV1	Isolated gastric varices in the fundus
	IGV2	Isolated non-fundic varices

with suspected portal hypertension. Spleen size and the state of the liver parenchyma can be assessed together with portal and hepatic vein patency and flow velocity, and the presence or absence of varices can often be determined. Computed tomography (CT) and magnetic resonance imaging (MRI) now give detailed road-maps of vascular anatomy prior to any surgical intervention with no need for invasive angiography in most cases.

Management of varices

The management of oesophageal varices will be considered in three sections: the prevention of bleeding in patients with varices who have never bled; the longer-term management of patients who have bled to prevent future bleeding episodes; and the emergency resuscitation and initial control of the acute bleeding episode. Though the emergency management of many patients will be in a district general hospital, patients may require referral to specialised centres with expertise in liver diseases and where recourse to specialised radiological intervention is available. As pharmacological therapy is employed in the majority of cases, the treatment aims of this will be discussed first.

Therapeutic aims for pharmacological therapy in portal hypertension

The hepatic venous pressure gradient (HVPG) reflects accurately portal pressure in sinusoidal portal hypertension and is readily measured.

Varices do not develop until the HVPG increases to 10–12 mmHg and the HVPG must be greater than 12 mmHg for the appearance of complications such as variceal bleeding and ascites.[13] Longitudinal studies of patients with complications of portal hypertension have demonstrated that when an HVPG decreases to less than 12 mmHg with pharmacological therapy, TIPS or an improvement in liver function, variceal bleeding is prevented and varices may decrease in size or disappear altogether.[14] When this target isn't reached, a substantial reduction in portal pressure by more than 20% still offers protection against variceal bleeding[15] and thus these two parameters are regarded as the end-points to therapeutic strategies to lower portal pressure.

Recent evidence suggests that these therapeutic end-points may also reduce the risk of other complications of portal hypertension, including ascites, spontaneous bacterial peritonitis and hepatorenal syndrome.[16,17]

Oesophageal varices

Primary prophylaxis for the prevention of variceal haemorrhage

All patients with cirrhosis should be screened for varices at the time of the first diagnosis of their cirrhosis. In patients with grade I varices at index endoscopy, a follow-up endoscopy should be performed after 12 months to detect the progression from grade II to III varices. Patients without varices should be re-evaluated in 2–3 years after their index endoscopy.

The mainstay of primary prophylactic therapy in the prevention of variceal haemorrhage is the non-selective β-adrenergic receptor blocker (beta-blocker). Twelve trials using beta-blockers in this context have been reported.

A meta-analysis has indicated that indefinite treatment with propanolol or nadolol significantly reduces the bleeding risk from 25% with non-active treatment or placebo to 15% with beta-blockers over a median follow-up period of 24 months; there was no significant reduction in mortality.[3] The benefit of therapy was only proven in those patients with grade II (or larger) varices; there was no evidence to support the use of primary prophylactic therapy in patients with grade I varices.

Withdrawal of therapy was associated with a return to the same bleeding risk (25%) as the untreated subpopulation; indeed, there may also be an increased risk of mortality over untreated patients in those individuals who stop therapy.[18,19]

Assessment of the success of primary prophylactic therapy is ideally undertaken by measurement of the HVPG before and after initiating therapy, with the aim being to reduce the HVPG <12 mmHg or to reduce it by >20% from its baseline value.[14] In practice, however, measurement of HVPG does require specific training and is probably not cost-effective for assessing primary prophylactic therapy. Thus, the clinician faces the question of how to adjust the dose of beta-blocker to maximise its beneficial effects. Traditional practice has recommended a stepwise increase in dose until the heart rate decreases by 25% or is <55 beats per minute, or there is arterial hypotension or clinical intolerance. This means that the dose of the beta-blocker is titrated against its β_1 effects (cardiac) and clinical tolerance; however, a fall in portal pressure results from blockade of both β_1 and β_2 receptors, and the fall in portal pressure does not readily correlate with the fall in heart rate or blood pressure. Therefore, titration solely against clinical tolerance may be the most useful surrogate marker of the maximal dose of beta-blocker in the absence of HVPG measurement.

There appears to be no advantage of one non-selective beta-blocker over another. However, the newest approach to increase response to beta-blockers has been the use of carvedilol, a drug which combines a non-selective beta-blocker action with an α_1-adrenoceptor blocker action. This causes a marked decrease in portal pressure, but has the side-effect of systemic hypotension.

When compared with propanolol, carvedilol significantly increased the number of patients achieving a target reduction of HVPG (<12 mmHg or >20% reduction from baseline HVPG).[19] There is considerable controversy about how to give the carvedilol because of its hypotensive side-effects; however, the above study demonstrated that lower doses (12.5 mg/day) or careful titration result in good tolerance.

In patients who are unable to tolerate beta-blockers (15–20%) because of side-effects or relative/absolute contraindications, treatment with nitrates is ineffective, despite its portal pressure-lowering properties.[20] Therefore, variceal band ligation (VBL) therapy is the only option for patients with high-risk varices (grade II or above) and contraindications to beta-blockers. More controversially, a meta-analysis has suggested that VBL is a more effective mode of treatment than beta-blockers for primary prophylaxis.[21] However, this analysis included four trials, only two of which have been published in full; therefore, it seems reasonable to recommend that, for the time being, beta-blockers remain the primary prophylactic therapy of choice in terms of cost and convenience. Of course, VBL does not reduce portal pressure (and therefore measurement of HVPG following endoscopic monotherapy is of no value) and this may leave the patient at risk of developing other complications of portal hypertension. An algorithm for the primary prevention of variceal bleeding is given in **Fig. 8.1**.

Prevention of re-bleeding from oesophageal varices

Following a variceal bleed, patients with cirrhosis should be assessed in two ways: firstly, they should receive urgent and active treatment for the prevention of re-bleeding; secondly, they should be examined for signs of physiological stress following their bleed, which might indicate a need for an elective liver transplant assessment (**Fig. 8.2**). Management of non-cirrhotic patients is discussed later in this chapter.

Endoscopic variceal band ligation therapy or beta-blocker therapy are the treatments of choice for the prevention of re-bleeding from oesophageal varices.

Meta-analyses of studies using beta-blocker therapy to prevent re-bleeding have demonstrated both a significantly decreased mortality (27% in controls to 20% in beta-blocker-treated individuals) and a decreased incidence of re-bleeding (63% to 42%).[3]

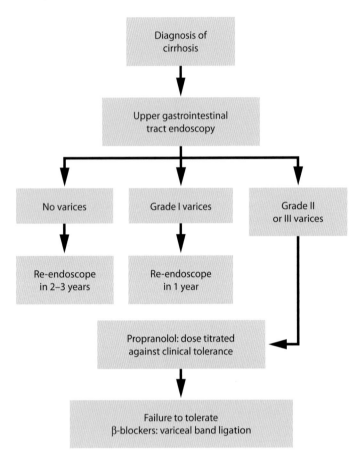

Figure 8.1 • Algorithm for primary prevention of variceal bleeding.

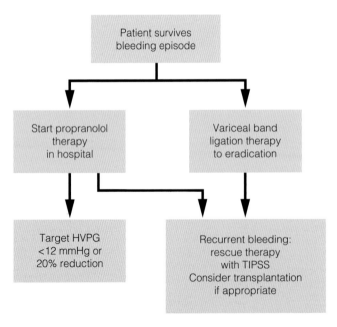

Figure 8.2 • Algorithm for secondary prevention of variceal bleeding.

VBL also both improves survival and significantly decreases re-bleeding rates; it is superior to endoscopic sclerotherapy since it is associated with significantly fewer complications.[22,23] Currently, it is unclear whether pharmacological therapy is better than VBL or vice versa; studies have demonstrated a variety of outcomes with reference to re-bleeding rates, but none have indicated any clear difference in survival.[15,24,25] A combination of pharmacological therapy and endoscopic therapy is commonly used, but evidence suggesting a better outcome with this combination compared with monotherapy is hard to find. Likewise, combination therapy of nitrates and beta-blockers has not been consistently shown to be more effective than beta-blockers alone or to VBL.[15,26]

Re-bleeding is still common with pharmacological or endoscopic therapy (30–50% at 2 years) and in these cases second-line therapies should be offered. This will depend on the underlying aetiology and fitness and age of the patient, and may be TIPS, shunt surgery or liver transplantation; these are considered later in this chapter.

Treatment for bleeding oesophageal varices

Variceal bleeding is a medical emergency and the first priority is to achieve adequate resuscitation of the patient in a safe environment, preferably a high-dependency or intensive care unit. On presentation, airway protection is essential, especially for intoxicated patients or those withdrawing from alcohol. Subsequent therapy is aimed at correcting hypovolaemic shock; blood volume replacement should maintain the haematocrit between 25% and 30% and preferably a pulmonary artery capillary wedge pressure of 10–15 mmHg. Over-transfusion should be avoided because of the risk of a rebound increase in portal pressure with continued bleeding or re-bleeding.

> Antibiotics should be instituted from admission, since these increase the survival of bleeding patients; norfloxacin 400 mg/12 hours or ciprofloxacin 250 mg/12 hours are the antibiotics of choice.[27,28]

Finally, early therapy should also involve starting a vasoactive drug from admission (usually, terlipressin or octreotide); a number of randomised, controlled trials demonstrate that early administration of vasoactive drugs facilitates endoscopy, improves control of bleeding and reduces 5 day re-bleeding rate.[29,30] Initiation of these measures in association with endoscopic therapy at the time of diagnostic endoscopy will control bleeding in about 75% of patients. However, as in most trials, in acute variceal bleeding, this combined approach failed to improve overall mortality compared with drug or endoscopic therapy alone. The optimal duration of vasoactive drug therapy is not well established and requires evaluation; current recommendations are to continue the drug for 5 days, since this covers the period of maximum risk of re-bleeding.

Endoscopic therapy should be performed at the time of diagnostic endoscopy, within 12 hours of admission in a resuscitated patient. However, if the patient is stable, endoscopic therapy can probably be postponed until within normal working hours. There are multiple randomised controlled trials examining modes of endoscopic therapy in acute variceal bleeding. These have compared: endoscopic therapy with no therapy; endoscopic therapy with vasoactive drug therapy; endoscopic sclerotherapy with variceal band ligation therapy; combined endoscopic therapy with variceal band ligation therapy; and endoscopic therapy with TIPS. Endoscopic therapy is certainly superior to no therapy;[31] of the two endoscopic therapies, variceal band ligation therapy should be considered the treatment of choice since it is associated with significantly fewer complications (oesophageal stricturing or oesophageal ulcer formation) and significantly fewer sessions of therapy to eradicate the varices. However, there is probably no difference in re-bleeding or mortality rates between the two therapies. Likewise, there is little evidence to support combined endoscopic therapy for the treatment of bleeding varices.[32] In practice, however, it is sometimes beneficial for the endoscopist to use a small volume of sclerosant initially to improve vision in order to place some variceal bands to achieve eventual haemostasis. If endoscopic therapy fails to control bleeding, balloon tamponade should be used as a 'bridge' until definitive therapy can be offered. In practice, this usually means a further attempt at endoscopic band ligation therapy followed by second-line therapies. An algorithm for the management of variceal bleeding in cirrhotics is given in **Fig. 8.3**.

Gastric varices

Gastric varices are most commonly caused by cirrhosis complicated by portal hypertension and are the source of 5–10% of all upper gastrointestinal bleeding episodes. Patients with pancreatic disease, especially inflammatory pancreatic disease, can also develop splenic vein thromboses with subsequent formation of isolated gastric varices. There have been sporadic reports of gastric varices developing after endoscopic therapy for bleeding oesophageal varices, particularly after endoscopic

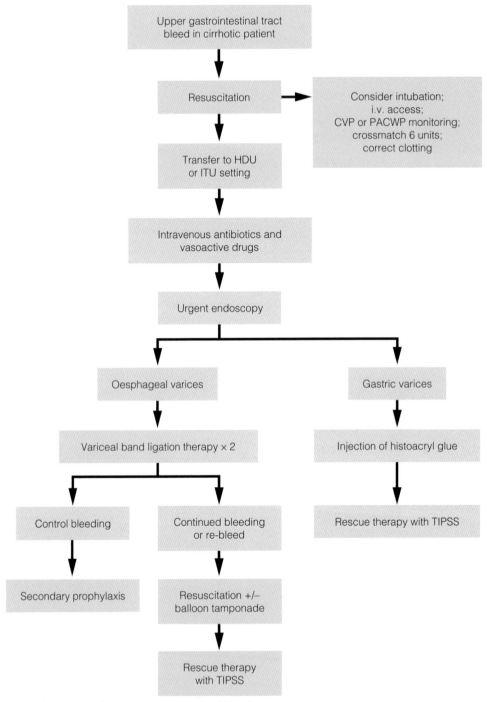

Figure 8.3 • Algorithm for the management of variceal bleeding.

sclerotherapy. The risk of bleeding from gastric varices is no greater than from oesophageal varices and it is probable that pharmacological therapy is equally as effective as primary prophylactic therapy in oesophageal varices, so patients with gastric varices should also receive non-selective beta-blockers as first-line therapy. There are no reports of primary attempts at prophylactic therapy using endoscopic-based therapy.

Treatment of acute gastric variceal bleeding is very challenging. Medical management is similar to the treatment of oesophageal varices. Terlipressin and octreotide are useful for control of acute bleeding, while beta-blockers may also be as effective as secondary prophylactic therapy. The Sengstaken–Blakemore tube may have some utility for controlling bleeding from junctional (GOV1 or GOV2) varices but has little effect on controlling bleeding varices in the fundus or further down the stomach. Some endoscopic therapies are promising, but quality data are scarce; sclerotherapy, glue injection, thrombin and variceal band ligation therapy have all been reported. Control of bleeding using sclerotherapy with cyanoacrylate has been reported as efficacious in 62–100% of cases with successful obliteration of varices in 0–94%.[33,34]

A randomised controlled trial from Taiwan has confirmed that endoscopic sclerotherapy with cyanoacrylate was more effective and also safer than band ligation in the management of bleeding gastric varices.[35]

The major rescue therapy (indeed, some may consider it the primary therapy) for bleeding gastric varices used in the UK is TIPS, which has a greater than 90% success rate for initial haemostasis and re-bleeding rates of 20–30%.

Recently, the first prospective, randomised controlled trial comparing TIPS with cyanoacrylate injection in the prevention of gastric re-bleeding has been published. This concluded that TIPS was more effective than glue injection in preventing re-bleeding from gastric varices, although the two modalities shared a similar mortality rate and frequency of complications.[36]

It is imperative that all patients treated with any of the above-mentioned interventions (for bleeding oesophageal and gastric varices), except medical management, also receive treatment with a proton pump inhibitor (PPI) to suppress acid secretion and to prevent complications related to acid interaction with bands, injection sites and treatment-related ulcers.

Portal hypertensive gastropathy

The presence of portal hypertensive gastropathy (PHG) is strongly correlated with the severity of cirrhosis, its overall prevalence in cirrhosis being about 80%.[37] However, the incidence of acute bleeding is low, occurring in about 2.5% of patients over an 18-month follow-up period, with an associated mortality of 12.5%; the incidence of chronic bleeding is significantly higher at 12%. Propanolol, octreotide and terlipressin have all been proposed for the treatment of acute bleeding from PHG based on their ability to decrease portal blood flow. In a randomised controlled trial, propanolol was found to reduce recurrent bleeding from PHG.[38] Once again, TIPS is considered as the rescue therapy of choice in patients who have repeated bleeding from PHG despite propanolol therapy.

Second-line therapies

Second-line therapies include the less invasive radiological techniques of TIPS or open surgery, which can range from direct oversewing of bleeding veins to surgical shunts and ultimately liver replacement.

TIPS (transjugular intrahepatic portosystemic shunt)

TIPS is a non-surgical method of creating a portocaval shunt. Its principal use is in treating active variceal bleeding or prevention of re-bleeding not controlled by medical and endoscopic means. It therefore has a role in both elective and emergency situations. TIPS is appropriate in selected cases of refractory ascites, hepatic hydrothorax, portal hypertensive gastropathy, Budd–Chiari syndrome and hepatorenal syndrome. TIPS may facilitate surgery in patients with portal hypertension requiring hepatic or other abdominal surgery, although it is not generally used prior to liver transplant without other specific indications.

TIPS is created by needle puncture from a hepatic vein to a major intrahepatic portal vein branch. The track is maintained by a stent.

The degree of shunting can be tailored to some extent by adjusting the diameter of the balloon-dilated shunt against the resulting pressure gradient, directly measured through the catheter.[39]

Occasionally there are severe and life-threatening complications but in the majority of cases few and only minor complications occur. Simpler radiological interventions can restore and maintain most narrowed or occluded TIPS, providing satisfactory secondary patency. Patients require regular follow-up by Doppler ultrasound and elective venography may be performed to treat stenoses before significant bleeding recurs. As with any shunt there is a risk of encephalopathy. This is greater in older patients, wider diameter shunts and in those with prior encephalopathy or more advanced liver disease. Patients with precarious liver function may deteriorate into liver failure as a result of reduced portal perfusion.

An early disadvantage of TIPS was the poor primary patency rate but this can be significantly improved by the use covered stents, as demonstrated in a recent randomised trial.[40]

TIPS has been compared unfavourably with surgery (see later section on surgical shunts) because of the high rate of reintervention, yet overall survival has been similar in randomised trials of both H-graft portocaval shunts and distal splenorenal shunts versus TIPS.[41,42] However, TIPS is usually preferred in patients with more advanced liver disease and in those likely to need future transplantation. Patients with more severe liver disease may be candidates for liver transplantation but TIPS can stabilise some to enable survival long enough to receive a successful transplant. Moreover, the MELD score can be used to predict likely survival following TIPS.[43]

TIPS for variceal bleeding

Uncontrolled bleeding from oesophagogastric or ectopic varices in the presence of a patent portal vein can usually be controlled by TIPS. The procedure can be performed on patients considered too sick for surgery. The mortality of these patients is due more to their general condition rather than the TIPS procedure. The 30-day mortality after TIPS in the UK National Confidential Enquiry into Perioperative Death study was 17%.[44] In this study 80% of patients dying after TIPS had the procedure performed urgently or as an emergency for bleeding varices.

TIPS can be combined with embolisation of varices as there is direct access to the portal system. This is done particularly in acute bleeding to further reduce the risk of haemorrhage. Reduction of extrahepatic portosystemic shunting may also improve portal venous flow towards the liver and the TIPS. In some cases this may counter encephalopathy as well as helping to maintain flow in the TIPS.

Meta-analyses of several trials[45,46] compare TIPS with endoscopic sclerotherapy and/or banding for prevention of recurrent variceal bleeding. Additional medical therapy was included in some.

TIPS was more successful at preventing re-bleeding but with no overall improvement in mortality. Encephalopathy was overall more frequent in the TIPS patients, but not in every trial. In some studies patients in the endoscopic groups were rescued by TIPS because of significant recurrent bleeding. General consensus is that endoscopic and medical therapy should be the primary treatment and TIPS reserved for those cases where control is not achieved. TIPS may be combined effectively with medical treatment or endoscopic variceal eradication after bleeding has been controlled. Long-term TIPS surveillance and reintervention may then be less necessary.[47,48]

Other procedures have been used to control bleeding from varices when venous anatomy permits catheter access. Retrograde balloon occlusion of gastric varices has been mainly used in Asia as an alternative to TIPS when there is a patent gastrorenal venous connection.[49,50]

Surgical options

Until endoscopic sclerotherapy was introduced in the early 1970s, the only practical options were surgical. These ranged from oesophageal transection and devascularisation procedures, portosystemic shunt procedures and, more recently, liver transplantation which is the treatment of choice for patients with variceal bleeding who meet the acceptance criteria.

Devascularisation procedures have been popular in Japan but were rarely used in the West and have been largely superseded by TIPS.

Portal systemic shunts

The variety of surgical shunts described for portal hypertension is perhaps a testament to the ingenuity of surgeons (**Fig. 8.4**). With the passing of the 'shunt era' most surgical trainees will not have seen a shunt, which now has a limited application for a selected group of patients. These are mainly those with non-cirrhotic portal hypertension and patients living in areas where newer therapies are not available.

A controlled crossover trial comparing DSRS with endoscopic sclerotherapy showed that shunting produced better control of bleeding but did not produce any survival advantage.[51]

Shunt operations can be classified into selective or non-selective shunts. The latter carry lower rates of hepatic encephalopathy but are less successful in controlling acute bleeding situations. The two main procedures which have achieved popularity are the distal splenorenal (Warren) shunt (DSRS) and the interposition portocaval or mesocaval shunt utilising a small-diameter prosthetic H-graft

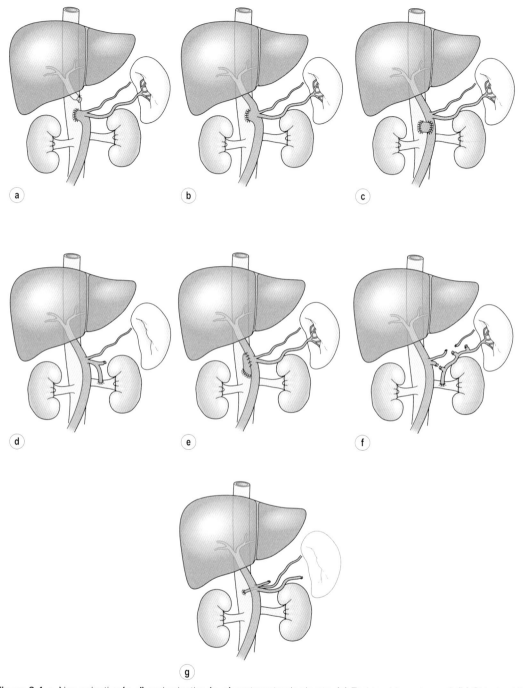

Figure 8.4 • Non-selective **(a–d)** and selective **(e–g)** portosystemic shunts. **(a)** End-to-side portocaval. **(b)** Side-to-side portocaval. **(c)** Mesocaval (jugular vein graft or prosthesis). **(d)** Proximal splenorenal. **(e)** Small-diameter PTFE H-graft portocaval. **(f)** Distal splenorenal (Warren). **(g)** Left gastric-IVC (Inokuchi).

(see Fig. 8.4e,f). Direct primary portocaval anastomosis produces the most effective lowering of portal pressure but with the highest encephalopathy rates, and the advantage of the small-diameter portocaval H-graft is that it is selective and main-

tains some portal flow. This shunt has been compared to TIPS in a single-centre randomised trial in which the entry criterion was variceal bleeding in patients who had failed or 'were not amenable to' sclerotherapy or banding; recruitment was rapid, which suggests a low threshold to proceed with second-line therapies.[52] There was a higher 30-day mortality in shunt patients but a better long-term control of bleeding than that seen in the TIPS patients. It should be recognised that the expertise needed for TIPS insertion and the protocols for subsequent surveillance will vary between centres, such that results should be interpreted with caution as they may reflect local interest and expertise. It had previously been established that shunt surgery for cirrhotics carries significant postoperative mortality rates, being as high as 26.1% for Child C patients even in specialised centres.[53] Furthermore 5-year survival rates in patients with advanced liver disease are poor and shunt surgery carries an additional burden due to the risks of hepatic encephalopathy.

 A recently reported multicentre randomised trial of TIPS versus DSRS showed no overall difference in survival and a tendency for TIPS to be more cost-effective in terms of lives saved.[42,54]

On current evidence there is no role for routine shunting in cirrhotic patients. Shunts should be avoided in patients in whom transplantation is an option as they significantly increase the risk of surgery. If endoscopic and radiological approaches fail, surgery away from the liver hilum is recommended either as a splenorenal or interposition mesocaval shunt.[55]

Liver transplantation

With the improved results and wider application of liver transplantation, this has become the definitive treatment for many patients with variceal bleeding. However, results are inferior for patients transplanted around the time of an acute bleed. Furthermore, there are reports of oesophageal complications including perforation in grafted patients who have undergone recent endoscopic therapy. Thus the indications for liver replacement are more to do with the stage of the underlying liver disease, although the priority for grafting will be influenced by a history of recent bleeding or a high risk for re-bleeding.

In 1997, minimal selection criteria, based on studies of the natural history of compensated chronic liver diseases, were developed to aid such a process.[56] The minimal listing criteria were: an estimated 1-year survival ≤90%; Child–Pugh score ≥7 (Class B or C) or portal hypertensive bleeding, or an episode of spontaneous bacterial peritonitis regardless of the Child–Pugh score. The basis of these criteria is that the expected outcome of the untreated patient would be significantly worse than that of the outcomes from liver transplanta-tion. This recognises the significantly worse prognosis of decompensated cirrhosis, which in those with hepatitis C, for example, dramatically reduces from a 91% 5-year survival to 50%.[57] Spontaneous bacterial peritonitis carries an adverse outcome in these patients with 1-year survival falling from 66% to 38% in one report,[58] and despite the many therapeutic modalities available for treatment, the only definitive therapy for recurrent variceal bleeding is liver transplantation.[59]

Broadly, liver transplantation should be considered in any patient who is able to cooperate with the treatment and in whom an anticipated survival rate of at least 50% at 5 years postgrafting is likely to be achieved. The decisions to proceed to liver replacement should be made by a multidisciplinary team including an experienced hepatologist.

Selection of second-line therapy

Non-cirrhotic

The easiest groups to consider are those without cirrhosis. If such patients fail with pharmacological or endoscopic therapy then a surgical shunt is the treatment of choice. For those with portal vein thrombosis a distal splenorenal shunt is recommended and has the advantage of preserving the spleen. For non-cirrhotics with patent portal veins the choice rests between a portocaval or distal splenorenal depending on local expertise.

Cirrhotic

It is clear that if the patient is a potential transplant candidate they should be assessed for this once the initial bleeding problem has been controlled. If the bleeding cannot be controlled they should be considered for urgent TIPS insertion and then consideration for liver replacement. Patients who are unsuitable for transplantation may be candidates for TIPS provided they do not have significant encephalopathy as this may worsen following the procedure. Once the transplant candidates, patients who are high risk because of comorbidity, and uncooperative patients who are actively drinking are identified as unsuitable for shunting, this leaves few potential candidates for this procedure. Clearly, in areas where transplantation is not available as an option, patients should be considered for shunting provided they are Child A or B.

Management of ascites

Ascites is a common feature of portal hypertension, although the exact mechanisms remain under debate.[60] Ascites in chronic liver disease can be effectively treated by a number of medical, surgical or radiological techniques. The new development of ascites should be investigated for the development of bacterial peritonitis, portal vein thrombosis or hepatic malignancy. Initial treatment involves dietary sodium restriction and diuretic therapy. Unresponsive patients may benefit from regular large-volume paracentesis with concurrent intravenous administration of 20% human albumin.[61] Though peritoneo-venous shunting is effective in controlling ascites, potential risks include disseminated intravascular coagulation, sepsis and cardiac failure. It has few advantages over large-volume paracentesis and is not recommended for patients who are transplant candidates.[62] Refractory ascites is an indication for transplant assessment.

TIPS can also be very effective in controlling ascites refractory to medical treatment, but many such patients have very advanced liver disease with poor prognosis. The immediate risk is worsening liver failure and hepatic encephalopathy, and advice from a skilled hepatologist should be sought before TIPS. Older patients and those with renal dysfunction fare worse, and if patients with severe ascites are liver transplant candidates this may be a better option than TIPS. Patients with better liver function and disproportionate ascites, especially those with liver disease that can improve, e.g. by withdrawal from alcohol, respond well to TIPS. Some trials have shown TIPS to be more effective than medical treatment plus paracentesis, but patient selection is most important. Some studies have shown an improved survival and quality of life in patients having TIPS for ascites whereas others have not.[63–65] Surgical shunts are no longer recommended for resistant ascites due to high perioperative mortality and encephalopathy rates.

Budd–Chiari syndrome

Budd–Chiari syndrome is a rare condition resulting from the occlusion of the hepatic veins. Presenting features include acute abdominal pain, ascites, acute fulminant liver failure or chronic liver failure, and can mimic many other conditions. Ultrasonography (US) will show absent or abnormal hepatic venous drainage. CT will often reveal abnormal liver perfusion which can be difficult to interpret and cases may be initially misdiagnosed as advanced hepatic malignancy. One common feature is the compensatory hypertrophy of the caudate lobe of the liver. This occurs as it has venous drainage separate from the three main hepatic veins. This regenerated liver is clearly life preserving, although pressure from the caudate may compound a tendency to caval throm-

bosis, which is seen in a proportion of patients. The majority of patients will have or will develop evidence of a thrombophilic state and should all be assessed by an expert haematologist. Given the lifetime risks of further thromboses, all patients will require long-term anticoagulation. Referral to a specialised centre with suitable hepatology, radiology and surgical skills is advised.

Acute Budd–Chiari syndrome

In the acute presentation there will usually be abdominal pain and swelling. If there is a short stenosis or occlusion of the hepatic vein(s) and/or inferior vena cava (IVC), balloon dilatation or stenting is very effective. Transjugular, transfemoral or transhepatic access may be required. Occlusion or stenosis of the IVC (sometimes a web) may similarly respond to balloon dilatation. If the dilated or recanalised segment of hepatic vein is not satisfactorily maintained after balloon inflation, a metal stent can be inserted to maintain the patent lumen.[66] These approaches have the benefit of restoring physiological hepatic vein outflow in at least one of the main hepatic veins. Adjunctive pharmacological or mechanical thombolysis may assist these procedures in selected cases, especially when acute thrombosis complicates an otherwise successful vein recanalisation. There are individual case reports of systemic thrombolysis producing improvement but these are rare.[67]

 TIPS can be used in both acute and chronic Budd–Chiari, and would now be regarded as the treatment of choice for those not responding to medical therapy and/or hepatic vein recanalisation.[68,69]

A recent study has shown that TIPS was the most frequent treatment modality applied in a 2-year multicentre European study of new Budd–Chiari presentations.[70] The advantage of TIPS is decompression of the portal vein above the compressed part of the IVC within the caudate lobe and avoidance of laparotomy. With their tendency to thrombosis, Budd–Chiari patients have a greater need for reintervention than other TIPS patients but covered stents have shown an improvement patency here as well.[71]

Extended TIPS can be successful treatment for Budd–Chiari syndrome complicated by portal and mesenteric vein thrombosis. A few cases have been described in which TIPS was a stabilising factor before liver transplantation, but most patients improve sufficiently after TIPS to avoid the need for transplantation. If TIPS cannot be achieved then surgical shunt can be performed or liver transplant when there is significant liver failure. In summary, there is a progressive hierarchy of radiological procedures that can manage a majority of Budd–Chiari patients according to their individual venous anatomy. These procedures are effective in combination with appropriate medical therapy.[72]

If the radiological approach fails, the type of surgical shunt will depend on the patency of the vena cava. If the cava is patent a mesocaval shunt using a length of autologous internal jugular vein between the superior mesenteric vein and the infrarenal vena cava is recommended. For cases with caval occlusion, a meso-atrial shunt using a graft of reinforced polytetrafluoroethylene (PTFE) between the superior mesenteric vein and the right atrium can be performed. Selection of patients for shunting is not easy and our experience suggests that patients with jaundice as an early symptom are at risk of decompensation and should be considered for liver grafting. If the patient develops fulminant hepatic failure, then emergency liver transplantation is the only potential option. High success rates are reported but recurrence can occur and all patients will require long-term anticoagulation.

Chronic Budd–Chiari syndrome

Many patients present with significant ascites and marked changes on liver biopsy, which include significant fibrosis or even cirrhosis. It is likely that for some patients the hepatic venous obstruction is sequential and that the condition is asymptomatic until a second or final (third) hepatic vein is occluded. Either hepatic vein dilatation or TIPS should be performed based on the presence of identifiable hepatic veins within the liver.[69,72] Shunt procedures should be reserved for radiological approach failures. Our local experience is that significant jaundice is an adverse prognostic sign and in these cases liver transplantation may be required.

Non-cirrhotic portal hypertension

Portal hypertension is uncommon in the absence of cirrhosis. The causes are mainly portal vein thrombosis, periportal fibrosis and segmental, usually left upper quadrant portal hypertension associated with splenic vein thrombosis.

Portal vein thrombosis

Portal vein thrombosis is rare in the West but is seen more frequently in Third World countries and is thought to be the result of umbilical sepsis in the neonatal period. Presentation can be in early childhood but is usually delayed to the early teenage years. The symptoms are usually that of a sudden variceal bleed, although some patients may be picked up by the presence of significant splenomegaly with or without haematological features of hypersplenism. The management of the acute bleed is similar to the patients with cirrhosis. Re-bleeding or the presence of large gastric varices should be considered as a clear indication for a surgical shunt. Given the risks of splenectomy in the young, a spleen-preserving procedure is recommended. In a small child, splenorenal shunts are less practical because of the small size of the vessels and interposition mesocaval shunts using autologous jugular vein have high success rates with good long-term patency.[73] In larger children, the distal splenorenal (Warren) shunt is usually favoured, although side-to-side splenorenal shunts have been reported in significant numbers from centres with a high prevalence of portal vein thrombosis.[74] The natural history of these patients is interesting in that as they grow the varices become less symptomatic, and certainly shunting is not indicated unless bleeding episodes have occurred.

Extensive mesenteric venous thrombosis is a potentially lethal complication seen in a few patients with portal vein thrombosis. Many patients will present with gut infarction but those presenting late pose major management problems. Careful angiography may reveal particularly dilated mesenteric collaterals, which might allow ad hoc shunts to the cava, but currently only medical therapies to lower portal pressure can be recommended.

Segmental portal hypertension

Segmental portal hypertension should always be considered as the potential cause of bleeding in patients with pancreatic pathology as they may have splenic vein thrombosis. Those with advanced pancreatic malignancy can usually be controlled with medical therapy or sclerotherapy. Patients with chronic pancreatitis who develop variceal bleeding secondary to splenic vein thrombosis should be considered for splenectomy, which will usually be curative.

TIPS and portal vein thrombosis

Interventions have extended into the portal venous system by percutaneous transhepatic, transjugular and even the transplenic routes in selected cases.[75] Limited acute portal vein thrombus is relatively easily treated by TIPS combined with thrombolysis, including clot disruption by balloon or other devices.[76] Patients with normal liver may only require transhepatic portal vein procedures for success, but those with hepatic portal hypertension benefit from TIPS improved outflow as well.

Chronic portal vein thrombosis is often associated with extensive portal collaterals forming a portal vein cavernoma. If there is an appropriate clinical indication, then these can be traversed and the main portal vein flow can be restored by balloon dilatation and/or stent insertion.[77] More extensive occlusion involving the splenic and superior mesenteric veins may respond but with more difficulty, and those with underlying liver disease fare worse.

Key points

- Patients with grade II varices or worse who have not bled should be treated with beta-blockers unless there are medical contraindications.
- Endoscopic band ligation is the initial treatment of choice for acute variceal bleeding.
- After bleeding patients should enter a programme of variceal ligation or beta-blockade to prevent recurrent bleeding.
- TIPS should be considered in patients in whom endoscopic therapy is unsuccessful.
- Liver transplantation should be considered in appropriate cases once variceal bleeding is problematic.
- Shunt surgery should be considered for non-cirrhotic patients with recurrent variceal bleeding and for Child–Pugh stage A and B patients who live in areas where TIPS or transplantation is unavailable.

References

1. Rodríguez-Vilarrupla A, Fernández M, Bosch J et al. Current concepts on the pathophysiology of portal hypertension. Ann Hepatol 2007; 6:28–36.

2. Schepis F, Camma C, Nicefero D et al. Which patients should undergo endoscopic screening for esophageal varices detection? Hepatology 2001; 33:333–8.

3. D'Amico G, Pagliaro L, Bosch J. Pharmacological treatment of portal hypertension: an evidence based approach. Semin Liver Dis 1999; 19:475–505.

   Meta-analysis illustrating the benefits of treating patients with beta-blockers after an episode of bleeding oesophageal varices both in terms of decreasing risk of re-bleeding and decreasing mortality.

4. Zoli M, Merkel C, Magalotti D et al. Natural history of cirrhotic patients with small esophageal varices: a prospective study. Am J Gastroenterol 2000; 95:503–8.

5. Vorobioff J, Grozmann RJ, Picabea E et al. Prognostic value of hepatic venous pressure gradient measurements in alcoholic cirrhosis: a 10 year prospective study. Gastroenterology 1996; 111:701–9.

6. The North Italian Endoscopic Club for the Study and Treatment of Esophageal Varices. Prediction of the first variceal haemorrhage in patients with cirrhosis of the liver and esophageal varices: a prospective multicenter study. N Engl J Med 1988; 319:983–9.

7. Albers I, Hartmann H, Bircher J et al. Superiority of the Child–Pugh classification to quantitative liver function tests for assessing prognosis of liver cirrhosis. Scand J Gastroenterol 1989; 24:269–76.

8. Kamath PS, Wiesner RH, Malinchoc M et al. A model to predict survival in patients with end-stage liver disease. Hepatology 2001; 33:464–70.

9. D'Amico G, Luca A. Natural history. Clinical–haemodynamic correlations. Prediction of the risk of bleeding. Baillière's Best Pract Res Clin Gastroenterol 1997; 11:243–56.

10. Ben Ari Z, Cardin F, McCormik AP et al. A predictive model for failure to control bleeding during acute variceal haemorrhage. J Hepatol 1999; 31:443–50.

11. Goulis J, Armonis A, Patch D et al. Bacterial infection is independently associated with failure to control bleeding in cirrhotic patients with gastrointestinal haemorrhage. Hepatology 1998; 27:1207–12.

12. Moitinho E, Escorsell A, Bandi JC et al. Prognostic value of early measurements of portal pressure in acute variceal bleeding. Gastroenterology 1999; 117:626–31.

13. Garcia-Tsao G, Grozsmann RJ, Fisher RL et al. Portal pressure, presence of gastroesophageal varices and variceal bleeding. Hepatology 1985; 5:419–24.

14. Feu F, Garcia-Pagan JC, Bosch J et al. Relation between portal pressure response to pharmacotherapy and risk of recurrent variceal bleeding in patients with cirrhosis. Lancet 1995; 346:1056–9.

15. Villaneuva C, Minana J, Ortiz J et al. Endoscopic ligation compared with combined treatment with nadolol and isosorbide mononitrate to prevent variceal bleeding. N Engl J Med 2001; 345:647–55.

   References 13–15 provide the rationale for the therapeutic aim of pharmacological therapy to decrease the HVPG to <12 mmHg or reduce it to 20% of its baseline value.

16. Tarantino I, Abraldes JG, Turnes J et al. The HVPG response to pharmacological treatment of portal hypertension predicts prognosis and the risk of developing complications of cirrhosis. J Hepatol 2002; 36(Suppl 1):15A.

17. Bosch J, Abraldes JG, Groszmann R. Current management of portal hypertension. J Hepatol 2003; 38:S54–68.

18. Abraczinskas DR, Ookubo R, Grace ND et al. Propanolol for the prevention of first esophageal haemorrhage: a lifetime commitment? Hepatology 2001; 34:1096–102.

19. Banares R, Moitinho E, Matilla A et al. Randomised comparison of long-term carvedilol and propanolol administration in the treatment of portal hypertension in cirrhosis. Hepatology 2002; 36:1367–73.

References 18 and 19 provide the rationale for the use of long-term beta-blockade to reduce the risk of bleeding in grade II or III varices.

20. Borroni G, Salerno F, Cazzaniga M et al. Nadolol is superior to isosorbide mononitrate for the prevention of the first variceal bleeding in cirrhotic patients with ascites. J Hepatol 2002; 37:315–21.

21. Imperiale TF, Chalasani N. A meta-analysis of endoscopic variceal ligation for primary prophylaxis of esophageal variceal bleeding. Hepatology 2001; 33:908–14.

22. De Franchis R, Primignami M. Endoscopic treatments for portal hypertension. Semin Liver Dis 1999; 19:439–55.

23. Laine L, El Newihi HM, Migikovsky B et al. Endoscopic ligation compared with sclerotherapy for the treatment of bleeding esophageal varices. Ann Intern Med 1993; 119:1–7.

24. Patch D, Sabin CA, Goulis J et al. A randomised, controlled trial of medical therapy versus endoscopic ligation for the prevention of variceal rebleeding in patients with cirrhosis. Gastroenterology 2002; 123:1013–9.

25. Lo GH, Chen WC, Chen MH et al. Banding ligation versus nadolol and isosorbide mononitrate for the prevention of esophageal rebleeding. Gastroenterology 2002; 123:728–34.

26. Gournay J, Masliah C, Martin T et al. Isosorbide mononitrate and propanolol compared with propanolol alone for the prevention of variceal re-bleeding. Hepatology 2000; 31:1239–45.

27. Bernard B, Grange JD, Khac EN et al. Antibiotic prophylaxis for the prevention of bacterial infections in cirrhotic patients with gastrointestinal bleeding: a meta-analysis. Hepatology 1999; 29:1655–61.

28. Rimola A, Garcia-Tsao G, Navasa M et al. Diagnosis, treatment and prophylaxis of spontaneous bacterial peritonitis: a consensus document. International ascites club. J Hepatol 2000; 32:142–53.

References 27 and 28 illustrate the benefit to cirrhotic patients of prophylactic antibiotics following a variceal bleed by decreasing mortality.

29. Avgerinos A, Nevens F, Raptis S et al. Early administration of somatostatin and efficacy of sclerotherapy in acute variceal bleeds: the European acute bleeding oesophageal variceal episodes (ABOVE) randomised trial. Lancet 1997; 350:1495–9.

30. Cales P, Masliah C, Bernard B et al. Early administration of vapreotide for variceal bleeding in patients with cirrhosis. French club for the study of portal hypertension. N Engl J Med 2001; 344:23–8.

31. Infante-Rivard C, Esnaola S, Villeneuve JP. Role of endoscopic variceal sclerotherapy in the long-term management of variceal bleeding: a meta-analysis. Gastroenterology 1989; 96:1087–92.

32. Singh P, Pooran N, Indaram A et al. Combined ligation and sclerotherapy versus ligation alone for secondary prophylaxis of esophageal variceal bleeding: a meta-analysis. Am J Gastroenterol 2002; 97:623–9.

33. Huang YH, Yeh HZ, Chen GH et al. Endoscopic treatment of bleeding gastric varices by N-butyl-2-cyanoacrylate (Histoacryl) injection: long-term efficacy and safety. Gastrointest Endosc 2000; 52:512–9.

34. Kind R, Guglielmi A, Rodella L et al. Bucrylate treatment of bleeding gastric varices: 12 years' experience. Endoscopy 2000; 32:512–9.

35. Lo GH, Lai KH, Cheng JS et al. A prospective randomised trial of butyl cyanoacrylate injection versus band ligation in the management of bleeding gastric varices. Hepatology 2001; 33:1060–4.

This was the first study to compare banding with the injection of 'glue' in the treatment of gastric varices as a prospective randomised trial.

36. Lo GH, Liang HL, Chen WC et al. A prospective, randomised controlled trial of transjugular intrahepatic portosystemic shunt versus cyanoacrylate injection in the prevention of gastric variceal rebleeding. Endoscopy 2007; 39:679–85.

A further rare, randomised controlled trial in gastric variceal bleeding from the same institution. This study compared the efficacy and complications of TIPS with glue injections in preventing re-bleeding from gastric varices. TIPS was more effective than glue injection in preventing re-bleeding, but was associated with a similar risk of mortality and frequency of complications.

37. Primignani M, Carpinelli L, Preatoni P et al. Natural history of portal hypertensive gastropathy in patients with liver cirrhosis. The new Italian endoscopic club for the study and treatment of esophageal varices (NIEC). Gastroenterology 2000; 119:181–7.

38. Perez-Ayuso RM, Pique JM, Bosch J et al. Propanolol in the prevention of recurrent bleeding from severe portal hypertensive gastropathy in cirrhosis. Lancet 1991; 337:1431–4.

39. Rossle M, Siegerstetter V, Olchewski M et al. How much reduction in portal pressure is necessary to prevent variceal rebleeding? A longitudinal study

in 225 patients with transjugular intrahepatic portosystemic shunts. Am J Gastoenterol 2001; 96:3379–83.

Observations on 225 patients having TIPS follow-up. Reduction of pressure gradient by 25–50% of original may be sufficient to prevent re-bleeding rather than the target of 12 mmHg.

40. Bureau C, Pagan JC, Layrargues GP et al. Patency of stents covered with polytetrafluoroethylene in patients treated by transjugular intrahepatic porto-systemic shunts: long-term results of a randomized multicentre study. Liver Int 2007; 27:742–7.

PTFE-covered stents require less reintervention with no disadvantage at 2 years.

41. Rosemurgy AS, Zervos EE, Blooston M et al. Post shunt resource consumption favors small-diameter prosthetic H-graft portocaval shunt over TIPS for patients with poor hepatic reserve. Ann Surg 2003; 237:820–5.

42. Henderson JM, Boyer TD, Kutner MH et al. Distal splenorenal shunt versus transjugular intra-hepatic portal systematic shunt for variceal bleed-ing: a randomized trial. Gastroenterology 2006; 130:1643–51.

43. Ferral H, Gamboa P, Postoak DW et al. Survival after elective transjugular intrahepatic portosys-temic shunt creation: prediction with model for end-stage liver disease score. Radiology 2004; 231:231–6.

44. NCEPOD report on Vascular Interventional Radiology 2000; www.ncepod.org.uk.

45. Burroughs AK, Vangeli M. Transjugular intra-hepatic portosystemic shunt versus endoscopic ther-apy: randomized trials for secondary prophylaxis of variceal bleeding: an updated meta-analysis. Scand J Gastroenterol 2002; 37:249–52.

46. Khan S, Tudur Smith C, Williamson P et al. Portosystemic shunts versus endoscopic therapy for variceal rebleeding in patients with cirrhosis. Cochrane Database Syst Rev 2006; 18:CD000553.

47. Brensing KA, Horsch M, Textor J et al. Hemodynamic effects of propranolol and nitrates in cirrhotic patients with transjugular intrahepatic portosystemic stent-shunt. Scand J Gastorenterol 2002; 37:1070–6.

48. Tripathi D, Lui HF, Helmy A et al. Randomised controlled trial of long term portographic follow up versus variceal band ligation following transjugu-lar intrahepatic portosystemic stent shunt for pre-venting oesophageal variceal rebleeding. Gut 2004; 53:431–7.

49. Hiraga N, Aikata H, Takaki S et al. The long-term outcome of patients with bleeding gastric vari-ces after balloon-occluded retrograde transvenous obliteration. J Gastroenterol 2007; 42:663–72.

50. Cho SK, Shin SW, Lee IH et al. Balloon-occluded retrograde transvenous obliteration of gastric vari-ces: outcomes and complications in 49 patients. Am J Roentgenol 2007; 189:W365–72.

51. Henderson JM, Kutner MH, Millikan WJ Jr et al. Endoscopic variceal sclerosis compared with dis-tal splenorenal shunt to prevent recurrent variceal bleeding in cirrhosis. A prospective, randomized trial. Ann Intern Med 1990; 112:262–9.

Shunting produced better control of bleeding but did not produce any survival advantage.

52. Rosemurgy A, Serafini F, Zweibel B et al. Transjugular intrahepatic portosystemic shunt vs. small-diameter prosthetic H-graft portacaval shunt: extended follow-up of an expanded randomized prospective trial. J Gastroint Surg 2000; 4:589–97.

53. Rikkers LF. The changing spectrum of treatment for variceal bleeding. Ann Surg 1998; 228:536–46.

54. Boyer TD, Henderson JM, Heerey AM et al. Cost of preventing variceal rebleeding with transjugular intrahepatic portal systemic shunt and distal spleno-renal shunt. J Hepatol 2008; 48:407–14.

55. Dell'Era A, Grande L, Barros-Schelotto P et al. Impact of prior portosystemic shunt procedures on outcome of liver transplantation. Surgery 2005; 137:620–5.

56. Lucey MR, Brown KA, Everson GT et al. Minimal criteria for placement of adults on liver transplant waiting list: a report of a national conference orga-nized by the American Association for the Study of Liver Diseases. Liver Transpl Surg 1997; 3:628–37.

57. Fattovich G, Giustina G, Degos F et al. Morbidity and mortality in compensated cirrhosis type C: a retrospective follow up study of 384 patients. Gastroenterology 1997; 112:463–72.

58. Andreu M, Sola R, Sitges-Serra A et al. Risks for spontaneous bacterial peritonitis in cirrhotic patients with ascites. Gastroenterology 1993; 104:1133–8.

59. D'Amico G, Pagliaro L, Bosch J. The treatment of portal hypertension: a meta-analytic review. Hepatology 1995; 22:332–54.

60. Jalan R, Hayes PC. Hepatic encephalopathy and ascites. Lancet 1997; 350:1309–15.

61. Gines A, Fernandez-Esparrach G, Monescillo A et al. Randomized trial comparing albumin, dextran 70, and polygeline in cirrhotic patients with asci-tes treated by paracentesis. Gastroenterology 1996; 111:1002–10.

62. Gines P, Arroyo V, Vargas V et al. Paracentesis with intravenous infusion of albumin as compared with peritoneovenous shunting in cirrhosis with refrac-tory ascites. N Engl J Med 1991; 325:829–35.

63. Salerno F, Camma C, Enea M et al. Transjugular intrahepatic portosystemic shunt for refractory ascites: a meta-analysis of individual patient data. Gastroenterology 2007; 133:825–34.

64. Deltenre P, Mathurin P, Dharancy S et al. Transjugular intrahepatic portosystemic shunt in refractory asci-tes: a meta-analysis. Liver Int 2005; 25:349–56.

65. Saab S, Nieto JM, Lewis SK, Runyon BA. TIPS ver-sus paracentesis for cirrhotic patients with refrac-tory ascites. Cochrane Database Syst Rev 2006; 18:CD 004889.

66. Beckett D, Olliff S. Interventional radiology in the management of Budd Chiari syndrome. Cardiovasc Interv Radiol 2008; 31:839–47.

67. Sharma S, Texeira A, Texeira P et al. Pharmacological thrombolysis in Budd Chiari syndrome: a single centre experience and review of the literature. J Hepatol 2004; 40:172–80.

68. Perello A, Garcia Pagan JC et al. TIPS is a useful long-term derivative therapy for patients with Budd Chiari syndrome uncontrolled by medical therapy. Hepatology 2002; 35:132–9.

69. Eapen CE, Velissaris D, Heydtmann M et al. Favourable medium term outcome following hepatic vein recanalisation and/or transjugular intrahepatic portosystemic shunt for Budd Chiari syndrome. Gut 2006; 55:878–84.

70. Heydtmann M, Raffa S, Olliff S et al. One year survival in Budd–Chiari syndrome treated with TIPS: an international study. Gut 2007; 56(Suppl II):A2.

71. Hernández-Guerra M, Turnes J, Rubinstein P et al. PTFE-covered stents improve TIPS patency in Budd–Chiari syndrome. Hepatology 2004; 40:1197–202.

72. Olliff S. Transjugular intrahepatic portosystemic shunt in the management of Budd Chiari syndrome. Eur J Gastro Hepatol 2006; 18:1151–4.

73. Gauthier F, De Dreuzy O, Valayer J et al. H-type shunt with an autologous venous graft for treatment of portal hypertension in children. J Pediatr Surg 1989; 24:1041–3.

74. Mitra SK, Rao KL, Narasimhan KL et al. Side-to-side lienorenal shunt without splenectomy in non-cirrhotic portal hypertension in children. J Pediatr Surg 1993; 28:398–401.

75. Tuite D J, Rehman J, Davies MH et al. Percutaneous transsplenic access in the management of bleeding varices from chronic portal vein thrombosis. J Vasc Interv Radiol 2007; 18:1571–5.

76. Uflacker R. Applications of percutaneous mechanical thrombectomy in transjugular intrahepatic portosystemic shunt and portal vein thrombosis. Tech Vasc Interv Radiol 2003; 6:59–69.

77. Bilbao JI, Elorz M, Vivas I et al. Transjugular intrahepatic portosystemic shunt (TIPS) in the treatment of venous symptomatic chronic portal thrombosis in non-cirrhotic patients. Cardiovasc Interv Radiol 2004; 27:474–80.

9

The spleen

Richard T. Schlinkert

Introduction

The history of splenic surgery, anatomy and physiology has been nicely detailed by McClusky et al. and will not be reviewed here.[1,2] The spleen lies in the left upper quadrant superior to the level of the costal margin. It is attached to adjacent structures via a series of ligaments, including the splenophrenic, splenorenal, splenocolic and gastrosplenic. Minor attachments to the spleen also include the presplenic fold located anterior to the gastrosplenic ligament, the pancreaticosplenic fold and the phrenicocolic ligament. The splenic vessels run in the splenorenal ligament at the level of the hilum.

Poulin et al.[3] have provided a review of splenic arterial anatomy. Essentially the splenic artery usually arises from the coeliac trunk but may arise from the aorta, the superior mesenteric, middle colic, left gastric or other arteries. The splenic artery gives off pancreatic branches (the largest of which is the pancreatic magna) as well as the left gastroepiploic artery before branching and entering the spleen. The splenic hilum may be characterised by a single, long splenic artery which branches late into the spleen. Alternatively, the artery may branch further from the spleen, making hilar dissection more tedious. Transverse connections exist between the splenic arterial branches. Each artery ends in the sinusoids of a segment of the spleen. The spleen also receives blood flow from the short gastric vessels.

The splenic vein leaves the hilum and runs along the posterior aspect of the pancreas. It receives several pairs of veins from the pancreas. It is joined by the inferior mesenteric vein before merging with the superior mesenteric vein to form the portal vein.

The spleen is composed of two or three lobes and two to ten segments with unique arterial supplies.

This pattern makes partial splenectomy feasible for selected patients. Accessory spleens occur in appropriately 10–15% of patients and are most commonly located near the splenic hilum, but may also be located at distant sites. Accessory spleens must be identified and removed when operating for excessive cellular destruction or sequestration.

The spleen plays significant roles in the fight against infection, particularly infections of encapsulated organisms. It also serves to filter aged blood cellular elements and removes intracellular inclusions, a process known as pitting. Presence of intraerythrocyte inclusions in the peripheral blood suggests either decreased splenic function or asplenia. There are extensive T cell and dendritic cell populations located primarily in the periarterial lymphatic sheaths. B cells are located in the lymphoid nodules while macrophages are distributed widely.

The immune and housekeeping functions of the spleen make splenic preservation desirable whenever feasible; however, massive blood loss from trauma, excessive cellular destruction or sequestration, certain lymphomatous or myeloid diseases, symptomatic splenomegaly, or tumours may require partial or total splenectomy.

Postsplenectomy sepsis

The loss of the spleen's ability to clear encapsulated organisms places splenectomised patients at risk of overwhelming sepsis throughout their life. Mortality from this complication is high. This lifetime risk of postsplenectomy sepsis is approximately 0.02% for adults.[4] In a recent large population-based study from Scotland, Kyaw et al.

report on 1648 splenectomised patients.[5] The study included 7337 years of follow-up and a mean follow-up of 4.45 years per patient. Severe infection, defined as need for hospitalisation, occurred with an incidence of 7 per 100 person-years. Higher risks were seen in older patients (>50) and the highest risk was seen in patients undergoing therapeutic splenectomy for malignancy followed by iatrogenic splenectomy in the setting of malignancy. The risk of overwhelming infection, defined as septicaemia or meningitis, was 0.89 per 100 person-years. Too few instances of this were encountered to define underlying risk factors.

Davies et al.[6] in 2002 revised the guidelines of the British Committee for Standards in Haematology published in 1996.[7] Ideally, vaccinations should be given more than 2 weeks prior to splenectomy. Vaccinations should include polyvalent pneumococcal, haemophilus influenza type B and meningococcal C vaccines (Box 9.1). A 23-valent pneumococcal vaccine has been the standard and protects against 88% of bacteraemic pneumococcal diseases in the USA. The clinical effectiveness is 60–70%.[8] A newer seven-valent vaccine may be more immunogenic but more restrictive in its coverage. Shatz et al.[9] studied prospectively 59 patients in a randomised fashion in an attempt to determine the ideal timing of postoperative immunisation in patients who did not receive preoperative vaccines. Improved functional antibody responses to certain serotypes and serogroups were identified if immunisations were delayed for 14 days. Pneumococcal vaccines should be repeated once at about 5 years.[8] A review of 974 splenectomised patients in Scotland revealed inadequate compliance with vaccination guidelines[10] and surgeons globally need to be more fastidious regarding this measure.

Patients should carry a medical alert card or tag and should be prepared to take antibiotic therapy should early symptoms of a febrile illness develop.

Box 9.1 • Immunisation recommendations

Vaccine recommendations:
• Polyvalent pneumococcus
• Haemophilus influenza B
• Meningococcus

Timing:

Ideal:	>2 weeks preop
If post-op:	Delay 2 weeks if possible
	Better to give sooner than 2 weeks
	if follow-up is unlikely

Repeat pneumococcus vaccine one time at 5 years.

Trauma

Splenic rupture may occur from diseases such as mononucleosis and typhoid; however, rupture is usually secondary to injury, either iatrogenic or traumatic. It has been estimated that 10–40% of splenectomies in adults are secondary to iatrogenic injuries at surgery.[11] Such injuries of the spleen usually result from excess traction against either the splenic ligaments or adhesions to the spleen.

Experience suggests that laparoscopic procedures are associated with lower risk of splenic injury and splenectomy than their open counterparts. Some potential causes of this finding include better visualisation, application of less traction, improved instrumentation for perisplenic dissection, and better control of capsular haemorrhage by the pressure of the pneumoperitoneum. This appears to be one further benefit of laparoscopic surgery in general.

Should iatrogenic splenic injury occur, steps to control this begin with direct pressure. Haemostatic agents such as microfibrillar collagen may be applied to aid haemostasis.[11] New agents such as microporous polysaccharide hemispheres,[12] which are currently under evaluation, may play a role in the future. Pressure on the bleeding site after application of such agents is best performed with biological tissues (i.e. adjacent structure such as omentum) rather than swabs or sponges. When these are removed, the haemostatic agent is often removed with them and rebleeding ensues. Haemostatic instruments such as argon-beam coagulators may be helpful. Ligation of select arteries in the hilum may help control bleeding and partial splenectomy may be required. Pachter et al.[11] detail the results of splenorrhaphy for splenic trauma and again this technique may be useful in iatrogenic injuries. Splenectomy, while not desirable, is preferable to significant blood loss and should be considered when bleeding is excessive, if the patient cannot tolerate prolonged procedures, or if there are other factors which would make rebleeding a greater risk than splenectomy.

Traumatic splenic injury may range from mild to severe and management options of the splenic injury range from observation to emergent splenectomy. Most recommendations regarding management of adult splenic trauma are based on level III and IV evidence.[13] Patients who are haemodynamically unstable should undergo rapid focused assessment by sonography for trauma (FAST).[13,14] If FAST is not available or if it is inconclusive, diagnostic peritoneal lavage is used to document intra-abdominal haemorrhage. Scant fluid on the FAST scan should prompt a search for other causes of shock. A large amount of intraperitoneal blood on FAST is an indication for emergent coeliotomy. Procedures for splenic trauma are performed open

Table 9.1 • American Association for the Study of Trauma (AAST) splenic injury scale based on CT criteria

Grade		Injury description
I	Haematoma	Subcapsular, <10% surface area
	Laceration	Capsular tear, <1 cm parenchymal depth
II	Haematoma	Subcapsular, 10–50% surface area
		Intraparenchymal, <5 cm in diameter
	Laceration	1–3 cm parenchymal depth, which does not involve a trabecular vessel
III	Haematoma	Subcapsular, >50% surface area or expanding; ruptured subcapsular or parenchymal haematoma Intraparenchymal haematoma >5 cm or expanding
	Laceration	>3 cm parenchymal depth, or involving trabecular vessels
IV	Laceration	Laceration involving segmental or hilar vessels producing major devascularisation (>25% of spleen)
V	Laceration	Completely shattered spleen
	Vascular	Hilar vascular injury that devascularises spleen

Advance one grade for multiple injuries, up to grade III.

at present and new technology will need to be developed before laparoscopic splenectomy for trauma will be considered.

Stable patients with physical findings of abdominal trauma should undergo abdominal computed tomography (CT) to assess their injuries, including those to the spleen. A grading system has been developed by the American Association for the Surgery of Trauma (AAST)[15] based on CT findings and is presented in Table 9.1. The decision to operate, however, is not based solely upon these grades and all grades of injuries have undergone successful non-operative management (NOM). Society for Surgery of the Alimentary Tract Patient Care Guidelines[16] are shown in Box 9.2. Indications for operative intervention in splenic trauma include haemodynamic instability, bleeding of more than 1000 ml, transfusion of more than 2 units of blood or other evidence of blood loss. They also suggest a more aggressive non-operative approach for children <14 years of age. Approximately 60–80% of splenic injuries now undergo NOM with success rates of 95%[13] but this

approach has been shown in several studies to be less successful in patients over 55 years of age.[17–19]

The use of selective arterial embolisation (SAE) in the management of splenic trauma was described by Sclafani et al.[20] but remains somewhat controversial. Protocol-driven strategies for its use in splenic trauma have yielded excellent results. Cooney et al.[21] found that a protocol employing SAE conservatively limited its use while providing high success rates for NOM. Haan et al.[22] used a more aggressive SAE strategy with 100% success of NOM and a length of stay of only 3.3 days, which was substantially shorter than historical controls. Others, however, have highlighted the difficulties in using CT grading systems and SAE.[23,24]

The decisions implicit in NOM are difficult and protocols will be useful to aid this process. Ultimately decisions will be determined by clinical acumen and resources available at the centre treating the patient. The risk of postsplenectomy-related sepsis of 0.02% in adults[4] will need to be weighed against the risks of transfusions, ongoing haemorrhage and late rebleeding.

Box 9.2 • Accepted indications for operative intervention in trauma of the spleen based on Society for Surgery of the Alimentary Tract (SSAT) Patient Care Guidelines

- Haemodynamic instability
- Bleeding >1000 ml
- Transfusion of more than 2 units of blood
- Other evidence of ongoing blood loss

More aggressive non-operative approach in children <14 years of age

Elective indications for splenectomy

Most recommendations for elective splenic surgery are based on level III or IV evidence. This is likely due to the relative rarity of diseases requiring splenectomy and the length of follow-up required to assess results. Recent literature reviews are referenced in this chapter when the supporting literature is composed largely of smaller non-prospective studies regarding a particular disease.

Immune thrombocytopenic purpura (ITP)

The most common non-traumatic indication for splenectomy is immune thrombocytopenic purpura. The disease is characterised by low platelet count, normal bone marrow and absence of other causes of thrombocytopenia. The destruction of platelets in this condition is mediated by platelet antibodies. The splenic B cells are a significant source of this antibody and the spleen is also the site of destruction of the platelets in many patients. Platelets may also be destroyed in the liver. ITP remains a diagnosis of exclusion as tests for antiplatelet antibodies are not reliable indicators of the disease. Bone marrow aspirate, if performed, will be normal with perhaps increased numbers of megakaryocytes. The spleen is normal to small in size. A palpable spleen should draw questions regarding the diagnosis. Importantly, platelet function is normal and while spontaneous bruising is common, severe haemorrhage is less likely, even with relatively low platelet counts. With platelet counts of 30 000–50 000, bruising may occur with minor trauma. Spontaneous bleeding may occur at levels less than 10 000 and therapy is frequently instituted with counts of 20 000–30 000.[25] In a retrospective study of 152 patients with ITP, Portielje et al.[26] found little difference in morbidity or mortality in patients with platelet counts greater than 30 000. Using a Markov analysis of retrospective studies from the literature, Cohen et al.[27] found a significant increase in mortality with counts less than 30 000. Most patients will respond to medical therapy, at least initially. Typically, prednisone is the first agent used but if counts respond and do not drop again after the treatment is stopped, observation is warranted. Patients who require prolonged treatment with prednisone, particularly if this is at higher doses, or patients who do not respond to prednisone should be considered for laparoscopic splenectomy. Intravenous immunoglobulin may be used to increase platelet counts temporarily, but the response lasts days to weeks only. Several authors have attempted to define predictors of success for splenectomy for ITP. Response to intravenous immunoglobulin[28,29] and patient age[30] are the only preoperative predictors. Fenaux et al.[30] also found postoperative platelet count to be predictive of long-term success.

Overall, about 85% of patients respond to splenectomy and, in the long term, about 65–85% of patients maintain their platelet counts.[28,31,32] Consideration should be given to screening failures for absence of nuclear inclusions such as Howell–Jolly bodies on peripheral smears which could

indicate residual splenic tissue. Liver spleen scans, magnetic resonance imaging (MRI) or CT may help localise such remnants and removal may result in cure.[32] Mild to moderate degrees of thrombocytopenia without symptoms of purpura or bleeding may be observed without resuming medical therapy.

Evan's syndrome

Rarely, patients develop autoimmune haemolytic anaemia in addition to autoimmune thrombocytopenia, as in Evan's syndrome. Splenectomy may be curative in up to 40% of patients and improve the situation in up to 60%; however, failures are common.[33]

Hereditary spherocytosis

Smedley and Bellingham[34] provide a review of hereditary spherocytosis which is caused by abnormalities of membrane proteins, the most important of which is spectrin. The degree of spectrin deficiency varies, as does the pattern of inheritance. Approximately 75% of cases demonstrate an autosomal dominant pattern. Autosomal recessive patients have a greater degree of spectrin deficiency and unlike the autosomal dominant patients do not respond to splenectomy. The disease is characterised by extravascular destruction of red cells, particularly in the spleen.

Patients with severe disease presenting in childhood require splenectomy. Surgery should be delayed until after 6 years of age if possible to allow maturation of the immune system.[34] Older patients with mild disease may be safely observed. Patients with intermediate disease may be observed with concomitant risk of transfusions, gallstone formation and haemolytic crisis (often triggered by infection), or operated with risk of postsplenectomy sepsis. Obviously, treatment must be tailored to the individual patient.

Cholecystectomy should be performed if gallstones are present at the time of splenectomy. Both laparoscopic splenectomy and cholecystectomy may be safely performed during the same operation.[35]

Stoehr et al.[36] and Bader-Meunier et al.[37] have reported on the use of subtotal splenectomy for the treatment of hereditary spherocytosis. The surgery successfully improved anaemia and maintained splenic function in most patients. However, mild to moderate haemolysis persisted and gallstone formation and aplastic crises still developed in some patients.

Elliptocytosis

The protein spectrin is also abnormal in elliptocytosis. Many mild cases require no therapy; however, if greater than 90% of cells are affected anaemia is substantive, and splenectomy should be considered.

Thallassaemias

Genetic abnormalities resulting in abnormal haemoglobin structure such as thalassaemias may require splenectomy. The haemoglobin tetramer contains alpha and beta subunits. Defective alpha chains lead to alpha thalassaemia and defective beta chains to beta thalassaemia. The alpha chains precipitate in the absence of the beta chain and create the more severe beta thalassaemia. Blood transfusions and chelation therapy are the mainstays of treatment and stem cell transplantation is playing a greater role in the management of this disease.[38] Splenectomy is rarely required. Thalassaemia patients are at increased risk of infective complications postoperatively.

Sickle cell anaemia

Sickle cell anaemia is characterised by high HgF levels. Al-Salem[39] recently reported a large series of patients and detailed the major indications for splenectomy as recurrent acute splenic sequestration crisis, hypersplenism, splenic abscess and massive splenic infarction. There was no mortality and 6% morbidity. Again cholecystectomy is recommended if stones are present and this can simplify the diagnosis if abdominal crisis occurs in the future.

Autoimmune haemolytic anaemia

Autoimmune haemolytic anaemia caused by IgG may respond to splenectomy in perhaps 50% of cases. Failure of medical therapy or need for high-dose steroids should prompt consideration of splenectomy. IgM haemolytic anaemias are not splenic driven and will not respond to splenectomy.

Lymphoma

Hodgkin's disease, for years, required laparotomy for staging and/or diagnosis. Treatment algorithms have changed, radiological scans have improved, and non-operative strategies have advanced to the point where surgical staging procedures are rarely if ever indicated.

Surgery plays essentially no role in the treatment of non-Hodgkin lymphoma. However, splenectomy may be required for symptomatic massive splenomegaly, hypersplenism, diagnosis (in cases of isolated splenic disease) or 'debulking' of splenic predominant disease.

Myeloid disease

Splenectomy plays little or no role in the treatment of chronic myelogenous leukaemias (Philadelphia chromosome translocations). Treatment of hairy cell leukaemia conversely may require splenectomy, although systemic therapy is playing a greater role in the management of the disease.[40]

The spleen may reach truly massive proportions, extending across the midline or into the pelvis or both in primary myelofibrosis (formerly called agnogenic myeloid metaplasia). This may lead to symptomatic splenomegaly, thrombocytopenia, hypercatabolic state with resultant high output heart failure, and forward flow portal hypertension. Life expectancy is perhaps 24 months, but splenectomy can yield significant symptomatic improvement.[41] Mortality rates are high due to bleeding diathesis, disseminated intravascular coagulation, and concomitant metabolic and physiological derangements. Surgery should occur at centres prepared to deal with these eventualities.

Volvulus

Some spleens have elongated or absent ligamentous attachments, leading to a 'wandering' spleen. These spleens may undergo torsion on their vascular pedicle. Patients present with severe abdominal pain and a right lower quadrant mass (the mobile spleen). In some patients, this occurs intermittently. The spleen should be returned to the left upper quadrant and fixed in place there. A mesh sac may be created for the spleen which is then tacked to the diaphragm.[42] A necrotic spleen requires resection.

Haemangiomas

Haemangiomas are the most common benign neoplasm in the spleen. Small lesions (less than 4 cm) may be safely watched.[43] It is unclear what risks larger haemangiomas present and options include splenectomy or observation.

Cysts

Hansen and Moller have recently reviewed the literature regarding splenic cysts.[44] Cystic lesions of the spleen may be classified as parasitic or non-parasitic. Cysts which are smooth walled without septations and asymptomatic may be observed only. Some authors recommend treatment for all cysts greater than 5 cm in diameter although this is somewhat arbitrary. Symptomatic cysts may be laparoscopically unroofed or resected. Percutaneous drainage and alcohol ablation have also been used with unreliable results. Bacterial abscesses may be drained either by percutaneous or surgical means. Splenectomy may be required.

Parasitic cysts are usually echinococcal in origin and the diagnosis is often confirmed by serological studies. Splenic conserving techniques may be appropriate for early disease or disease located at the perimeter of the spleen.[45] Spillage of hydatid cyst contents must be meticulously avoided as anaphylactic shock may occur.

Malignant non-lymphomatous

Primary angiosarcoma is a rare but highly aggressive tumour. Rupture is common and present in about 30% of cases. Lesions often present as multiple nodules and liver metastases are common.[46] Splenectomy is indicated if the lesion is resectable.

Portal hypertension

Forward flow portal hypertension from primary myelofibrosis has already been discussed. Sinistral (left-sided) portal hypertension secondary to splenic vein thrombosis may lead to bleeding gastric varices. Splenectomy is curative. This is the only situation where we currently consider preoperative splenic artery embolisation to decrease venous pressure in the splenic collaterals to increase the safety of surgery. The embolisation is performed under the same anaesthesia as the splenectomy as splenic embolisation is extremely painful to the patient.

Preparation for splenectomy

Preoperative preparation for splenectomy, as for other procedures, is designed to prevent or minimise complications. Splenectomy carries the usual risk of other abdominal operations and, depending on the disease, increased risks such as bleeding, coagulopathies including disseminated intravascular coagulation, and infection (both immediate and delayed). Altered cardiovascular performance may also be seen in the hypercatabolic state of primary myelofibrosis.

Efforts should be made to correct all coagulopathies preoperatively. Thrombocytopenia may require correction. In patients with ITP, laparoscopic splenectomy can be performed safely with very low platelet counts (in our experience as low as 9000). Bruising is increased; however, we have not seen significant bleeding. If platelets are to be given in destructive or consumptive states, transfusion should be held if possible until the splenic artery is controlled to prevent the rapid breakdown of the transfused platelets. Disseminated intravascular coagulation may be present in some states, particularly primary myelofibrosis, and should be treated prior to surgery.

Each patient presents a unique set of physiological parameters and challenges. Blood counts must be adequate for the given patient's cardiovascular risk factors. Red cells should be transfused preoperatively to meet a patient's given cardiovascular need. These cells may be broken down relatively rapidly and so the timing of transfusion is crucial.

Patients with massive splenomegaly second to primary myelofibrosis may have hypertrophied cardiac dysfunction, pulmonary hypertension, ascites and pleural effusions. The patient's condition should be optimised and this may require the assistance of the cardiologist preoperatively. Conditions which lower the patient's white blood cell count or conditions such as thalassaemia may be associated with increased risk of infections immediately following surgery. Appropriate antibiotics should be given preoperatively. Pulmonary function should be optimised and meticulous haemostasis maintained during surgery.

Technique

Open splenectomy

Open splenectomy remains the standard for trauma surgery and surgery for massive splenomegaly such as seen in primary myelofibrosis. The patient is placed in the supine position and prepped from nipples to pubis. An upper midline or left subcostal incision may be used. Our preference is for an upper midline approach. In trauma, four-quadrant packing can control bleeding temporarily. Packs are removed sequentially and bleeding controlled and the spleen is mobilised from its lateral attachments. The hilum may be compressed by the surgeon's hands to secure haemostasis while the remaining vessels are controlled. The remaining vascular attachments are divided and the spleen removed. Haemostasis is checked, in particular by inspecting the ligated short gastric vessels. Inspection is carried out to be sure that there is not another short gastric vessel superior to the highest one visualised.

Massive splenomegaly is approached through a long midline incision. The lesser sac is opened early in the dissection and the splenic artery is ligated. Platelet transfusions are given following this manoeuvre if necessary. The splenic ligaments are divided sequentially and the hilar vessels are divided between clamps and ligated or divided with a linear stapler. The latter is very secure on enlarged splenic veins, which are often encountered in splenomegaly. Accessory spleens should be sought and removed if surgery is designed to correct a destructive or sequestration state.

Laparoscopic splenectomy

 Laparoscopic splenectomy has been shown to be safe, provide comparative haematological results, and carry decreased risks of postoperative complications when compared to open splenectomy. Hospital stay is short. Laparoscopic splenectomy is the preferred procedure for non-traumatic splenectomy in patients with normal to mildly enlarged spleens.[11,47,48]

The operative goal of laparoscopic splenectomy is circumferential mobilisation of the splenic hilum for transection. Reported techniques vary in the sequence in which the ligaments are divided, but all procedures involve the same steps.[47,49] The patient is placed in the right lateral semi-decubitus position and is rolled back slightly from full lateral decubitus so that the midline is exposed should urgent conversion to open surgery be required. The surgeon and camera operator stand in front of the patient and one assistant stands behind the patient. We prefer a five-port technique but others report a four-port technique.[11,47] We begin by examining the omentum to the degree feasible and the inferior aspect of the left side of the transverse mesocolon for accessory spleens. Throughout the procedure, a wary eye is kept to identify accessory spleens. Steps of dissection are illustrated in **Figs. 9.1–9.6**.[49] Dissection begins by dividing the splenocolic ligament and then proceeds anteriorly. The lesser sac is opened and the gastrosplenic ligament including the short gastric vessels is divided. Modern energy sources which seal and divide tissues facilitate dissection. The main splenic artery is isolated if feasible and ligated. This facilitates later hilar transection and seems to decrease bleeding at the staple line. The lateral attachments (splenorenal and splenophrenic ligaments) are divided. Some will leave the highest end of the splenophrenic ligament attached until after hilar transection, the hanged spleen technique.[50] This helps prevent the spleen

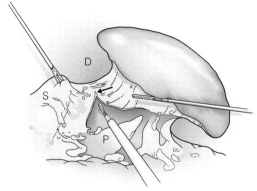

Figure 9.2 • The gastrosplenic ligament is divided (arrow). Dissection is begun at the inferior aspect and continued until all short gastric vessels are divided. The superior medial aspect of the splenophrenic ligament is also divided. D, diaphragm; H, hilum; P, pancreas; S, stomach. Reprinted with permission from Schlinkert RT, Teotia SS. Laparoscopic splenectomy. Arch Surg 1999; 134:100–1. Copyright © 1999, American Medical Association. All rights reserved.

from rotating while the hilum is controlled. We usually prefer complete division for full access to the splenic hilum; however, we do find the hanged spleen technique is useful in select cases.

The hilum may be controlled with staples, clips or energy devices; however, our preference is to use linear staplers. The hilar vessels should be clearly freed from the pancreas prior to transection. The spleen is placed into a bag and morcellated after the open end of the bag is brought through a trocar site.

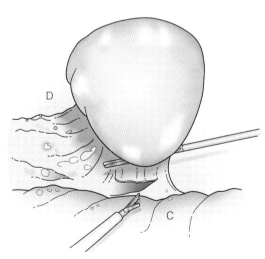

Figure 9.1 • After exploration, the dissection of the splenic attachments is begun with the splenocolic ligament (arrow). Traction is always placed toward the spleen with countertraction, if necessary. C, colon; D, diaphragm. Reprinted with permission from Schlinkert RT, Teotia SS. Laparoscopic splenectomy. Arch Surg 1999; 134:100–1. Copyright © 1999, American Medical Association. All rights reserved.

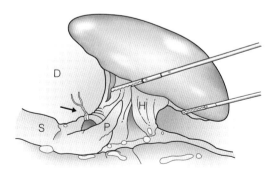

Figure 9.3 • If the splenic artery can be identified superior to the tail of the pancreas, it is ligated (arrow). D, diaphragm; H, hilum; P, pancreas; S, stomach. Reprinted with permission from Schlinkert RT, Teotia SS. Laparoscopic splenectomy. Arch Surg 1999; 134:100–1. Copyright © 1999, American Medical Association. All rights reserved.

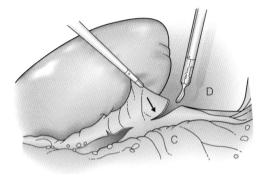

Figure 9.4 • The splenorenal ligament (arrow) is divided, retracting the spleen anteriorly. Areolar connective tissue between this ligament and the splenic hilum is gently divided. C, colon; D, diaphragm. Reprinted with permission from Schlinkert RT, Teotia SS. Laparoscopic splenectomy. Arch Surg 1999; 134:100–1. Copyright © 1999, American Medical Association. All rights reserved.

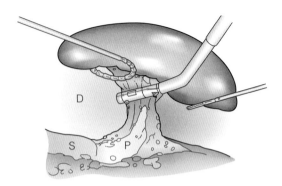

Figure 9.6 • The splenic hilum is now divided with the spleen retracted far into the left upper quadrant. After transection, the spleen is placed in a bag, morcellated and removed. D, diaphragm; P, pancreas; S, stomach. Reprinted with permission from Schlinkert RT, Teotia SS. Laparoscopic splenectomy. Arch Surg 1999; 134:100–1. Copyright © 1999, American Medical Association. All rights reserved.

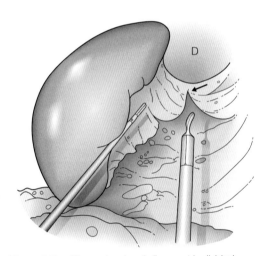

Figure 9.5 • The gastrophrenic ligament is divided (arrow) and areolar connective tissue again is dissected. At the completion of this step, the splenic hilum has been mobilised circumferentially. D, diaphragm; H, hilum. Reprinted with permission from Schlinkert RT, Teotia SS. Laparoscopic splenectomy. Arch Surg 1999; 134:100–1. Copyright © 1999, American Medical Association. All rights reserved.

Moderately enlarged spleens may be removed with similar techniques. The larger the spleen, the more the patient is rotated towards a supine position. This positional modification facilitates exposure of the splenic artery since large spleens are difficult to lift. The length of the spleen is often a misleading indicator of the success of the laparoscopic approach. More often the bulk of the spleen, as assessed by its anterior–posterior and lateral–medial dimensions, has a greater effect on exposure. For moderately enlarged spleens, hand-assisted techniques are valuable. This allows greater ability to move the large spleen, safer dissection of the hilum and easier vascular control should trouble arise. The spleen may be removed intact through the hand incision. Even if this incision needs to be enlarged for splenic removal, it is a lower abdominal incision which results in less respiratory compromise than the standard upper abdominal incisions. We use a lower midline for the hand port for this technique.

Massively enlarged spleens are treated with an open approach.

Approximately 75% of our patients undergoing laparoscopic splenectomy for ITP leave the hospital on the day following surgery. With greater degrees of splenomegaly or hypersplenism, patient recovery varies.

Summary

Laparoscopic splenectomy is the preferred method of splenic removal for most haematological conditions. Open splenectomy is reserved for trauma and massive splenomegaly. Careful attention to preoperative preparation, meticulous technique and careful postoperative care allow excellent results for these procedures.

Key points

- Most splenic injuries can be safely managed non-operatively. Management protocols may improve success.
- Vaccinations are mandatory for patients undergoing splenectomy and are ideally administered more than 2 weeks preoperatively.
- ITP is the most common haematological indication for splenectomy, with response rates of approximately 85%.
- Laparoscopic splenectomy is the procedure of choice for haematological diseases when the spleen is normal to moderately enlarged. Hand-assisted techniques may improve success rates for moderately enlarged spleens.
- Open splenectomy is preferred for trauma and massive splenomegaly.

References

1. McClusky DA, 3rd Skandalakis LJ, Colborn GL et al. Tribute to a triad: history of splenic anatomy, physiology, and surgery – part 1. World J Surg 1999; 23:311–25.

2. McClusky DA 3rd, Skandalakis LJ, Colborn GL et al. Tribute to a triad: history of splenic anatomy, physiology, and surgery – part 2. World J Surg 1999; 23:514–26.

3. Poulin EC, Schlachta CM, Mamazza J. Surgical anatomy in surgical diseases of the spleen. In: Katkhouda N, Soper N (eds) Problems in general surgery. Philadelphia: Lippincott Williams & Wilkins, 2002; pp. 16–23.

4. Galvan DA, Peitzman AB. Failure of nonoperative management of abdominal solid organ injuries. Curr Opin Crit Care 2006; 12:590–4.

5. Kyaw MH, Holmes EM, Toolis F et al. Evaluation of severe infection and survival after splenectomy. Am J Med 2006; 276(119):271–7.

6. Davies JM, Barnes R, Milligan D. Update of guidelines for the prevention and treatment of infection in patients with an absent or dysfunctional spleen. Clin Med 2002; 2:440–3.

7. Working Party of the British Committee for Standards in Haematology Clinical Haematology Task Force. Guidelines for the prevention and treatment of infection in patients with an absent or dysfunctional spleen. BMJ 1996; 312:430–4.
   Evidence based guidelines outlining prevention of sepsis in splenectomised patient.

8. Taylor MD, Genuit T, Napolitano LM. Overwhelming postsplenectomy sepsis and trauma: time to consider revaccination? J Trauma 2005; 59:1482–5.

9. Shatz DV, Schinsky MF, Pais LB et al. Immune responses of splenectomized trauma patients to the 23-valent pneumococcal polysaccharide vaccine at 1 versus 7 versus 14 days after splenectomy. J Trauma 1998; 44:760–5; discussion 765–6.

10. Kyaw MH, Holmes EM, Chalmers J et al. A survey of vaccine coverage and antibiotic prophylaxis in splenectomised patients in Scotland. J Clin Pathol 2002; 55:472–4.

11. Pachter HL, Hofstetter SR, Spencer FC. Evolving concepts in splenic surgery: splenorrhaphy versus splenectomy and postsplenectomy drainage: experience in 105 patients. Ann Surg 1981; 194:262–9.

12. Humphreys MR, Castle EP, Andrews PE et al. Microporous polysaccharide hemospheres for management of laparoscopic trocar injury to the spleen. Am J Surg 2008; 195:99–103.

13. Schroeppel TJ, Croce MA. Diagnosis and management of blunt abdominal solid organ injury. Curr Opin Crit Care 2007; 13:399–404.

14. Rozycki GS. Surgeon-performed ultrasound: its use in clinical practice. Ann Surg 1998; 228:16–28.

15. Moore EE, Cogbill TH, Jurkovich GJ et al. Organ injury scaling: spleen and liver (1994 revision). J Trauma 1995; 38:323–4.

16. Surgical treatment of injuries and diseases of the spleen. J Gastrointest Surg 2005; 9:453–4.

17. Harbrecht BG, Peitzman AB, Rivera L et al. Contribution of age and gender to outcome of blunt splenic injury in adults: multicenter study of the eastern association for the surgery of trauma. J Trauma 2001; 51:887–95.

18. McIntyre LK, Schiff M, Jurkovich GJ. Failure of nonoperative management of splenic injuries: causes and consequences. Arch Surg 2005; 140:563–8; discussion 568–9.

19. Smith JS Jr, Wengrovitz MA, DeLong BS. Prospective validation of criteria, including age, for safe, nonsurgical management of the ruptured spleen. J Trauma 1992; 33:363–8; discussion 368–9.

20. Sclafani SJ, Shaftan GW, Scalea TM et al. Nonoperative salvage of computed tomography-diagnosed splenic injuries: utilization of angiography for triage and embolization for hemostasis. J Trauma 1995; 39:818–25; discussion 826–7.

21. Cooney R, Ku J, Cherry R et al. Limitations of splenic angioembolization in treating blunt splenic injury. J Trauma 2005; 59:926–32; discussion 932.

22. Haan J, Ilahi ON, Kramer M et al. Protocol-driven nonoperative management in patients with blunt splenic trauma and minimal associated injury decreases length of stay. J Trauma 2003; 55:317–21; discussion 321–2.

23. Barquist ES, Pizano LR, Feuer W et al. Inter- and intrarater reliability in computed axial tomographic grading of splenic injury: why so many grading scales? J Trauma 2004; 56:334–8.

24. Harbrecht BG, Ko SH, Watson GA et al. Angiography for blunt splenic trauma does not improve the success rate of nonoperative management. J Trauma 2007; 63:44–9.

25. Ruggeri M, Rodeghiero F, Tosetto A. Steroids and intravenous immune globulins for the treatment of acute idiopathic thrombocytopenic purpura in adults. Cochrane Database Systemic Rev 2007; 4.

Evidence base for medical therapy of ITP.

26. Portielje JE, Westendorp RG, Kluin-Nelemans HC et al. Morbidity and mortality in adults with idiopathic thrombocytopenic purpura. Blood 2001; 97:2549–54.

27. Cohen YC, Djulbegovic B, Shamai-Lubovitz O et al. The bleeding risk and natural history of idiopathic thrombocytopenic purpura in patients with persistent low platelet counts. Arch Intern Med 2000; 160:1630–8.

28. Chirletti P, Cardi M, Barillari P et al. Surgical treatment of immune thrombocytopenic purpura. World J Surg 1992; 16:1001–4; discussion 1004–5.

29. Law C, Marcaccio M, Tam P et al. High-dose intravenous immune globulin and the response to splenectomy in patients with idiopathic thrombocytopenic purpura. N Engl J Med 1997; 336:1494–8.

30. Fenaux P, Caulier MT. Hirschauer MC et al. Reevaluation of the prognostic factors for splenectomy in chronic idiopathic thrombocytopenic purpura (ITP): a report on 181 cases. Eur J Haematol 1989; 42:259–64.

31. Pizzuto J, Ambriz R. Therapeutic experience on 934 adults with idiopathic thrombocytopenic purpura: Multicentric Trial of the Cooperative Latin American group on Hemostasis and Thrombosis. Blood 1984; 64:1179–83.

Evidence to support splenectomy in long-term management of ITP.

32. Watson DI, Coventry BJ, Chin T et al. Laparoscopic versus open splenectomy for immune thrombocytopenic purpura. Surgery 1997; 121:18–22.

33. Duperier T, Felsher J, Brody F. Laparoscopic splenectomy for Evans syndrome. Surg Laparosc Endosc Percutan Tech 2003; 13:45–7.

34. Smedley JC, Bellingham AJ. Current problems in haematology. 2: Hereditary spherocytosis. J Clin Pathol 1991; 44:441–4.

35. Caprotti R, Franciosi C, Romano F et al. Combined laparoscopic splenectomy and cholecystectomy for the treatment of hereditary spherocytosis: is it safe and effective? Surg Laparosc Endosc Percutan Tech 1999; 9:203–6.

36. Stoehr GA, Stauffer UG, Eber SW. Near-total splenectomy: a new technique for the management of hereditary spherocytosis. Ann Surg 2005; 241:40–7.

37. Bader-Meunier B, Gauthier F, Archambaud F et al. Long-term evaluation of the beneficial effect of subtotal splenectomy for management of hereditary spherocytosis. Blood 2001; 97:399–403.

38. Locatelli F, De Stefano P. Innovative approaches to hematopoietic stem cell transplantation for patients with thalassaemia. Haematologica 2005; 90:1592–4.

39. Al-Salem AH. Indications and complications of splenectomy for children with sickle cell disease. J Pediatr Surg 2006; 41:1909–15.

40. Saven A, Piro LD. Treatment of hairy cell leukemia. Blood 1992; 79:1111–20.

41. Tefferi A. Prognosis and treatment of primary myelofibrosis (agnogenic myeloid metaplasia). Up to Date Patient Information. Available from: http://patients.uptodate.com/topic.asp?file=leukemia/6366, 2007.

42. Rescorla FJ, West KW, Engum SA et al. Laparoscopic splenic procedures in children: experience in 231 children. Ann Surg 2007; 246:683–7; discussion 687–8.

43. Willcox TM, Speer RW, Schlinkert RT et al. Hemangioma of the spleen: presentation, diagnosis, and management. J Gastrointest Surg 2000; 4:611–3.

44. Hansen MB, Moller AC. Splenic cysts. Surg Laparosc Endosc Percutan Tech 2004; 14:316–22.

45. Kalinova K, Stefanova P, Bosheva M. Surgery in children with hydatid disease of the spleen. J Pediatr Surg 2006; 41:1264–6.

46. Chen KT, Bolles JC, Gilbert EF. Angiosarcoma of the spleen: a report of two cases and review of the literature. Arch Pathol Lab Med 1979; 103:122–4.

47. Katkhouda N, Hurwitz MB, Rivera RT et al. Laparoscopic splenectomy: outcome and efficacy in 103 consecutive patients. Ann Surg 1998; 228:568–78.

48. Park AE, Birgisson G, Mastrangelo MJ et al. Laparoscopic splenectomy: outcomes and lessons learned from over 200 cases. Surgery 2000; 128:660–7.

49. Schlinkert RT, Teotia SS. Laparoscopic splenectomy. Arch Surg 1999; 134:99–103.

50. Delaitre B. Laparoscopic splenectomy. The "hanged spleen" technique. Surg Endosc 1995; 9:528–9.

10

Gallstones

Leslie K. Nathanson

Introduction

In the UK it has been estimated from autopsy studies that approximately 12% of men and 24% of women of all ages have gallstones present.[1] The prevalence in North America is comparable to that in the UK, and it is believed that 10–30% of gallstones become symptomatic. There is a high prevalence in native Americans, who have an incidence of 50% in men and 75% in women in the age group 25–44 years, and this points to the importance of genetic factors in the aetiology of gallstones. In the UK more than 40 000 cholecystectomies are performed each year,[2] whereas in the USA approximately 500 000 operations are performed annually.[3] The incidence of common bile duct stones found before or during cholecystectomy is approximately 12%,[4] indicating that in the UK alone more than 4000 common bile ducts require stone clearance annually.

Composition, formation and risk factors

Gallstones are usually designated as cholesterol stones, mixed stones or pigment stones.[5] Pure cholesterol and pure pigment stones account for only 20% of gallstones, and mixed stones are considered as variants of cholesterol stones as they usually contain over 50% cholesterol and account for about 80% of gallstones in Western countries. Chemical analysis shows a continuous spectrum of stone composition rather than three mutually exclusive stone types, and 10–20% contain enough calcium to be rendered radio-opaque.

The two most important determinants of gallstone frequency in any population are age and gender; gallstones become more common with increasing age and are at least twice as common in women.[6] The increased frequency in women becomes manifest at puberty, and an increased risk of gallstones is conferred by parity and by the ingestion of oral contraceptives.[7] Other factors related to the development of cholesterol gallstones include obesity, ileal disease or resection, cirrhosis, cystic fibrosis, diabetes mellitus, long-term parenteral nutrition, impaired gallbladder emptying, ingestion of clofibrate,[8] heart transplant,[9] and periods of dieting on a very low fat diet.[10] A positive family history of previous cholecystectomy also increases the risk of developing symptomatic gallstone disease.[11] Increasing evidence is emerging that impaired colonic motility contributes to stone formation, and speculation arises for this as a means of prevention.[12]

Little is known of the epidemiology and cause of bilirubin stones. They are especially common in the Far East and become more frequent with increasing age, although occurring with equal frequency in men and women. They may be associated with haemolytic anaemia, cirrhosis and infection of bile with β-glucuronidase-producing bacteria such as *Escherichia coli* and *Bacteroides* species, and occur in diseases affecting the ileum due to increased enterohepatic cycling of bilirubin.[13] The metabolic mechanisms responsible for the formation of cholesterol gallstones centre on the solubility of the main constituents of bile.[14] The bile acid conjugates have detergent-like properties and form micelles in aqueous solution. Lecithin is incorporated with bile acids into micelles, and these also incorporate cholesterol, thereby promoting its solubility in the aqueous environment of bile. The capacity of this solubilising system may, under certain circumstances, be exceeded and bile is then converted into a state of cholesterol supersaturate, thereby favouring the nidation of cholesterol microcrystals. There is evidence to suggest that factors responsible for cholesterol microcrystal nucleation and for its inhibition are present in bile.[15] Excessive secretion of cholesterol in the bile may account for the increased predisposition to gallstones in obese patients, those ingesting oestrogens, and during pregnancy.

Biliary stasis, diminished gallbladder function and diet have similarly been implicated. Suture material has been identified in almost one-third of patients with ductal stones following open cholecystectomy and may be an important nidus for stone formation.[16]

Presentation

Gallstones present with symptoms related to the site of the gallstones and are therefore considered according to site.

Cholecystolithiasis

Gallstones confined to the gallbladder may present with an acute episode of pain from acute cholecystitis, biliary colic, chronic recurrent abdominal discomfort from repeated episodes of mild biliary colic, or from a vague collection of symptoms usually referred to as flatulent dyspepsia.

Pathophysiology

Impaction of a stone in the neck of the gallbladder is thought to result in gallbladder spasm, which produces biliary colic. As the stone falls back, the gallbladder empties and the pain stops, whereas continuing impaction of the stone in the gallbladder neck produces continuing pain. The trapped bile alters in composition producing local inflammation, which creates a more constant pain that may take several days to resolve. The gallbladder contents may become infected, adding to the patient's toxaemia, and may lead to the development of empyema or possible gangrene and perforation. An empyema will produce pain, right upper quadrant tenderness and a swinging pyrexia. Urgent intervention at this point is required since conservative measures rarely succeed in resolution. Increasing oedema and intramural vascular compromise may result in infarction of the gallbladder wall with consequent perforation of the organ.

The pathophysiology behind 'flatulent dyspepsia' is not understood. The gallbladder may be shrunken and contracted from episodes of subclinical inflammation but it is not unusual to find a normal-looking gallbladder at cholecystectomy in patients with gallstones causing 'flatulent dyspepsia'. Contraction of the gallbladder against stones is the traditional explanation for postprandial discomfort, but there is a poor correlation between such symptoms and the presence of gallstones in a general population. A mucocoele may develop when a gallstone impacts in Hartmann's pouch in an empty gallbladder. The gallbladder secretes mucus behind the obstructing stone, producing a steady increase in the size of the gallbladder, which may be easily palpable.

Clinical features

There is a poor correlation between pathological findings in the gallbladder wall and the presenting clinical features. Typically, acute cholecystitis presents with sharp, constant, right upper quadrant pain, which frequently is of sudden onset but may have been preceded by years of postprandial epigastric discomfort. It will be worse on inspiration or movement and frequently radiates to the back or to the tip of the right shoulder blade. It may be associated with nausea, vomiting or loss of appetite, and may persist for several days. Examination may reveal signs of toxaemia; the abdomen is tender in the right upper quadrant and classically a positive Murphy's sign is elicited. In more advanced cases, there may be a palpable inflammatory mass, which is usually due to an enlarged oedematous gallbladder surrounded by adherent omentum. Clinical signs of swinging pyrexia, tachycardia and impaired cardiorespiratory function should raise clinical suspicion of an empyema. The development of diffuse upper abdominal peritonism is a sign of perforation of the gallbladder. The presence of jaundice suggests choledocholithiasis, although the possibility of common bile duct compression from an inflamed and oedematous gallbladder may need to be considered (Mirizzi's syndrome).

Biliary colic presents in a similar fashion to acute cholecystitis but is usually not affected by movement and lasts only for several hours. It is often precipitated by ingestion of fatty foods but resolution is spontaneous. Chronic pain due to gallstones is attributed to the occurrence of 'flatulent dyspepsia' characterised by bouts of postprandial fullness, belching, nausea and a sensation of regurgitation of food. A family history of gallstone disease is not unusual, and factors predisposing to the development of gallstones may be present. Patients presenting with flatulent dyspepsia or recurrent episodes of biliary colic have little to find on examination.

Choledocholithiasis

Pathophysiology

It is uncertain whether all common bile duct (CBD) stones produce symptoms. It is traditionally held that the CBD cannot produce colicky pain as it does not contain smooth muscle, but pain in the right upper quadrant following cholecystectomy may be a sign of retained bile duct stones. A stone impacted in the lower end of the CBD may also be associated with nausea and vomiting, and undoubtedly the muscular spasms of the sphincter of Oddi or duodenum could account for the pain that is often felt radiating through to the back. Obstructive jaundice results when a stone becomes impacted within the CBD, in the tapered portion within the pancreas or ampulla. A stone may pass spontaneously or fall back into the CBD ('ball-valving') with spontaneous regression of the jaundice, or it may remain impacted until it is removed. A stone at the lower end of the CBD may also cause pancreatitis by temporary obstruction of the pancreatic duct, and this may be associated with transient jaundice (see Chapter 13). Ascending cholangitis results from infection within an obstructed or poorly draining biliary system. In patients with CBD stones, coliforms are identified within the bile in around 80% of cases.[17] The classic Charcot's triad of symptoms produced by bile duct stones with cholangitis consists of pain, obstructive jaundice and fever (with or without rigors). Acute cholangitis may progress to acute obstructive suppurative cholangitis with pain, obstructive jaundice, fever, hypotension and mental obtundation (Reynolds' pentad) requiring early recognition and prompt endoscopic retrograde cholangiopancreatography (ERCP) drainage to save life.[18]

Clinical features

Presentation of a patient with right upper quadrant pain some time after cholecystectomy may indicate choledocholithiasis. However, CBD stones are more likely to be either silent and found at the time of cholecystectomy or present due to one of the complications of obstructive jaundice, pancreatitis or ascending cholangitis. Pain is associated more frequently with obstructive jaundice due to gallstones as opposed to an underlying malignancy. In addition to the presence of bilirubin in the urine and pale stool, obstructive jaundice may be associated with pruritus and steatorrhoea. Examination will not normally reveal a palpable gallbladder, and features of pancreatitis should be sought. Ascending cholangitis should be suspected in the presence of rigors and swinging pyrexia associated with jaundice. The patient may demonstrate signs of bacteraemia or septicaemia with a flushed appearance, tachycardia and hypotension.

Investigation

The diagnosis of gallstone disease is suspected on clinical grounds but relies on the relevant laboratory or radiological investigations for confirmation. The differentiation between gallstone causes for pain and other intra-abdominal disease should

include an erect chest radiograph, and may require a plain radiograph of the abdomen. Less than 10% of gallstones are radio-opaque and therefore the yield from abdominal radiographs is low. Occasionally, in cases of intestinal obstruction, air is seen in the biliary tree, suggesting a cholecyst-enteric fistula and gallstone ileus.

Blood tests

Liver function tests (LFTs) should be performed routinely in patients with suspected gallstones. Although these may not be affected by the presence of cholecystolithiasis, they may be abnormal in the presence of choledocholithiasis. An isolated increase of unconjugated bilirubin is present in prehepatic jaundice such as is seen with excessive haemolysis. The biochemical picture of hepatic jaundice, as seen with hepatitis, is one of raised conjugated and unconjugated bilirubin, high aspartate (AST) and alanine (ALT) transaminase levels, but associated with a relatively normal or slightly raised alkaline phosphatase (ALP). Posthepatic (obstructive) jaundice is associated with a raised conjugated bilirubin only, high ALP and normal AST and ALT. In late cases of obstructive jaundice or in acute cholangitis, the transaminase levels will rise as hepatocellular damage proceeds. Minor abnormalities in the LFTs occur with non-obstructing stones in the CBD. These minor abnormalities may prompt the undertaking of an operative cholangiogram at the time of surgery if a selective operative cholangiogram policy is being pursued.[19,20]

Approximately 60% of patients with CBD stones (including asymptomatic stones) will have one or more abnormal liver function tests, although a substantial number of patients with an abnormal liver function test will not have CBD stones. Bilirubin, ALP and γ-glutamyl transpeptidase (GGT) are the most sensitive tests routinely used.[21] In the acute situation, a serum amylase or lipase level should also be ascertained to exclude a diagnosis of pancreatitis, and a raised white blood cell count may support a clinical diagnosis of acute cholecystitis.

Ultrasonography

Ultrasound is the investigation used most widely to confirm the diagnosis of cholelithiasis. It is easy to perform, causes little discomfort to the patient, avoids irradiation and potentially toxic contrast media, and may be useful in demonstrating and assessing other structures in the upper abdomen. The gallbladder wall, as well as its contents, can be assessed and this may give additional information useful for planning management. CBD stones may be harder to identify, although the presence of a dilated CBD and small stones within the gallbladder give clues as to their presence. If the gallbladder cannot be identified, the presence of an echogenic focus in the gallbladder area is nearly as specific a finding as that of calculi in a distended gallbladder. With high-quality ultrasound scanning, gallstones should be detected in at least 95% of patients with stones. Its reliability in detecting CBD stones varies between 23% and 80% depending on body habitus and experience of the ultrasonographer.[22]

Endoscopic ultrasound (EUS)

Prat and colleagues have reported EUS with a sensitivity of 93% and specificity of 97% in detecting CBD stones, showing some promise of approaching values achieved by ERCP (89% and 100%).[23] Endoscopic ultrasound has also been reported as more sensitive than the transabdominal approach. Norton and Alderson reported confirmation of gallstone disease in 15 of 44 patients with 'idiopathic' pancreatitis who underwent EUS.[24]

Computed tomography (CT) scanning

CT may be more accurate than ultrasound in identifying CBD stones, with a sensitivity of 75% for CBD stones causing obstructive jaundice.[25] However, the relatively low rate of gallbladder stone detection may be due, in part, to cholesterol stones being isodense with bile on CT scanning. The newer generation spiral CT and magnetic resonance imaging (MRI) may be better but their potential advantage over abdominal ultrasound scanning is not readily apparent. Spiral CT following intravenous infusion cholangiography has been shown to allow accurate reconstruction of cystic duct/CBD anatomy.[26]

Radioisotope scanning

Technetium-labelled hydroxy-imino-diacetic acid (HIDA) is excreted in the bile after intravenous injection. It may be useful for demonstrating the patency of the biliary tree or of biliary-enteric anastomoses but its use with gallstones is limited. Failure to demonstrate a gallbladder due to blocked cystic duct may assist in the diagnosis of acute cholecystitis but images are too poor to reveal CBD stones. HIDA scanning may be helpful in patients with right upper quarter pain, fever, gallstones and right lower lobe pneumonia. Referred pain and tenderness can give confusing clinical signs, and the presence of a functional gallbladder makes the diagnosis of cholecystitis much less likely. HIDA scanning is of no value in cases of severe jaundice, since the isotope is not excreted into an obstructed system.

Intravenous cholangiography (IVC)

The advent of laparoscopic cholecystectomy has ensured a revival in the use of IVC as a means of identifying suspected CBD stones. Failure to opacify the biliary tree, however, arises in 3–10% of cases.[27,28] Although improvements in IVC make it a useful occasional alternative to ultrasonographic assessment of the bile duct, factors such as time, cost and occasional failure, together with a low risk of allergic reaction, make it less attractive. The adoption of infusional cholangiography improves the safety of the investigation, and tomography improves imaging of the bile duct, although anatomical delineation is not as clear as peroperative cholangiography.[29] The use of IVC is therefore limited in that it cannot be employed in patients who are allergic to iodine or in those patients with biliary obstruction, as secretion of the contrast into the biliary tree does not occur.

Magnetic resonance cholangiography (MRCP)

Emerging developments of fast image acquisition in a few seconds and improving software have allowed imaging of the biliary and pancreatic tree in enough detail to approach the resolution of ERCP.[30] The technique relies on the principle of imaging fluid columns that are static and so give detail of bile and static fluid in the duodenum and stomach. Better images are obtained with dilated ducts, and bile flow can be a source of error in false-positive stone detection. The presence of CBD calculi can be detected with a sensitivity of 95%, specificity of 89% and accuracy of 92%. The ability to detect anatomical variation of the extrahepatic bile ducts is less established.[31] Following standard non-invasive tests, Liu et al. stratified suspicion of CBD stones into four categories. Patients at extremely high risk of CBD stone underwent ERCP. Patients at high risk underwent MRCP followed by ERCP if stones were seen. With diagnostic accuracies greater than 90% many patients were spared unnecessary ERCP.[32] The strength of this system lies in accurate triage and minimised redundant use of MRCP. However, the capital expense and running costs of MRI still limit widespread availability in all but the most affluent of medical environments.

Percutaneous transhepatic cholangiography (PTC)

PTC is best performed in patients who have a dilated biliary tree, but is not employed routinely in patients with suspected gallstone biliary obstruction. Despite the use of a fine-gauge needle, there is a risk of bile leakage and haemorrhage in patients with abnormal clotting.

Endoscopic retrograde cholangiopancreatography (ERCP)

ERCP is considered the gold standard in preoperative CBD imaging. With direct visualisation of the papilla using a side-viewing duodenoscope, the papilla can be cannulated selectively to provide images of both the pancreatic and common bile ducts. Water-soluble contrast medium is injected to outline the biliary tree, and offers the advantage over other biliary tree imaging techniques of therapeutic intervention with sphincterotomy and stone extraction at the time of examination (**Fig. 10.1**). The role of ERCP in the management of CBD stones is discussed later in this chapter.

Management of gallbladder stones

Asymptomatic stones

There has been much debate regarding the need for surgical intervention in patients with asymptomatic gallstones. In one American study, which assessed the natural history of subjects with asymptomatic stones, individuals with gallstones were diagnosed by ultrasound scan on entry to a large university health care plan.[33] Only 2% of patients with incidentally diagnosed gallstones became symptomatic each year and presented with biliary colic or cholecystitis rather than the more serious complications of jaundice, empyema or cholangitis.[33] Only 10% of the asymptomatic patients, followed for a mean of almost 5 years by McSherry and Glenn, developed symptoms, and only 7% required operation.[34] Although stones are undoubtedly associated with an increased risk of gallbladder cancer, only one of the 691 gallstone patients followed in this study was found eventually to have an incidental carcinoma at operation, and further data are required to clarify this issue.

 There is no evidence to support interventional treatment of patients with asymptomatic gallstones since natural history studies have shown that symptoms develop at a rate of less than 2% per year.

Non-operative treatments for gallstones

Dissolution

In the early 1970s there was great interest in the use of dissolution agents, principally chenodeoxycholic acid (CDCA), in the treatment of gallstones.[35] Prerequisites for attempting dissolution therapy were a functioning gallbladder, multiple small stones (which have a greater total surface area for contact with the dissolution agent rather than a smaller number of larger stones) and radiolucency (indicative of pure cholesterol stones without a calcium or pigment matrix to impede dissolution). Success was slow to be achieved in most subjects, usually taking 6–12 months as judged by the disappearance of stones on ultrasound. Side-effects of treatment included abdominal cramps, diarrhoea and occasional liver function test abnormalities. Ursodeoxycholate (UDCA) has been shown to be equally effective as CDCA in dissolving gallstones. In patients administered dissolution agents, O'Donnell and Heaton[36] found that recurrence rates increased rapidly in the first few years, with rates of 13% at 1 year, 31% at 3 years, 43% at 4 years and 49% at 11 years. Although recurrent stones were readily redissolved, they generally recurred when therapy ceased.

Lithotripsy

Success with lithotripsy for renal stones led to the use of the same techniques for gallbladder stones. Early lithotripters, with immersion in large water baths,

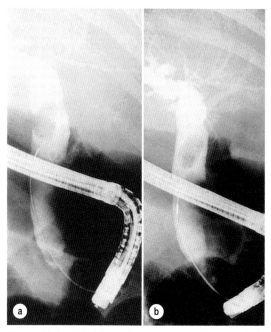

Figure 10.1 • (a) A large stone has been demonstrated by endoscopic retrograde cholangiography within the common bile duct. **(b)** The common bile duct stone has been snared by a Dormia basket ready for extraction.

were soon succeeded by smaller devices with a limited area of contact via a water-filled cushion. Biliary anatomy, however, did not lend itself to a repeat of the success observed with renal stones. The tidal flow of bile into and out of the gallbladder, along with the presence of multiple gallstones, were factors that contributed to the failure of the technique. Ahmed et al. reported 45% of patients undergoing lithotripsy required subsequent cholecystectomy.[37] Lithotripsy has therefore been retained only for the management of ductal stones resistant to endoscopic removal.[38]

 The potential role of oral dissolution therapy and lithotripsy has been superseded by the advent of laparoscopic cholecystectomy.

Operative treatment of gallbladder stones

Open cholecystectomy

The operative mortality of open cholecystectomy for cholelithiasis had fallen in the years before the introduction of laparoscopic surgery, with many series reporting operative mortality rates of less than 1%.[39] Common duct exploration was regarded as increasing the risk of open cholecystectomy by four- to eight-fold.[40] In a comparative study between a North American and a European centre, 12–14% of patients developed complications, and the bile duct was explored in 8.6% of the patients in Toronto as opposed to 17.9% in Geneva, the incidences of positive exploration being 61% and 73% respectively. Factors increasing the risk of postoperative mortality were advancing age, acute admission, admission to hospital within 3 months of the index admission, and the number of discharge diagnoses.[40] Only 18% of postoperative deaths in this study were related to the gallstone disease or the surgery, with underlying cardiovascular or respiratory disease contributing to 48% of deaths.

There has been considerable uncertainty regarding the true incidence of bile duct injury at open cholecystectomy, and the surveys available cite figures of one injury per 300–1000 operations.[41] At cholecystectomy, injury results from imprecise dissection and inadequate demonstration of the anatomical structures.[42] Although some patients do have anatomical anomalies or pathological changes that increase the risk of duct injury, it is noteworthy that in the extensive Swedish review, the patients most at risk appeared to be young, slim females who have not undergone previous surgery.[41]

In a detailed analysis of a consecutive group of patients undergoing cholecystectomy for presumed biliary pain in a District General Hospital between 1980 and 1985, Bates and colleagues compared the outcome of an age- and sex-matched control group of surgical patients without gallstone disease.[43] Flatulent dyspepsia was more frequent in gallstone patients but operation markedly reduced these symptoms to an incidence almost identical to that of the control group.

However, within 1 year of cholecystectomy, no less than 34% of patients still suffered some abdominal pain and none of the 35 patients referred back to hospital for investigation had evidence of retained ductal stones. Multivariate analysis showed that preoperative flatulence and long durations of attacks of pain were risk factors for postoperative dissatisfaction.

 Given that the basis for symptoms before cholecystectomy often remains uncertain, it is evident that a substantial number of patients continue to experience problems after operation.

Minilaparotomy cholecystectomy

In the few years before the advent of laparoscopic cholecystectomy, there had been a resurgence of interest in open cholecystectomy through a small incision, the so-called minilaparotomy cholecystectomy, in an effort to reduce the trauma of open surgery.

There have been few controlled trials; of those that have been performed, one showed laparoscopic cholecystectomy to be superior and the other showed mini-laparotomy cholecystectomy as superior.[44,45] The most recent randomised trial has again confirmed a smoother convalescence for laparoscopic cholecystectomy although operating times remained longer.[46]

The technique relies on retractors to provide exposure for a fundus-first cholecystectomy carried out without the surgeon's hands entering the abdominal cavity. Cholangiography is possible but not performed in most reports of the technique. The author's limited first-hand experience of the technique has not persuaded him that the view of the cystic duct/CBD junction is comparable to that achieved by laparoscopic cholecystectomy. The true incidence of bile duct injury with this technique is unknown and cannot be equated to the open era of large incisions.

 There is no evidence to support the routine use of minicholecystectomy in the treatment of symptomatic gallstone disease.

Laparoscopic cholecystectomy

Despite the paucity of randomised controlled trials, enthusiasm for the technique of laparoscopic cholecystectomy continues unabated, driven predominantly by patient satisfaction, with less pain and an earlier return to normal activities. Surgeons are attracted by the excellent view of the gallbladder and biliary tree afforded by the laparoscope, and health providers and purchasers are attracted by the short hospital stay, which offers significant cost savings.

Symptomatic gallstones

The laparoscopic procedure can be offered to all patients with symptomatic gallstones, providing their cardiorespiratory status did not preclude laparoscopy. Of all patients presenting for operation, 95% can be completed successfully by laparoscopic means. Obesity, acute inflammation, adhesions and previous abdominal surgery do not usually prevent a laparoscopic cholecystectomy, but may require some adaptations of technique to complete the procedure.[47–55] Techniques of laparoscopic cholecystectomy have been previously well described,[47,48] including cases performed under regional anaesthesia in patients with chronic pulmonary disease.[49] Laparoscopic cholecystectomy has been widely reported in pregnancy,[50] and in patients with cirrhosis.[51] In a substantial audit of seven European centres,[52,53] 96% of procedures were completed successfully in the 1236 patients and only four bile duct injuries were reported. There were no postoperative deaths and a median hospital stay of 3 days, with a median return to normal activities of only 11 days observed.

Acute cholecystitis

Fears that laparoscopic cholecystectomy in the management of acute cholecystitis could carry an unacceptable risk of disseminating infection or of perpetrating an injury to the bile duct appear unfounded.[55] Several large series report success and safety with this procedure, although the incidence of bile duct injury and conversion to open operation remain slightly higher.[56] In difficult cases, improvement in the exposure of Calot's triangle may require additional or different positioning of the laparoscopic cannulas, the use of oblique viewing telescopes and placement of endoscopic retractors. Decompression of a distended or inflamed gallbladder may also improve access.

Complications

The mortality rate in a good-risk patient undergoing elective operation is less than 1%, and operative risks usually arise from comorbid conditions. The laparoscopic technique is associated with lower wound infection rates than open surgery.[57] Furthermore, a recent meta-analysis has shown that antibiotic prophylaxis is not warranted in low-risk patients undergoing laparoscopic cholecystectomy.[58]

Day-case laparoscopic cholecystectomy

Worldwide, laparoscopic cholecystectomy is being performed in the day-case setting with good preoperative patient selection, improved techniques, and improved postoperative control of pain, nausea and vomiting.[59]

Needlescopic cholecystectomy

This technique has been described using 2- and 3-mm instruments and a 3-mm laparoscope. A randomised trial has shown less pain and smaller scars when this technique was used in patients with chronic cholecystitis.[60]

Bile duct injury

Anxieties regarding an increased incidence of bile duct injury with the introduction of laparoscopic cholecystectomy have not been substantiated by multicentre studies from Europe[52] and the USA,[53] with a reported incidence of injury to the CBD of 1 in 200–300 cases. In a study in the West of Scotland, a prospective audit of laparoscopic cholecystectomy was undertaken.[61] A total of 5913 laparoscopic cholecystectomies were undertaken by 48 surgeons, and 37 laparoscopic bile duct injuries were reported. Major bile duct injuries were defined as those where laceration to more than 25% of the bile duct diameter occurred, where the common hepatic duct or CBD was transected, or in those instances when a bile duct stricture developed in the postoperative period. Of the 37 injuries, 20 were classified in this way, giving an incidence of 0.3%. Delayed identification of bile duct injury occurred in 19 patients and, although it was noted by the author that cholangiography did not play a part in the identification of bile duct injuries, it was noteworthy that imaging was used in only 8.8% of all laparoscopic procedures. During the course of this 5-year study, the annual incidence of bile duct injury peaked at 0.8% in the third year but had fallen to 0.4% in the final year of audit. A meta-analysis of more than 100 000 cases reported an injury rate of 0.5%.[62] Archer et al. emphasised the importance of supervised surgical training to allow attenuation of the trainee surgeon's learning curve by the experience of his/her proctoring surgeon. The importance of cholangiography in the early detection of bile duct injury was also emphasised.[63] Way et al. analysed bile duct injuries from a cognitive psychological perspective and concluded that errors that led to bile duct injury stemmed from anatomical misperceptions as opposed to errors of skill or judgement (**Fig. 10.2**). This analysis concluded with a list of rules to help prevent injuries.[64]

Cholecystostomy

For patients whose symptoms of acute cholecystitis did not settle in the past, cholecystostomy was often undertaken in those cases where open cholecystectomy was thought to carry an unacceptable risk of injury to the biliary tree. The procedure could be undertaken under local anaesthesia and, following decompression of the gallbladder and

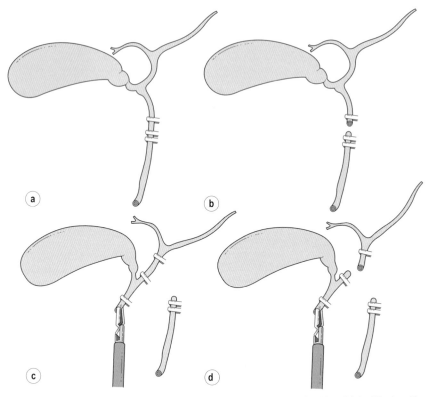

Figure 10.2 • The 'classical' laparoscopic bile duct injury. **(a)** The common duct is misidentified as the cystic duct and is doubly clipped. **(b)** The common duct is then divided. **(c)** The gallbladder is retracted to the right, stretching the common hepatic duct and placing it in contact with the gallbladder. This is identified as an accessory duct, and double clipped. **(d)** A high transection of the common hepatic duct results in the excision of most of the extrahepatic biliary tree.

stone removal, a drain could be left in situ. With the demonstration that acute cholecystectomy could be undertaken safely,[56] cholecystostomy has become an infrequent surgical procedure. The technique now is most often undertaken percutaneously under ultrasound or CT guidance and is most used in the frail patient with cardiorespiratory instability requiring time to control or when anticoagulation precludes surgery. It may rarely be of value during a difficult laparoscopic cholecystectomy when the risk of conversion to an open procedure may be considered unacceptable in the frail patient. In such instances, a drain can be inserted through one of the 5-mm cannulas, which can be introduced directly into the gallbladder by reinsertion of a trocar.

Subtotal cholecystectomy

This is another strategy to consider if dense fibrosis or large vessels are present in the area of Calot's triangle and the cystic duct is clearly identified and confirmed by cholecystogram. The cystic duct is ligated and excision of the gallbladder is undertaken

leaving its posterior wall intact on the liver. This situation probably arises most in those patients with cirrhosis and portal hypertension.

 Laparoscopic cholecystectomy is associated with less pain, shorter hospital stay, faster return to normal activity and less abdominal scarring than open surgery, and is therefore preferred to open surgery in the management of symptomatic gallstone disease.[65]

Intraoperative cholangiography (IOC)

The debate over the potential benefit of operative cholangiography has spanned the open and laparoscopic eras.

Routine IOC

Many surgeons who had previously performed the technique routinely at the time of open cholecystectomy abandoned cholangiography during laparoscopic cholecystectomy, since it was thought to be too difficult to undertake. In a large population-based study in Western Australia, Fletcher et al. concluded that operative cholangiography had a protective effect for complications of cholecystectomy.[66] In a large study of over 1.5 million Medicare patients undergoing cholecystectomy, Flum and colleagues demonstrated that surgeons performing operative cholangiography routinely had a lower rate of bile duct injuries than those who did not, and this difference disappeared when IOC was not used.[67] The author believes that operative cholangiography has an important role in laparoscopic cholecystectomy, not only to detect CBD stones but also to confirm, beyond doubt, the anatomy of the biliary tree, since the severity of bile duct injury appears far greater in laparoscopic surgery. The addition of cholangiography to the total dissection time of laparoscopic cholecystectomy is relatively short. On the basis that the time to learn operative cholangiography is not during the management of a difficult case, it is recommended that it should be performed as a routine but should not be seen as a substitute for careful dissection of the infundibulum of the gallbladder and the cystic duct close to the gallbladder. By dissecting these structures both anteriorly and posteriorly, the gallbladder is displaced (sometimes called the 'flag' technique) to enable the surgeon to see behind the gallbladder and thus minimise the risk of injury to the portal structures. Routine IOC also improves the surgeon's skills to enable successful transcystic exploration of the CBD.

Selective IOC

There are data supporting a selective approach to IOC at open[20] and laparoscopic cholecystectomy.[68] Unsuspected stones on routine cholangiography at laparoscopic cholecystectomy occurred in only 2.9%, and residual CBD stones causing symptoms in patients not undergoing routine cholangiography were found in only 0.30%. The strength of any selective policy for IOC will depend on the predictive values of preoperative investigations. Numerous studies have examined risk factors for choledocholithiasis but, from multivariate analysis, it would appear that an increased diameter of the CBD and the presence of multiple (>10) gallstones are the only significant independent indicators.[20]

Bile duct injury

The principal cause of damage is due to misidentification of the CBD as the cystic duct. As dissection proceeds an 'accessory duct' (in reality the common hepatic duct) is visualised, clipped and divided, resulting in resection of most of the extrahepatic biliary tree (Fig. 10.2). Operative cholangiography adds to the certainty that the cannula is in the cystic duct. If only the distal biliary tree is filled, the surgeon is alerted to the error before any duct is completely divided. Although critics of operative cholangiography will argue that the CBD has been injured by the incision through which the cholangiogram catheter is introduced, the injury at this point is recoverable, either by direct suture or insertion of a T-tube (**Fig. 10.3**). In the rarer situation when the

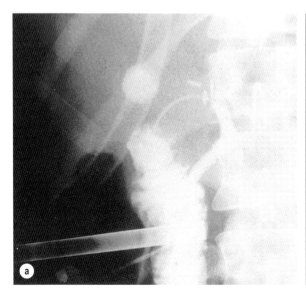
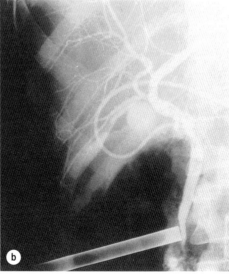

Figure 10.3 • **(a)** The small-diameter common bile duct has been mistaken for the cystic duct. Only the distal common bile duct and duodenum are shown, with no proximal filling of the ducts. Recognition of the error at this stage averts a major injury to the common duct. **(b)** After further dissection, the cystic duct was identified and a T-tube placed in the incision in the common duct. A subsequent T-tube cholangiogram confirms the normal anatomy, and laparoscopic cholecystectomy was completed successfully.

cystic duct arises from the right hepatic duct, and dissection has not progressed correctly, cholangiography identifies such anomalies and helps to avert more major injury (**Fig. 10.4**).

Laparoscopic ultrasound (LUS)

The emergence of ultrasound probes that can be passed down the laparoscopic ports has further improved the accurate measurement of CBD diameter, as well as the stone load within the gallbladder.

Both mechanical sectoral and linear array laparoscopic ultrasound probes have been shown to be as useful as cholangiography in the detection of CBD stones.[69-70] LUS is less invasive, less time-consuming, allows less radiation exposure and has similar failure rates to IOC when performed in well-trained hands. In a large series the common hepatic duct and the CBD were identified in 93% and 99% of cases respectively. Sensitivity and specificity for identifying bile duct stones were 92%

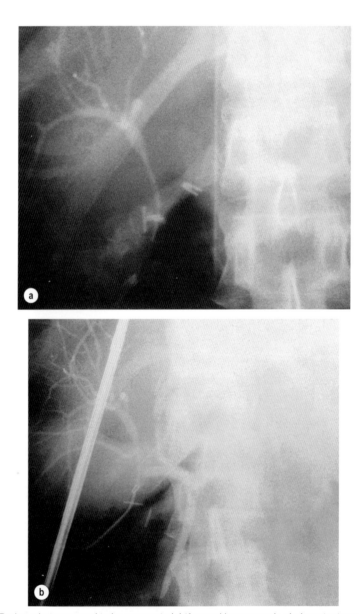

Figure 10.4 • (a) During what appeared to be a very straightforward laparoscopic cholecystectomy, the routine operative cholangiogram showed only the right hepatic duct and right hepatic biliary tree. **(b)** Repositioning of the catheter and the LigaClip showed the remainder of the biliary tree and made clear that the structure initially thought to be the cystic duct was the distal right hepatic duct below an anomalous origin of the cystic duct.

and 100% respectively. A normal CBD diameter at LUS was also an excellent negative predictor of CBD stones.[71] The same authors later concluded that LUS could replace IOC.[72] Others feel IOC and LUS should be seen as complementary tests rather than competitive.[73] Laparoscopic ultrasonography may facilitate a policy of selective cholangiography. Despite reports of accurate identification of anatomy it remains to be seen whether this will translate to prevention of bile duct injury. A cost benefit also remains to be demonstrated given the capital outlay for the equipment.

The use of intraoperative cholangiography allows detection of CBD stones during cholecystectomy and when interpreted appropriately is associated with a lower risk of CBD injury.

Management of common bile duct stones

The natural history of a given common bile duct (CBD) stone remains difficult to predict. In a prospective study of 1000 cases of symptomatic gallstones it was found that 73% of cases that presented with features suggestive of CBD stones had no CBD stone at the time of operation and were therefore considered to have passed the stone spontaneously. Cases of cholangitis or jaundice were less likely to pass stones spontaneously.[74]

Primary bile duct stones form within the CBD usually due to ampullary stenosis, diverticula or impaired bile duct motility. Management of these stones will often require choledochojejunostomy depending on the circumstances and patient age.[75,76] Treatment of primary duct stones with choledochotomy and T-tube drainage alone is associated with recurrence rates up to 41%.[77] Laparoscopic choledochoduodenostomy remains an option for the advanced laparoscopic surgeon,[78,79] although there may be concerns regarding the longer-term consequences of bilioenteric reflux.

Secondary bile duct stones are stones that originate within the gallbladder and are found in the CBD prior to, at the time of, or within 2 years of cholecystectomy. Approximately 12% of patients undergoing surgery for symptomatic gallbladder stones will also have stones in the CBD. More than 90% of these patients will have preoperative indications such as a history of jaundice or pancreatitis or abnormal liver function tests, but 5–10% have no indication of stones in the bile duct other than a positive finding (filling defect, absence of filling of the terminal segment of the common duct, delay or absence of flow into the duodenum) on the peroperative cholangiogram.

The best management of CBD stones is still a matter of debate. Discussion of different practices is presented here in the order the author considers most practical, and a suggested algorithm is presented.

Laparoscopic transcystic common bile duct exploration

Laparoscopic CBD exploration has been described through the cystic duct or common duct using either fibreoptic instruments or radiologically guided wire baskets or balloons.[80–83] The laparoscopic approach to the common duct was developed with increased emphasis on the transcystic route because of the ease of closure without the added need for intracorporeal suture technique, combined with postoperative recovery similar to cholecystectomy alone. Careful evaluation of the CBD diameter and stone load from the cholangiogram is required to determine the best approach.

The author's preferred initial method of laparoscopic exploration is by fluoroscopic means using a C-arm image intensifier, which is mobile and provides dynamic images with angulation. We employ a 5.5-Fr 70-cm radio-opaque nylon catheter with soft tip and end hole along with a side arm that connects to a catheter for injection of contrast (**Fig. 10.5**). Once the cystic duct is opened for insertion of the cholangiogram catheter, absence of bile backflow is a signal to milk the cystic duct backwards to extrude stones caught in transit to the CBD, rather than push them onwards into the CBD. A cholangiogram is performed (**Fig. 10.6a**), note being taken of the cystic duct and bile duct diameter, stone numbers, diameter and their distribution in the biliary tree. CBD stones which appear to be of a size able to be removed out via the cystic duct and are not too numerous indicates transcystic clearance has a high chance of success. Transcystic clearance proceeds by passing a 75-cm-long stone extractor (Cook®, Wilson-Cook Medical GI Endoscopy Inc., North Carolina). The basket tip should be positioned well back from the cannula tip to avoid perforation of the duct. Once the cannula tip is progressed, under image intensification, the basket is advanced within the cannula to allow engagement of the stone, which is withdrawn into the basket and extracted via the cystic duct (**Fig. 10.6b**). It is useful to remove the proximal stones first, and vital to avoid opening the basket within the duodenum or withdrawing through the ampulla with the basket wires open. Any impacted stones can be dislodged by passing a 4-Fr Fogarty catheter beyond the stone and withdrawing the catheter with the balloon inflated. Failed disimpaction may require choledochoscopy and lithotripsy (**Fig. 10.6c–f**, Box 10.1).

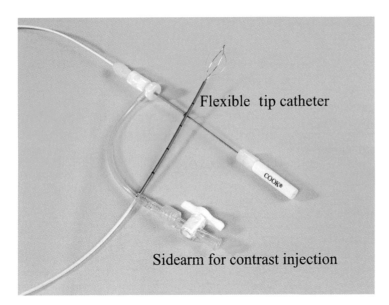

Figure 10.5 • Composite cholangiogram catheter and stone extraction basket used for laparoscopic transcystic exploration of the common bile duct. Reproduced with permission of Cook Australia.

Flexible tip catheter

Sidearm for contrast injection

Traditionally at open surgery, the common duct was decompressed postoperatively with a T-tube until it was known that the bile was draining satisfactorily through the ampulla and there was no bile leak. Most series of laparoscopic transcystic common duct explorations do not report the routine use of drainage of the common duct. A subhepatic drain is routine.

There is accumulating evidence, including three randomised trials, that 60–70% of patients are able to have their calculi cleared via the cystic duct.[84–89]

Laparoscopic choledochotomy

In up to 35% of patients laparoscopic transcystic exploration of the CBD will fail to clear the CBD.[84–89] Choledochotomy then needs to be considered. The only absolute contraindication to choledochotomy is a CBD diameter of less than 8 mm (Box 10.2). It should also be borne in mind that approximately one-third of stones detected at cholangiography may be passed spontaneously, and that exploration of a small duct may result in increased morbidity for the patient.[90] Therefore, laparoscopic choledochotomy is only an option for appropriately trained surgeons (Box 10.3).

Once clearance of the duct has been confirmed by choledochoscopy (see below), a T-tube is inserted or primary closure can be considered with the insertion of an antegrade stent across the ampulla.[84] Antegrade stenting, placement of a T-tube or cystic duct tube decompression of the CBD is wise where doubt exists about free postoperative bile drainage through the ampulla. This is most likely where a stone was impacted, ampullary manipulation has

been extensive or with established cholangitis. Placement of a subhepatic drain is essential.

Open choledochotomy

Successful exploration of the CBD can only be achieved through an adequately sized choledochotomy to facilitate both removal of any obvious stones and choledochoscopy. The gradual adoption of operative choledochoscopy during the 1970s and 1980s saw a decline in the incidence of retained CBD stones following surgery, from about 10% to 1.2%, with a number of surgeons reporting large series of patients with no retained stones.[91] On initial examination of the proximal ducts, it is normally possible to visualise several generations of ducts when these are dilated. Once it has been ascertained that the upper ducts are clear, the distal biliary tree can be examined. It is mandatory to clearly visualise the rather ragged appearance of the ampulla of Vater and then withdraw the choledochoscope. If a stone is visualised it can be retrieved with a stone basket and the procedure repeated until the duct is clear. The common duct is closed with or without a T-tube.[92] The latter is probably unnecessary for an experienced choledochoscopist but, for the less experienced surgeon, it allows access to the biliary tree for postoperative cholangiography to confirm ductal clearance and to allow re-exploration of the duct without the need for re-operation.

With the advent of laparoscopic cholecystectomy, ERCP and endoscopic sphincterotomy (ES) have become the usual procedure for treating common duct stones, since laparoscopic common duct exploration is not yet a widely practised technique (Box 10.4). Moreover, cholecystectomy without

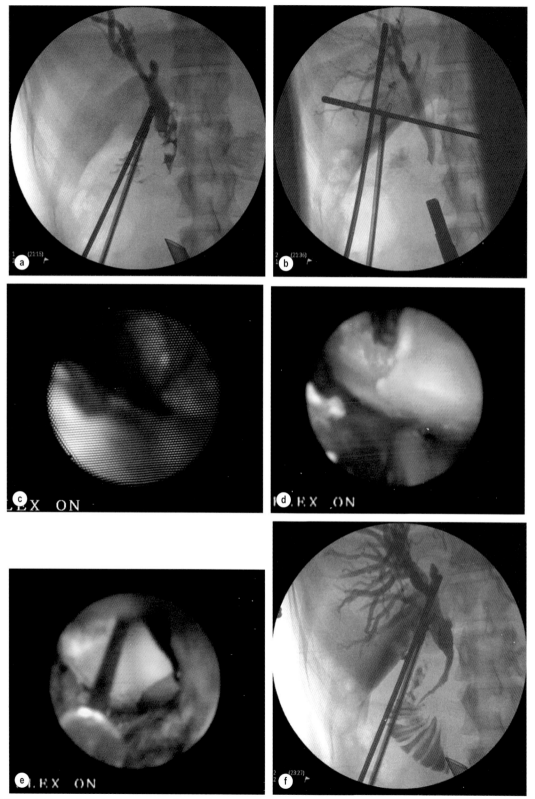

Figure 10.6 • **(a)** Cholangiogram of a 21-year jaundiced patient demonstrating multiple CBD stones with one impacted 3 cm proximal to ampulla. **(b)** Fluoroscopic view of bile duct showing after rapid transcystic four-wire basket retrieval of all except the impacted stone. **(c)** Transcystic choledochoscopic view of impacted stone, unable to be dislodged with a balloon catheter. **(d)** Transcystic ureteroscopic lithoclast stone fragmentation. **(e)** Wire basket stone retrieval under vision. **(f)** Fluoroscopic view of cleared bile duct.

Box 10.1 • Techniques for improving transcystic clearance

- Careful dissection of cystic duct/CBD junction
- Avoidance of the spiral valves when incising cystic duct
- Careful examination of cholangiogram ('did that stone pass through the cystic duct?')
- Approach cystic duct from different or extra ports
- Choledochoscopy via cystic duct, with lithotripsy if required
- Vary retraction on fundus

Box 10.2 • Indications for choledochotomy

- Unsuccessful transcystic exploration
- Cystic duct diameter smaller than size of stones
- CBD diameter >8 mm
- Multiple large stones
- Ampullary diverticulum on IOC
- Previous Billroth II gastrectomy
- Previous failed ERCP
- Contraindication to postoperative ERCP
- ERCP unavailable

Box 10.3 • Useful tips in performing laparoscopic choledochotomy

- Deflate duodenum with nasogastric tube (NGT)
- Extra port to retract duodenum
- Leave cholangiocatheter in to prevent deflation
- Sharp scissors choledochotomy
- Intraoperative lithotripsy preferably by lithoclast

Box 10.4 • Reasons to consider converting to open choledochotomy

- Unsuccessful transcystic CBD exploration
- Unsuccessful laparoscopic choledochotomy
- Multiple (>10) CBD stones
- Large CBD stones
- Intrahepatic or proximal ductal stones
- Impacted stones
- Failed or unavailable ERCP

cholangiography is commonly performed in the expectation that ERCP and ES will be effective in dealing with unrecognised retained common duct stones at a later date. Such a policy, however, does expose the patient to an additional and often unnecessary procedure. Laparoscopic common duct exploration by whatever route has the advantage for the patient of being able to deal with both gallbladder and CBD stones at the same time.[93]

Endoscopic retrograde cholangiopancreatography (ERCP)

There is general agreement that endoscopic removal of bile duct stones is preferable to surgery in post-cholecystectomy patients, and in high-risk surgical patients when the gallbladder is still present – that is, patients with severe acute cholangitis and selected patients with acute biliary pancreatitis.[94–96] The author believes ERCP becomes an option when transcystic CBD exploration has failed, but should not be considered the first-line management of all CBD stones.

Duct clearance can be expected in 90–95% of patients undergoing successful sphincterotomy, and this results in an overall success rate for endoscopic stone clearance of 80–95%, the highest success rates being recorded as experience increases.[94,96,97] Major complications occur in up to 10% of patients, and include haemorrhage, acute pancreatitis, cholangitis and retroduodenal perforation, but the overall procedure-related mortality is less than 1%.[94] However, the 30-day mortality can reach 15%, reflecting the severity of the underlying disease. In selected patients with calculi less than 15 mm in diameter, morbidity may be reduced by papillary dilatation rather than sphincterotomy.[95] Difficulties in removing CBD stones endoscopically may be due to unfavourable or abnormal anatomy, such as periampullary diverticulum or previous surgery. Stones larger than 15 mm and those situated intrahepatically or proximal to a biliary stricture may be difficult to remove (Box 10.5). Adjuvant techniques include mechanical lithotripsy, extracorporeal shockwave lithotripsy and chemical dissolution.[96,98,99] Although successful stone fragmentation has been reported in up to 80% of patients, the major drawback is the need for multiple treatment sessions and at least one subsequent ERCP to extract stone fragments.

The establishment of ERCP in the prelaparoscopic era was based on the avoidance of an open exploration of the CBD, a procedure that was believed to have significant morbidity.[100] ERCP was therefore generally reserved for the high-risk surgical patients

Box 10.5 • Difficult bile duct stones at ERCP

- Stones greater than 15 mm
- Intrahepatic stones
- Multiple stones
- Impacted stones
- Stone proximal to a biliary stricture
- Tortuous bile duct
- Disproportionate size of the bile duct stone
- Duodenal diverticulum
- Billroth II reconstruction
- Surgical duodenotomy

but open cholecystectomy and exploration of the CBD was reserved for the younger patient. In the laparoscopic era, management strategies vary considerably and are based on local endoscopic and laparoscopic resources and expertise.

ERCP stent insertion

In the 5% or less of situations where extraction of CBD stones is incomplete or impossible, a nasobiliary tube or stent should be inserted to provide biliary decompression and prevent stone impaction of the distal CBD (**Fig. 10.7**).[101] Such manoeuvres may allow improvement of the patient's clinical condition until complete stone clearance can be achieved by further endoscopic manoeuvres or subsequent surgery. Temporary biliary endoprosthesis placement avoids accidental or intentional dislodgement of the nasobiliary catheter by a confused or uncooperative patient. The stent may become blocked after a few months, but bile drainage often continues around the stent, and the presence of the stent alone may be sufficient to prevent stones from becoming impacted at the lower end of the CBD. In the surgically unfit patient, a change of stent may be required if jaundice recurs. Recurrent episodes of cholangitis may result in secondary biliary cirrhosis in the long term, and careful consideration of the patient's level of fitness must be made before surgery is totally discounted.

Preoperative ERCP

For some, ERCP is the chosen method of preoperative CBD stone detection for any patient with suspected CBD stones. The advantage of this strategy is that duct clearance preoperatively removes the dilemma as to how to manage CBD stones found at operation. This management policy, however, will expose a substantial number of patients to an unnecessary endoscopic intervention.

A randomised study has shown no significant advantage for patients treated by preoperative sphincterotomy as opposed to open cholecystectomy and exploration of CBD alone.[102] Despite this, ERCP and ES have become popular practice in the management of CBD stones, with an increased reliance on ERCP and a reluctance among surgeons to perform surgical exploration of the CBD.[103]

Cholecystectomy should routinely follow clearance of the CBD except in those considered too frail or unfit for general anaesthetic. It can be expected that if the gallbladder is left intact following ERCP and ES, up to 47% of patients will develop at least one recurrent biliary event, with many requiring cholecystectomy.[87]

Intraoperative ERCP

There have been several reports over the years describing this technique with success but few centres consider this the most appropriate use of resource.[104]

Postoperative ERCP

If ductal stones are not suspected preoperatively, their presence can be determined at laparoscopic cholecystectomy by intraoperative cholangiography (IOC). CBD stones identified in this way could be referred for postoperative endoscopic clearance if the surgeon was unable to explore the duct. Such a policy would reduce dramatically the number of ERCPs undertaken by a policy of routine or selective preoperative ERCP. This would leave only a small proportion of patients in whom stones could not be cleared by ERCP, requiring a second operation.[105] If the surgeon is trained in laparoscopic exploration of the CBD, ERCP should be reserved for the few patients in whom laparoscopic ductal clearance fails. A recent randomised trial lends some evidence that this approach is safe and represents an effective management plan.[89]

At the present time, the precise role of ERCP remains to be defined but is likely to be dictated by local expertise and practice (see 'Laparoscopic choledochotomy' above). A number of acceptable algorithms have been proposed to manage the laparoscopic cholecystectomy patients suspected of harbouring CBD stones.

There is argument for leaving small stones (<5 mm) found intraoperatively. On follow-up for up to 33 months in a small group of patients, 29% in this category developed symptoms, but were safely managed with ERCP.[106]

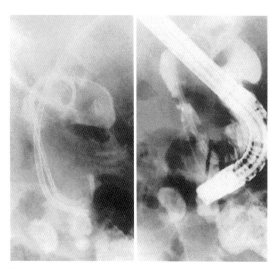

Figure 10.7 • Multiple common bile duct stones lying above a mid-common bile duct stricture and not amenable to endoscopic extraction. Biliary drainage is maintained with two endoscopically placed stents.

Transcystic exploration of the CBD versus preoperative or postoperative ERCP

At present, the array of management strategies for common duct stones requires data to guide us, with the techniques employed depending on local circumstances. In hospitals with ready access to ERCP, a surgeon may see little need for ascending the learning curve of laparoscopic CBD exploration, whereas those units with less ready access to ERCP see many attractions in dealing with common duct stones by laparoscopic means.

Preoperative ERCP and laparoscopic clearance of the CBD have been shown to be equivalent in overall outcomes.[85] However, those patients whose ductal stones were cleared transcystically experienced a far shorter hospital stay.

Postoperative ERCP clearance in a small single-surgeon study showed equivalent overall outcome to laparoscopic CBD clearance.[86] However, the number of choledochotomies was small and the retained stone rate high. Placement of biliary stents at the time of operation may improve the success of postoperative ERCP and stone clearance.

With experience, the majority of CBD stones can be treated at the time of surgery provided a flexible approach is employed. No single technique will be applicable to the management of all stones. In general, if the stones are few in number, small (<1 cm) in size, situated in the common duct or distal to cystic duct entry, then transcystic exploration has a high chance of success. If the stone or stones are large and numerous, or if the stones are situated in the common hepatic duct or intrahepatic biliary tree, a choledochotomy and exploration with the larger 5-mm choledochoscope is the preferred option. For those embarking on laparoscopic exploration, careful consideration of the strategies to be employed, equipment required and adequacy of assistance will go a long way to simplifying what can be a complex procedure. When laparoscopic transcystic exploration fails, the surgeon has three options:

- to ligate the cystic duct, complete the cholecystectomy and rely on postoperative ERCP;
- to perform a laparoscopic choledochotomy;
- to perform a laparotomy and open exploration of the CBD.

If laparoscopic choledochotomy fails, the options include insertion of a T-tube and subsequent extraction of the retained stones via the T-tube track after 6 weeks; postoperative ERCP and sphincterotomy; or conversion to open exploration CBD. Individual circumstances will dictate which option is the most suitable, although this should be discussed carefully with the patient before a management strategy is implemented.

It has been suggested that preoperative ERCP is the most cost-effective management of patients at high risk for CBD stone.[107] There is evidence accumulating, however, that where transcystic clearance is successful this leads to less morbidity and more rapid recovery.[85,89] Intraoperative stone fragmentation remains an option for stones found at operation that are unable to be dislodged at laparoscopic or open surgery. The author believes the most cost-effective approach is laparoscopic cholecystectomy, IOC and transcystic clearance of CBD stones, preserving ERCP for retained stones. Learning the techniques to achieve this seems worthwhile.

In a recent extensive review of the literature, it was concluded that laparoscopic CBD exploration is safe and effective for all patients presenting with gallstones and may be a better way of removing CBD stones than ERCP.[108,109]

Recurrent or retained CBD stones

Recurrent CBD stones occur in up to 10% of cases. In a retrospective series of 169 patients followed for up to 19 years, recurrences were more common in patients with primary duct stones, large CBD diameters (around 16 mm) and periampullary diverticula. Lowest recurrence rates were found in those patients undergoing choledochoduodenostomy.[76]

Retained CBD stones found at postoperative T-tube cholangiography are best dealt with by ERCP. If ERCP is unsuccessful or not available, exploration of the CBD via the T-tube tract is indicated. It usually takes approximately 6 weeks for the T-tube track to mature, at which time percutaneous choledochoscopy or radiologically guided extraction can be performed. A cholangiogram is obtained immediately prior to the procedure as a proportion of stones will have passed spontaneously.

The T-tube is removed, a guidewire is left in situ, and either a steerable catheter or choledochoscope is advanced down the track and into the CBD. With choledochoscopy, the remainder of the technique is identical to that carried out at open operation.[110] With the steerable catheter technique, fluoroscopy and further cholangiograms are taken as the stones are retrieved with a stone basket.[111]

If there is uncertainty as to the completeness of clearance, a straight tube may be inserted to keep the track open for a further attempt a few days later.

Both techniques are successful in more than 95% of cases and carry less risk of complications such as pancreatitis or haemorrhage than ERCP. Providing there are no time constraints and the patient is happy to be managed as an outpatient with a T-tube, the technique is effective.

 Transcystic exploration of the common bile duct at the time of cholecystectomy is an effective means of managing choledocholithiasis with low morbidity and cost.

 ERCP is effective in managing the remaining patients in whom this is not achievable and is the accepted means of managing the patient presenting with acute cholangitis.

Transhepatic stone retrieval

In a few patients, particularly those who have previously undergone a Pólya gastrectomy, the ampulla will not be readily accessible for ERCP. Access to the common duct can be achieved using a percutaneous transhepatic technique. Over a percutaneously inserted guidewire, a series of dilators are advanced into the biliary tree, so as to develop a transhepatic tract. Following insertion of a sheath, a choledochoscope or steerable catheter can be inserted and stones retrieved.[112]

Acalculous biliary pain

Given the poor understanding of the mechanisms of pain production in patients with acalculous biliary disease, the outcome for patients following cholecystectomy is uncertain. There is gathering evidence that some patients have abnormal motility of the sphincter of Oddi, in addition to the gallbladder. Some authors have reported improvement in symptoms in as many as 85–95% of patients with acalculous biliary pain after cholecystectomy,[113] but it is conceivable that surgery confers a placebo effect. Controversy exists over the use of cholecystokinin (CCK) provocation tests as a means of reproducing symptoms and predicting which patients might benefit from cholecystectomy. In one study, all 26 patients with positive CCK tests showed improvement after removal of the gallbladder,[114] whereas 10 of the 16 patients with negative tests were found to have other pathology accounting for their pain. Despite these encouraging results, other investigators have failed to demonstrate differences in outcome in patients with positive CCK tests when compared to those with negative tests.[115] Objective criteria on which to base the decision to recommend cholecystectomy in such patients are difficult to define. It is clear, however, that, despite the minimally invasive nature of laparoscopic cholecystectomy, there should be no relaxation in the indications for cholecystectomy with patients with acalculous biliary pain.

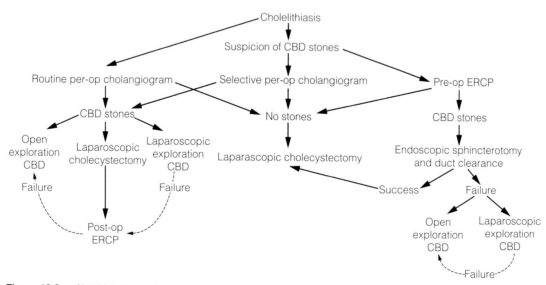

Figure 10.8 • Algorithm showing the available strategies for management of common bile duct stones.

Key points

- Asymptomatic gallstones do not require surgical intervention.
- The standard treatment for symptomatic gallstones is now laparoscopic, and there are few exceptions to a trial of a laparoscopic approach in all comers.
- All surgeons undertaking cholecystectomy, by whatever technique, should be capable of performing operative cholangiography.
- The use of operative cholangiography appears to be associated with a lower incidence of bile duct injury.
- Experience is accumulating that transcystic clearance of the CBD at the time of cholecystectomy is effective, with low morbidity and cost. In the one-third of patients where this is not achievable, ERCP is probably the best means of clearance.
- An algorithm for the management of common bile duct stones is shown in Fig. 10.8. The management strategy chosen will depend on personal experience, equipment availability, time and the availability of other departmental expertise. There is no consensus as to the ideal approach.

References

1. Godfrey PJ, Bates T, Harrison M et al. Gallstones and mortality: a study of all gallstone related deaths in a single health district. Gut 1984; 25:1029–33.

2. Hospital In-patient Inquiry, 1980: Main tables. Department of Health and Social Security/Office of Population Census and Surveys. London: HMSO, 1989.

3. Socio-economic fact book for surgery. Socioeconomic Affairs Department, American College of Surgeons, Chicago, 1988.

4. Motson RW. Operative cholangiography. In: Motson RW (ed.) Retained common duct stones. Prevention and treatment. London: Grune & Stratton, 1985; pp. 8–9.

5. Neoptolemos JP, Hofmann AF, Moossa AR. Chemical treatment of stones in the biliary tree. Br J Surg 1986; 73:515–24.

6. Bennion LJ, Grundy SM. Risk factors for the development of cholelithiasis in man. N Engl J Med 1978; 299:1161–221.

7. Scragg RKR, McMichael AJ, Seamark RF. Oral contraceptives, pregnancy and endogenous oestrogen in gallstone disease – a case controlled study. Br Med J 1984; 288:1795–9.

8. Scragg RKR, McMichael AJ, Paghurst PA. Diet, alcohol and relative weight in gallstone disease: a case controlled study. Br Med J 1984; 288:1113–18.

9. Richardson WS, Surowiec WJ, Carter KM et al. Gallstone disease in heart transplant recipients. Ann Surg 2003; 237:273–6.

10. Festi D, Colecchia A, Orsini M et al. Gallbladder motility and gallstone formation in obese patients following very low calorie diets. Int J Obes Relat Metab Disord 1998; 22(6):592–600.

11. Nakeeb A, Comuzzie AG, Martin L et al. Gallstones: genetics versus environment. Ann Surg 2002; 235(6):842–9.

12. Dowling RH, Veysey MJ, Pereira SP et al. Role of intestinal transit in the pathogenesis of gallbladder stones. Can J Gastroenterol 1997; 11(1):57–64.

   Recent case-controlled study implicating impaired colonic motility as a cause of gallstone formation.

13. Brink MA, Slors JF, Keuleman YC et al. Enterohepatic cycling of bilirubin: a putatative mechanism for pigment gallstone formation in ileal Crohn's disease. Gastroenterology 1999; 116(6):1420–7.

14. Smith BF, LaMont JT. The central issue of cholesterol gallstones. Hepatology 1986; 6:529–31.

15. Dowling RH. Review: pathogenesis of gallstones. Aliment Pharmacol Ther 2000; May 14, Suppl 2:39–47.

16. Wosiewitz U, Schenk J, Sabinski F et al. Investigations on common bile duct stones. Digestion 1983; 26:43–52.

17. Keighley MRB. Micro-organisms in the bile. A preventable cause of sepsis after biliary surgery. Ann R Coll Surg Eng 1977; 59:328–34.

18. Glenn F, Moody FG. Acute obstructive suppurative cholangitis. Surg Gynecol Obstet 1961; 113:265–73.

19. Taylor TV, Torrance B, Rimmer S et al. Operative cholangiography: is there a statistical alternative? Am J Surg 1983; 145:640–3.

20. Wilson TG, Hall JC, Watts JM. Is operative cholangiography always necessary? Br J Surg 1986; 73:637–40.

Two studies that have sought to identify which patients undergoing open cholecystectomy might benefit from a policy of selective cholangiography.

21. Prat F, Meduri B, Ducot B et al. Prediction of common bile duct stones by noninvasive tests. Ann Surg 1999; 229(3):362–8.

22. Lindsel DRM. Ultrasound imaging of pancreas and biliary tract. Lancet 1990; 335:390–3.

 23. Prat F, Amouyal G, Amouyal P et al. Prospective controlled study of endoscopic ultrasonography and endoscopic retrograde cholangiography in patients with suspected common bile duct lithiasis. Lancet 1996; 347(8994):75–9.

A study making the case for endoscopic ultrasonography as an alternative to ERCP for the detection of common bile duct stones.

24. Norton SA, Alderson D. Endoscopic ultrasonography in the evaluation of idiopathic acute pancreatitis. Br J Surg 2000; 87:1650–5.

25. Baroll RL. Common bile duct stones. Reassessment of criteria for CT diagnosis. Radiology 1987; 162:419–24.

26. Ichii H, Takada M, Kashiwagi R et al. Three-dimensional reconstruction of biliary tract using spiral computed tomography for laparoscopic cholecystectomy. World J Surg 2002; 26:608–11.

27. Hammerstrom L-E, Holmin T, Stridbeck H et al. Routine preoperative infusion cholangiography at elective cholecystectomy: a prospective study in 694 patients. Br J Surg 1996; 83:750–4.

28. Bloom ITM, Gibbs SL, Keeling-Roberts CS et al. Intravenous infusion cholangiography for investigation of the bile duct – a direct comparison with ERCP. Br J Surg 1996; 83:755–7.

29. Joyce WP, Keane R, Burke GJ et al. Identification of bile duct stones in patients undergoing laparoscopic cholecystectomy. Br J Surg 1991; 78:1174–6.

30. Hochwalk SN, Dobransky MBA, Rofsky NM et al. Magnetic resonance cholangiopancreatography occurately practics the presence or absence of choledocholithiasis. J Gastrointest Surg 1998; 2(6):573–9.

31. Masui T, Takehara Y, Fujiwara T et al. MR and CT cholangiography in evaluation of the biliary tract. Acta Radiol 1998; 39(5):557–63.

 32. Liu TH, Consorti ET, Kawashima A et al. Patient evaluation and management with selective use of magnetic resonance cholangiography and endoscopic retrograde cholangiopancreatography before laparoscopic cholecystectomy. Ann Surg 2001; 234(1):33–40.

This article outlines a simple system to allow stratification of the risk of CBD stones based on routine blood tests. With selective use and accurate reporting of MRCP many patients are saved unnecessary ERCP.

33. Gracie WA, Ransahoff DF. The natural history of silent gallstones: the innocent gallstone is not a myth. N Engl J Med 1982; 307:798–800.

34. McSherry CK, Glenn F. The incidence and causes of death following surgery for non-malignant biliary tract disease. Ann Surg 1980; 191:271–5.

Two important studies that have documented the natural history of asymptomatic gallstones.

35. Iser JH, Dowling RH, Mok HYI et al. Chenodeoxycholic acid treatment of gallstones. N Engl J Med 1975; 293:333–78.

36. O'Donnell LDJ, Heaton KW. Recurrence and re-recurrence of gallstones after medical dissolution: a long-term follow-up. Gut 1988; 29:655–8.

A study highlighting the limitation of oral dissolution therapy of gallstones.

37. Ahmed R, Freeman JV, Ross B et al. Long term response to gallstone treatment – problems and surprises. Eur J Surg 2000; 166:447–54.

38. Sauerbruch T, Stern M. Fragmentation of bile duct stones by extracorporeal shockwaves. A new approach to biliary calculi after failure of routine endoscopic measures. Gastroenterology 1989; 96:146–52.

39. Clavien PA, Sanabria JR, Mentha G et al. Recent results of elective open cholecystectomy in a North American and a European centre – comparison of complications and risk factors. Ann Surg 1992; 216:618–26.

40. Bredesen J, Jorgensen T, Andersen TF et al. Early postoperative mortality following cholecystectomy in the entire female population of Denmark – 1977–1991. World J Surg 1992; 16:530–5.

Both these papers document the results of open cholecystectomy prior to the advent of laparoscopic cholecystectomy.

41. Andren-Sandberg A, Alinder A, Bengmark S. Accidental lesions of the common bile duct at cholecystectomy: pre- and peroperative factors of importance. Ann Surg 1985; 201:328–33.

Frequently cited study that documents risk factors implicated in injury to the common bile duct during open cholecystectomy.

42. Connor S, Garden OJ. Bile duct injury in the era of laparoscopic cholecystectomy. Br J Surg 2006; 93:158–68.

43. Bates T, Ebbs SR, Harrison M et al. Influence of cholecystectomy on symptoms. Br J Surg 1991; 78:964–7.

44. MacMahon AJ, Russell IT, Baxter JN et al. Laparoscopic versus minilaparotomy cholecystectomy: a randomised trial. Lancet 1994; 343:135–8.

45. Majeed AW, Troy G, Nicholl JP et al. Randomised, prospective, single-blind comparison of laparoscopic versus small-incision cholecystectomy. Lancet 1996; 347:989–94.

46. Ros A, Gustafsson L, Krook H et al. Laparoscopic cholecystectomy versus mini-laparotomy cholecystectomy: a prospective, randomised, single-blind study. Ann Surg 2001; 234(6):741–9.

No evidence to support routine minicholecystectomy.

47. Dubois F, Icard P, Berthelot G et al. Coelioscopic cholecystectomy. Ann Surg 1990; 211:60–2.

48. Nathanson LK, Shimi S, Cuschieri A. Laparoscopic cholecystectomy: the Dundee technique. Br J Surg 1991; 78:155–9.

49. Gramatica L, Brasesco OE, Mercado LA et al. Laparoscopic cholecystectomy performed under regional anaesthesia in patients with chronic obstructive pulmonary disease. Surg Endosc 2002; 16:472–5.

50. Ghumman E, Barry M, Grace PA. Management of gallstones in pregnancy. Br J Surg 1997; 84:1646–50.

51. Yeh CN, Chen MF, Jan YY. Laparoscopic cholecystectomy in 226 cirrhotic patients. Experience of a single centre in Taiwan. Surg Endosc 2002; 16:1583–7.

52. Cuschieri A, Dubois F, Mouiel J et al. The European experience of laparoscopic cholecystectomy. Am J Surg 1991; 161:385–7.

53. The Southern Surgeons Club. A prospective analysis of 1518 laparoscopic cholecystectomies. N Engl J Med 1991; 324:1073–8.

54. Wilson P, Leese T, Morgan WP et al. Elective laparoscopic cholecystectomy for 'all comers'. Lancet 1991; 338:795–7.

55. Unger SW, Rosenbaum G, Unger HM et al. A comparison of laparoscopic and open treatment of acute cholecystitis. Surg Endosc 1993; 7:408–11.

56. Navez B, Mutter D, Russier Y et al. Safety of laparoscopic approach for acute cholecystitis: retrospective study of 609 cases. World J Surg 2001; 25(10):1352–6.

57. Richards C, Edwards J, Culver D et al. Does using a laparoscopic approach to cholecystectomy decrease the risk of surgical site infection? Ann Surg 2003; 3:358–62.

58. Al-Ghnaniem R, Benjamin IS, Patel AG. Meta-analysis suggests antibiotic prophylaxis is not warranted in low-risk patients undergoing laparoscopic cholecystectomy. Br J Surg 2003; 90:365–6.

59. Lau H, Brooks DC. Contemporary outcomes of ambulatory laparoscopic cholecystectomy in a major teaching hospital. World J Surg 2002; 26:1117–21.

60. Cheah WK, Lenzi JE, So BY et al. Randomised trial of needlescopic versus laparoscopic cholecystectomy. Br J Surg 2001; 88:45–7.

61. Richardson MC, Bell G, Fullarton GM and The West of Scotland Laparoscopic Cholecystectomy Audit Group. Incidence and nature of bile duct injuries following laparoscopic cholecystectomy: an audit of 5913 cases. Br J Surg 1996; 83:1356–60.

   Large audit of UK practice of laparoscopic cholecystectomy attempting to assess the causation and incidence of common bile duct injuries during laparoscopic cholecystectomy.

62. MacFadyen BV, Vecchio R, Ricardo AE et al. Bile duct injury after laparoscopic cholecystectomy. Surg Endosc 1998; 12:315–21.

63. Archer SB, Brown DW, Hunter JG et al. Bile duct injury during laparoscopic cholecystectomy: results of a national survey. Ann Surg 2001; 234(4):549–59.

64. Way LW, Stewart L, Hunter JG et al. Causes and prevention of laparoscopic bile duct injuries. Analysis of 252 cases from a human factors and cognitive psychology perspective. Ann Surg 2003; 4:460–9.

65. Keus F, de Jong JAF, Gooszen HG, Van Laarhoven, GJHM. Laparoscopic versus open cholecystectomy for patients with symptomatic cholecystolithiasis. Cochrane Database of Systematic Reviews 2006, Issue 4. Art No.: CD006231.

66. Fletcher DR, Hobbs M, Tan P et al. Complications of cholecystectomy. Risks of the laparoscopic approach and protective effects of operative cholangiography: a population-based study. Ann Surg 1999; 229(4):449–57.

67. Flum DR, Dellinger EP, Cheadle A et al. Intraoperative cholangiography and risk of common bile duct injury during cholecystectomy. JAMA 2003; 289:1639–44.

   Large study on 1.5 million patients demonstrating an increased risk of common bile duct injury when intraoperative cholangiography was not used during laparoscopic cholecystectomy.

68. Snow LL. Evaluation of operative cholangiography in 2043 patients undergoing laparoscopic cholecystectomy. A case for the selective operative cholangiogram. Surg Endosc 2001; 15:14–20.

69. John TG, Banting SW, Pye S et al. Preliminary experience with intracorporeal laparoscopic ultrasonography using a sector scanning probe. A prospective comparison with intraoperative cholangiography in the detection of choledocholithiasis. Surg Endosc 1994; 8:1176–81.

70. Greig JD, John TG, Mahadaven M et al. Laparoscopic ultrasonography in the evaluation of the biliary tree during laparoscopic cholecystectomy. Br J Surg 1994; 84:1202–6.

71. Tranter SE, Thompson MH. Potential of laparoscopic ultrasonography as an alternative to operative cholangiography in the detection of bile duct stones. Br J Surg 2001; 88:65–9.

72. Tranter SE, Thompson MH. A prospective single-blinded controlled study comparing laparoscopic ultrasound of the common bile duct with operative cholangiography. Surg Endosc 2003; 17:216–19.

73. Catheline JM, Turner R, Paries J. Laparoscopic ultrasonography is a complement to cholangiography for the detection of choledocholithiasis at laparoscopic cholecystectomy. Br J Surg 2002; 89:1235–9.

74. Tranter SE, Thompson MH. Spontaneous passage of bile duct stones: frequency of occurrence and relation to clinical presentation. Ann R Coll Surg Engl 2003; 85:174–7.

75. LygidakisNJ. A prospective randomised study of recurrent choledocholithiasis. Surg Gynecol Obstet 1982; 155(5):679–84.

76. Panis Y, Fagniez PL, Brisset D et al. Long-term results of choledochoduodenostomy versus choledochojejunostomy for choledocholithiasis. Surg Gynecol Obstet 1993; 177(1):33–7.

Two studies stressing the need to consider a surgical drainage procedure if ductal stones are thought to represent primary calculi.

77. Uchiyama K, Onishi H, Tani M et al. Long-term prognosis after treatment of patients with choledocholithiasis. Ann Surg 2003; 238(1):97–102.

78. Jeyapalan M, Almeida JA, Michaelson RL et al. Laparoscopic choledochoduodenostomy: review of a 4-year experience with an uncommon problem. Surg Laparosc Endosc 2002; 12(3):148–53.

79. Rhodes M, Nathanson L. Laparoscopic choledochoduodenostomy. Surg Laparosc Endosc 1996; 6(4):318–21.

80. Petelin JB. Clinical results of common bile duct exploration. Endosc Surg Allied Technol 1993; 1(3):125–9.

81. Berci G, Morgenstern L. Laparoscopic management of common bile duct stones. A multi-institutional SAGES study. Society of American Gastrointestinal Endoscopic Surgeons. Surg Endosc 1994; 8:1168–74.

82. Rhodes M, Nathanson L, O'Rourke N et al. Laparoscopic exploration of the common bile duct: lessons learned from 129 consecutive cases. Br J Surg 1995; 82:666–8.

83. Khoo D, Walsh CJ, Murphy C et al. Laparoscopic common bile duct exploration: evolution of a new technique. Br J Surg 1996; 83:341–6.

84. Martin IJ, Bailey IS, Rhodes M et al. Towards T-tube free laparoscopic bile duct exploration: a methodologic evolution during 300 consecutive procedures. Ann Surg 1998; 228(1):29–34.

85. Cuschieri A, Lezoche E, Morino M et al. E.A.E.S. multicentre prospective randomised trial comparing two-stage vs. single-stage management of patients with gallstone disease and ductal calculi. Surg Endoscopy 1999; 13(10):952–7.

86. Rhodes M, Sussman L, Cohen L et al. Randomised trial of laparoscopic exploration of common bile duct versus postoperative endoscopic retrograde cholangiography for common bile duct stones. Lancet 1998; 351:159–61.

Two important randomised studies indicating success of laparoscopic bile duct exploration.

87. Boerma D, Rauws EAJ, Keulemans YCA et al. Wait-and-see policy of laparoscopic cholecystectomy after endoscopic sphincterotomy for bile-duct stones: a randomised trial. Lancet 2002; 360:761–5.

88. Riciardi R, Islam S, Canete JJ et al. Effectiveness and long-term results of laparoscopic common bile duct exploration. Surg Endosc 2003; 17:19–22.

89. Nathanson LK, O'Rourke NA, Martin IJ et al. Postoperative ERCP versus laparoscopic choledochotomy for clearance of selected bile duct calculi: a randomized trial. Ann Surg 2005; 242(2):188–92.

The author's own experience indicating that laparoscopic bile duct exploration is as effective as ERCP in clearing ductal calculi.

90. Collins C, Maguire D, Ireland A et al. A prospective study of common bile duct calculi in patients undergoing laparoscopic cholecystectomy: natural history of choledocholithiasis revisited. Ann Surg 2004; 239(1):28–33.

A small study showing that a third of incidental common bile duct stones pass spontaneously following laparoscopic cholecystectomy.

91. Finnis D, Rowntree T. Choledochoscopy in exploration of the common bile duct. Br J Surg 1977; 64:661–4.

92. Williams JA, Treacy PJ, Sidey P et al. Primary duct closure versus T-tube drainage following exploration of the common bile duct. Aust NZ J Surg 1994; 64(12):823–6.

93. Tanaka M. Bile duct clearance, endoscopic or laparoscopic? J Hepatobil Pancreat Surg 2002; 9:729–32.

94. Leese T, Neoptolemos JP, Carr-Locke DL. Successes, failures, early complications and their management: results of 394 consecutive patients from a single centre. Br J Surg 1985; 72:215–19.

95. Ochi Y, Mukawa K, Kiyosawa K et al. Comparing the treatment outcomes of endoscopic papillary dilation and endoscopic sphincterotomy for removal of bile duct stones. J Gastroenterol Hepatol 1999; 14(1):90–6.

96. Vaira D, Ainley C, Williams S et al. Endoscopic sphincterotomy in 1000 consecutive patients. Lancet 1989; ii:431–4.

Three reports supporting use of endoscopic removal of common bile duct stones in high-risk surgical patients.

97. Lambert ME, Betts CD, Hill J et al. Endoscopic sphincterotomy – the whole truth. Br J Surg 1991; 78:473–6.

98. Webber J, Ademak HE, Riemann JF. Extracorporeal piezo-electric lithotripsy for retained bile duct stones. Endoscopy 1992; 24:239–43.

99. Shaw MJ, Mackie RD, Moore JP et al. Results of a multi-centre trial using a mechanical lithotriptor for the treatment of large bile duct stones. Am J Gastroenterol 1993; 88:730–3.

100. Leese T, Neoptolemos JP, Baker AR et al. Management of acute cholangitis and the impact of endoscopic sphincterotomy Br J Surg 1986; 73:988–92.

101. Leung JWC, Cotton PB. Endoscopic nasobiliary catheter drainage in biliary and pancreatic disease. Am J Gastroenterol 1991; 86:389–94.

102. Neoptolemos JP, Carr-Locke DL, Fossard NP. A prospective randomised study of pre-operative endoscopic sphincterotomy versus surgery alone for common bile duct stones. Br Med J 1987; 294:470–4.

103. Barwood NT, Valinsky LJ, Hobbs M et al. Changing methods of imaging the common bile duct in the laparoscopic cholecystectomy era in Western Australia. Implications for surgical practice. Ann Surg 2002; 235(1):41–50.

104. Tatulli F, Cuttitta A. Laparoendoscopic approach to treatment of common bile duct stones. J Laparoendosc Adv Surg Tech 2000; 10(6):315–17.

105. Ng T, Amaral J. Timing of endoscopic retrograde cholangio-pancreatography and laparoscopic cholecystectomy in the treatment of choledocholithiasis. J Laparoendosc Adv Surg Tech 1999; Part A, 9(1):31–7.

106. Ammori BJ, Birbas K, Davides D et al. Routine vs 'on demand' postoperative ERCP for small bile duct calculi detected at intraoperative cholangiography. Surg Endosc 2000; 14:1123–6.

107. Urbach DR, Khanjanchee YS, Jobe BA et al. Cost-effective management of common bile duct stones. Surg Endosc 2001; 15:4–13.

108. Tranter SE, Thompson MH. Comparison of endoscopic sphincterotomy and laparoscopic exploration of the common bile duct. Br J Surg 2002; 89:1495–1504.

109. Martin DJ, Vernon DR, Toouli J. Surgical versus endoscopic treatment of bile duct stones. Cochrane Database of Systematic Reviews 2006; Issue 2. Art No.: CD003327.
     Similar clearance rates and more procedures with ERCP.

110. Menzies D, Motson RW. Percutaneous flexible choledochoscopy: a simple method for retained common bile duct stone removal. Br J Surg 1991; 78(8):959–60.

111. Mason R. Percutaneous extraction of retained gallstones via the T-tube track – British experience of 131 cases. Clin Radiol 1980; 31:587–97.

112. Nussinson E, Cairns SR, Vaira D et al. A 10-year single centre experience of percutaneous and endoscopic extraction of bile duct stones with T-tube in situ. Gut 1991; 32:1040–3.

113. Nathan MH, Newman MA, Murray DJ et al. Cholecystokinin cholecystography. Four years evaluation. Am J Roentgenol 1970; 110:240–51.

114. Lennard TWJ, Farndon JR, Taylor RMR. Acalculous biliary pain: diagnosis and selection for cholecystectomy using the cholecystokinin test for pain reproduction. Br J Surg 1984; 71:368–70.

115. Sunderland GT, Carter DC. Clinical application of the cholecystokinin provocation test. Br J Surg 1988; 75:444–9.

11

Benign biliary tract diseases

Benjamin N.J. Thomson
O. James Garden

Introduction

Apart from those disorders related to choledocho-lithiasis, benign diseases of the biliary tree are relatively uncommon (Box 11.1). The most challenging issues are in patients who present with symptoms associated with biliary strictures, which arise more commonly following iatrogenic injury during cholecystectomy. Congenital abnormalities such as choledochal cysts and biliary atresia are usually in the domain of the paediatric surgeon, although later presentation of cysts may occur after missed diagnosis or when revisional surgery is required. Most of the published literature regarding benign non-gallstone biliary disease is retrospective or at best prospectively gathered, non-randomised data, but clear guidelines can be followed based upon observation.

Congenital anomalies

Biliary atresia

Biliary atresia occurs in approximately 1 per 10 000 live births but its aetiology remains unclear. There is experimental evidence for a primary perinatal infection as well as cellular and humoral autoimmunity. An inflammatory process before birth may result in failure of the biliary lumen to develop in all or part of the extrahepatic biliary tree.

Presentation is usually in the early neonatal period with prolongation of neonatal jaundice. Most patients are treated in specialist neonatal surgical units; however, occasionally patients may be referred to adult units for assessment for liver transplantation following previous unsuccessful treatment. Management in the neonate is by porto-enterostomy (Kasai's operation), which involves anastomosis of a Roux limb of jejunum to the tissue of the hilum. Restoration of bile flow has been reported in 86% of infants treated before 8 weeks of age, but only 36% in older children.[1] Four-year survival is dependent on the timing of surgery. Of 349 North American children with biliary atresia, 210 (60%) required later liver transplantation with a 4-year transplantation survival of 82%.[2]

Choledochal cysts

The earliest description of a choledochal cyst was by Douglas in 1952,[3] who described a 17-year-old girl with jaundice, fever and a painful mass in the right hypochondrium. However, presentation is usually in childhood and around 25% are diagnosed in the first year, although prenatal diagnosis is now possible with improvements in antenatal ultrasonography. Adult centres treat a small proportion of those presenting with delayed diagnosis as well as those with complications from previous cyst surgery.

The incidence of choledochal cysts in Western countries is around 1 in 200 000 live births but it is much higher in Asia. There is frequent association with other hepatobiliary disease such as hepatic fibrosis as well as an aberrant pancreatico-biliary duct junction.[4]

Magnetic resonance cholangiopancreatography (MRCP) now allows images that are superior to traditional cholangiography (**Fig. 11.1**), and it should be recommended due to its non-invasive nature.[5]

Strictures of the extrahepatic biliary tree

Iatrogenic biliary injury
  Postcholecystectomy
  Trauma
  Other
Gallstone related
  Mirizzi's syndrome
Inflammatory
  Recurrent pyogenic cholangitis
  Parasitic infestation
    Clonorchis sinensis
    Opisthorchis viverrini
    Echinococcus
Ascaris
  Primary sclerosing cholangitis
  Benign strictures imitating malignancy
    Pancreatitis
      Lymphoplasmacytic pancreatitis
    Inflammatory pseudotumour
    Idiopathic strictures
HIV cholangiopathy

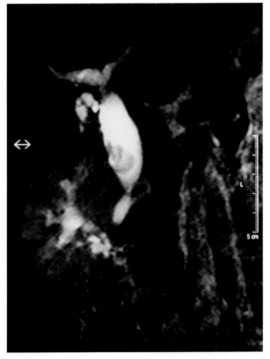

Figure 11.1 • MRCP demonstrating a type I choledochal cyst.

Classification

The modified Todani classification is employed to describe the various forms of choledochal cyst[6] (**Fig. 11.2**). Type I, the most common, represents a solitary cyst characterised by fusiform dilatation of the common bile duct. Type II comprises a diverticulum of the common bile duct, whilst type III cysts are choledochocoeles. Type IV is the second most common, with extension of cysts into the intrahepatic ducts. Lastly, type V involves intrahepatic cystic disease with no choledochal cyst, which merges into the syndrome of Caroli's disease.

Risk of malignancy

In the Western literature, the incidence of cholangiocarcinoma is reported to be around 12%,[7] compared to Todani's Japanese experience of 16% of 1353 patients.[8] The incidence of malignancy is reported to be 2% at 20 years, increasing to 43% for those in their sixties.[9] Cyst drainage without cyst excision does not prevent later malignant change, and there is continuing debate regarding the precise ongoing risk following cyst resection.

Management

Surgical resection is required to prevent recurrent episodes of sepsis and pain, to prevent the risk of pancreatitis from passage of debris and calculi, and because of the association with cholangiocarcinoma. Complete cyst excision with preservation of the pancreatic duct is required, with hepatico-jejunostomy for reconstruction. Some authors advocate liver resection for type IV cysts with intrahepatic extension for complete removal of the cyst, although the advantage is debatable.[10] For those patients with Caroli's disease, resection may be feasible if the biliary involvement is localised to one part of the liver. For other patients, endoscopic or radiological techniques may be required to address biliary sepsis by improving biliary drainage, while others may need to be considered for hepatic replacement if liver failure develops.[11]

For extrahepatic cysts, cyst-enterostomy, or drainage of the cyst into the duodenum, should no longer be performed as the cyst epithelium remains unstable and malignant potential exists. If previous drainage has been performed, symptoms of cholangitis generally persist and conversion to a Roux-en-Y hepatico-jejunostomy is advisable.

Special operative techniques

During operative exposure, intraoperative ultrasound is very useful to identify the biliary confluence, the intrahepatic extension of the cyst and the relationship with the right hepatic artery above and to the pancreatic duct below (**Fig. 11.3**). Small aberrant hepatic ducts may enter the cyst below the biliary confluence and these are missed frequently

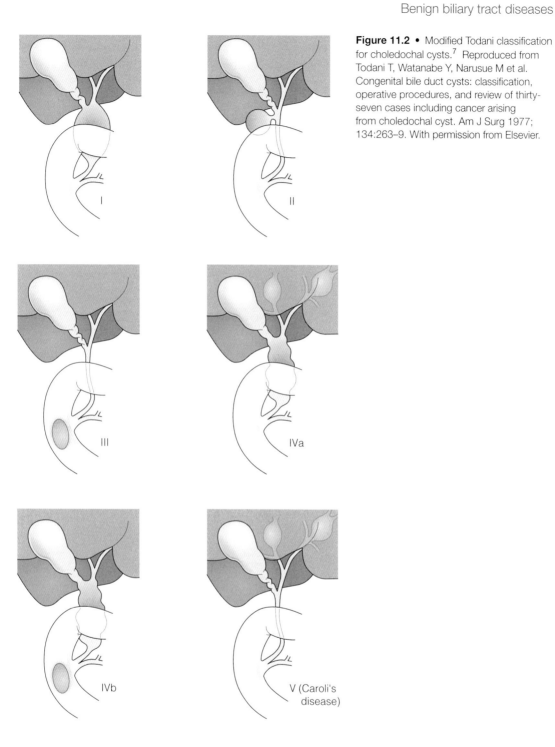

Figure 11.2 • Modified Todani classification for choledochal cysts.[7] Reproduced from Todani T, Watanabe Y, Narusue M et al. Congenital bile duct cysts: classification, operative procedures, and review of thirty-seven cases including cancer arising from choledochal cyst. Am J Surg 1977; 134:263–9. With permission from Elsevier.

on preoperative imaging.[12] Such aberrant ducts are usually identified once the cyst has been opened. The cyst is normally best excised in its entirety and this is facilitated by opening it along its anterior length. This aids identification of the vessels from which the cyst is freed. Early identification of the biliary confluence aids the surgeon in planning the incorporation of any segmental duct into the eventual hepatico-jejunal Roux-en-Y anastomosis. Dissection into the head of the pancreas is made easier by use of bipolar scissors and the CUSA™ (ultrasonic surgical aspiration system, ValleyLab, Boulder, CO) if the plane of dissection is obscured by fibrosis or inflammation. It may be necessary

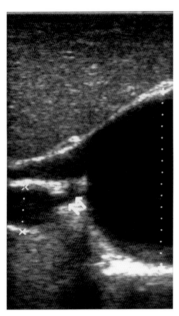

Figure 11.3 • Operative ultrasound scan of a type I choledochal cyst. The junction of the undilated proximal biliary tree with the cyst (long dotted line) is demonstrated. The right hepatic artery is posterior (two arrows), as is the right branch of the portal vein (short dotted line).

to leave a small oversewn lower common bile duct stump to avoid compromise to the pancreatic duct lumen.

 There is an accepted association between choledochal cyst and cholangiocarcinoma. The cyst should be excised and the biliary tree reconstructed by means of a hepatico-jejunostomy Roux-en-Y.

Iatrogenic biliary injury

The commonest cause of an injury to the extrahepatic biliary tree is as a result of an iatrogenic injury at the time of cholecystectomy. Although it is recognised that injury may also occur during other gastric or pancreatic procedures, this is much less common with the reduction in ulcer surgery and increasing specialisation in pancreatico-biliary surgery. Rarely, the injury may be related to abdominal trauma, injection of scolicidal agents in the management of hydatid cyst, or radiotherapy.

The true incidence of biliary injury following laparoscopic cholecystectomy remains obscure. It has been suggested that there was a slight decrease in the incidence of injuries following initial introduction of the laparoscopic technique,[13] with a reported incidence of 0.3–0.7%.[14–16] Open cholecystectomy is said to have a lower incidence of biliary injury, with a rate of 0.13%.[17,18]

Aetiology

Previous reports of injury during laparoscopic cholecystectomy suggested that injury was more likely to occur when performed for pancreatitis, cholangitis or acute cholecystitis.[19] However, in a prospective analysis of patients referred following biliary injury, 71% occurred in patients in whom the indication for cholecystectomy was biliary colic alone,[20] and thus surgeons should always be vigilant regardless of the indication.

In the majority of patients the problem is misinterpretation of the biliary anatomy, with the common bile duct confused with the cystic duct. Associated injury to the right hepatic artery often occurs as it is mistaken for the cystic artery. Partial injury may occur to the common bile duct after a diathermy burn or due to rigorous traction on the cystic duct, leading to its avulsion from the bile duct.

Techniques to avoid injury

Many techniques have been described to decrease the risk of injury to the common bile duct during cholecystectomy. The main risk factors are thought to be inexperience, aberrant anatomy and inflammation.[21] However, in a recent analysis of 252 laparoscopic bile duct injuries, the authors suggested that the primary cause of error was a visual perceptual illusion in 97% of cases, whilst faults in technical skill were thought to have been present in only 3% of injuries.[22]

Correct identification of the biliary anatomy is essential in avoiding injury to the extrahepatic bile duct. Dissection of Hartmann's pouch should start at the junction of the gallbladder and cystic duct and continue lateral to the cystic lymph node, thus staying as close as possible to the gallbladder. The biliary tree and hepatic arterial anatomy is highly variable and therefore great care must be taken in identifying all structures within Calot's triangle before ligation. In Couinaud's published study of biliary anatomy, 25% had drainage of a right sectoral duct directly into the common hepatic duct.[23] Sometimes this structure may follow a prolonged extrahepatic course, where it can be at greater risk from cholecystectomy. The right hepatic artery may also course through this area. All structures should be traced into the gallbladder to minimise the risk of injury (**Fig. 11.4**).

Extensive dissection should be avoided in Calot's triangle as diathermy injury may occur to the lateral wall of the common hepatic duct. Furthermore, arterial bleeding in this area should not be cauterised or clipped blindly. Most bleeding can be controlled with several minutes of direct pressure with a laparoscopic forceps compressing Hartmann's pouch onto the bleed point. During the era of open cholecystectomy many advocated complete excision

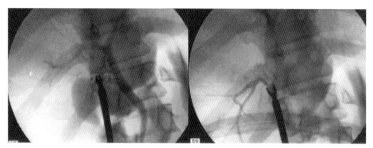

Figure 11.4 • Operative cholangiography of an aberrant right sectoral duct. The injury was recognised after division of the duct following cholangiography. The cholangiogram catheter was used to obtain a cholangiogram of the aberrant duct. The surgeon obtained advice by telephone and a decision was made to ligate the duct. The patient remains asymptomatic.

of the cystic duct to its insertion into the common bile duct to avoid a cystic duct stump syndrome. However, extensive dissection around the common bile duct with or without diathermy may cause an ischaemic stricture due to damage to the intricate blood supply of the common hepatic duct.

Many authors argue that operative cholangiography is essential to avoid biliary injury.[14,19] Fletcher et al. reported an overall twofold reduction in biliary injuries with the use of operative cholangiography, with an eightfold decrease in complex cases.[19] Flum and colleagues analysed retrospectively the Medicare database in the USA and identified 7911 common bile duct injuries following cholecystectomy. After adjusting for patient-level factors and surgeon-level factors the adjusted relative risk was 1.49 when intraoperative cholangiography was not used.[14] When the use of intraoperative cholangiography has undergone cost analysis, routine cholangiography has been found to be the most cost effective during high-risk operations when employed by less experienced surgeons.[24]

Unfortunately, many operative cholangiograms are interpreted incorrectly and injuries are missed. Although this event should be less frequent with the use of modern C-arm imaging, in recent reported series of biliary injuries, only 6–33% of operative cholangiograms were interpreted correctly.[25,26] For correct anatomical interpretation of the proximal biliary tree, both right sectoral/sectional ducts and the left hepatic duct should be visualised. In the presence of an endoscopic sphincterotomy contrast will preferentially flow into the duodenum and the patient may need to be placed in a head-down position to fill the intrahepatic ducts. If the anatomy is unclear no proximal clip should be placed on what is presumed to be the cystic duct, to avoid a crush injury to what may be the common hepatic duct.

Retrograde cholecystectomy has been described previously as a safe technique when inflammation around Calot's triangle makes identification of the anatomy difficult. Nonetheless, care still needs to

be exercised during dissection to avoid injury to the right hepatic artery and common hepatic duct, which may be adherent to an inflamed gallbladder. If identification remains impossible then the gallbladder can be opened to facilitate identification of the cystic duct. A subtotal cholecystectomy should be considered if a safe plane of dissection cannot be established, thus avoiding injury to the common hepatic or left hepatic ducts. Originally described for open cholecystectomy, these techniques have now also been performed laparoscopically.[27,28]

Bile duct injury can be avoided by careful identification of the biliary anatomy, dissection close to the gallbladder and avoidance of diathermy in Calot's triangle. The use of operative cholangiography and its correct interpretation is associated with a reduced incidence of bile duct injury.

Classification

Injury to the distal biliary tree is less technically demanding to repair than involvement of the biliary confluence. The success of reconstruction depends on the type of injury and the anatomical location.[29] Bismuth first described a classification system for biliary strictures reflecting the relationship of the injury to the biliary confluence (Table 11.1).[30] Strasberg and colleagues further proposed a broader classification to include a number of biliary complications including cystic stump leaks, biliary leaks and partial injuries to the biliary tree (**Fig. 11.5**).[18]

Presentation

It is preferable that injuries are recognised at the time of surgery to allow the best chance of repair, but this occurs in less than a third of patients. An unrecognised injury may present early with a postoperative biliary fistula, symptoms of biliary peritonitis or

Table 11.1 • Bismuth classification of biliary strictures

Bismuth classification	Definition
Bismuth 1	Low common hepatic duct stricture – hepatic duct stump >2 cm
Bismuth 2	Proximal common hepatic duct stricture – hepatic duct stump <2 cm
Bismuth 3	Hilar stricture with no residual common hepatic duct – hepatic duct confluence intact
Bismuth 4	Destruction of hepatic duct confluence – right and left hepatic ducts separated
Bismuth 5	Involvement of aberrant right sectoral hepatic duct alone or with concomitant stricture of the common hepatic duct

jaundice. Early symptoms or signs may be lacking but ductal injury should be suspected in the patient whose recovery is not immediate or is complicated by symptoms of peritoneal or diaphragmatic irritation and/or associated with deranged liver function tests in the first 24–48 hours of surgery. Signs may range from localised abdominal tenderness through to generalised peritonitis with overwhelming sepsis. Ligation of the bile duct will present early with jaundice; however, later presentation may occur as a result of stricture formation from a partial injury, localised inflammation or ischaemic insult.

Ligation of sectoral ducts may cause subsequent or late atrophy of the drained liver segments, which may become infected secondarily. Occasionally, injuries may present late with secondary biliary cirrhosis, which may require liver transplantation when liver failure results.[31]

In many patients there is a delay until referral, despite evidence of a biliary injury. In a report by Mirza et al., the median interval until referral was 26 days.[32] This delay is not inconsequential as the opportunity for an early repair is lost and results in the liver sustaining further damage.[33]

Management

Intraoperative recognition

In a review by Carroll et al., only 27% of patients underwent a successful repair by the primary surgeon responsible for the injury, whilst 79% of repairs performed following referral had a successful outcome.[34] If experienced help is not at hand, no attempt should be made to remedy the situation since this may compromise subsequent successful management. A T-tube or similar drain should be placed to the biliary injury and drains left in the subhepatic space followed by referral to a specialist centre. No attempt should be made to repair a transection or excision of the bile duct.

A partial injury to the bile duct may sometimes be managed with direct closure with placement of a T-tube through a separate choledochotomy. Primary repair with or without a T-tube for complete transection of the common bile duct is nearly always unsuccessful. This may result from unappreciated loss of common duct or arterial injury, or result from local diathermy injury or devascularisation of the duct from overzealous dissection of the common bile duct[35] (**Fig. 11.6a,b**). Recently de Reuver et al. have reported 43 patients managed with endoscopic (40) or percutaneous (3) stents for stricture formation after end-to-end repair. At 7 years follow-up 66% have been successfully managed without further surgery.[36]

 If an injury to the biliary tree is suspected during cholecystectomy, help must be sought from an experienced hepatobiliary surgeon. A successful repair by the surgeon who has caused the injury is far less likely than one performed by a surgeon experienced in performing a hepatico-jejunostomy.

Postoperative recognition: biliary fistula

Any patient who is not fit for discharge at 24 hours due to ongoing abdominal pain, vomiting, fever or bile in an abdominal drain should be considered to have a biliary leak. The lack of bile in an abdominal drain does not exclude the possibility of a biliary leak, particularly if there is liver function test derangement. Symptoms and signs vary widely, and widespread soiling of the abdominal cavity may be present with few signs.

Initial investigation should include full blood examination and determination of serum levels of urea, electrolytes, creatinine and liver function tests. Ultrasound is usually the initial investigation but it cannot readily differentiate bile and blood from a residual fluid collection following uneventful cholecystectomy. It may provide important information about the presence of intra-abdominal or pelvic fluid, biliary dilatation or retained stones within the bile duct.

If there is evidence of significant peritoneal irritation from widespread biliary peritonitis, laparoscopy allows confirmation of this and provides an opportunity for abdominal lavage. The porta hepatis can be inspected to determine the cause of the bile leak. Whilst dislodged clips from the cystic duct can be managed by application of further clips or suture, any other form of bile leak should lead to specialist referral. Drains can be placed to the subhepatic space as well as the subdiaphragmatic space

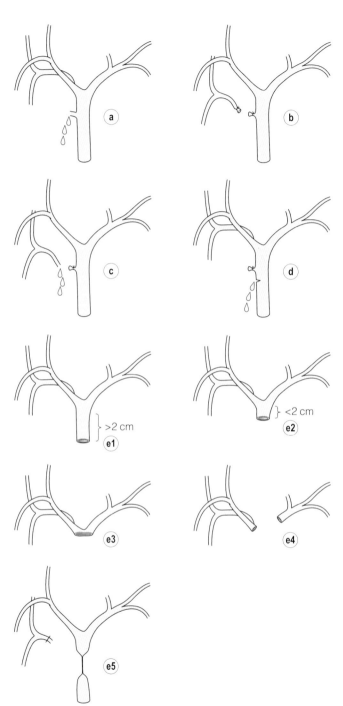

Figure 11.5 • Strasberg classification. Type A injuries include leakage from the cystic duct or subvesical ducts. Type B involves occlusion of part of the biliary tree, most usually an aberrant right hepatic duct. If the former injury involves transection without ligation this is termed a type C injury. A lateral injury to the biliary tree is a type D injury. Type E injuries are those described by Bismuth and subdivided into his classification (Table 11.1). Adapted from Strasberg SM et al. An analysis of the problem of biliary injury during laparoscopic chole cystectomy. J Am Coll Surg 1995; 180:102–25. With permission from the American College of Surgeons.

and pelvis if required. No attempt should be made to repair an injury laparoscopically. If laparotomy is required, this should be considered in conjunction with specialist assistance if bile duct injury is suspected.

Further assessment depends on the clinical situation. The majority of biliary fistulas are due to leaks from the cystic duct stump or subvesicle ducts, and endoscopic retrograde cholangiopancreatography (ERCP) allows anatomical definition, endoscopic

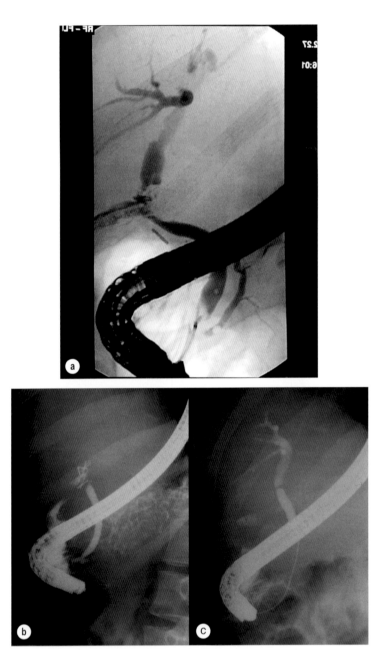

Figure 11.6 • **(a)** Failure of primary repair with T-tube. Primary repair was performed for an injury to the common bile duct presenting with biliary peritonitis. A T-tube was inserted through the anastomosis and this was removed at 4 weeks. An anastomotic stricture developed and the patient required a hepatico-jejunostomy 2 months later. **(b)** Failure of primary repair for ligation of the common bile duct. A complete transection of the common bile duct identified at postoperative endoscopic retrograde cholangiopancreatography (ERCP). Immediate repair was performed with a direct duct-to-duct repair. **(c)** A tight anastomotic stricture is demonstrated at a later ERCP.

sphincterotomy or stent placement. As complete transection of the bile duct precludes ERCP, computed tomography (CT) intravenous cholangiography or MRCP can determine continuity of the biliary tree prior to endoscopy. Occasionally, persistent bile drainage is associated with choledo-

cholithiasis requiring sphincterotomy and stone extraction. Most simple cystic duct stump leaks can be resolved by endoscopic stenting if cannulation is possible at ERCP[37] and occasionally side injury to the biliary tree can be controlled with endoscopic stent placement.[38]

If ERCP is unsuccessful or the bile duct is ligated or occluded by clips, percutaneous transhepatic cholangiography may facilitate biliary decompression but it is less frequently employed for diagnosis or delineation of the biliary anatomy. Occasionally, both sides of the liver may need to be externally drained to gain control of a biliary fistula, especially with E4 injuries to the biliary confluence. However, injury to the biliary tree detected in this way may allow surgical repair to be considered within the first week of injury in the stable non-septic patient, and again such further investigation or management decisions should only be considered following specialist referral.

Where the diagnosis of bile duct injury has been delayed, the aim should be to control the biliary fistula with external drainage using surgical or radiologically placed drains. Further control may be required with endoscopic stenting or external biliary drainage. Delayed repair can be considered subsequently once sepsis and intra-abdominal soiling have resolved, as a planned elective procedure in a specialist unit usually 2–3 months following injury. Such an initial conservative approach renders a potentially difficult operation into a repair, which will be considerably easier.

Diagnosis of a bile duct injury in the postoperative period should lead to immediate referral to a specialist centre since inappropriate attempts to manage this outwith a specialist centre will compromise the outcome.

Postoperative recognition: biliary obstruction

Ligation or inadvertent clipping of the biliary tree presents early in the postoperative period with jaundice. Later, stricture formation may occur as a result of direct trauma during dissection, clips placed inadvertently on the cystic duct but compromising the bile duct, or from damage to the intricate vascular supply of the bile duct by extensive mobilisation or diathermy. Initial investigation should include haematology, assessment of coagulation by estimation of prothrombin time, and by liver function tests. Ultrasound may indicate the level of obstruction or exclude the presence of a correctable cause of obstructive jaundice, such as a retained stone in the common bile duct.

ERCP will identify a stricture or complete transection of the bile duct. Overzealous instillation of contrast should be avoided, and placement of an endoscopic stent should only be considered after consultation with a specialist unit since this may introduce sepsis into the biliary tree and compromise further management. Furthermore, an undrained biliary tree may allow proximal biliary dilatation, thereby facilitating later reconstruction. Although some have reported satisfactory resolution of biliary strictures with endoscopic stenting alone, the follow-up has usually been short and almost all patients require later surgery in our experience. Partial occlusion of the duct by a clip may be remedied by balloon dilatation with or without placement of a stent; however, delay in diagnosis may result in subsequent recurrent stricture formation. Nonetheless, de Reuver et al. reported 110 patients with bile duct strictures following cholecystectomy that were treated with endoscopic stenting, 48 (44%) of which had already undergone attempted surgical repair. At a mean follow-up of 7.6 years, 74% of patients had a successful outcome.[37]

If the diagnosis of ductal obstruction is made early within the first week postsurgery, if the bilirubin level is only moderately elevated and there is no coexisting coagulopathy or sepsis, immediate repair offers the best chance of a successful outcome.

If repair needs to be delayed, stent placement may still be avoidable and a decision will generally be made based on the individual patient circumstances. Suspicion or evidence of arterial injury may influence the management decision.

For strictures that declare late, appropriate indications for stent placement are the presence of sepsis, severe itch resistant to medical therapy, or significant hepatic dysfunction.

The timing of repair

Early repair

When an injury is recognised in the early postoperative period and there is minimal peritoneal contamination or sepsis, a definitive repair by an experienced surgeon can be successful (**Fig. 11.7**). In our series of 123 patients referred with injury to the biliary tree, 22 patients underwent primary biliary repair in the first 2 weeks following injury and three had revision of a failed biliary repair. Between 2 weeks and 6 months, a further 22 injuries were repaired selectively. Successful repair was possible in 22 of 25 early repairs compared with 20 of 22 delayed repairs.[20]

Delayed repair

Many injuries continue to be unrecognised or referral delayed. In a recent prospective audit of major bile duct injuries from Australia, the median delay before referral was 9 days (2–28 days), and this included five patients with generalised peritonitis.[25]

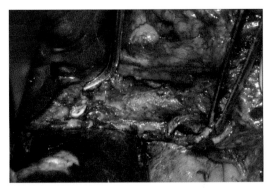

Figure 11.7 • Operative picture of an early repair of an E4 injury. A right-angle forceps is placed in the opening of the left hepatic duct whilst the open right hepatic duct is visible below. The portal vein is skeletonised with ligation and excision of both the extrahepatic biliary tree and right hepatic artery (held by forceps).

Controlling the biliary injury and associated sepsis is the first treatment aim, which may require endoscopic or percutaneous biliary decompression, allowing jaundice to settle or biliary sepsis to be drained. Intra-abdominal collections may be drained percutaneously, or in the early postoperative period this may be better achieved by laparoscopic means. It is accepted, however, that bile collections are frequently loculated and difficult to eradicate in patients with intra-abdominal sepsis or widespread biliary contamination or peritonitis. The most effective treatment may be laparotomy with extensive lavage and the placement of large intra-abdominal drains. Definitive repair should not be contemplated if there is severe peritoneal soiling since injudicious attempts to repair the injury may aggravate the injury and result in a poor outcome.

Once these objectives have been met, the patient should be allowed to recover from the combined insult of surgery and sepsis. A period of rehabilitation at home is generally required before repair is contemplated in these compromised patients. Abdominal and biliary drainage can be managed on an outpatient basis with community nursing support. Nutritional supplementation may be required, particularly in those who have required a prolonged admission to the intensive care unit and hospital. Attention should be paid to the consequences of prolonged external biliary drainage and consideration given to recycling of bile.

Associated vascular injury

Abdominal CT is required to ensure resolution of intra-abdominal collections and before repair to exclude the presence of liver atrophy. Atrophy can occur from prolonged obstruction to the segmental, sectional or hepatic ducts, but is generally associated with the presence of a vascular injury, most usually of the right hepatic artery. Liver resection may occasionally be needed at the time of definitive repair to remove a source of ongoing sepsis or if satisfactory and secure reconstruction to the left or right duct is not possible.

Buell et al. identified associated vascular injury as an independent predictor of mortality, with 38% of patients dying compared to 3% ($P < 0.001$) where no arterial injury was present.[39] Some authors advocate arteriography before repair to identify such associated vascular injury as a repair is less likely to be successful,[40] or for consideration of hepatic arterial reconstruction at the time of hepatico-jejunostomy.[40,41] However, a recent paper described 55 patients with postcholecystectomy strictures who underwent surgical reconstruction with a left duct approach and preoperative coeliac axis and superior mesenteric artery angiography.[42] Twenty-six patients (47%) had an associated vascular injury, of which 20 (36%) were of the right hepatic artery. In this series only one patient in each group (vascular injury vs. no injury) developed a recurrent stricture after repair.[42] A proximal anastomosis may offer a better blood supply, minimising the risk of anastomotic stricturing. In support of this theory, Mercado et al. demonstrated that an anastomosis fashioned below the biliary confluence was more likely to require revisional surgery (16%) compared to an anastomosis performed at the biliary confluence (0%; $P < 0.05$).[43] Recent improvements in magnetic resonance imaging (MRI) and spiral CT are producing impressive arterial and venous anatomical reconstructions, which may negate the need for invasive arteriography (**Fig. 11.8**).

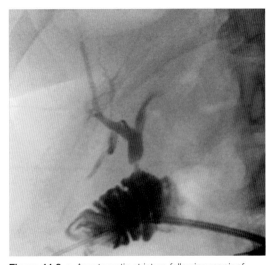

Figure 11.8 • Anastomotic stricture following repair of biliary injury. Percutaneous transjejunal cholangiogram (PTJC) of a Bismuth 1 injury repaired by hepatico-jejunostomy at the level of the transection of the common bile duct (not to the left hepatic duct). Three months later the patient required reconstruction of the anastomotic stricture.

Injury to the hepatic arterial supply may present with haemobilia or intra-abdominal haemorrhage from a false aneurysm, usually associated with ongoing subhepatic sepsis and most frequently of the right hepatic arteries. If suspected, urgent angiography is required (**Fig. 11.9**). Haemorrhage may be controlled by embolisation of the feeding vessel, although re-bleeding can occur and necessitate further embolisation. However, in our experience, further bleeding in the presence of ongoing sepsis usually requires laparotomy for control of bleeding and drainage of any subhepatic collection.

Further imaging

For patients with injury to the biliary confluence (E3 and E4), preoperative imaging will help in the planning of future repair. In the presence of a biliary stricture, invasive cholangiography by ERCP or percutaneous transhepatic cholangiogram (PTC) risks introducing sepsis. However, if PTC is required for external biliary drainage, an adequate cholangiogram may be obtained at this time. The quality of MRCP continues to improve, and detailed biliary anatomical reconstructions can be produced, thereby negating the need for more invasive imaging.

Operative techniques

Biliary reconstruction should be performed under optimal circumstances at the time of injury or soon thereafter. Once this opportunity has been lost, repair should only be considered when the patient has been optimised, in the absence of intra-abdominal sepsis

and when sufficient time has elapsed to allow for maturation of adhesions and the tissues at the porta hepatis.

We use a right subcostal incision for access, which can be extended across the midline if required. Retraction is provided with Doyen's blades and the Omni-tract® (Omni-tract surgical, St Paul, MN) mechanical retractor. Laparotomy is undertaken to assess the liver and to allow adhesiolysis, thereby freeing the small bowel for reconstruction. Frequently the omentum, hepatic flexure, duodenum and hepatoduodenal ligament are involved in a dense inflammatory mass, and occasionally an unsuspected fistula between bile duct and duodenum or colon is identified. Dissection is often easier if commenced laterally and then directed towards the biliary structures. The common bile duct can be difficult to identify, particularly in the presence of extensive fibrosis, and intraoperative ultrasound is a useful tool in allowing its location and relationship to vessels to be determined.

For injuries that involve the biliary confluence, lowering of the hilar plate allows easier identification of the left and right hepatic ducts. This may be aided by the use of an ultrasonic dissector (CUSA), which is also employed to break down the contracted fibrotic tissue in the gallbladder bed and facilitate the division of any bridge of liver tissue between segments 3 and 4. Opening these two planes on the right and left sides facilitates identification of and access to the biliary confluence.

Since the blood supply to the bile duct is often damaged at the time of injury, the common hepatic

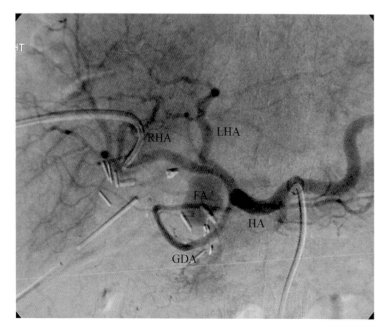

Figure 11.9 • Digital subtraction angiogram demonstrating a false aneurysm of the common hepatic artery. Embolisation was required for control. The patient has undergone a primary repair for a complete transection of the common bile duct. FA, false aneurysm; GDA, gastroduodenal artery; HA, common hepatic artery; LHA, left hepatic artery; RHA, right hepatic artery.

duct should be opened as proximally as possible, although frequently there has been retraction of the fibrotic remnant superiorly. Extension of the incision into the left hepatic duct allows a wide anastomosis to be fashioned with adequate views of the left- and right-sided ducts. Care should be taken since there may be a small superficial arterial branch crossing the left duct anteriorly and running above to segment 4. For injuries with separation of the confluence, the right and left hepatic ducts can be anastomosed together before formation of a hepatico-jejunostomy, allowing a single biliary anastomosis. If possible injuries to an isolated right sectoral duct are best repaired or drained into a Roux limb of bowel (Fig. 11.4). Simple ligation may lead to atrophy of the drained segments, which may become a nidus for sepsis.

Repair should be effected by a hepatico-jejunostomy with a 70-cm Roux limb of jejunum, thereby minimising the risk of enteric reflux and chronic damage to the biliary tree. Moraca et al. advocate hepatico-duodenostomy for biliary injury on the basis that it is more physiological, quicker to perform, and allows later ERCP for imaging and intervention.[44] They found no difference in outcome following hepatico-duodenostomy when compared with hepatico-jejunostomy, although median follow-up was only 54 months. Hepatico-duodenostomy has largely been abandoned in the treatment of other benign biliary disease due to ongoing enteric reflux. There have been anecdotal reports of the late development of cholangiocarcinoma,[45] as well as the need to undertake liver transplantation in patients so managed when secondary biliary cirrhosis due to enteric reflux has resulted. Our own view is that hepatico-duodenostomy has no role in the management of bile duct injury.

Fine absorbable interrupted sutures of 4/0 or 5/0 polydioxanone sulphate (PDS II) should be used to fashion an end-to-side hepatico-jejunostomy, with care being taken to produce good mucosal apposition. Some authors advocate the use of an access limb, particularly for E3 and E4 injuries, to allow subsequent radiological intervention for dilatation of recurrent strictures.[46] However, others believe that advances in percutaneous transhepatic techniques have made this unnecessary and have achieved satisfactory results without using this surgical approach.

Partial injury to the biliary tree can be repaired with fine interrupted sutures, although when resulting from diathermy dissection, formal hepatico-jejunostomy may be necessary as conduction of the thermal injury may cause later stricture formation. If a T-tube is placed to protect a primary duct repair, this should be placed through a separate choledochotomy.

Management of complications related to repair

Revisional surgery

Many patients with biliary injury continue to suffer from complications despite reconstruction. Factors such as the experience of the initial surgeon, the level of injury, the associated sepsis and liver atrophy all increase the chance of an unsuccessful repair. Following primary repair of a ductal tear or laceration, further stricture formation may result if there has been extensive dissection around the common hepatic duct. In such instances, surgical revision with the formation of a Roux-en-Y hepatico-jejunostomy is indicated.

The majority of patients requiring revisional surgery will have undergone a previous biliary enteric drainage procedure. Anastomotic stricturing will require revision of the anastomosis, with extension of the choledochotomy into the left hepatic duct (Fig. 11.8). Choledocho-duodenotomy will require conversion to a Roux-en-Y hepatico-jejunostomy to avoid ongoing problems with biliary enteric reflux.

Liver resection and transplantation

In the acute setting of bile duct injury, long-term damage to the hepatic parenchyma is difficult to predict. Major vascular injury or unrecognised segmental biliary obstruction may lead to atrophy of the liver, chronic intrahepatic infection, abscess formation or secondary biliary cirrhosis. In such patients, careful operative assessment is required; CT should be performed to identify areas of associated liver atrophy and to exclude portal vein thrombosis.

In our experience, the majority of patients requiring liver resection are those with ongoing sepsis in an obstructed segment or those where drainage of the extrahepatic biliary tree is not possible due to sectoral duct damage or fibrosis.[31] Very rarely, resection may be needed to gain access to the biliary tree, especially when the injury involves the biliary confluence (E4). The right lobe is most commonly affected by sepsis and atrophy as the right-sided sectoral ducts and arterial supply are more likely to be damaged during cholecystectomy, although both left- and right-sided hepatic resections have been reported in patients with severe biliary injury. Resection of the right liver can be performed, for example, at the time of delayed reconstruction if there is any doubt regarding the integrity of the anastomosis to the right sectoral or hepatic duct and when a satisfactory anastomosis can be achieved to the long extrahepatic left duct.

Failed reconstruction and persistent cholangitis may lead to end-stage liver failure within a few years and this may require liver transplantation[31] (**Fig. 11.10**). A long interval between injury and referral

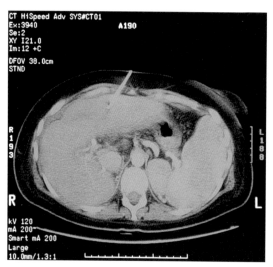

Figure 11.10 • Contrast-enhanced CT of the liver after unsuccessful revisional hepatico-jejunostomy. The surgeon who performed the laparoscopic cholecystectomy performed the hepatico-jejunostomy for an E4 injury. A revisional hepatico-jejunostomy was performed before referral, which was complicated by an anastomotic stricture and portal vein thrombosis. The CT shows evidence of right lobe atrophy and splenomegaly as well as a percutaneous biliary drain.

is known to be associated with end-stage liver disease.[47] Rarely, liver transplantation may be needed when the combined biliary and vascular injury is so severe as to preclude attempted reconstruction, although the results are universally poor.[31]

Prognosis

Success of repair

Successful repair has been well described and can be achieved in 90% of patients in a specialised unit.[20,26] However, anastomotic strictures, liver atrophy and cirrhosis may occur many years following repair. Predictors of a poor outcome include involvement of the biliary confluence,[29,47] repair by the injuring surgeon,[34,48,49] three or more previous attempted repairs,[29] and recent active inflammation.[49]

Survival

Mortality following injury to the biliary tree is significant. Death may follow the acute injury itself, following the biliary repair, or occur later as a result of biliary sepsis or cirrhosis. In a recent report of a nationwide analysis of survival following biliary injury after cholecystectomy, Flum et al. identified 7911 (0.5%) injuries from 1 570 361 cholecystectomies.[48] Within the first year after cholecystectomy the mortality rate was 6.6% in the uninjured group and 26.1% in those with injury to the common bile duct. The adjusted hazard ratio for death during follow-up

was higher for those with an injury (2.79; 95% CI 2.71–2.88). The risk of death increased significantly with advancing age and comorbidities. If the initial repair was performed by the injuring surgeon then the adjusted hazard of death increased by 11%.

Quality of life

Boerma et al. first undertook an assessment of quality of life in patients who had sustained biliary injury or leak that required additional intervention.[50] Five years after injury, quality of life in the physical and mental domains was significantly worse than controls, despite a successful outcome in 84% of treated patients and regardless of the type of treatment or severity of injury. However, the length of treatment was an independent predictor of a poor mental quality of life. Melton et al. report that quality of life in 89 patients who had undergone biliary repair following laparoscopic cholecystectomy showed no difference in the physical or social domains when compared to controls.[51] However, in the psychological domain, patients were significantly worse, particularly in the 31% of patients who sought legal recourse for their injury.

Associated malignancy

A small number of reports exist about the development of cholangiocarcinoma at the site of anastomosis 20–30 years following repair.[45] It is possible that enteric reflux into the biliary tree with sepsis and the production of mutagenic secondary bile salts may be responsible. Furthermore, hepatocellular carcinoma may develop due to secondary biliary cirrhosis (**Fig. 11.11**).

Benign biliary strictures

Mirizzi's syndrome

Mirizzi first described the syndrome of extrahepatic biliary stricture in association with cholelithiasis in 1948,[52] a condition that occurs in fewer than 0.5% of cholecystectomies.[53] Obstruction of the common hepatic duct may occur for two reasons: (i) a stone impacted in the cystic duct may cause direct pressure or oedema (Mirizzi type I) (**Fig 11.12**), or (ii) occasionally the stone may erode through the wall of the gallbladder or cystic duct and into the common hepatic duct (Mirizzi type II).

Presentation

Diagnosis can be difficult as symptoms may be the same as for acute cholecystitis, but all patients with the disease process will have abnormal liver function tests and some may present with jaundice. Occasionally the diagnosis is made at the time of laparoscopic cholecystectomy.

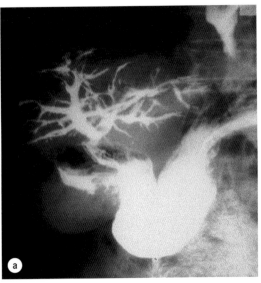

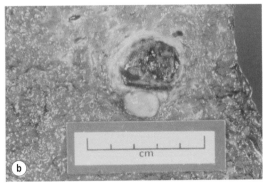

Figure 11.11 • Hepatocellular carcinoma as a consequence of biliary injury. This patient required a liver transplant for secondary biliary cirrhosis, which developed following hepato-duodenostomy for a biliary injury **(a)**. At pathological examination a hepatocellular carcinoma was detected in the explanted liver **(b)**.

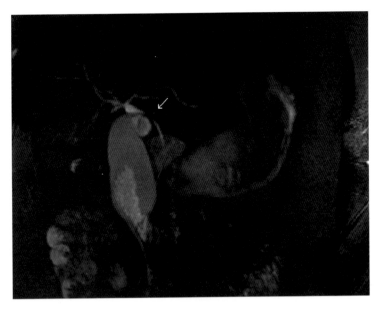

Figure 11.12 • Mirizzi syndrome (type 1). Magnetic resonance cholangiopancreatography (MRCP) demonstrating compression of the common bile duct (single arrow) secondary to acute cholecystitis from a stone impacted in Hartmann's pouch.

Management

The investigations may be aimed at excluding a diagnosis of bile duct or gallbladder cancer. Ultrasound assessment will identify dilatation of the biliary tree proximal to the stricture and may even have features suggestive of a Mirizzi syndrome. An ultrasound finding of a decompressed gallbladder with stones involving the common hepatic duct would be more suggestive of a Mirizzi syndrome. An associated mass or lymphadenopathy would be more in keeping with biliary malignancy, but associated sepsis or an empyema of the gallbladder may lead the operator to diagnose Mirizzi's syndrome as cancer. Both conditions may coexist. ERCP allows endoscopic stent placement to relieve jaundice and may demonstrate a fistula between the gallbladder and common hepatic duct (type II). A smooth, tapered stricture is more typical of a benign rather than malignant cause of jaundice. Endoscopic stenting provides resolution of jaundice, an anatomical roadmap and also may help with identification of the common hepatic duct at operation. Occasionally a stone impacted in the cystic duct may produce a distal biliary stricture. This occurs when there is a low insertion of the cystic duct with stone impaction at the cystic duct/common bile duct junction. It can be difficult to visualise or extract the stone at ERCP and therefore MRCP will be required to confirm the diagnosis.

When Mirizzi's syndrome is difficult to distinguish from a malignant stricture, CT may aid in the diagnosis. Occasionally laparoscopic ultrasound may be necessary to further delineate the stricture and exclude tumour dissemination. Although the two conditions may appear similar, vascular invasion may be seen and targeted biopsy may confirm a malignant diagnosis.[54]

Successful completion of cholecystectomy by laparoscopic means has been reported for apparent type I Mirizzi's syndrome,[55] although this would be inappropriate where there was a clear fistulous communication between gallbladder and common hepatic duct. One of these reported patients has subsequently developed a biliary stricture (O.J. Garden, personal communication). The conventional approach for type I strictures is to perform an open cholecystectomy or to convert from a laparoscopic procedure to allow adequate assessment of the associated biliary stricture. Operative cholangiography should be performed, and in those with persistent strictures a hepatico-jejunostomy should be performed. For type II, where a defect results from the removal of the gallbladder and stent, the common bile duct should be explored. The majority of patients will require a hepatico-jejunostomy, although apparently successful reconstructions using grafts of Hartmann's pouch have been described.[56] Long-term results of this innovative approach are awaited.

In a recent report, Schafer et al. identified Mirizzi's syndrome in 39 (0.3%) of 13 023 patients undergoing a laparoscopic cholecystectomy.[57] Thirty-four (87%) patients had a type I Mirrizi syndrome. Of these, 23 patients underwent cholecystectomy alone, 10 patients required bile duct exploration and T-tube insertion, and one patient had a Roux-en-Y reconstruction. Twenty-four (74%) of the 34 patients had required open conversion. Of the remaining five patients with a type II Mirizzi syndrome, three underwent a hepatico-jejunostomy and two had simple closure with a T-tube drainage. All had required open conversion and, interestingly, four (10%) patients were found to have a gallbladder carcinoma on histopathology.

 Mirizzi's syndrome is an uncommon cause of obstructive jaundice secondary to gallstone disease. This condition will normally necessitate conversion to open surgery if a laparoscopic cholecystectomy is attempted, and a hepatico-jejunostomy will normally be required for a type II lesion.

Hepatolithiasis

Intrahepatic gallstone disease (hepatolithiasis) is also known as oriental cholangiohepatitis or recurrent pyogenic cholangitis. It is most common in Taiwan, South-East Asia and Hong Kong. Symptoms include abdominal pain, jaundice as well as cholangitis.

Recently there has been a decline in incidence, possibly related to improved economic conditions and changes in diet.[58] The cause is unknown, although *Clonorchis sinensis*, ascariasis and nutritional insufficiency have been suggested as associated factors in its causation.

Pathologically there is gross irregular dilatation and intrahepatic stricture formation of the biliary tree, which frequently contains stones, debris and pus. Bile duct proliferation, and portal and periportal inflammation and fibrosis are seen, and occasionally there is liver abscess formation. Stone formation is frequently associated with bacterial superinfection and the bile is infected in 96% of patients with hepatolithiasis, most usually with *E. coli*.[59] There is a strong association between hepatolithiasis and cholangiocarcinoma.[60] Diagnosis is based on history and demographic features, and investigation includes liver biochemistry and abdominal ultrasonography. Ultrasound is usually diagnostic, although abdominal CT may add further information regarding associated liver atrophy or abscess formation. ERCP will provide important anatomical detail and will allow endoscopic stenting if required. If stricture formation or stones prevent filling of the intrahepatic ducts, MRCP should provide further information, avoiding the risk of PTC.

Management

In an acute attack, treatment of cholangitis is initiated with broad-spectrum antibiotics. A third-generation cephalosporin and metronidazole with the addition of ampicillin for resistant enterococci will provide broad cover for most biliary pathogens. Intravenous fluid resuscitation and analgesia are required. Conservative treatment fails in around 30% of cases, and is more likely in those with obstruction of the extrahepatic biliary tree rather than an isolated segment.[61] When conservative treatment fails, biliary decompression is required by either an endoscopic, radiological or surgical approach.

Following resolution of an acute attack definitive surgery is required. A multidisciplinary approach is required involving radiologists, surgeons and gastro-enterologists. A full spectrum of interventions from simple exploration and stone removal, hepatico-jejunostomy or liver resection through to liver transplantation may be required. Of 97 Japanese patients treated for hepatolithiasis, 49% undergoing hepaticojejunostomy, 25% drained with T-tube and 10% treated with percutaneous transhepatic cholangioscopic lithotripsy were found to have residual stones. No patients treated with hepatic resection had residual stone disease. Furthermore, recurrent stones were found in 14% of hepatectomy patients compared to 25% or more for the other treatment options.[62]

Parasitic infestation causing jaundice

Liver flukes (trematodes)

Infestation with liver flukes is caused through consuming inadequately cooked, pickled or salted infected fish. The immature fluke passes into the biliary tree, where it grows to maturity. Ova are passed into the gastrointestinal tract and subsequently to water supplies, infecting molluscs and fish. Infection with *Clonorchis sinensis* occurs in China, Japan and South-East Asia, whilst *Opisthorchis viverrini* is found in parts of eastern Europe and Siberia. Infection may be asymptomatic or the patient may present with an acute febrile illness or chronic symptoms. Chronic infestation results in hepatolithiasis and should be managed as detailed above.

Diagnosis is possible by the detection of ova within the stool or in duodenal aspirates, and an eosinophilia may also be present on blood film. ERCP may demonstrate slender filling defects within the bile duct as well as associated changes of fibrosis and calculus formation.

Echinococcus

Hydatid cysts involving the liver remain endemic in parts of the Mediterranean and Far East, as well as sheep farming areas of Australia, New Zealand, South America and South Africa. Infection is from *Echinococcus granulosus*, and less commonly *Echinococcus multilocularis* in central Europe.

Biliary obstruction can occur due to local compression of the common hepatic duct by the expanding cyst, or when daughter cysts pass down the common hepatic duct following rupture of the cyst into intrahepatic radicles. Secondary sclerosing cholangitis has been described following inappropriate injection of scolicidal agents into the hepatic cyst when there is communication with the biliary tree.[63]

Treatment

Preoperative endoscopic cholangiography may identify debris within the biliary tree, and endoscopic sphincterotomy may prevent further episodes of biliary obstruction. Endoscopic stenting may also allow resolution of obstruction secondary to a large intrahepatic cyst.

The secondary sclerosing cholangitis produced by inappropriate instillation of a scolicidal agent into the biliary tree will often only be amenable to hepatic replacement. Surgical bypass may be possible for localised strictures.

Ascaris lumbricoides

The roundworm *Ascaris lumbricoides* is the commonest worm to infect humans. Rarely, an infected patient can present with obstructive jaundice due to migration of the worm into the biliary tree and this is difficult to distinguish from stone disease. The more frequent presentation is from cholangitis due to the worm traversing the ampulla. *Ascaris* has also been associated with recurrent pyogenic cholangitis.[64]

Ultrasound sometimes identifies a long, linear filling defect within the biliary tree. Identification may occur at the time of ERCP where endoscopic extraction may be possible. Medical treatment exists with the anthelmintics mebendazole or albendazole, which are often curative. The late complication of papillary stenosis can be treated with endoscopic sphincterotomy.

Primary sclerosing cholangitis

Aetiology

Primary sclerosing cholangitis is a rare condition, and although the precise cause has yet to be determined there is increasing evidence of an immunological basis. Around 70% of patients will have ulcerative colitis, or more rarely Crohn's disease. There are other reports of association with Riedel's thryoiditis, retroperitoneal fibrosis, lymphoplasmacytic sclerosing pancreatitis[65] as well as a strong association with a number of HLA antigens.[66]

Presentation

Primary sclerosing cholangitis is a progressive obliterative fibrosis of the intrahepatic and extrahepatic biliary tree with a wide clinical spectrum and frequent remissions and relapses. In the early stages of disease most patients are asymptomatic but later in the disease process patients may have pruritus, ill-defined pain, fever, jaundice and weight loss. Many asymptomatic patients are diagnosed by detection of abnormal liver function tests during the investigation of inflammatory bowel disease. Although some patients may present at an advanced stage, signs of liver failure develop over a period of time.

Sudden deterioration may suggest the development of cholangiocarcinoma, with which there is a strong association.

Investigation

Liver biochemistry demonstrates a cholestatic picture. Although antineutrophil cytoplasmic antibodies are present in the serum of around 80% of patients,[67] testing for autoantibodies is usually performed to exclude primary biliary cirrhosis, a condition with which it can be difficult to differentiate.

The mainstay of investigation is cholangiography, which usually demonstrates a diffuse picture of stricturing and attenuated intrahepatic bile ducts. As well as providing anatomical details of the biliary tree, ERCP enables endoscopic therapy and the opportunity for brush cytology if malignancy is suspected. MRCP is highly sensitive, with a diagnostic accuracy comparable to ERCP, and is now preferred as a means of both diagnosing and assessing the extent of disease to avoid the introduction of bacteria, possibly causing severe biliary sepsis.

Management

The prognosis of primary sclerosing cholangitis is poor, with a median survival of only 9.6 years from diagnosis to death or liver transplantation.[68] Survival may improve with earlier diagnosis and liver transplantation. The use of ursodeoxycholic acid in the treatment of pruritus has been associated with improvements in biochemical function and histological appearance.[69] Episodes of cholangitis can be treated with antibiotics covering biliary pathogens. There is no evidence that colectomy for inflammatory bowel disease alters disease progression.

Endoscopic or transhepatic dilatation of short dominant strictures has been described as effective, safe and well tolerated.[70] The addition of endoscopic or percutaneous stents following biliary dilatation is more likely to cause procedure-related complications,[71] and there is a considerable risk that endoscopic treatment may introduce infection leading to cholangitis, liver abscess formation or precipitation of liver failure. In those patients without cirrhosis but with jaundice secondary to a dominant stricture, surgical drainage with an access limb has been described. However, adhesions and cholangitis following surgery may compromise later liver transplantation and liver disease may progress following an apparently successful drainage procedure.[72]

Liver transplantation is necessary to treat end-stage liver disease. However, it is now more usual for patients to be considered if there is persistent jaundice, intractable pruritus, recurrent cholangitis, malnutrition or fatigue. Many patients are now transplanted before liver failure, with survival rates of greater than 80% at 5 years.[73]

Exclusion of associated malignant stricture

Cholangiocarcinoma and gallbladder cancer complicates 10–36% of patients with primary sclerosing cholangitis,[68,74] and needs to be excluded before liver transplantation. The majority of patients have recurrence of cholangiocarcinoma following transplantation, with only a 30% survival at 1 year and no 6-year survivors.[74]

In the majority of patients, concern regarding occult cholangiocarcinoma is small, and liver transplantation is undertaken in the absence of a dominant stricture. Serum carbohydrate antigen (CA) 19-9 has been used in an attempt to identify cases with an occult biliary malignancy. In patients with a level >100 U/mL, the test had a 75% sensitivity and an 80% specificity in identifying cholangiocarcinoma.[75]

Patients with a sudden rapid deterioration in their clinical state or with a dominant stricture must be considered to have a cholangiocarcinoma and be investigated extensively. Brush cytology at ERCP may provide the diagnosis if a malignant smear is obtained. In a recent prospective study of biliary brush cytology at ERCP the sensitivity for diagnosing cholangiocarcinoma was found to be 80%.[76] CT or MRI may demonstrate a mass lesion in association with the biliary tree, although the usual appearance is of a stricture indistinguishable from a benign disease. Positron emission tomography (PET) scanning is superior to conventional radiological investigations to differentiate primary sclerosing cholangitis and cholangiocarcinoma.[77]

Laparoscopy identifies the majority of patients with unresectable biliary tract cancer,[78] and may be of use in assessing those considered for transplantation in whom a cholangiocarcinoma is suspected since tumour dissemination often occurs early. Laparoscopic ultrasound may further aid assessment, and occasionally laparotomy may be required if there is diagnostic doubt regarding cholangiocarcinoma.

Biliary strictures imitating malignancy

It is not unusual for benign biliary pathology to be found in resected specimens of the pancreatic head that had been thought to be malignant. Around 10% of Whipple resections for malignancy will be found to have benign pathology.[79] Most commonly the pathology is chronic pancreatitis related to alcohol or gallstone disease. However, other confounding pathologies include lymphoplasmacytic sclerosing pancreatitis, primary sclerosing cholangitis, choledocholithiasis and inflammatory pseudotumours.

Up to 14% of patients undergoing surgery for presumed malignant hilar obstruction are found to have a benign fibrotic stricture of the bile duct.[80] It is usually impossible to differentiate them from malignancy preoperatively and thus resection is often attempted and nearly always feasible. Successful treatment has been described with the use of steroids.[81]

Lymphoplasmacytic sclerosing pancreatitis

Lymphoplasmacytic sclerosing pancreatitis is also known as autoimmune pancreatitis, sclerosing pancreatitis or primary inflammatory pancreatitis. The disease is associated with other autoimmune diseases such as Sjögren's syndrome, Riedel's thyroiditis, retroperitoneal fibrosis, ulcerative colitis and primary sclerosing cholangitis.[82] Although only accounting for about 2.4% of pancreatic resections, the condition is important since a proportion of patients will develop either biliary anastomotic strictures or intrahepatic strictures following resection. In a series of 31 patients, eight (28%) went on to develop recurrent jaundice after resection.[82]

Recently, increased levels of IgG4 have been described in association with the disease, and successful treatment with steroids has been described, although disease recurrence is reported.[83] As yet the value of steroid treatment in the prevention and treatment of recurrent strictures is not well described.

HIV cholangiopathy (AIDS cholangiopathy)

Human immunodeficiency virus (HIV) cholangiopathy is a secondary sclerosing cholangitis caused by opportunistic infections that can affect the entire biliary tree. Causative organisms include cytomegalovirus, *Cryptosporidium*, *Mycobacterium avium* complex, microsporidia, herpes simplex virus[84] and giardiasis. Up to 50% of patients will not have a causative organism isolated.[84]

Most patients with HIV will have abnormal liver function tests during the course of their disease, most commonly as a result of drug interactions or viral hepatitis. For those with obstructive or mixed liver function tests, initial investigation should include abdominal ultrasonography to identify areas of biliary dilatation.

ERCP allows identification of biliary strictures and has the ability to facilitate biliary biopsies and sample bile for culture.

Biliary strictures may respond to endoscopic stenting, and surgical treatment is rarely warranted as the 1-year survival for HIV cholangiopathy is only 41%.[85]

Functional biliary disorders

Most patients who present for investigation of sphincter of Oddi dysfunction have already undergone cholecystectomy for presumed gallbladder pain. However, up to 39–90% of patients with idiopathic recurrent pancreatitis may also have sphincter of Oddi dysfunction.[86] In those patients with postcholecystectomy pain, the presentation and investigation identifies three types:[87]

- Type 1 – Abdominal pain, obstructive liver function tests, biliary dilatation and delayed emptying of contrast at ERCP.
- Type 2 – Pain with only one or two of the above-mentioned criteria.
- Type 3 – Recurrent biliary pain only.

Between 65% and 95% of group 1 patients will be found on biliary manometry to have sphincter of Oddi dysfunction compared to only 12–28% of type 3.[86] Diagnosis is usually by exclusion of other causes of abdominal pain such as peptic ulcer disease and irritable bowel syndrome. Liver function tests, abdominal ultrasonography, CT, endoscopy and MRCP have often been already performed.

At ERCP, biliary manometry is not required if there is delayed drainage of contrast in type 1 or 2 patients. This investigation should be reserved for those patients in whom the diagnosis remains unclear.

Medical therapy with calcium channel blockers, nitrates and botulinum toxin is available but long-term results are unknown. Avoidance of opiate analgesia may prevent the onset of pain. Endoscopic sphincterotomy is the usual treatment; however, 5–16% of patients will develop postprocedural pancreatitis[88] and good or excellent responses are only reported in 69% of patients at long-term follow-up.[89] Surgical sphincterotomy is now indicated rarely due to the lower cost and lower morbidity of endoscopic sphincterotomy but it may be required if the endoscopic approach has been unsuccessful.

Key points

- Choledochal cysts should be treated with complete cyst excision and hepatico-jejunostomy due to the risk of malignancy in the remaining biliary epithelium.
- Identification of the biliary anatomy and minimisation of diathermy near the common bile duct are essential during laparoscopic cholecystectomy to avoid biliary injury.
- Operative cholangiography is useful for delineating the biliary anatomy during cholecystectomy; however, many cholangiograms are not interpreted correctly at the time of biliary injury.
- Following laparoscopic cholecystectomy, any patient who is not fit for discharge at 24 hours due to ongoing abdominal pain, vomiting, fever or bile in an abdominal drain should be considered to have a biliary leak.
- Diagnosis of a bile duct injury in the postoperative period should lead to immediate referral to a specialist centre since inappropriate attempts to manage this outwith a specialist centre will compromise the outcome.
- In the absence of sepsis, repair of injuries to the biliary tree can be performed successfully within the first week.

References

1. Mieli-Vergani G, Howard ER, Portmann B et al. Late referral for biliary atresia: missed opportunities for effective surgery. Lancet 1989; i:421–3.

2. Schreiber RA, Barker CC, Roberts EA et al. Canadian Pediatric Hepatology Research Group. Biliary atresia: the Canadian experience. J Pediatr 2007; 151:659–65.

3. Douglas AH. Case of dilatation of the common bile duct. Monthly J M Sci 1952; 14:97–101.

4. Suda K, Miyano T, Suzuki F et al. Clinicopathologic and experimental studies on cases of abnormal pancreatico-choledocho-ductal junction. Acta Pathol Jpn 1987; 37:1549–62.

5. Kim SH, Lim JH, Yoon HK et al. Choledochal cyst: comparison of MR and conventional cholangiography. Clin Radiol 2000; 55:378–83.

6. Todani T, Watanabe Y, Narusue M et al. Congenital bile duct cysts: classification, operative procedures, and review of thirty-seven cases including cancer arising from choledochal cyst. Am J Surg 1977; 134:263–9.

7. Lenriot JP, Gigot JF, Segol P et al. Bile duct cysts in adults: a multi-institutional retrospective study. French Associations for Surgical Research. Ann Surg 1998; 228:159–66.

8. Todani T, Watanabe Y, Toki A et al. Carcinoma related choledochal cysts with internal drainage operations. Surg Gynecol Obstet 1987; 164:61–4.

9. Voyles CR, Smadja C, Shands WC et al. Carcinoma in choledochal cysts. Age-related incidence. Arch Surg 1983; 118:986–8.

10. Nakayama H, Masuda H, Ugajin W et al. Left hepatic lobectomy for type IV-A choledochal cyst. Am Surg 2000; 66:1020–2.

11. Ulrich F, Pratschke J, Pascher A et al. Long-term outcome of liver resection and transplantation for Caroli disease and syndrome. Ann Surg 2008; 247:357–64.

12. Narasimhan KL, Chowdhary SK, Rao KL. Management of accessory hepatic ducts in choledochal cysts. J Pediatr Surg 2001; 36:1092–3.

13. Morgenstern L, McGrath MF, Carroll BJ et al. Continuing hazards of the learning curve in laparoscopic cholecystectomy. Am Surg 1995; 61:914–18.

14. Flum DR, Dellinger EP, Cheadle A et al. Intraoperative cholangiography and risk of common bile duct injury during cholecystectomy. JAMA 2003; 289:1691–2.

    A retrospective analysis of more than 1.5 million cholecystectomies detailing the risk of injury and the decreased risk if operative cholangiography is used.

15. Richardson MC, Bell G, Fullarton GM and the West of Scotland Laparoscopic Cholecystectomy Audit Group. Incidence and nature of bile duct injuries following laparoscopic cholecystectomy: an audit of 5913 cases. Br J Surg 1996; 83:1356–60.

A prospective audit of biliary injury following cholecystectomy in Scotland. One of the first studies to record the rate of biliary injury and the more severe nature of the injuries at laparoscopic surgery.

16. Waage A, Nilsson M. Iatrogenic bile duct injury: a population-based study of 152 776 cholecystectomies in the Swedish Inpatient Registry. Arch Surg 2006; 141:1207–13.

Population-based study in Sweden of 152 776 cholecystectomies with 613 (0.40%) requiring biliary reconstruction.

17. Moore MJ, Bennett CL. The learning curve for laparoscopic cholecystectomy. The Southern Surgeon's Club. Am J Surg 1995; 170:55–9.

18. Strasberg SM, Hertl M, Soper NJ. An analysis of the problem of biliary injury during laparoscopic cholecystectomy. J Am Coll Surg 1995; 180:102–25.

This paper describes a very useful classification system for biliary injury that includes the Bismuth classification as well as other less major injuries.

19. Fletcher DR, Hobbs MS, Tan P et al. Complications of cholecystectomy: risks of the laparoscopic approach and protective effects of operative cholangiography: a population-based study. Ann Surg 1999; 229:449–57.

A retrospective audit of biliary injury in Western Australia that identified the increased risk of biliary injury after laparoscopic cholecystectomy compared to open cholecystectomy. This study also identified a significantly reduced risk of injury if operative cholangiography was performed.

20. Thomson BN, Parks RW, Madhavan KK et al. Early specialist repair of biliary injury. Br J Surg 2006; 93:216–20.

21. Strasberg SM. Avoidance of biliary injury during laparoscopic cholecystectomy. J Hepatobil Pancreat Surg 2002; 9:543–7.

22. Way LW, Stewart L, Gantert W et al. Causes and prevention of laparoscopic bile duct injuries: analysis of 252 cases from a human factors and cognitive psychology perspective. Ann Surg 2003; 237:460–9.

Analysis of 252 bile duct injuries according to the principles of the cognitive science of visual perception judgement and human error showing that the majority of errors result from misperception, not errors of skill, knowledge or judgement.

23. Couinaud C. Le Foi. Etudes anatomigues et chirurgicales. Paris: Masson, 1957.

24. Flum DR, Flowers C, Veenstra DL. A cost-effectiveness analysis of intra-operative cholangiography in the prevention of bile duct injury during laparoscopic cholecystectomy. J Am Coll Surg 2003; 196:385–93.

25. Thomson BNJ, Cullinan MJ, Banting SW et al. Recognition and management of biliary complications after laparoscopic cholecystectomy. Aust NZ J Surg 2003; 73:183–8.

26. Slater K, Strong RW, Wall DR et al. Iatrogenic bile duct injury: the scourge of laparoscopic cholecystectomy. Aust NZ J Surg 2002; 72:83–8.

27. Mahmud S, Masuad M, Canna K et al. Fundus-first laparoscopic cholecystectomy. Surg Endosc 2002; 16:581–4.

28. Philips JA, Lawes DA, Cook AJ et al. The use of laparoscopic subtotal cholecystectomy for complicated cholelithiasis. Surg Endosc 2007 (Epub ahead of print).

29. Chapman WC, Halevy A, Blumgart LH et al. Postcholecystectomy bile duct strictures. Arch Surg 1995; 130:597–604.

30. Bismuth H. Postoperative strictures of the bile duct. In: Blumgart LH (ed.) The biliary tract. Clinical surgery international. Edinburgh: Churchill Livingstone, 1982; pp. 209–18.

31. Thomson BN, Parks RW, Madhavan KK et al. Liver resection and transplantation in the management of iatrogenic biliary injury. World J Surg 2007; 31:2363–9.

32. Mirza DF, Narsimhan KL, Ferras Neto BH et al. Bile duct injury following laparoscopic cholecystectomy: referral pattern and management. Br J Surg 1997; 84:786–90.

33. Johnson SR, Koehler A, Pennington LK et al. Long-term results of surgical repair of bile duct injuries following laparoscopic cholecystectomy. Surgery 2000; 128:668–77.

34. Carroll BJ, Birth M, Phillips EH. Common bile duct injuries during laparoscopic cholecystectomy that result in litigation. Surg Endosc 1998; 12:310–13.

35. Stewart L, Way LW. Bile duct injuries during laparoscopic cholecystectomy: factors that influence the results of treatment. Arch Surg 1995; 130:1123–9.

36. de Reuver PR, Busch OR, Rauws EA et al. Long-term results of a primary end-to-end anastomosis in peroperative detected bile duct injury. J Gastrointest Surg 2007; 11:296–302.

37. de Reuver PR, Rauws EA, Vermeulen M et al. Endoscopic treatment of post-surgical bile duct injuries: long term outcome and predictors of success. Gut 2007; 56:1599–605.

38. Sandha GS, Bourke MJ, Haber GB et al. Endoscopic therapy for bile leak based on a new classification: results in 207 patients. Gastrointest Endosc 2004; 60:567–74.

39. Buell JF, Cronin DC, Funakii B. Devastating and fatal complications associated with combined vascular and bile duct injuries during cholecystectomy. Arch Surg 2002; 137:703–8.

40. Schmidt SC, Settmacher U, Langrehr JM et al. Management and outcome of patients with combined bile duct and hepatic arterial injuries after laparoscopic cholecystectomy. Surgery 2004; 135:613–18.

41. Li J, Frilling A, Nadalin S et al. Management of concomitant hepatic artery injury in patients with

iatrogenic major bile duct injury after laparoscopic cholecystectomy. Br J Surg 2008; 95:460–5.

42. Alves A, Farges O, Nicolet J et al. Incidence and consequence of an hepatic artery injury in patients with postcholecystectomy bile duct strictures. Ann Surg 2003; 238:93–6.

43. Mercado MA, Chan C, Orozco H et al. Acute bile duct injury. The need for a high repair. Surg Endosc 2003; 17:1351–5.

44. Moraca RJ, Lee FT, Ryan JA et al. Long-term biliary function after reconstruction of major bile duct injuries with hepaticoduodenostomy or hepaticojejunostomy. Arch Surg 2002; 137:889–93.

45. Bettschart V, Clayton RA, Parks RW et al. Cholangiocarcinoma arising after biliary-enteric drainage procedures for benign disease. Gut 2002; 51:128–9.

46. Al-Ghnaniem R, Benjamin IS. Long-term outcome of hepaticojejunostomy with routine access loop formation following iatrogenic bile duct injury. Br J Surg 2002; 89:1118–24.

47. Nordin A, Halme L, Makisalo H et al. Management and outcome of major bile duct injuries after laparoscopic cholecystectomy: from therapeutic endoscopy to liver transplantation. Liver Transpl 2002; 8:1036–43.

48. Flum DR, Cheadle A, Prela C et al. Bile duct injury during cholecystectomy and survival in medicare beneficiaries. JAMA 2003; 290:2168–74.

A retrospective analysis of survival following bile duct injury among Medicare beneficiaries in the USA. This study demonstrates the increased hazard ratio of death following injury in comparison to a control group of routine cholecystectomy patients.

49. Huang CS, Lien HH, Tai FC et al. Long-term results of major bile duct injury associated with laparoscopic cholecystectomy. Surg Endosc 2003; 17:1362–7.

50. Boerma D, Rauws EA, Keulemans YC et al. Impaired quality of life 5 years after bile duct injury during laparoscopic cholecystectomy: a propsective analysis. Ann Surg 2001; 234:750–7.

A prospective analysis of quality of life that demonstrated a poor outcome at 5 years, despite successful repair.

51. Melton GB, Lillemoe KD, Cameron JL et al. Major bile duct injuries associated with laparoscopic cholecystectomy: effect of surgical repair on quality of life. Ann Surg 2002; 235:888–95.

A study of the impact of biliary injury on quality of life that demonstrated a significantly worse psychological domain, especially in those pursuing legal action.

52. Mirizzi PL. Sindrome del conducto hepatico. J Int Chir 1948; 8:731–77.

53. Johnson LW, Sehon JK, Lee WC et al. Mirizzi's syndrome: experience from a multi-institutional review. Am Surg 2001; 67:11–14.

54. Garden OJ, Paterson-Brown S. The gallbladder and bile ducts. In: Garden OJ (ed.) Intraoperative and laparoscopic ultrasonography. Oxford: Blackwell Science, 1995; pp. 17–43.

55. Binnie NR, Nixon SJ, Palmer KR. Mirizzi syndrome managed by endoscopic stenting and laparoscopic cholecystectomy. Br J Surg 1992; 79:647.

56. Shah OJ, Dar MA, Wani MA et al. Management of Mirizzi syndrome: a new surgical approach. Aust NZ J Surg 2001; 71:423–7.

57. Schafer M, Schneiter R, Krahenbuhl L. Incidence and management of Mirizzi syndrome during laparoscopic cholecystectomy. Surg Endosc 2003; 17:1186–90.

58. Lo CM, Fan ST, Wong J. The changing epidemiology of recurrent pyogenic cholangitis. Hong Kong Med J 1997; 3:302–4.

59. Tabata M, Nakayama F. Bacteriology of hepatolithiasis. Prog Clin Biol Res 1984; 152:163–74.

60. Chen DW, Tung-Ping Poon R, Liu CL et al. Immediate and long-term outcomes of hepatectomy for hepatolithiasis. Surgery 2004; 135:386–93.

61. Fan ST, Lai ECS, Mok FPT et al. Acute cholangitis secondary to hepatolithiasis. Arch Surg 1991; 126:1027–31.

62. Uchiyama K, Kawai M, Ueno M et al. Reducing residual and recurrent stones by hepatectomy for hepatolithiasis. J Gastrointest Surg 2007; 11:626–30.

63. Belghiti J, Benhamou JP, Houry S et al. Caustic sclerosing cholangitis. A complication of the surgical treatment of hydatid disease of the liver. Arch Surg 1986; 121:1162–5.

64. Khuroo MS, Sarjar SA, Mahajan R. Hepatobiliary and pancreatic ascariasis in India. Lancet 1990; 335:1503–6.

65. Montefusco PP, Geiss AC, Bronzo RL et al. Sclerosing cholangitis, chronic pancreatitis, and Sjögren's syndrome: a syndrome complex. Am J Surg 1984; 147:822–6.

66. Chapman RW, Kelly PM, Heryet A et al. Expression of HLA-DR antigens on bile duct epithelium in primary sclerosing cholangitis. Gut 1988; 29:422–7.

67. Duerr RH, Targan SR, Labders CJ et al. Neutrophil cytoplasmic antibodies: a link between primary sclerosing cholangitis and ulcerative colitis. Gastroenterology 1991; 100:1385–91.

68. Tischendorf JJ, Hecker H, Krüger M et al. Characterization, outcome, and prognosis in 273 patients with primary sclerosing cholangitis: a single center study. Am J Gastroenterol 2007; 102:107–14.

69. Beuers U, Spengler U, Kruis W et al. Ursodeoxycholic acid for treatment of primary sclerosing cholangitis: a placebo-controlled trial. Hepatology 1992; 16:707–14.

A prospective randomised double-blind trial that demonstrated the efficacy of ursodeoxycholic acid in the treatment of primary sclerosing cholangitis.

70. Wagner S, Gebel M, Meier P et al. Endoscopic management of biliary tract strictures in primary sclerosing cholangitis. Endoscopy 1996; 28:576–7.

71. Kaya M, Petersen BT, Angulo P et al. Balloon dilation compared to stenting of dominant strictures in primary sclerosing cholangitis. Am J Gastroenterol 2001; 96:1059–66.

72. Lemmer ER, Borman PC, Krige JE et al. Primary sclerosing cholangitis. Requiem for biliary drainage operations? Arch Surg 1994; 129:723–8.

73. Roberts MS, Angus DC, Bryce CL et al. Survival after liver transplantation in the United States: a disease-specific analysis of the UNOS database. Liver Transpl 2004; 10:886–97.

74. Nashan B, Schlitt HJ, Tusch G et al. Biliary malignancies in primary sclerosing cholangitis: timing for liver transplantation. Hepatology 1996; 23:1105–11.

75. Chalasani N, Baluyut A, Ismail A et al. Cholangiocarcinoma in patients with primary sclerosing cholangitis: a multicenter case-control study. Hepatology 2000; 31:247–8.

76. Glassbrenner B, Ardan M, Boeck W et al. Prospective evaluation of brush cytology of biliary strictures during endoscopic retrograde cholangiopancreatography. Endoscopy 1999; 31:758–60.

77. Prytz H, Keiding S, Björnsson E et al. Dynamic FDG-PET is useful for detection of cholangiocarcinoma in patients with PSC listed for liver transplantation. Hepatology 2006; 44:1572–80.

78. Weber SM, DeMatteo RP, Fong Y et al. Staging laparoscopy in patients with extrahepatic biliary carcinoma. Analysis of 100 patients. Ann Surg 2002; 235:392–9.

79. Powell JJ, Parks RW, Pleass H et al. Whipple's resection of non-neoplastic pathology in patients with presumed malignancy. Br J Surg 2003; 90:49.

80. Uhlmann D, Wiedmann M, Schmidt F et al. Management and outcome in patients with Klatskin-mimicking lesions of the biliary tree. J Gastrointest Surg 2006; 10:1144–50.

81. Saint-Paul MC, Hastier P, Baldini E et al. Inflammatory pseudotumor of the intrahepatic biliary tract. Gastroenterol Clin Biol 1999; 23:581–4.

82. Weber SM, Cubukcu-Dimopulo O, Palesty JA et al. Lymphoplasmacytic sclerosing pancreatitis: inflammatory mimic of pancreatic carcinoma. J Gastrointest Surg 2003; 7:129–37.

83. Church NI, Pereira SP, Deheragoda MG et al. Autoimmune pancreatitis: clinical and radiological features and objective response to steroid therapy in a UK series. Am J Gastroenterol 2007; 102:2417–25.

84. Keaveny AP, Karasik MS. Hepatobiliary and pancreatic infections in AIDS: Part II. AIDS Patient Care STDs 1998; 12:451–6.

85. Ducreux M, Buffet C, Lamy P et al. Diagnosis and prognosis of AIDS-related cholangitis. AIDS 1995; 9:875–80.

86. Corazziari E. Sphincter of Oddi dysfunction. Dig Liver Dis 2003; 35:S26–9.

87. Geenen JE, Hogan WJ, Dodds WJ et al. The efficacy of endoscopic sphincterotomy after cholecystectomy in patients with sphincter of Oddi dysfunction. N Engl J Med 1989; 320:82–7.

88. Lehman GY, Sherman S. Sphincter of Oddi dysfunction. Int J Pancreatol 1996; 20:11–25.

89. Freeman ML, Gill M, Overby C et al. Predictors of outcomes after biliary and pancreatic sphincterotomy for sphincter of oddi dysfunction. J Clin Gastroenterol 2007; 41:94–102.

12

Malignant lesions of the biliary tract

Shishir K. Maithel
William R. Jarnagin

Introduction

Malignant lesions of the biliary tract, specifically arising from the gallbladder or biliary epithelium, are rare and only account for approximately 15% of hepatobiliary neoplasms. Gallbladder cancer is the most common site, accounting for 60% of all biliary tract cancers, while the remaining 40% are distributed throughout the extrahepatic and intrahepatic biliary tree, with the next most common site occurring at the extrahepatic biliary confluence.[1] Complete resection is associated with the best survival and is the most effective therapy, but is usually only possible in a minority of patients. Palliating the effects of biliary obstruction is thus often the primary therapeutic goal. Chemotherapy and radiation therapy have not been proven to reduce the incidence of recurrence after resection nor to improve survival. Unfortunately, due to the rarity of these tumours and their frequently advanced stage at presentation, randomised prospective trials assessing different treatment regimens have not been performed but management recommendations will be made based on available evidence.

Cholangiocarcinoma

General considerations

Epidemiology

Cholangiocarcinoma is an uncommon cancer with an incidence of 1–2 per 100 000 in the USA and approximately 5000 new cases diagnosed each year.[2] Overall, men are affected 1.5 times as much as women and the majority of patients are greater than 65 years of age, with the peak incidence occurring in the eighth decade.[2] Tumours are classified according to their site of origin within the biliary tree, with those involving the biliary confluence, or hilar cholangiocarcinoma, being the most common and accounting for approximately 60% of all cases.[3–6] Twenty to thirty percent originate in the distal bile duct, while approximately 10% arise within the intrahepatic biliary tree.[7–9] Rarely, patients will present with multifocal or diffuse involvement of the biliary tree.[10] These proportions are based on older data, however, and more recent studies have documented a marked increase in incidence of intrahepatic cholangiocarcinoma.[11–14]

Natural history

Most patients with unresectable bile duct cancer die within 6 months to a year of diagnosis, usually from liver failure or infectious complications secondary to biliary obstruction.[3,15–17] The prognosis is often worse for hilar lesions and better for lesions of the distal bile duct, which probably reflects the greater complexity and difficulty in effectively managing proximal lesions more so than differences in tumour biology. Indeed, it has been shown that location within the biliary tree (proximal versus distal) has no impact on survival provided that complete resection is performed.[4] However, patients with intrahepatic cholangiocarcinoma often present with advanced lesions due to the absence of symptoms, such as jaundice or biliary tract-related sepsis.

Aetiology

Most cases of cholangiocarcinoma in the West are sporadic and have no obvious risk factors. Certain conditions are associated with an increased incidence, the most common of which is primary sclerosing cholangitis (PSC). The majority of patients (70–80%) with PSC have associated ulcerative colitis while a minority with ulcerative colitis develop PSC.[18] The natural history of PSC is variable, and the true incidence of cholangiocarcinoma is unknown. In a Swedish series of 305 patients followed for several years, 8% of patients eventually developed cancer. However, occult cholangiocarcinoma has been reported in up to 40% of autopsy specimens and in up to 36% of liver explants from patients with PSC.[18,19] Patients with cholangiocarcinoma associated with PSC are often not candidates for resection because of multifocal disease or severe underlying hepatic dysfunction.

Congenital biliary cystic disease (i.e. choledochal cysts) is also associated with an increased risk for the development of biliary tract cancer.[20,21] This appears to be related to the finding of an abnormal choledocho-pancreatic duct junction, which predisposes to reflux of pancreatic secretions into the biliary tree, chronic inflammation and bacterial contamination.[21–24] A similar mechanism may also explain the increased incidence of cholangiocarcinoma reported in patients subjected to transduodenal sphincteroplasty or endoscopic sphincterotomy. In 119 patients subjected to this procedure for benign conditions, Hakamada et al. found a 7.4% incidence of cholangiocarcinoma over 18 years.[25]

Hepatolithiasis is a well-known risk factor for the development of cholangiocarcinoma in Japan and parts of South-East Asia, arising in 10% of those affected. Chronic portal bacteraemia and portal phlebitis lead to intrahepatic pigment stone formation, obstruction of intrahepatic ducts, and recurrent episodes of cholangitis and stricture formation.[26,27] This recurrent inflammatory state is likely the main contributing factor to cholangiocarcinogenesis. Biliary parasites (*Clonorchis sinensis, Opisthorchis viverrini*) are also endemic in parts of Asia, such as Thailand, and are similarly associated with an increased risk of cholangiocarcinoma.[19] Finally, exposure to several radionuclides and chemical carcinogens, such as thorium, radon, nitrosamines, dioxin and asbestos, may also increase the risk of cholangiocarcinoma.

Histopathology

Three macroscopic subtypes of extrahepatic cholangiocarcinoma are described: sclerosing, nodular and papillary, of which the first two are often combined into one (i.e. nodular-sclerosing) since features of both types are often seen together.[28] The histopathology

is distinct between cholangiocarcinomas arising from the extrahepatic and intrahepatic biliary system. For extrahepatic cholangiocarcinoma, the overwhelming majority are adenocarcinomas, and most are firm, sclerotic tumours with a paucity of cellular components within a dense fibrotic, desmoplastic background. As a consequence, a non-diagnostic preoperative biopsy is not uncommon.[2,28,29] Papillary tumours represent a less common morphologic variant, accounting for approximately 10% of tumours arising from the extrahepatic biliary tree.[28] Papillary tumours are soft and friable, may be associated with little transmural invasion and are characterised by a mass that expands rather than contracts the duct (**Fig. 12.1**). Although papillary tumours may grow to significant size, they often arise from a well-defined stalk, with the bulk of the tumour mobile within the ductal lumen. Despite this histological variant being the minority of cases, recognition of this entity is important since they are more often resectable and have a more favourable prognosis than the other types.[19,30]

 The prognosis related to papillary bile duct tumours is related to the extent of the invasive component. Tumours with ≤10% invasive cancer have a much more favourable outcome after resection, while those with >10% behave similarly to the more common nodular-sclerosing lesions.

Hilar cholangiocarcinoma is typically highly invasive within the hepatoduodenal ligament. Direct invasion of the liver or perihepatic structures, such as the portal vein or hepatic artery, is a common feature and has important clinical implications regarding resectability.[28] The liver is also a common site of metastatic disease, as are the regional lymph node basins, but spread to distant extra-abdominal sites is uncommon at initial presentation.[3,31] These tumours also have a propensity for longitudinal spread along the duct wall and periductal tissues, which is an important pathological feature as it pertains to the margin of resection.[28] There may be substantial extension of tumour beneath an intact epithelial lining, as much as 2 cm proximally and 1 cm distally, thus predisposing to a radiographic underestimation of tumour extent.[32] This predilection for submucosal extension underscores the difficulty in achieving a complete resection. Frozen section analysis of the duct margin during operation may be helpful in this regard but caution must be used when interpreting the results. In our experience with intraoperative frozen sections, we found a substantial false-negative rate and the benefits of extending the resection with a positive frozen section result were questionable.[33]

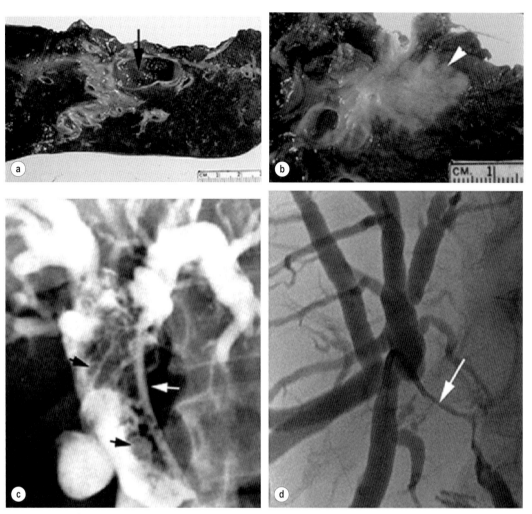

Figure 12.1 • Gross and cholangiographic appearance of a papillary cholangiocarcinoma **(a,c)** and a nodular-sclerosing tumour **(b,d)**. In **(a)** and **(c)**, note that the papillary tumour occupies the lumen and expands the duct (black arrow). A biliary stent is visualised (white arrow). In **(b)** and **(d)**, the nodular-sclerosing variant constricts the lumen, nearly obliterating it (white arrow). Reprinted with permission from Blumgart LH (ed.) Surgery of the liver, biliary tract, and pancreas, 4th edn. Saunders, 2007.

 A frozen section evaluation of the bile duct margins may help guide the extent of resection but caution should be used when interpreting the results.

Gross examination of intrahepatic cholangiocarcinoma reveals a grey scirrhous mass, often infiltrative into the liver parenchyma.[34] These tumours are adenocarcinomas and the diagnosis of intrahepatic or peripheral cholangiocarcinoma should be considered in all patients presenting with a presumptive diagnosis of metastatic adenocarcinoma with an unknown primary, particularly in the setting of a large, solitary hepatic mass. A small number show different patterns with focal areas of papillary carcinoma with mucous production, signet ring cells, squamous cell, mucoepidermoid and spindle cell variants.[35] The Liver Cancer Study Group of Japan established a subclassification of these tumours based on morphology: mass-forming, periductal-infiltrating and intraductal growth types.[36] Although some studies have suggested a correlation with outcome based on morphological subtype, this classification scheme has not gained wide acceptance. Positive immunohistochemical staining usually includes carcinoembryonic antigen (CEA), tumour markers CA50 and CA19-9. K-ras mutations have also been detected in 70% of intrahepatic cholangiocarcinomas.[37,38] Metastatic disease at the time of exploration is not an infrequent finding. Tumours with both hepatocellular and cholangiocellular differentiation (combined tumours) are rare but well described, and their clinical behaviour more closely approximates that of cholangiocarcinoma rather than hepatocellular carcinoma.[39]

Cholangiocarcinoma involving the proximal bile ducts (hilar cholangiocarcinoma)

Clinical presentation and diagnosis

The early symptoms of hilar cholangiocarcinoma are often non-specific, with abdominal pain, discomfort, anorexia, weight loss and/or pruritus seen in about one-third of patients.[6,19,40,41] Most patients present with jaundice or incidentally discovered abnormal liver function tests. Pruritus may precede jaundice by some weeks, and this symptom should prompt an evaluation, especially if associated with abnormal liver function tests. Patients with papillary tumours of the hilus may give a history of intermittent jaundice, perhaps due to the ball-valve effect of a pedunculated mass within the lumen or, more likely, small fragments of tumour having passed into the common bile duct. Physical exam findings are often non-specific but may provide some useful information. Jaundice is usually obvious, and patients with pruritus often have multiple excoriations of the skin. The liver may be enlarged and firm as a result of biliary tract obstruction. The gallbladder is usually decompressed and non-palpable with hilar obstruction. Rarely, patients with longstanding biliary obstruction and/or portal vein involvement may have findings consistent with portal hypertension.

In patients with no previous biliary intervention, cholangitis is rare at initial presentation, despite a 30% incidence of bacterial contamination.[42,43] Endoscopic or percutaneous instrumentation increases significantly the incidence of bacterial contamination and the subsequent risk of clinical infection. The incidence of bacterobilia approaches 100% after endoscopic biliary intubation, thus making cholangitis more common.[43] Bacterial contamination of the biliary tract in partial obstruction is not always clinically apparent. The presence of overt or subclinical infection at the time of surgery is a major source of postoperative morbidity and mortality. Thus, endoscopic and percutaneous intubations are both associated with greater morbidity and mortality following surgical resection or palliative bypass for hilar cholangiocarcinoma. In an analysis of 71 patients who underwent either resection or palliative biliary bypass for proximal cholangiocarcinoma, all patients stented endoscopically and 62% of those stented percutaneously had bactibilia. Postoperative infectious complications were doubly increased in patients stented before operation compared to non-stented patients, while non-infectious complications were equal in both groups.[43] *Enterococcus, Klebsiella, Escherichia coli, Streptococcus viridans* and *Enterobacter aerogenes* are the most common organisms, and this spectrum of bacteria must be considered when administrating perioperative antibiotics; it is imperative to take intraoperative bile specimens for culture in order to guide selection of postoperative antibiotic therapy.

While gallstones or even common bile duct stones may coexist with bile duct cancer, in the absence of certain predisposing conditions (e.g. primary sclerosing cholangitis, Oriental cholangiohepatitis), it is uncommon for choledocholithiasis to cause obstruction at the biliary confluence. Furthermore, the degree of bilirubin elevation tends to be higher for malignant obstruction compared to benign stone disease. Other conditions may mimic hilar cholangiocarcinoma on imaging studies such as benign idiopathic focal stenosis of the hepatic ducts (malignant masquerade), Mirizzi's syndrome resulting from a large stone impacted in the neck of the gallbladder, and gallbladder cancer.[44] Nevertheless, it is imperative to fully investigate and delineate the level and nature of any obstructing lesion causing jaundice to avoid missing the diagnosis of carcinoma.

However, the histopathological diagnosis of hilar cholangiocarcinoma is often not made until the specimen is removed at operation since non-diagnostic preoperative biopsies or brushings are the norm. In the authors' view, histological confirmation of malignancy is not mandatory prior to exploration. With no prior suggestive history (i.e. prior biliary tract operation, PSC, hepatolithiasis), the finding of a focal stenotic lesion combined with the appropriate clinical presentation are sufficient for a presumptive diagnosis of hilar cholangiocarcinoma, which is correct in most instances.[45] Furthermore, the alternative conditions are often best assessed and treated at operation. Reliance on negative preoperative biopsy or cytology is dangerous, particularly in the face of compelling radiographic evidence of malignant disease.[46] Once a diagnosis of cholangiocarcinoma is suggested, radiographic studies are crucial to determine the extent of the tumour to appropriately design a therapeutic plan.

One should not rely on preoperative biopsies or intraluminal brushings to make a diagnosis of cholangiocarcinoma, as these are not always reliable, and negative results may delay significantly appropriate treatment.

Radiographic studies

High-quality radiographic studies are necessary to select accurately patients for resection. Until recently, computed tomography (CT), percutaneous transhepatic cholangiography (PTC) and angiography were considered standard investigations. With improvement in the quality of non-invasive modalities, the authors' current practice relies almost exclusively on magnetic resonance cholangiopancreatography (MRCP) and duplex ultrasonography (US) for preoperative assessment, which provide similar information with less risk to the patient.

Direct cholangiography

Cholangiography demonstrates the location of the tumour and the extent of biliary disease, both of which are critical in surgical planning. Although endoscopic retrograde cholangiography (ERC) may provide helpful information, PTC displays the intrahepatic bile ducts more reliably and has been the preferred approach. However, there is often a knee-jerk reflex to proceed with invasive cholangiography before a complete radiographic assessment has been made, which can lead to unnecessary patient morbidity and infectious complications.

Computed tomography

Cross-sectional imaging provided by CT remains an important study for evaluating patients with biliary obstruction by providing valuable information regarding the level of obstruction, vascular involvement and liver atrophy. As portal venous inflow and bile flow are important in the maintenance of liver cell size and mass, segmental or lobar atrophy may be evident on CT that would suggest portal venous occlusion or biliary obstruction.[47] CT angiography is helpful for assessing portal venous and hepatic arterial involvement. However, CT imaging tends to underestimate the proximal extent of tumour within the bile duct and is thus not ideal as the primary determinant of resectability.[48]

Duplex ultrasonography

Ultrasonography is a non-invasive but operator-dependent study that often delineates precisely the level of the tumour within the bile duct (**Fig. 12.2**), and can also provide information regarding tumour extension within the bile duct and in the periductal tissues.[49-51] In a series of 19 consecutive patients with malignant hilar obstruction, ultrasonography with colour spectral Doppler technique was equivalent to angiography and CT portography in diagnosing lobar atrophy, level of biliary obstruction, hepatic parenchymal involvement and venous invasion.[51] Duplex ultrasonography is particularly useful for assessing portal venous invasion. In a series of 63 consecutive patients from the Memorial Sloan-Kettering Cancer Center (MSKCC), duplex ultrasonography predicted portal vein involvement in 93% of the cases with a specificity of 99% and

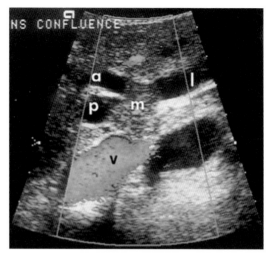

Figure 12.2 • Ultrasonographic view of a hilar cholangiocarcinoma showing a papillary tumour (m) extending into the right anterior (a) and posterior (p) sectoral ducts and the origin of the left duct (l). The adjacent portal vein (v) is not involved and has normal flow. Reprinted with permission from Blumgart LH (ed.) Surgery of the liver, biliary tract, and pancreas, 4th edn. Saunders, 2007.

a 97% positive predictive value. In the same series, angiography with CT angioportography had a 90% sensitivity, 99% specificity and a 95% positive predictive value.[52]

Magnetic resonance cholangiopancreatography (MRCP)

In the authors' practice, MRCP has largely replaced endoscopic and percutaneous studies. Several studies have demonstrated its utility in evaluating patients with biliary obstruction.[53-56] MRCP may not only identify the tumour and the level of biliary obstruction, but may also reveal obstructed and isolated ducts not appreciated at endoscopic or percutaneous study. By virtue of being an axial imaging modality, MRCP has further advantages over standard cholangiography by also providing information regarding the patency of hilar vascular structures, the presence of nodal or distant metastases, and the presence of lobar atrophy (**Fig. 12.3**). Furthermore, it is not associated with the same incidence of bactibilia and infectious complications as standard cholangiography.[43]

 Perform non-invasive imaging with MRCP, US and CT prior to proceeding with preoperative invasive cholangiography in order to avoid unnecessary interventions that may increase patient morbidity and infectious complications.

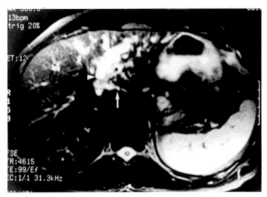

Figure 12.3 • Cross-sectional MRCP from a patient with hilar cholangiocarcinoma extending into the left hepatic duct and left lobe atrophy. The bile ducts appear white. The left lobe is small with dilated and crowded ducts (arrowhead). The principal caudate lobe duct, seen joining the left hepatic duct, is also dilated (arrow). Reprinted with permission from Blumgart LH (ed.) Surgery of the liver, biliary tract, and pancreas, 4th edn. Saunders, 2007.

Preoperative evaluation and assessment of resectability

Evaluation of patients with hilar cholangiocarcinoma is principally an assessment of resectability, since resection is the only effective therapy. First and foremost, the surgeon must assess the patient's general condition, fitness for operation and liver function, since a complete resection usually includes a partial hepatectomy. The presence of significant comorbid conditions, chronic liver disease and/or portal hypertension generally precludes resection. In these patients, biliary drainage is the most appropriate intervention, and the diagnosis should be confirmed histologically if chemotherapy or radiation therapy is planned.

The preoperative evaluation must address four critical determinants of resectability: extent of tumour within the biliary tree, vascular invasion, hepatic lobar atrophy and the presence of metastatic disease.[3] The presence of lobar atrophy is often overlooked; however, its importance in determining resectability cannot be overemphasised, since it implies portal venous involvement, suggests a more locally advanced lesion, and compels the surgeon to perform a partial hepatectomy, if the tumour is indeed resectable.[47] While longstanding biliary obstruction may cause moderate atrophy, concomitant portal venous compromise results in rapid and severe atrophy of the involved segments.

Appreciation of gross atrophy on preoperative imaging often influences both operative and non-operative therapy.[47] If the tumour is not resectable, percutaneous biliary drainage through an atrophic lobe should be avoided unless to control sepsis, since it will not reduce bilirubin levels. Atrophy is apparent on cross-sectional imaging as a small, often hypoperfused lobe with crowding of the dilated intrahepatic ducts (Fig. 12.3). Tumour involvement of the portal vein is usually present if there is compression/narrowing, encasement or occlusion seen on imaging studies.[3,57]

The staging systems currently used for hilar cholangiocarcinoma do not account fully for all tumour-related variables influencing resectability, namely biliary tumour extent, lobar atrophy and vascular involvement. The modified Bismuth–Corlette classification stratifies patients solely based on the extent of biliary duct involvement by tumour,[58] but it is not indicative of resectability or survival. Similarly, the current American Joint Committee on Cancer (AJCC) T-stage system is based largely on pathological criteria and has little applicability for preoperative staging. The ideal staging system should predict accurately resectability, the need for hepatic resection, and correlate with survival. Our preoperative staging system places the finding of portal venous involvement and lobar atrophy into the proper context for determining resectability,[3,57] especially when partial hepatectomy is an important component of the operative approach (Table 12.1). For example, a tumour with unilateral extension into second-order bile ducts that is associated with ipsilateral portal vein involvement and/or lobar atrophy would still be considered potentially resectable, while such involvement on the contralateral side would preclude a resection. This staging system correlates well

Table 12.1 • Proposed T-stage criteria for hilar cholangiocarcinoma

Stage	Criteria
T1	Tumour involving biliary confluence ± unilateral extension to second-order biliary radicles
T2	Tumour involving biliary confluence ± unilateral extension to second-order biliary radicles
	AND *ipsilateral* portal vein involvement ± *ipsilateral* hepatic lobar atrophy
T3	Tumour involving biliary confluence + bilateral extension to second-order biliary radicles
	OR unilateral extension to second-order biliary radicles with *contralateral* portal vein involvement
	OR unilateral extension to second-order biliary radicles with *contralateral* hepatic lobar atrophy
	OR main or bilateral portal venous involvement

Reprinted with permission from Jarnagin WR et al. Staging, resectability, and outcome in 225 patients with hilar cholangiocarcinoma. Ann Surg 2001; 234:507–19.

Table 12.2 • Resectability, incidence of metastatic disease, and survival stratified by T stage

T stage	n	Explored with curative intent	Resected	Negative margins	Hepatic resection	Portal vein resection	Metastatic disease	Median survival (months)
1	87	73 (84%)	51 (59%)	38	33	2	18 (21%)	20
2	95	79 (83%)	29 (31%)	24	29	7	40 (43%)	13
3	37	8 (22%)	0	0	0	0	15 (41%)	8
Total	219	160 (71%)	80 (37%)	62	62	9	73 (33%)	16

Reprinted with permission from Jarnagin WR et al. Staging, resectability, and outcome in 225 patients with hilar cholangiocarcinoma. Ann Surg 2001; 234:507–19.

with resectability, the likelihood of associated distant metastatic disease, and median survival (Table 12.2).[57] Independent confirmation of the utility of this classification scheme (the Blumgart clinical staging system) was recently reported in a series of 85 patients from China.[59] The authors' criteria for unresectability are detailed in Box 12.1.

 The current AJCC staging and Bismuth–Corlette classification systems are minimally helpful in guiding preoperative decision-making. A modified system (the Blumgart clinical staging system) reclassifies the T stage based on the extent of bile duct and portal vein involvement, as well as the presence or absence of lobar atrophy, which is highly correlated with tumour resectability and survival. This proposed system can aid with preoperative decision-making.

Treatment options

In patients with operable disease, the principal objective is complete resection, obtaining negative histological margins with subsequent restoration of biliary-enteric continuity. Complete resection is associated with 5-year survival rates of approximately 25–40%, which is far superior to that obtainable with non-operative therapies. Clearly, patient selection contributes largely to this finding, as patients treated non-operatively typically have more advanced disease, and no comparative trials have been performed equating stage for stage. Nevertheless, given the relatively poor response rates with chemotherapy and chemoradiation therapy, resection has emerged as the most effective treatment.

Orthotopic liver transplantation has been attempted for unresectable hilar tumours. Klempnauer et al. reported four long-term survivors out of 32 patients who underwent transplantation for hilar cholangiocarcinoma.[60] The same group also reported a 17.1%

Box 12.1 • Criteria of unresectability

Patient factors

Medically unfit or otherwise unable to tolerate a major operation

Hepatic cirrhosis

Local tumour-related factors

Tumour extension to secondary biliary radicles bilaterally

Encasement or occlusion of the main portal vein proximal to its bifurcation

Atrophy of one hepatic lobe with contralateral portal vein branch encasement or occlusion

Atrophy of one hepatic lobe with contralateral tumour extension to secondary biliary radicles

Unilateral tumour extension to secondary biliary radicles with contralateral portal vein branch encasement or occlusion

Metastatic disease

Histologicalally proven metastases to distant lymph node basins*

Lung, liver, or peritoneal metastases

*Includes peripancreatic, periduodenal, coeliac, superior mesenteric or posterior pancreatico-duodenal lymph nodes. Reprinted with permission from Jarnagin WR et al. Staging, resectability, and outcome in 225 patients with hilar cholangiocarcinoma. Ann Surg 2001; 234:507–19.

5-year survival for their overall transplant group.[61] Comparable results were reported by Iwatsuki et al.[62] The results of transplantation have previously not been sufficiently adequate to justify its use, and most centres now do not perform liver transplantation for cholangiocarcinoma. More recently, data from the Mayo Clinic has emerged suggesting good results with transplantation in highly selected patients with low-volume unresectable disease and combined with an intensive pre-transplant treatment regimen.[63,64] Although the data are compelling, this approach is applicable to a very small fraction of patients and remains experimental.

Resection

Resection is the most effective therapy for patients with potentially resectable tumours based on pre-operative imaging, with the primary objective being complete removal of all gross disease with clear histological margins. The importance of an R0 resection is clear from previous studies showing that incomplete (R1 or R2) resections do not improve survival beyond that of patients with unresectable tumours (**Fig. 12.4**).[3,57] There is now overwhelming evidence to support the fact that partial hepatectomy, combined with excision of the extrahepatic biliary system, is usually required to achieve this goal (Table 12.3). A review of several series in the literature shows a close correlation between the proportion of patients who underwent concomitant partial hepatectomy and the proportion of R0 resections achieved. For tumours extending into the left hepatic duct, en bloc caudate lobectomy is usually necessary to obtain a complete resection, since the principal biliary drainage of the caudate lobe is via the left hepatic duct.[65,66] A dilated caudate duct, suggesting tumour involvement, may occasionally be visualised on preoperative imaging (Fig. 12.3).

Despite improvements in preoperative imaging, a considerable number of patients are still found to have unresectable disease at the time of exploration. In a recent report from the MSKCC, this number approached 50% of patients with cholangiocarcinoma explored with curative intent.[30] In an effort to minimise the number of non-curative laparotomies performed, staging laparoscopy has been utilised. Two recent studies specifically analysing patients with biliary cancer have shown that laparoscopy can identify a large proportion of patients with unresectable disease primarily in the form

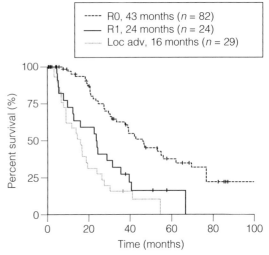

Figure 12.4 • Survival curves after resection of hilar cholangiocarcinoma. R0 indicates complete resection with histologically negative resection margins (median survival 43 months). R1 indicates histologically involved resection margins (median survival 24 months; $P < 0.001$, R0 versus R1). Loc Adv indicates patients explored, but found to have unresectable tumours owing to local invasion (no metastatic disease; median survival 16 months; $P < 0.19$, R1 versus Loc Adv). Reprinted with permission from Blumgart LH (ed.) Surgery of the liver, biliary tract, and pancreas, 4th edn. Saunders, 2007.

of radiographically occult metastases, the yield of which is greatest in locally advanced tumours.[67,68] Weber et al. evaluated 56 patients with potentially resectable hilar cholangiocarcinomas; 33 were ultimately determined to have unresectable disease, of which 14 (42%) were identified at laparoscopy and spared an unnecessary laparotomy. Additionally, recent reports have suggested a potential role for fluorodeoxyglucose positron emission tomography (FDG-PET) scanning as a means of identifying occult

Table 12.3 • Summary of selected studies showing the relationship between the rate of partial hepatectomy and proportion of negative histological margins achieved

Author	Complete gross resection (n)	Partial hepatectomy (%)	Negative margin (%)
Tsao (2000)	25	16	28
Cameron (1990)	39	20	15
Gerhards (2000)	112	29	14
Hadjis (1990)	27	60	56
Jarnagin (2001)	80	78	78
Klempnauer (1997)	147	79	79
Neuhaus (2000)	95	85	61
Nimura (1990)	55	98	83

metastatic disease; however, most of these studies include small numbers of patients, and further evaluation is needed before PET can be recommended routinely.[69–71] In our experience with FDG-PET for all biliary tract cancer, the information provided influenced management in 24% of patients.[72]

To achieve an R0 resection, a concomitant partial hepatectomy is almost always necessary due to tumour extension into second-order biliary radicles or ipsilateral portal vein involvement. A caudate lobe resection in particular is often necessary, especially for left-sided tumours, in order to obtain negative margins. Staging laparoscopy should be liberally utilised prior to open exploration in an effort to minimise the number of non-curative laparotomies performed.

Technical aspects of intraoperative tumour assessment, exposure and resection are outside the scope of this chapter. The reader is referred to specialty texts for a detailed description of surgical techniques.[73] The authors' general approach involves the liberal use of staging laparoscopy, followed by a full exploration of the abdomen and pelvis, including intraoperative ultrasonography. Resection of the tumour involves, at a minimum, removal of the entire extrahepatic biliary apparatus from just above the pancreas distally to beyond the biliary confluence with a complete porta hepatis lymphadenectomy. En bloc partial hepatectomy is required in nearly every case in order to achieve complete tumour clearance. Tumour involvement of the main portal vein proximal to its bifurcation additionally requires a vascular resection and reconstruction if technically feasible.

The extent of lymphadenectomy that should be performed remains an area of controversy. Some surgeons advocate an extended nodal dissection as some studies have demonstrated measurable 5-year actuarial survival in the presence of metastatic disease to distant nodal basins (e.g. para-aortic).[74,75] However, an analysis of studies specifically reporting 5-year survival in patients would suggest that any nodal involvement is a powerful adverse factor and that very few patients benefit from such an aggressive approach (Table 12.4). Thus, while a complete porta hepatis lymphadenectomy should be routinely performed when attempting complete resection, the authors do not advocate an extended lymph node dissection.

Results of resection

Long-term survival after resection of hilar cholangiocarcinoma can be achieved and has improved over recent years.[3,4,6,65,76,77] It is clear, however, that the results of resection depend critically on the status of the resection margins. We believe that increased use of hepatic resection is responsible for the increase in the percentage of R0 resections (negative histological margins) and the observed improvement in survival after resection. These observations have been emphasised by a reported series of 269 patients accumulated over a 20-year interval.[78] A more recent study from the MSKCC in 106 consecutive patients showed a median survival of 43 months in patients following R0 resection compared to 24 months in those with involved resection margins.[30] Multivariate analysis showed that an R0 resection, a concomitant hepatic resection, well-differentiated histology and papillary tumour phenotype were independent predictors of long-term survival.

Adjuvant therapy

The rarity of cholangiocarcinoma has prevented any meaningful clinical trials evaluating the use of adjuvant therapy. Several small, single-centre studies have attempted to investigate the benefit of

Table 12.4 • Summary of selected series showing proportion of number of patients surviving 5 years after resection of hilar cholangiocarcinoma with metastatic disease to regional lymph nodes

Author	Resections (*n*)	Node positive (%)	Five-year survivors with positive nodes (*n*)
Sugiura (1994)	83	51	3
Klempnauer (1997)	151	29	2
Nakeeb (1996)	109	–	0
Ogura (1998)	66	52	0
Iwatsuki (1998)	72	35	0
Kosuge (1999)	65	46	4
Jarnagin (2001)	80	24	3
Kitagawa (2001)	110	53	5
Total	802	–	17 (2.1%)

postoperative adjuvant chemo-radiation therapy. Two studies from Johns Hopkins suggested no benefit of adjuvant external beam or intraluminal radiation therapy.[79,80] In contrast, Kamada et al. suggested that radiation may improve survival in patients with histologically positive hepatic duct margins.[81] In a small study of five patients, resectability was reportedly greater in patients given neoadjuvant radiation therapy prior to exploration.[82] However, none of these studies was randomised and most consist of a small, heterogeneous group of patients.

The only phase III trial investigating adjuvant chemotherapy, which used mitomycin/5-fluorouracil (5-FU), included 508 patients with resected bile duct tumours ($n = 139$), gallbladder cancers ($n = 140$), pancreatic cancers ($n = 173$) and ampullary tumours ($n = 56$).[83] On subset analysis, there were no significant differences in overall or disease-free survival for bile duct tumours. As with radiation therapy, there are no data to support the routine use of chemotherapy in the adjuvant setting, until newer agents, such as oxaliplatin, are tested in a randomised controlled fashion.

Adjuvant chemotherapy or radiation therapy has not been shown to prolong survival beyond that of complete surgical resection alone for hilar cholangiocarcinoma. Large prospective randomised controlled trials have not been performed. However, patients at high risk for recurrence (i.e. node positive, margin positive) may benefit from treatment, and the authors usually recommend consultation with a medical oncologist in such cases.

Palliation

All patients should be assessed properly for possible resection but unfortunately the majority are not candidates for resection. Management goals therefore include biliary decompression and/or supportive care. Given the associated morbidity and mortality, jaundice alone is not necessarily an indication for biliary decompression, the indications for which include intractable pruritus, recurrent cholangitis and the need for access for intraluminal radiotherapy. Such intervention may also allow recovery of hepatic parenchymal function in patients receiving chemotherapeutic agents. Supportive care alone is probably the best approach for elderly patients with significant comorbid conditions and in the absence of intractable pruritus. In patients who are found to be unresectable at operation, an operative biliary decompression can be performed and can be so constructed as to provide access to the biliary tree for postoperative irradiation.[3,84]

If the patient is deemed unresectable, the diagnosis should be confirmed by biopsy. Biliary decompression can be obtained either by a percutaneous transhepatic route or by endoscopic stent placement, although hilar tumours are more difficult to transverse endoscopically. Moreover, the failure rates and incidence of subsequent cholangitis associated with endoscopic decompression are high.[85] Thus, most are probably better palliated via a percutaneous approach.

Percutaneous biliary drainage

Although more difficult than in those with distal bile duct tumours, percutaneous transhepatic biliary drainage and placement of a self-expandable metallic endoprosthesis (Wallstent) can be performed successfully in most patients with hilar obstruction.[86–88] Frequently, hilar tumours involve all three major hilar ducts (left hepatic, right anterior sectoral hepatic and right posterior sectoral hepatic), and thus require several stents for adequate drainage.[89] Jaundice secondary to portal vein occlusion without intrahepatic biliary dilatation, however, is not correctable with biliary stents. In addition, the presence of lobar atrophy is an important factor and biliary decompression of an atrophic lobe does not usually provide much palliative benefit.

The median patency of metallic endoprostheses placed at the hilus is approximately 6 months and is less for similar distal bile duct stents.[90] Becker et al. reported 1-year patency rates of 46% and 89% for Wallstents placed at the hilus and the distal bile duct respectively, with 25% of patients requiring re-intervention.[86] This concurs with our findings of a mean patency of 6.1 months in 35 patients similarly palliated. The periprocedural mortality was 14% at 30 days and seven patients (24%) had documented stent occlusion requiring repeated intervention.[90]

Intrahepatic biliary-enteric bypass

Patients found to be unresectable at operation, particularly after the bile duct has been divided, may be candidates for intrahepatic biliary-enteric bypass. The segment III duct is usually the most accessible and is our preferred approach, but the right anterior or posterior sectoral hepatic ducts can also be used.[91] Segment III bypass provides excellent biliary drainage and is less prone to occlusion since the anastomosis can be placed remote from the tumour. The 1-year bypass patency can approach 80% without any perioperative deaths.[91] Decompression of only one-third of the functioning hepatic parenchyma is usually sufficient to relieve jaundice. Furthermore, provided that the undrained lobe has not been percutaneously drained or otherwise contaminated, communication between the right and left hepatic ducts is not necessary.[92] As discussed for stenting, bypass to an atrophic lobe or a lobe heavily involved with tumour is generally not effective.

Radiation therapy

Patients with locally unresectable tumours without evidence of widespread disease may be candidates for palliative radiation therapy. Typically, external beam radiation (EBRT) alone is used, although a combination of EBRT (5000–6000 cGy) and intra-luminal iridium-192 (2000 cGy) delivered percutaneously can be administered safely and may be more effective. However, there was no improved duration of survival compared to biliary decompression alone in a controlled study.[79,84,93,94] In a group of 12 patients treated with this regimen over a 3-year period at the MSKCC, the median survival was 14.5 months. Cholangitis and intermittent jaundice were relatively common but serious complications was uncommon and there were no treatment-related deaths.[84] Given the increased morbidity and minimal benefit associated with radiation therapy, it is clearly not indicated for most patients with unresectable hilar cholangiocarcinoma.

Photodynamic therapy

Ortner has recently evaluated the efficacy of photodynamic therapy in unresectable hilar cholangiocarcinoma and has reported a median survival of 439 days.[95,96] The technique involves direct illumination via cholangioscopy that activates a photosensitiser which results in tumour cell death. Ortner treated nine patients in this fashion who had failed endoscopic stenting. No mortality was reported for the procedure but there was a 25% mortality related to the initial endoscopic stenting. Their indication for biliary drainage or specific reasons for tumour unresectability were unclear, thus making it difficult to interpret the extended duration in survival with this palliative therapy. Two small further randomised studies have reported an improvement in duration of survival for patients with unresectable tumours treated with stenting and photodynamic therapy compared to stenting alone.[97,98]

Chemotherapy

In cases of advanced biliary tract cancers, palliative chemotherapy has been used to potentially improve quality of life, reduce symptoms and increase survival. In the only randomised study, 37 patients with advanced biliary tract cancers received chemotherapy (5-FU/leucovorin with or without etoposide) or best supportive care.[99] Short-term improvements in survival (6.5 vs 2.5 months) and quality of life, as measured by the EORTC QLQ-C30 instrument, were noted among the chemotherapy group.

Cholangiocarcinoma involving the distal bile duct

Tumours of the lower bile duct, namely the mid- and distal bile duct, are classified according to their anatomical location, although there may be considerable overlap. Mid-bile duct tumours arise between the upper border of the duodenum and the cystic duct (below the bile duct bifurcation), while distal bile duct tumours are those arising anywhere from the duodenum to the papilla of Vater.[5] Tumours of the distal bile duct may represent approximately 20–30% of all cholangiocarcinomas and 5–10% of all periampullary tumours.[6,101–103] True mid-duct tumours are distinctly uncommon, and thus Nakeeb et al. have proposed an alternative classification scheme that divides cholangiocarcinomas into intrahepatic, perihilar and distal subgroups, thereby eliminating the mid-duct group, which is often difficult to accurately classify.[6] As is true throughout the biliary tree, adenocarcinoma is the principal histological type in the lower bile duct, and it has previously been suggested that the papillary variant is more common at this location compared to the biliary confluence.[5]

Clinical presentation and diagnosis

The clinical presentation of distal bile duct cancer is generally indistinguishable from that of hilar cholangiocarcinoma or other periampullary malignancies. Progressive jaundice is seen in 75–90% of patients,[104] with abdominal pain, weight loss, fever or pruritus occurring in less than one-third.[6,101] Distal bile duct tumours are frequently mistaken for the more common adenocarcinoma of the pancreas. Endoscopic retrograde cholangiopancreatography (ERCP) can provide valuable information regarding the level of obstruction, may show that the obstruction is arising from the bile duct without involvement of the pancreatic duct, and can be both diagnostic and therapeutic in cases of choledocholithiasis. Percutaneous transhepatic cholangiography is generally less useful for tumours of the distal bile duct. Good quality cross-sectional imaging is required, usually CT with CT angiography, to assess for vascular involvement and/or metastatic disease. It is not uncommon that CT does not reveal a mass given the frequent small tumour size at presentation. Increasingly, magnetic resonance cholangiopancreatography (MRCP) is being used to evaluate periampullary tumours. As is true for hilar lesions, MRCP can provide information of the distal bile duct previously obtainable only with the combination of ERCP and CT.[105]

In patients with a stricture of the distal bile duct and a clinical presentation consistent with cholangiocarcinoma (or any other periampullary malignancy), histological confirmation of malignancy is generally unnecessary, unless non-operative therapy is planned. Benign strictures do occur in the lower bile duct but these are difficult to differentiate definitively from malignant strictures without resection. In addition, endoscopic brushings of the bile duct have an unacceptably low sensitivity, making a negative result virtually useless.[106] Excessive reliance on the results of percutaneous or brush biopsies serves only to delay therapy.

 The decision of whether or not to attempt resection of a presumed distal cholangiocarcinoma should not be delayed waiting for a preoperative histological diagnosis, as current methods of obtaining a preoperative tissue diagnosis are not reliable.

Staging and assessment of resectability

Carcinomas of the distal common bile duct are staged according to the AJCC system (6th edition) for tumours of the extrahepatic bile ducts. This system is of limited clinical use, as it is based on pathological information and does not provide any information pertaining to factors that define resectability. The most important of these is the presence of tumour involvement of the portal vein, superior mesenteric artery or common hepatic artery. Tumours involving a short segment of the portal vein (<2 cm) may be resected with reconstruction of the vein. Metastatic disease to distant sites, such as the liver or peritoneum, represent an absolute contraindication to proceeding with resection; the involvement of regional nodal basins should perhaps be viewed as a relative contraindication, given the poor survival in patients with node-positive disease. Along with good quality preoperative imaging, staging laparoscopy may help to reduce the number of non-curative laparotomies performed. Endoscopic ultrasonography (EUS) can provide additional staging information (nodal or vascular involvement) and allows an opportunity to biopsy the lesion, if necessary; however, EUS is generally not required if resection is planned based on the results of high-quality cross-sectional imaging studies.

Treatment options

Complete resection is the only effective therapy for cancers of the distal bile duct.[4–6,101–103] Reported 5-year survival rates are 14–40% after complete resection and survival beyond 1 year was uncommon in patients with tumours not amenable to resection.[5,38,101,102] Nearly all distal bile duct cancers require pancreatico-duodenectomy for complete excision. In our unit, 13% of patients (6 of 45) underwent bile duct excision alone, while in the Veterans Hospital study this figure was only 8% (3 of 34).[101,102] In addition to resection margin status (i.e. an R0 resection), metastatic disease to regional lymph nodes is a critical determinant of outcome.

Lymph node status was the only independent predictor of long-term survival after complete resection, with positive nodes conferring a 6.7 times greater likelihood of recurrence and death.[101]

Survival after resection of distal bile duct tumours is comparable, and may be better, than that for pancreatic cancer.[6,101,102] Furthermore, it has been erroneously assumed that survival is greater than that after resection of hilar cholangiocarcinomas as well.[5] However, if adjusted for stage and completeness of resection, the survival rates between the two are similar.[4] Adjuvant therapy after resection (chemotherapy and radiation therapy) has not been proven to improve survival, although this issue has not been evaluated in a prospective fashion.[6]

Surgically created bypasses (hepatico-jejunostomy or choledocho-jejunostomy) or biliary endoprostheses can be used for palliation of symptomatic biliary obstruction. Endoprostheses for distal biliary obstruction are easier to place and have a greater long-term patency than those placed for hilar obstruction.[86] Surgical bypass provides excellent relief of jaundice, but is typically used when irresectability is found at laparotomy. The authors generally use biliary endoprostheses in patients with clear-cut unresectable disease, discovered preoperatively or at staging laparoscopy, and in those unfit for operation. Laparoscopic biliary enteric bypass is also possible, but the expertise needed to perform this procedure is not widely available.

Cholangiocarcinoma involving the intrahepatic bile ducts

Clinical presentation

Intrahepatic cholangiocarcinoma (IHC), also referred to as peripheral cholangiocarcinoma, originates from the intrahepatic biliary radicles. IHC is rare in Western countries, only accounts for approximately 10% of all cholangiocarcinomas and is less frequently associated with underlying liver parenchymal disease than is hepatocellular carcinoma, although an association appears to exist. Recently, a marked increase in the incidence and age-adjusted mortality have been identified, the reasons for which are unclear but may be related to the rising incidence of obesity-related non-alcoholic fatty liver disease or chronic hepatitis C infection.[12,13] The presenting symptoms are subtle and often only include pain either directly or indirectly related to a large lesion. Malaise, weight loss and fever are uncommon, but jaundice and pruritus may be seen in up to one-third of cases, which is generally indicative of compression or invasion of the biliary confluence. Small lesions often present as incidental findings on imaging studies undertaken for unrelated symptoms.

Diagnosis

A solitary, intrahepatic tissue mass at first raises concern for hepatocellular carcinoma, a more common disease than IHC. However, in the absence of chronic hepatic parenchymal disease, chronic hepatitis or an elevated serum α-fetoprotein level, IHC must be considered. Percutaneous needle biopsy is often performed and will demonstrate adenocarcinoma; however, a definitive diagnosis often cannot be made based on needle biopsy alone. Patients should be investigated for evidence of a primary tumour elsewhere, since the most common diagnosis for adenocarcinoma in the liver is metastatic disease. In the absence of an extrahepatic primary site, patients with biopsy-proven adenocarcinoma in the liver should be considered to have an intrahepatic cholangiocarcinoma. Immunohistochemical staining of the biopsy specimen may further support the diagnosis by demonstrating a lesion of pancreaticobiliary origin.

Radiological investigations

The radiographic features of IHC on cross-sectional imaging are well described, and when combined with histological findings from a needle biopsy can be virtually diagnostic. On MRI, these tumours are generally hypointense on T1-weighted images and heterogeneously hyperintense on T2-weighted images. These lesions demonstrate initial rim enhancement characterised by progressive and concentric enhancement post-administration of contrast material. Generally the lesions do not completely enhance post-contrast. On contrast-enhanced CT, variable rim-like enhancement is also seen, predominantly on the arterial phase images with gradual centripetal enhancement on delayed imaging (**Fig. 12.5**). Intrahepatic cholangiocarcinomas

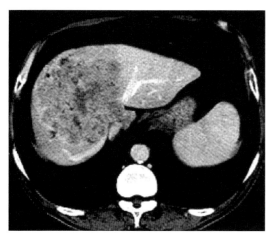

Figure 12.5 • Characteristic CT appearance of intrahepatic cholangiocarcinoma demonstrating heterogenous enhancement.

may only enhance completely on delayed imaging obtained hours after contrast administration, a finding related to the desmoplastic nature of the tumour. Capsular retraction may also be seen.[107,108]

Staging and assessment of resectability

Currently, there is no useful clinical staging system for intrahepatic cholangiocarcinoma. The AJCC TNM classification for primary liver cancers is applied both to hepatocellular carcinoma and IHC, but is of little clinical value. Because IHCs tend to be relatively silent lesions, they are often large at presentation. Thirty percent of patients will have peritoneal or hepatic metastases at presentation and many of these will not be detected until staging laparoscopy or exploratory laparotomy is performed. In a review of 53 peripheral cholangiocarcinomas treated at the MSKCC over an 8-year period, the median tumour diameter was 7.1 cm at presentation.[109] Twenty patients were found to be unresectable at exploration for a 62% overall resectability rate. Operative findings precluding resection were intrahepatic metastases (35%), peritoneal metastases (30%), coeliac lymph node metastases (25%) and portal vein involvement (10%). Staging laparoscopy was conducted in 22 patients, of whom six were spared laparotomy secondary to findings of peritoneal and intrahepatic metastases. In a more recent review at the authors' institution, a total of 270 IHC patients were seen over a 16-year period, representing an average annual increase of 14% in patients with this diagnosis over the study period. Of the patients treated at the MSKCC, 54% had unresectable disease at presentation; ultimately, 34% of the entire cohort underwent a potentially curative resection (70% of those explored with curative intent).[14]

Treatment options

Hepatic resection with negative histological margins remains the only potentially curative treatment for this disease. Unfortunately, less than half of patients have potentially resectable lesions at presentation and many of these will have findings at operation that preclude resection.[14,109] Median survival after resection was approximately 36 months in a recent study by Endo et al., compared to 9 months for patients with irresectable disease.[14] Unfortunately, even after a complete resection, recurrence was common and was predicted by tumour size >5 cm, the presence of multiple liver tumours, or metastatic disease to regional lymph nodes; the liver was the single most common site of recurrence.

Orthotopic liver transplantation has been utilised in the management of some patients.[110,111] However, many of these lesions are suitable for resection, which would likely produce similar results. Given the critical shortage of liver grafts, transplantation for intrahepatic cholangiocarcinoma is not performed in most centres, unless it is done in the context of a clinical trial. The use of chemotherapy has not been shown to improve survival, either as adjuvant therapy following resection or in patients with unresectable lesions.[112] External beam radiation therapy, intraoperative radiation and intraluminal radiation therapy have all been evaluated but in small, retrospective studies, and none has shown a significant survival benefit in patients with unresectable disease.

 Complete surgical resection is the best treatment for intrahepatic cholangiocarcinoma. Chemotherapy and/or radiation therapy, whether in an adjuvant or palliative setting, have not been shown to provide any significant survival benefit.

Gallbladder cancer

Gallbladder cancer is an uncommon malignancy with approximately 5000 new cases per year in the USA.[1] Historically, clinical attitudes towards gallbladder cancer have been largely based on pessimism and nihilism. This frustration spawns from the usual late presentation, lack of effective therapy and the resultant dismal prognosis. In fact, most older series reported a median survival of 2–5 months for untreated gallbladder cancers and less than 5% 5-year survival for treated gallbladder cancers. However, improved understanding of the disease and its treatment has led to prolonged survival and cure in selected patients. Currently the only chance of cure is complete surgical extirpation of the cancer.

Epidemiology/aetiology

Worldwide, the highest incidence of gallbladder cancer is found among people indigenous to the Andes Mountains of South America. In North America, the incidence is approximately 1.2 per 100 000, the

highest being among native American Indians and Mexican Americans. It occurs in women almost three times more often than in men across all populations studied.[113]

As with other biliary tract tumours, chronic inflammation leading to high cellular turnover is a common denominator of associated risk factors. The most common risk factor is cholelithiasis; other factors include the presence of a cholecysto-enteric fistula, typhoid bacillus infection and an anomalous pancreatico-biliary junction.[113,114] As with other gastrointestinal malignancies, the adenoma to carcinoma sequence has been demonstrated within adenomatous polyps of the gallbladder.[115] Gallbladder polyps are noted in 3–6% of the population undergoing ultrasonography, although the vast majority are cholesterol polyps or adenomyomatosis, which have no malignant potential. However, about 1% of cholecystectomy specimens contain adenomatous polyps, which do have malignant potential.[116] Conditions that increase the risk of malignancy include polyp size >1 cm, patient age >50 years and the presence of multiple lesions.[117] The conservative recommendation is to perform a prophylactic cholecystectomy for polypoid lesions greater than 0.5 cm in size, although the likelihood of malignancy in polyps even up to 1 cm appears to be extremely low. This is in contrast to gallbladder polyps arising in the setting of primary sclerosing cholangitis, which are more often neoplastic.[118] The authors' practice is to recommend cholecystectomy for polyps >1 cm. Polypoid lesions <0.5 cm have a much lower likelihood of harbouring malignancy and are safe to follow with serial ultrasounds for evidence of growth or change in character.[115,116,119]

A gallbladder with a calcified wall, also known as a 'porcelain gallbladder', is associated with an increased risk of developing cancer (**Fig. 12.6**).

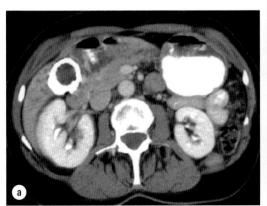 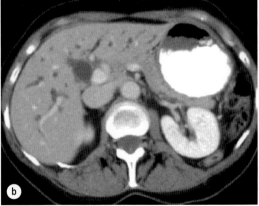

Figure 12.6 • Axial CT images of a porcelain gallbladder. Note the marked, circumferential calcification of the gallbladder wall **(a)** and the intrahepatic biliary ductal dilatation **(b)**. This patient had a gallbladder cancer arising in the setting of a porcelain gallbladder, which had progressed to involve the common hepatic duct.

The deposition of calcium most likely reflects a state of chronic inflammation. Although the risk of malignancy in a porcelain gallbladder previously was considered to be extremely high (10–50%), recent studies demonstrate a much lower incidence (<10%), with stippled calcification actually carrying a higher risk than diffuse intramural calcification.[120,121] Nevertheless, the current recommendation for patients with a porcelain gallbladder is to perform a cholecystectomy, which in most cases can be safely done laparoscopically.

Although most gallbladder polyps identified at ultrasonography are benign, true adenomatous polyps do have a malignant potential. Cholecystectomy should be performed for adenomatous polyps >1 cm in size, and those <1 cm should be followed closely with serial ultrasound to detect any growth or change. A calcified gallbladder wall, likely a reflection of chronic inflammation, is also an indication for cholecystectomy.

Clinical presentation and diagnosis

Many patients present late in the course of their disease, and 75% of patients present with unresectable disease.[122] Two-thirds of patients present with abdominal pain/biliary colic. Approximately one-third will present with jaundice and 10% will have significant weight loss.[123] For early stage cancers, the diagnosis is usually made upon pathological examination of a cholecystectomy specimen resected for symptoms presumed to be benign biliary colic. Preoperative diagnosis should be suspected for any mass or irregularity of the gallbladder wall noted on radiological exam (CT or ultrasound). In any patient suspected of having a gallbladder malignancy, a duplex ultrasound exam should be performed to evaluate the extent of disease and possible involvement of the portal vasculature. In addition, abdominal cross-sectional imaging (CT or MRI) should be performed to evaluate for nodal disease or M1 disease. For those patients suspected of having gallbladder cancer on preoperative imaging, a tissue diagnosis is not necessary prior to exploration, and both the surgeon and patient should be prepared for an appropriate resection, knowing that the final pathology may in fact reveal benign disease.

Imaging findings of asymmetric gallbladder wall thickening, intraluminal papillary projections or any other finding suggesting a mass must be taken very seriously, particularly when noted on ultrasonography. Any such findings should immediately raise concern for a possible gallbladder cancer and be treated accordingly.

Histopathology and staging

The overwhelming majority of gallbladder cancers are adenocarcinomas, with a papillary subtype being associated with a relatively better prognosis compared to others.[124] Other histological subtypes, such as adenosquamous carcinoma or pure squamous cell carcinoma, are seen in the gallbladder more commonly than at any other site within the biliary tree. The updated AJCC staging system (6th edition, 2002) is based on the standard TNM classification (Table 12.5). of which the T stage has the greatest clinical impact on the extent of surgery performed, because it is dependent on the depth of invasion into the gallbladder wall and adjacent organs. The wall of the gallbladder consists of a mucosa and lamina propria, a thin muscular layer, perimuscular connective tissue and a serosa, which lacks a serosal covering along its border with the liver. The perimuscular connective tissue is continuous with the liver connective tissue. T1a tumours are limited to the lamina propria and T1b lesions invade the muscle layer. T2 tumours invade through the muscle layer into the perimuscular connective tissue and T3 tumours penetrate the serosa and directly invade either the liver or another single extrahepatic organ. T4 tumours reflect locally unresectable tumours due to invasion into the main portal vein, hepatic artery or multiple extrahepatic organs. In patients with a new diagnosis of gallbladder cancer, the presence of jaundice is an ominous finding, generally implying advanced disease. Previously, the N stage was divided into locoregional and distant lymph node involvement, but due to the powerful adverse negative impact of any positive lymph node, the new staging system simply divides tumours into being either node negative or positive, i.e. N0 or N1 respectively. Metastatic disease refers to distant metastasis. It should be noted that the majority of studies referenced in this chapter utilise the previous edition of the staging system, where the major difference is that T4 tumours are not deemed as unresectable.

Preoperative staging should be aimed at assessing the local extent of disease and excluding distant metastases. Cross-sectional imaging (CT or MRCP) are the mainstays of investigation, while duplex ultrasonography is helpful to assess the gallbladder lesion and can provide some insight as to the likelihood of a malignancy; in addition, US may be helpful in assessing possible vascular involvement. FDG-PET has been shown to be helpful in identifying additional disease that changes management in one-quarter of patients.[72] Staging laparoscopy is helpful for identifying distant disease, thereby avoiding non-therapeutic laparotomies.[68]

Table 12.5 • TNM staging system (6th edition) for gallbladder cancer

Primary tumour (T)	
TX:	Primary tumour cannot be assessed
T0:	No evidence of primary tumour
Tis:	Carcinoma in situ
T1:	Tumour invades lamina propria or muscle layer
T1a:	Tumour invades lamina propria
T1b:	Tumour invades muscle layer
T2:	Tumour invades perimuscular connective tissue: no extension beyond serosa or into liver
T3:	Tumour perforates serosa (visceral peritoneum) or directly invades the liver and/or one other adjacent organ or structure, e.g. stomach, duodenum, colon pancreas, omentum, extrahepatic bile ducts
T4:	Tumour invades main portal vein or hepatic artery, or invades two or more extrahepatic organs or structures
Regional lymph nodes (N)	
NX:	Regional lymph nodes cannot be assessed
N0:	No regional lymph node metastasis
N1:	Regional lymph node metastasis
Distant metastasis (M)	
MX:	Presence of distant metastasis cannot be assessed
M0:	No distant metastasis
M1:	Distant metastasis
Stage grouping	
Stage 0:	Tis, N0, M0
Stage IA:	T1, N0, M0
Stage IB:	T2, N0, M0
Stage IIA:	T3, N0, M0
Stage IIB:	T1, N1, M0
	T2, N1, M0
	T3, N1, M0
Stage III:	T4, any N, M0
Stage IV:	Any T, any N, M1

Evidence for an aggressive surgical approach

Over the past three decades, decreasing morbidity and mortality associated with radical en bloc resections including hepatectomy, bile duct resection and regional lymphadenectomy have allowed for broader application of surgical resection in selected patients.[123,125] The current surgical approaches generally employ segmental resections (segments IVb/V) or major resections (hemihepatectomy or extended hepatectomy) when necessary. In most cases, it is the involvement of major hepatic vascular structures rather than actual depth of tumour invasion into the liver that dictates the extent of hepatic resection that must be performed.

Our group reported 149 cases in which complete surgical radical resection yielded an actuarial 5-year survival of 83% for stage II, 63% for stage III and 25% for stage IV.[123] Many contemporary studies have reported similar results, even for stage III and IV disease.[126–129] The improved survival reported in these studies relative to historical studies, in which the survival rates were dismal, demonstrates the importance of achieving negative margins.

Regional lymphadenectomy is currently employed as part of an aggressive surgical approach, but evidence to support an associated survival benefit is controversial. The chance of nodal involvement increases with increasing T stage. Bartlett et al. found nodal disease associated with 46% of resected T2 tumours and 54% of resected T3 tumours.[123] Node status was found to be the most powerful predictor of outcome and no patient with node-positive disease experienced long-term survival.

Surgical therapy

Patients with gallbladder cancer may present where malignancy is suspected preoperatively or found at the time of exploration and when it is diagnosed after simple cholecystectomy. Contraindications to resection include distant spread (peritoneum, discontiguous liver lesions), tumour involvement of the hepatic vasculature or biliary tree that would preclude a complete resection, and presence of disease in distant lymph node groups (peripancreatic, periduodenal, periportal, coeliac and/or superior mesenteric).

The goal of resection should always be complete tumour extirpation with negative histological margins (R0). Patients with cancer identified preoperatively typically have relatively larger tumours and more extensive disease than is seen in patients diagnosed postcholecystectomy. Gallbladder cancer identified intraoperatively is an uncommon but difficult situation, since one will have limited staging information; however, it is reasonable to proceed with definitive surgical management, since this is the only effective therapy. When the diagnosis is made after simple cholecystectomy, the need for further resection is primarily dictated by the T stage.

It is important to remember that the incidence of lymph node and distant metastases is directly related to the T stage. Fong et al. reported a progressive increase in distant and nodal metastases from 16% to 79% and from 33% to 69% respectively, in going from T2 to T4 tumours, which resulted in a progressive decline in resectability, from 58% to 13%.[130]

T1 tumours

T1a tumours, or those that are confined to the lamina propria, are most often discovered after, and adequately treated with, a simple cholecystectomy. Because nodal involvement is rare, cure rates approach 85–100% if negative margins are achieved.[131,132] T1b tumours should be cured by simple cholecystectomy, but there have been reports documenting recurrence and death following a simple cholecystectomy for T1b tumours.[133] Given the limited data regarding T1b gallbladder cancers

in the literature, the decision to perform a simple cholecystectomy versus a more radical procedure should be made on a case-by-case basis.

T2 tumours

T2 lesions should be treated with an aggressive resection, including removal of adjacent liver, lymphadenectomy of the hepatoduodenal ligament, and a bile duct resection only if necessary to obtain a negative margin on the cystic duct. In the absence of tumour involvement of the right portal pedicle, the authors prefer to perform a segmental resection of segments IVb and V, and most T2 tumours are amenable to such an approach. It should be noted that the normal plane of dissection of simple cholecystectomy, open or laparoscopic, is within the perimuscular connective tissue intimately associated with the liver. Thus, a simple cholecystectomy will not achieve tumour clearance with certainty. A lymphadenectomy is performed in the treatment of T2 tumours given that approximately 50% of these lesions have associated lymph node metastases.[123] de Aretxabala et al. reported 5-year survival rates of 70% with an extended resection compared with only 20% after simple cholecystectomy alone.[134]

T3 tumours

T3 tumours require hepatic resection and porta hepatis lymphadenectomy at a minimum. If a limited partial hepatectomy cannot be performed to achieve tumour clearance, a more extensive partial hepatectomy and/or bile duct resection may be required. When a complete resection is achieved, 5-year survival rates of 30–50% can be obtained in this patient population.[123,128,130]

T4 tumours

T4 lesions, as defined by the 6th edition staging system, generally reflect unresectable disease.

Preoperative suspicion of malignancy

If gallbladder cancer is suspected on preoperative imaging studies, a staging laparoscopy prior to laparotomy is helpful to assess the abdomen for evidence of peritoneal spread or discontiguous liver disease. In general, however, a laparoscopic cholecystectomy should be avoided[67,68,135] and the surgeon needs to be prepared to proceed with resection of an invasive malignancy, unless proven otherwise. It is not unreasonable to obtain intraoperative frozen section histology to prove malignancy before proceeding with hepatic resection.

Unsuspected malignancy at exploration

It should be routine to inspect the gallbladder mucosa after simple cholecystectomy. Suspicious lesions should be sent immediately for frozen section. If a carcinoma is diagnosed, the need to perform additional surgery is dictated by the T stage on frozen section, although the information will be limited since a full histopathological evaluation is not available at the time of operation. The authors prefer to perform an oncologically correct resection, suitable for an invasive lesion, at the time it is discovered, unless there are extenuating circumstances that mandate otherwise. However, if the surgeon is not comfortable with performing a radical cholecystectomy/hepatic resection, the patient is best served by transferring them to a specialist centre/surgeon. A delayed radical and appropriate resection does not negatively impact on the patient's outcome.[130]

Malignancy diagnosed postcholecystectomy

When the cancer is diagnosed by postoperative histology, the need for a more radical resection will be based on T stage as outlined above. Fong et al. demonstrated 5-year survival rates of 61% in patients who were re-resected compared to 19% for patients who did not undergo a radical second operation.[130] However, prior to undertaking a second operation, a high-quality cross-sectional imaging (CT/MRI) should be obtained to appropriately stage the disease. Postoperative inflammatory changes may be indistinguishable from tumour and thus may necessitate bile duct resection or a more aggressive hepatic resection to ensure complete tumour eradication.

Given that inadvertent cholecystotomy during cholecystectomy is rarely documented, it is difficult to predict who is at increased risk for peritoneal dissemination and, specifically, port site recurrence. In the past, routine resection of laparoscopic port sites was recommended, in an effort to ensure clearance of microscopic disease that may have implanted during the laparoscopic procedure. However, there is little evidence to support the efficacy of routine resection of all port sites at re-operation.[136] In the authors' experience, recurrence at the port sites is a harbinger of generalised peritoneal recurrence that will not be prevented with resection of these limited areas.

When exploring a patient for gallbladder cancer after a non-curative laparoscopic cholecystectomy has been performed, a finding of disease at the port sites is a sign of generalised peritoneal spread of disease.

Adjuvant therapy

We have investigated the initial pattern of recurrence after resection of biliary tract cancers to provide a rational framework upon which to develop adjuvant therapies for patients having undergone resection. Sixty-six percent of patients with gallbladder cancers who underwent a potentially curative resection recurred within a median follow-up of 24 months. Only 15% of patients developed a locoregional recurrence as the first site of failure, while the majority of patients (85%) had recurrence that involved a distant site.[137] Thus, local therapies targeted at locoregional disease, such as radiotherapy, are unlikely to significantly impact the course of this disease, further emphasising the importance of developing effective systemic adjuvant therapies.

Most studies evaluating adjuvant therapy comprise phase II trials and these are limited by small numbers, often combine chemotherapy with radiation treatment, and are confounded by inclusion of patients with less than an R0 resection.[138,139] Based on the paucity of good evidence, there remains a theoretical benefit to adding locoregional therapy such as external beam radiation therapy for disease control.

A Japanese phase III multi-institutional trial included 508 patients with biliary and pancreatic cancers.[83] Of the 140 gallbladder cancer patients randomised to receive surgical resection alone or resection plus adjuvant mitomycin and 5-flourouracil, the actuarial 5-year disease-free survival favoured the adjuvant chemotherapy group (20.3% vs. 11.6% for surgery alone). It is reasonable to offer such adjuvant chemotherapy to resected gallbladder patients but no consensus has been reached regarding routine use of adjuvant chemotherapy.[100]

Palliation

Patients with advanced, incurable disease may present with pain, jaundice or gastrointestinal obstruction. Given the dismal prognosis of approximately 2–5 months, non-surgical methods of palliation including both percutaneous and endoscopic techniques to relieve intestinal or biliary obstruction should be entertained first. If unresectable disease is discovered at the time of exploration, a segment III bypass can be performed to relieve jaundice, but in general patients are best served by avoiding a major operative procedure and proceeding with percutaneous biliary drainage postoperatively.[140] Intestinal bypass should be performed only in patients who have symptomatic obstruction.

Key points

Cholangiocarcinoma

Hilar

- Preoperative assessment is mainly a decision of resectability. Attention should be paid to the extent of bile duct involvement, portal vein involvement, and to the presence or absence of hepatic atrophy.
- Most complete resections for hilar disease necessitate a hepatectomy.
- Chemotherapy and radiotherapy have not been shown to be beneficial beyond complete surgical resection alone.

Distal

- The clinical presentation is similar to other periampullary tumours.
- Similar to hilar disease, a preoperative tissue diagnosis is not necessary to proceed with surgical resection.
- Endoscopic palliation is the preferred method to relieve symptomatic jaundice in the setting of unresectable disease.

Intrahepatic

- Hepatocellular carcinoma must be excluded in patients with an intrahepatic mass.
- Metastatic adenocarcinoma to the liver from a remote primary, such as lung, breast or gastrointestinal, must be excluded.
- Similar to all other locations of cholangiocarcinoma, complete surgical resection is the optimal treatment and only chance for cure.

Gallbladder cancer

- Duplex ultrasonography should be part of the preoperative imaging to properly assess the tumour within the gallbladder wall and its relation to the bile duct and hepatic vasculature.
- A cholecystectomy should be performed for adenomatous polyps greater than 1 cm or those that are smaller but growing and changing in character. Cholesterol polyps and adenomyomatosis are not premalignant conditions.
- Complete surgical resection is the goal, whether the diagnosis is made preoperatively, intraoperatively or after a non-curative laparoscopic cholecystectomy.

References

1. Landis SH, Murray T, Bolden S et al. Cancer statistics, 1998. Cancer J Clin 1998; 48:6–29.

2. Carriaga MT, Henson DE. Liver, gallbladder, extrahepatic bile ducts, and pancreas. Cancer 1995; 75:171–90.

3. Burke EC, Jarnagin WR, Hochwald SN et al. Hilar cholangiocarcinoma: patterns of spread, the importance of hepatic resection for curative operation, and a presurgical clinical staging system. Ann Surg 1998; 228:385–94.

4. Nagorney DM, Donohue JH, Farnell MB et al. Outcomes after curative resections of cholangiocarcinoma. Arch Surg 1993; 128:871–7; discussion 877–9.

5. Tompkins RK, Thomas D, Wile A et al. Prognostic factors in bile duct carcinoma: analysis of 96 cases. Ann Surg 1981; 194:447–57.

6. Nakeeb A, Pitt HA, Sohn TA et al. Cholangiocarcinoma. A spectrum of intrahepatic, perihilar, and distal tumors. Ann Surg 1996; 224:463–73; discussion 473–5.

7. Berdah SV, Delpero JR, Garcia S et al. A western surgical experience of peripheral cholangiocarcinoma. Br J Surg 1996; 83:1517–21.

8. Chu KM, Lai EC, Al-Hadeedi S et al. Intrahepatic cholangiocarcinoma. World J Surg 1997; 21:301–5; discussion 305–6.

9. Harrison LE, Fong Y, Klimstra DS et al. Surgical treatment of 32 patients with peripheral intrahepatic cholangiocarcinoma. Br J Surg 1998; 85:1068–70.

10. Saunders K, Longmire W Jr, Tompkins R et al. Diffuse bile duct tumors: guidelines for management. Am Surg 1991; 57:816–20.

11. Patel T, Steer CJ, Gores GJ. Apoptosis and the liver: a mechanism of disease, growth regulation, and carcinogenesis. Hepatology 1999; 30:811–5.

12. Welzel TM, Graubard BI, El-Serag HB et al. Risk factors for intrahepatic and extrahepatic cholangiocarcinoma in the United States: a population-based case–control study. Clin Gastroenterol Hepatol 2007; 5:1221–8.

13. Welzel TM, Mellemkjaer L, Gloria G et al. Risk factors for intrahepatic cholangiocarcinoma in a low-risk population: a nationwide case–control study. Int J Cancer 2007; 120:638–41.

14. Endo I, Gonen M, Yopp AC et al. Intrahepatic cholangiocarcinoma: rising frequency, improved survival, and determinants of outcome after resection. Ann Surg 2008; 248:84–96.

15. Kuwayti K, Baggenstoss AH, Stauffer MH et al. Carcinoma of the major intrahepatic and the extrahepatic bile ducts exclusive of the papilla of Vater. Gynecol Obstet 1957; 104:357–66.

16. Sako K, Seitzinger GL, Garside E. Carcinoma of the extrahepatic bile ducts; review of the literature and report of six cases. Surgery 1957; 41:416–37.

17. Okuda K, Kubo Y, Okazaki N et al. Clinical aspects of intrahepatic bile duct carcinoma including hilar carcinoma: a study of 57 autopsy-proven cases. Cancer 1977; 39:232–46.

18. Broome U, Olsson R, Loof L et al. Natural history and prognostic factors in 305 Swedish patients with primary sclerosing cholangitis. Gut 1996; 38:610–5.

19. Pitt HA, Dooley WC, Yeo CJ et al. Malignancies of the biliary tree. Curr Probl Surg 1995; 32:1–90.

20. Hewitt PM, Krige JE, Bornman PC et al. Choledochal cysts in adults. Br J Surg 1995; 82:382–5.

21. Vogt DP. Current management of cholangiocarcinoma. Oncology (Williston Park) 1988; 2(6):37–44, 54.

22. Lipsett PA, Pitt HA, Colombani PM. Choledochal cyst disease. A changing pattern of presentation. Ann Surg 1994; 220:644–52.

23. Tanaka K, Ikoma A, Hamada N et al. Biliary tract cancer accompanied by anomalous junction of pancreaticobiliary ductal system in adults. Am J Surg 1998; 175:218–20.

24. Jeng KS, Ohta I, Yang FS et al. Coexisting sharp ductal angulation with intrahepatic biliary strictures in right hepatolithiasis. Arch Surg 1994; 129:1097–102.

25. Hakamada K, Sasaki M, Endoh M et al. Late development of bile duct cancer after sphincteroplasty: a ten- to twenty-two-year follow-up study. Surgery 1997; 121:488–92.

26. Chu KM, Lo CM, Liu CL et al. Malignancy associated with hepatolithiasis. Hepatogastroenterology 1997; 44:352–7.

27. Kubo S, Kinoshita H, Hirohashi K et al. Hepatolithiasis associated with cholangiocarcinoma. World J Surg 1995; 19:637–41.

28. Weinbren K, Mutum SS. Pathological aspects of cholangiocarcinoma. J Pathol 1983; 139:217–38.

29. Rodgers CM, Adams JT, Schwartz SI. Carcinoma of the extrahepatic bile ducts. Surgery 1981; 90:596–601.

30. Jarnagin WR, Bowne W, Klimstra DS et al. Papillary phenotype confers improved survival after resection of hilar cholangiocarcinoma. Ann Surg 2005; 241:703–12; discussion 712–14.

31. Tsuzuki T, Ogata Y, Iida S et al. Carcinoma of the bifurcation of the hepatic ducts. Arch Surg 1983; 118:1147–51.

32. Shimada H, Niimoto S, Matsuba A et al. The infiltration of bile duct carcinoma along the bile duct wall. Int Surg 1988; 73:87–90.

33. Endo I, House MG, Klimstra DS et al. Clinical significance of intraoperative bile duct margin assessment for hilar cholangiocarcinoma. Ann Surg Oncol 2008; 15:2104–12.

34. Craig JR, Peters RL, Edmondson HA. Tumor liver and intrahepatic ducts. Armed Forces Institute of Pathology, 1989.

35. The Liver Cancer Study Group of Japan. Primary liver cancer in Japan. Sixth report. Cancer 1987; 60:1400–11.

36. Yamamoto J, Kosuge T, Shimada K et al. Intrahepatic cholangiocarcinoma: proposal of new macroscopic classification [in Japanese]. Nippon Geka Gakkai Zasshi 1993; 94:1194–200.

37. Levi S, Urbano-Ispizua A, Gill R et al. Multiple K-ras codon 12 mutations in cholangiocarcinomas demonstrated with a sensitive polymerase chain reaction technique. Cancer Res 1991; 51:3497–502.

38. Nakeeb A, Lipsett PA, Lillemoe KD et al. Biliary carcinoembryonic antigen levels are a marker for cholangiocarcinoma. Am J Surg 1996; 171:147–52; discussion 152–3.

39. Jarnagin WR, Weber S, Tickoo SK et al. Combined hepatocellular and cholangiocarcinoma: demo-

graphic, clinical, and prognostic factors. Cancer 2002; 94:2040–6.

40. Farley DR, Weaver AL, Nagorney DM. "Natural history" of unresected cholangiocarcinoma: patient outcome after noncurative intervention. Mayo Clin Proc 1995; 70:425–9.

41. Vatanasapt V, Uttaravichien T, Mairiang EO et al. Cholangiocarcinoma in north-east Thailand. Lancet 1990; 335:116–7.

42. McPherson GA, Benjamin IS, Hodgson HJ et al. Pre-operative percutaneous transhepatic biliary drainage: the results of a controlled trial. Br J Surg 1984; 71:371–5.

43. Heslin MJ, Brooks AD, Hochwald SN et al. A preoperative biliary stent is associated with increased complications after pancreatoduodenectomy. Arch Surg 1998; 133:149–54.

44. Corvera CU, Blumgart LH, Darvishian F et al. Clinical and pathologic features of proximal biliary strictures masquerading as hilar cholangiocarcinoma. J Am Coll Surg 2005; 201:862–9.

45. Wetter LA, Ring EJ, Pellegrini CA et al. Differential diagnosis of sclerosing cholangiocarcinomas of the common hepatic duct (Klatskin tumors). Am J Surg 1991; 161:57–62; discussion 62–3.

46. Rabinovitz M, Zajko AB, Hassanein T et al. Diagnostic value of brush cytology in the diagnosis of bile duct carcinoma: a study in 65 patients with bile duct strictures. Hepatology 1990; 12:747–52.

47. Hadjis NS, Blumgart LH. Role of liver atrophy, hepatic resection and hepatocyte hyperplasia in the development of portal hypertension in biliary disease. Gut 1987; 28:1022–8.

48. Tillich M, Mischinger HJ, Preisegger KH et al. Multiphasic helical CT in diagnosis and staging of hilar cholangiocarcinoma. Am J Roentgenol 1998; 171:651–8.

49. Gibson RN, Yeung E, Thompson JN et al. Bile duct obstruction: radiologic evaluation of level, cause, and tumor resectability. Radiology 1986; 160:43–7.

50. Okuda K, Ohto M, Tsuchiya Y. The role of ultrasound, percutaneous transhepatic cholangiography, computed tomographic scanning, and magnetic resonance imaging in the preoperative assessment of bile duct cancer. World J Surg 1988; 12:18–26.

51. Hann LE, Greatrex KV, Bach AM et al. Cholangiocarcinoma at the hepatic hilus: sonographic findings. Am J Roentgenol 1997; 168:985–9.

52. Bach AM, Hann LE, Brown KT et al. Portal vein evaluation with US: comparison to angiography combined with CT arterial portography. Radiology 1996; 201:149–54.

53. Itoh K, Fujita N, Kubo K et al. MR imaging of hilar cholangiocarcinoma – comparative study with CT [in Japanese]. Nippon Igaku Hoshasen Gakkai Zasshi 1992; 52:443–51.

54. Guthrie JA, Ward J, Robinson PJ. Hilar cholangiocarcinomas: T2-weighted spin-echo and gadolinium-enhanced FLASH MR imaging. Radiology 1996; 201:347–51.

55. Schwartz LH, Coakley FV, Sun Y et al. Neoplastic pancreaticobiliary duct obstruction: evaluation with breath-hold MR cholangiopancreatography. Am J Roentgenol 1998; 170:1491–5.

56. Lee MG, Lee HJ, Kim MH et al. Extrahepatic biliary diseases: 3D MR cholangiopancreatography compared with endoscopic retrograde cholangiopancreatography. Radiology 1997; 202:663–9.

57. Jarnagin WR, Fong Y, DeMatteo RP et al. Staging, resectability, and outcome in 225 patients with hilar cholangiocarcinoma. Ann Surg 2001; 234:507–17; discussion 517–19.

58. Bismuth H, Nakache R, Diamond T. Management strategies in resection for hilar cholangiocarcinoma. Ann Surg 1992; 215:31–8.

59. Chen RF, Li ZH, Zhou JJ et al. Preoperative evaluation with T-staging system for hilar cholangiocarcinoma. World J Gastroenterol 2007; 13:5754–9.

60. Klempnauer J, Ridder GJ, Werner M et al. What constitutes long-term survival after surgery for hilar cholangiocarcinoma? Cancer 1997; 79:26–34.

61. Pichlmayr R, Weimann A, Klempnauer J. Surgical treatment in proximal bile duct cancer. A single-center experience. Ann Surg 1996; 224:628–38.

62. Iwatsuki S, Todo S, Marsh JW et al. Treatment of hilar cholangiocarcinoma (Klatskin tumors) with hepatic resection or transplantation. J Am Coll Surg 1998; 187:358–64.

63. Heimbach JK, Haddock MG, Alberts SR et al. Transplantation for hilar cholangiocarcinoma. Liver Transpl 2004; 10:S65–8.

64. Lazaridis KN, Gores GJ. Cholangiocarcinoma. Gastroenterology 2005; 128:1655–67.

65. Nimura Y, Hayakawa N, Kamiya J et al. Hepatic segmentectomy with caudate lobe resection for bile duct carcinoma of the hepatic hilus. World J Surg 1990; 14:535–43; discussion 544.

66. Mizumoto R, Suzuki H. Surgical anatomy of the hepatic hilum with special reference to the caudate lobe. World J Surg 1988; 12:2–10.

67. Vollmer CM, Drebin JA, Middleton WD et al. Utility of staging laparoscopy in subsets of peripancreatic and biliary malignancies. Ann Surg 2002; 235:1–7.

68. Weber SM, DeMatteo RP, Fong Y et al. Staging laparoscopy in patients with extrahepatic biliary carcinoma. Analysis of 100 patients. Ann Surg 2002; 235:392–9.

69. Kluge R, Schmidt F, Caca K et al. Positron emission tomography with [18F]fluoro-2-deoxy-d-glucose for diagnosis and staging of bile duct cancer. Hepatology 2001; 33:1029–35.

70. Fritscher-Ravens A, Bohuslavizki KH, Broering DC et al. FDG-PET in the diagnosis of hilar cholangiocarcinoma. Nucl Med Commun 2001; 22:1277–85.

71. Anderson CD, Rice MH, Pinson CW et al. Fluorodeoxyglucose PET imaging in the evaluation of gallbladder carcinoma and cholangiocarcinoma. J Gastrointest Surg 2004; 8:90–7.

72. Corvera CU, Blumgart LH, Akhurst T et al. ^{18}F-fluorodeoxyglucose positron emission tomography influences management decisions in patients with biliary cancer. J Am Coll Surg 2008; 206:57–65.

73. Jarnagin WR, Blumgart LH, Saldinger P. Cancer of the bile ducts. In: Blumgart LH and Fong Y (eds) Surgery of the liver and biliary tract. Saunders 2000; p. 1017.

74. Kitagawa Y, Nagino M, Kamiya J et al. Lymph node metastasis from hilar cholangiocarcinoma: audit of 110 patients who underwent regional and para-aortic node dissection. Ann Surg 2001; 233:385–92.

75. Tojima Y, Nagino M, Ebata T et al. Immunohistochemically demonstrated lymph node micrometastasis and prognosis in patients with otherwise node-negative hilar cholangiocarcinoma. Ann Surg 2003; 237:201–7.

76. Hadjis NS, Blenkharn JI, Alexander N et al. Outcome of radical surgery in hilar cholangiocarcinoma. Surgery 1990; 107:597–604.

77. Baer HU, Stain SC, Dennison AR et al. Improvements in survival by aggressive resections of hilar cholangiocarcinoma. Ann Surg 1993; 217:20–7.

78. Saldinger PF, Blumgart LH. Resection of hilar cholangiocarcinoma – a European and United States experience. J Hepatobil Pancreat Surg 2000; 7:111–14.

79. Cameron JL, Pitt HA, Zinner MJ et al. Management of proximal cholangiocarcinomas by surgical resection and radiotherapy. Am J Surg 1990; 159:91–7; discussion 97–8.

80. Pitt HA, Nakeeb A, Abrams RA et al. Perihilar cholangiocarcinoma. Postoperative radiotherapy does not improve survival. Ann Surg 1995; 221:788–97; discussion 797–8.

81. Kamada T, Saitou H, Takamura A et al. The role of radiotherapy in the management of extrahepatic bile duct cancer: an analysis of 145 consecutive patients treated with intraluminal and/or external beam radiotherapy. Int J Radiat Oncol Biol Phys 1996; 34:767–74.

82. McMasters KM, Tuttle TM, Leach SD et al. Neoadjuvant chemoradiation for extrahepatic cholangiocarcinoma. Am J Surg 1997; 174:605–8; discussion 608–9.

83. Takada T, Amano H, Yasuda H et al. Is postoperative adjuvant chemotherapy useful for gallbladder carcinoma? A phase III multicenter prospective randomized controlled trial in patients with resected pancreaticobiliary carcinoma. Cancer 2002; 95:1685–95.

84. Kuvshinoff BW, Armstrong JG, Fong Y et al. Palliation of irresectable hilar cholangiocarcinoma with biliary drainage and radiotherapy. Br J Surg 1995; 82:1522–5.

85. Liu CL, Lo CM, Lai EC et al. Endoscopic retrograde cholangiopancreatography and endoscopic endoprosthesis insertion in patients with Klatskin tumors. Arch Surg 1998; 133:293–6.

86. Becker CD, Glattli A, Maibach R et al. Percutaneous palliation of malignant obstructive jaundice with the Wallstent endoprosthesis: follow-up and reintervention in patients with hilar and non-hilar obstruction. J Vasc Interv Radiol 1993; 4:597–604.

87. Cheung KL, Lai EC. Endoscopic stenting for malignant biliary obstruction. Arch Surg 1995; 130(2):204–7.

88. Miyazaki M, Ito H, Nakagawa K et al. Aggressive surgical approaches to hilar cholangiocarcinoma: hepatic or local resection? Surgery 1998; 123:131–6.

89. Schima E. Surgery of the biliary tract in geriatric patients [author's transl]. Zentralbl Chir 1977; 102:858–68.

90. Glattli A, Stain SC, Baer HU et al. Unresectable malignant biliary obstruction: treatment by self-expandable biliary endoprostheses. HPB Surg 1993; 6:175–84.

91. Jarnagin WR, Burke E, Powers C et al. Intrahepatic biliary enteric bypass provides effective palliation in selected patients with malignant obstruction at the hepatic duct confluence. Am J Surg 1998; 175:453–60.

92. Baer HU, Rhyner M, Stain SC et al. The effect of communication between the right and left liver on the outcome of surgical drainage for jaundice due to malignant obstruction at the hilus of the liver. HPB Surg 1994; 8:27–31.

93. Bowling TE, Galbraith SM, Hatfield AR et al. A retrospective comparison of endoscopic stenting alone with stenting and radiotherapy in non-resectable cholangiocarcinoma. Gut 1996; 39:852–5.

94. Vallis KA, Benjamin IS, Munro AJ et al. External beam and intraluminal radiotherapy for locally advanced bile duct cancer: role and tolerability. Radiother Oncol 1996; 41:61–6.

95. Ortner M. Photodynamic therapy for cholangiocarcinoma. J Hepatobil Pancreat Surg 2001; 8:137–9.

96. Ortner M. Photodynamic therapy in the biliary tract. Curr Gastroenterol Rep 2001; 3(2):154–9.

97. Ortner ME, Caca K, Berr F et al. Successful photodynamic therapy for nonresectable cholangiocarcinoma: a randomized prospective study. Gastroenterology 2003; 125:1355–63.

98. Zoepf T, Jakobs R, Arnold JC et al. Palliation of nonresectable bile duct cancer: improved survival after photodynamic therapy. Am J Gastroenterol 2005; 100:2426–30.

99. Glimelius B, Hoffman K, Sjoden PO et al. Chemotherapy improves survival and quality of life in advanced pancreatic and biliary cancer. Ann Oncol 1996; 7:593–600.

100. Daines WP, Rajagopalan V, Grossbard ML et al. Gallbladder and biliary tract carcinoma: a comprehensive update, Part 2. Oncology (Williston Park) 2004; 1:1049–59; discussion 1060, 1065–6, 1068.

101. Fong Y, Blumgart LH, Lin E. Outcome of treatment for distal bile duct cancer. Br J Surg 1996; 83:1712–5.

102. Wade TP, Prasad CN, Virgo KS et al. Experience with distal bile duct cancers in U.S. Veterans Affairs hospitals: 1987–1991. J Surg Oncol 1997; 64:242–5.

103. Yeo CJ, Cameron JL, Sohn TA et al. Six hundred fifty consecutive pancreaticoduodenectomies in the 1990s: pathology, complications, and outcomes. Ann Surg 1997; 226:248–57; discussion 257–60.

104. Way LW. Biliary tract. Current surgical diagnosis and treatment, 10th edn. Norwalk: Appleton & Lange, 1994; pp. 537–66.

105. Georgopoulos SK, Schwartz LH, Jarnagin WR et al. Comparison of magnetic resonance and endoscopic retrograde cholangiopancreatography in malignant pancreaticobiliary obstruction. Arch Surg 1999; 134:1002–7.

106. Ryan ME. Cytologic brushings of ductal lesions during ERCP. Gastrointest Endosc 1991; 37:139–42.

107. Maetani Y, Itoh K, Watanabe C et al. MR imaging of intrahepatic cholangiocarcinoma with pathologic correlation. Am J Roentgenol 2001; 176:1499–507.

108. Lim JH. Cholangiocarcinoma: morphologic classification according to growth pattern and imaging findings. Am J Roentgenol 2003; 181:819–27.

109. Weber SM, Jarnagin WR, Klimstra D et al. Intrahepatic cholangiocarcinoma: resectability, recurrence pattern, and outcomes. J Am Coll Surg 2001; 193:384–91.

110. Schlinkert RT, Nagorney DM, Van Heerden JA et al. Intrahepatic cholangiocarcinoma: clinical aspects, pathology and treatment. HPB Surg 1992; 5:95–101; discussion 101–2.

111. Ringe B, Canelo R, Lorf T. Liver transplantation for primary liver cancer. Transpl Proc 1996; 28:1174–5.

112. Falkson G, MacIntyre JM, Moertel CG. Eastern Cooperative Oncology Group experience with chemotherapy for inoperable gallbladder and bile duct cancer. Cancer 1984; 54:965–9.

113. Lazcano-Ponce EC, Miquel JF, Munoz N et al. Epidemiology and molecular pathology of gallbladder cancer. Cancer J Clin 2001; 51:349–64.

114. Serra I, Diehl AK. Number and size of stones in patients with asymptomatic and symptomatic gallstones and gallbladder carcinoma. J Gastrointest Surg 2002; 6:272–3; author reply 273.

115. Kozuka S, Tsubone N, Yasui A et al. Relation of adenoma to carcinoma in the gallbladder. Cancer 1982; 50:2226–34.

116. Fong Y, Malhotra S. Gallbladder cancer: recent advances and current guidelines for surgical therapy. Adv Surg 2001; 35:1–20.

117. Yeh CN, Jan YY, Chao TC et al. Laparoscopic cholecystectomy for polypoid lesions of the gallbladder: a clinicopathologic study. Surg Laparosc Endosc Percutan Tech 2001; 11:176–81.

118. Buckles DC, Lindor KD, Larusso NF et al. In primary sclerosing cholangitis, gallbladder polyps are frequently malignant. Am J Gastroenterol 2002; 97:1138–42.

119. Yang HL, Sun YG, Wang Z. Polypoid lesions of the gallbladder: diagnosis and indications for surgery. Br J Surg 1992; 79:227–9.

120. Stephen AE, Berger DL. Carcinoma in the porcelain gallbladder: a relationship revisited. Surgery 2001; 129:699–703.

121. Kwon AH, Inui H, Matsui Y et al. Laparoscopic cholecystectomy in patients with porcelain gallbladder based on the preoperative ultrasound findings. Hepatogastroenterology 2004; 51:950–3.

122. Adson M. Advances in diagnosis and surgical treatment of biliary tract disease. New York: Masson, 1983.

123. Bartlett DL, Fong Y, Fortner JG et al. Long-term results after resection for gallbladder cancer. Implications for staging and management. Ann Surg 1996; 224:639–46.

124. Henson DE, Albores-Saavedra J, Corle D. Carcinoma of the gallbladder. Histologic types, stage of disease, grade, and survival rates. Cancer 1992; 70:1493–7.

125. Nakamura S, Sakaguchi S, Suzuki S et al. Aggressive surgery for carcinoma of the gallbladder. Surgery 1989; 106:467–73.

126. Shirai Y, Yoshida K, Tsukada K et al. Radical surgery for gallbladder carcinoma. Long-term results. Ann Surg 1992; 216:565–8.

127. Donohue JH, Nagorney DM, Grant CS et al. Carcinoma of the gallbladder. Does radical resection improve outcome? Arch Surg 1990; 125:237–41.

128. Chijiiwa K, Tanaka M. Carcinoma of the gallbladder: an appraisal of surgical resection. Surgery 1994; 115:751–6.

129. Onoyama H, Yamamoto M, Tseng A et al. Extended cholecystectomy for carcinoma of the gallbladder. World J Surg 1995; 19:758–63.

130. Fong Y, Jarnagin W, Blumgart LH. Gallbladder cancer: comparison of patients presenting initially for definitive operation with those presenting after prior noncurative intervention. Ann Surg 2000; 232:557–69.

131. Shirai Y, Yoshida K, Tsukada K et al. Inapparent carcinoma of the gallbladder. An appraisal of a radical second operation after simple cholecystectomy. Ann Surg 1992; 215:326–31.

132. Yamaguchi K, Tsuneyoshi M. Subclinical gallbladder carcinoma. Am J Surg 1992; 163:382–6.

133. Kimura W, Shimada H. A case of gallbladder carcinoma with infiltration into the muscular layer that resulted in relapse and death from metastasis to the liver and lymph nodes. Hepatogastroenterology 1990; 37:86–9.

134. de Aretxabala XA, Roa IS, Burgos LA et al. Curative resection in potentially resectable tumours of the gallbladder. Eur J Surg 1997; 163:419–26.

135. Callery MP, Strasberg SM, Doherty GM et al. Staging laparoscopy with laparoscopic ultrasonography: optimizing resectability in hepatobiliary and pancreatic malignancy. J Am Coll Surg 1997; 185:33–9.

136. Shoup M, Fong Y. Surgical indications and extent of resection in gallbladder cancer. Surg Oncol Clin N Am 2002; 11:985–94.

137. Jarnagin WR, Ruo L, Little SA et al. Patterns of initial disease recurrence after resection of gallbladder carcinoma and hilar cholangiocarcinoma: implications for adjuvant therapeutic strategies. Cancer 2003; 9:1689–700.

138. Kresl JJ, Schild SE, Henning GT et al. Adjuvant external beam radiation therapy with concurrent chemotherapy in the management of gallbladder carcinoma. Int J Radiat Oncol Biol Phys 2002; 52:167–75.

139. Mahe M, Stampfli C, Romestaing P et al. Primary carcinoma of the gall-bladder: potential for external radiation therapy. Radiother Oncol 1994; 33:204–8.

140. Kapoor VK, Pradeep R, Haribhakti SP et al. Intrahepatic segment III cholangiojejunostomy in advanced carcinoma of the gallbladder. Br J Surg 1996; 83:1709–11.

13

Acute pancreatitis

C. Ross Carter
Colin J. McKay
Euan J. Dickson

General description

Acute pancreatitis is a common cause for emergency hospital admission, with approximately 40 cases per year for each 100 000 population in Scotland,[1] Norway and Sweden.[2,3] For unknown reasons, there has been a steady increase in the incidence and a slight reduction in case mortality over the period 1985–94.[1] In approximately 80% of patients, acute pancreatitis is a rapidly-resolving condition requiring little more than analgesia and a short period of intravenous fluid resuscitation with the remainder developing a multisystem illness characterised by a systemic inflammatory response with a variable degree of organ dysfunction.

Pathophysiology

The mechanism by which gallstones trigger an attack of acute pancreatitis has not been clearly defined. The bile reflux theory, proposed by Opie in 1901, suggested that obstruction of the common bile duct/pancreatic duct common channel by a gallstone-induced reflux of bile into the pancreatic duct causes acute pancreatitis. While there is no doubt that passage of and at least transient obstruction by a gallstone is the initial step in biliary acute pancreatitis, there is little evidence that bile reflux is involved. Studies in the opossum, which has a long common channel between common bile duct and pancreatic duct, have demonstrated that obstruction of the pancreatic duct alone, obstruction of the pancreatic duct and common

bile duct separately, and obstruction of the common channel all induce acute pancreatitis of similar severity.

Experimental models have shed some light on the mechanism by which pancreatic duct obstruction induces acute pancreatitis. Pancreatic duct obstruction has been shown to induce activation of pro-enzymes within the acinar cell by intracellular lysosomal enzymes.[4,5] These enzymes are normally segregated within the acinar cell but, in the presence of duct obstruction, mixing of these enzymes occurs by a process termed 'co-localisation'.[6] Hyperstimulation of pancreatic acinar cells with a cholecystokinin (CCK) analogue in vitro induces intracellular activation of trypsinogen by lysosomal enzymes, following which activated trypsin is released into the cytosolic compartment.[4] Recent evidence has demonstrated that these intracellular events are triggered by a rise in intracellular calcium.[7,8]

The mechanism of alcohol-induced acute pancreatitis is less clear, but alcohol has been shown to increase the sensitivity of acinar cells to CCK hyperstimulation, resulting in enhanced intracellular protease activation.[9] Alcohol also influences acinar cell calcium homeostasis, but several alternative theories have been proposed.

Natural history

Acute pancreatitis varies from a mild, self-limiting attack to a severe life-threatening illness and, for this reason, patients are often classified as having either mild or severe acute pancreatitis. This rather simplistic categorisation ignores the wide variety of clinical behaviour that can be observed in these patients but helps to focus attention on the subgroup of patients who develop complications. Several international consensus meetings have examined nomenclature of pancreatitis (Box 13.1),[10-13] the Atlanta meeting clarifying the terminology used in acute pancreatic inflammation with the rejection of terms such as 'phlegmon' and 'infected pseudocyst' in favour of inflammatory mass and abscess. Improved understanding of treatment concepts and the dynamic nature of the pathophysiology has rendered a number of the concepts outlined in the Altlanta Conference outdated and a revision is currently being undertaken.[14]

Within this framework there are different patterns of disease which have emerged. Recent multicentre trials in acute pancreatitis have enabled prospective study of severe acute pancreatitis and several important points have emerged. Firstly, the majority of patients who develop severe acute pancreatitis have evidence of early systemic organ dysfunction. It is exceptional for a patient to have no evidence of organ failure in the first week of illness and to subsequently develop a significant later local complication. Secondly, most patients who develop organ failure have evidence of this at the time of admission or very shortly thereafter.[15,16] Thirdly, while the tendency is for early organ dysfunction to recover without further problems, worsening organ failure is associated with a high mortality.[16,17]

These observations have important implications for patient management. The presence of early organ dysfunction identifies a high-risk group of patients who merit close observation for both early and late clinical complications. In particular, deteriorating organ failure carries a mortality of around 50% and should prompt early involvement of intensive care and consideration of transfer to a specialist unit if possible. The fact that organ dysfunction is present at or shortly after admission in the majority of patients in whom it develops means that efforts should be directed at early recognition of this rather than employing prediction systems of disease severity.

The majority of patients with severe early organ dysfunction will have pancreatic necrosis on computed tomography (CT) scan. A significant proportion (30–40%) of patients with pancreatic necrosis will develop secondary pancreatic infection, usually in the second to third week after admission,[18] which may be associated with a deterioration in organ failure. Patients who have infected pancreatic necrosis complicated by multiple organ failure have a particularly poor prognosis, even with surgical intervention.

Box 13.1 • Definitions

Acute pancreatitis

Acute pancreatitis is an acute inflammatory process of the pancreas, with variable involvement of other regional tissues or remote organ systems.

Mild acute pancreatitis

Mild acute pancreatitis is associated with minimal organ dysfunction and an uneventful recovery. The predominant feature is interstitial oedema of the gland.

Severe acute pancreatitis

Severe acute pancreatitis is associated with organ failure and/or local complication such as necrosis (with infection), pseudocyst or abscess. Most often this is an expression of the development of pancreatic necrosis although patients with oedematous pancreatitis may manifest clinical features of a severe attack.

Systemic inflammatory response syndrome[75]

Response to a variety of severe clinical insults, manifested by two or more of the following conditions:
- Temperature >38 or <360°C
- Heart rate >90 beats/min
- Respiratory rate >20/min or $PaCO_2$ <32 mmHg (<4.3 kPa)
- WBC >12 000 cells/mm^3, <4000 cells/mm^3, or >10% immature (band) forms

Multiple organ dysfunction syndrome[75]

Presence of altered organ function in an acutely ill patient such that homeostasis cannot be maintained without intervention.

An **acute pseudocyst** is a collection of pancreatic juice enclosed in a wall of fibrous or granulation tissue that arises following an attack of acute pancreatitis. Formation of pseudocyst requires 4 or more weeks from the onset of acute pancreatitis.

A **pancreatic abscess** is a circumscribed intra-abdominal collection of pus, usually in proximity to the pancreas, containing little or no pancreatic necrosis, which arises as a consequence of acute pancreatitis.

Diagnosis

In the majority of patients the diagnosis of acute pancreatitis is relatively easy, characterised by a clinical presentation of sudden severe epigastric pain radiating through to the back. Vomiting within the first 24 hours is very frequently severe and contributes to dehydration. The presence of other signs and symptoms such as tachycardia, tachypnoea and circulatory collapse are dependent on the severity of the attack. A raised serum amylase (at least three times upper limit normal) supports the diagnosis

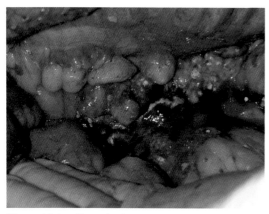

Figure 13.1 • Extensive fat necrosis in the infracolic compartment in a patient with severe acute pancreatitis.

in >95% of cases. Serum amylase estimation may be inaccurate in association with hyperlipidaemia, where a raised urinary amylase can be diagnostic. Serum lipase may be marginally more accurate; however, it is not frequently used in clinical practice. CT can confirm the diagnosis where doubt exists, or in patients with delayed presentation, and rarely the diagnosis is made at laparotomy (**Fig. 13.1**).

Aetiology

Obstructive factors

Biliary disease

The mechanism by which the migration of gallstones results in acute pancreatitis is not fully understood. Transient hold-up or impaction in the ampullary area is associated with between 35% and 65% of episodes of acute pancreatitis in most prospective studies.

Benign pancreatic duct stricture

Following a focal area of necrosis with secondary fibrosis can result in recurrent attacks of pancreatitis. Congenital or developmental anatomical abnormalities can occasionally present with pancreatitis (choledochal cyst, duodenal duplication, anomalous pancreaticobiliary junction). The role of pancreas divisum is probably overstated unless associated with ductal obstruction.

Tumours of the ampulla or pancreas

These can result in ductal obstruction and acute pancreatitis, and should be considered in an older patient where no other cause is identified, particularly if there is an antecedent history of weight loss.

Toxic factors

Alcohol is the second most common aetiology and may predominate in certain populations. The association is usually found in young males who drink in excess of 80 g alcohol per day, but unlike alcoholic liver disease there is no clear dose-dependent increase in risk, and it is likely that other genetic and environmental cofactors are important.

Viral infection, particularly mumps, coxsackie B and viral hepatitis, can cause acute pancreatitis. One clinical feature that may prove useful is prodromal diarrhoea, which is rare in all other types of acute pancreatitis.

Metabolic factors

Hyperparathyroidism may be associated with pancreatitis but is extremely rare (0.1%). Patients with hyperlipoproteinaemia (types I and V) may develop acute pancreatitis, but hyperlipidaemia is more commonly a secondary phenomenon seen during an acute attack.

Genetic defects

Genetic familial defects of the cationic trypsinogen gene[19] (*N29I*, *R117H*) and the cystic fibrosis gene (*CTFR*) may be associated with recurrent pancreatitis, but severe acute inflammatory changes are uncommon.

Trauma

Hyperamylasaemia may occur after blunt abdominal trauma, usually from a crush injury to the body of the pancreas against the vertebral column, and is suggestive of pancreatic injury. Investigation is by contrast-enhanced CT to determine the extent of pancreatic and associated visceral injury.

Iatrogenic causes

Hyperamylasaemia may follow surgical or endoscopic procedures on the panceas, and is usually self-limiting. The risk increases following a therapeutic endoscopic retrograde cholangiopancreatography (ERCP) (3%), especially when a sphincterotomy has been performed, and where a patient has significant symptoms the potential of iatrogenic duodenal perforation should be excluded by a CT scan.

Drug-induced acute pancreatitis[20] may occur following ingestion of a number of drugs; those most commonly implicated are valproic acid, azathioprine, L-asparaginase and corticosteroids. However, unless gallstone disease has been excluded with confidence it is unwise to ascribe acute pancreatitis to a particular drug. Repeat exposure to the same drug again causing acute pancreatitis is the strongest evidence of a direct association.

Inflammatory

Autoimmune pancreatitis is a rare condition, considered part of the IgG4-related autoimmune disease spectrum.[21] This presents as abdominal pain associated with homogeneous gland enlargement with a well-defined edge on CT, an increased IgG4/IgG ratio and a periductal lymphoplasmocytic infiltrate on biopsy. This may also be associated with abnormalities in the extrahepatic biliary tree resembling sclerosis cholangitis and a response to steroids is diagnostic. Focal autoimmune pancreatitis may prove difficult to differentiate from carcinoma. There are established associations with other autoimmune diseases (polyarteritis nodosa, systemic lupus erythematosus, vasculitis) and inflammatory bowel disease (Crohn's and ulcerative colitis), and many are now considered part of the autoimmune spectrum, although only a small proportion appear to have an association with IgG4 serum or tissue abnormalities.

Physiological

Sphincter manometric abnormalities

Type 1 pancreatic sphincter dysfunction[22] may be associated with hyperamylasaemia, associated with abnormalities on sphincter manometry, as part of the global gut dysmotility spectrum, and correction of sphincter spasm may only partly resolve the patient's symptoms. Traditional treatment involves endoscopic sphincterotomy, but the risk of post-ERCP pancreatitis in these patients is extremely high (30%).

Assessment of severity

We have previously described the dynamic nature of organ dysfunction in patients presenting with acute pancreatitis,[17] and for over 30 years, authors have explored ways of 'predicting' those patients with more severe disease. We have also shown that mortality is associated with the development and persistence of organ failure.[23] This had been indirectly shown, if not recognised, 25 years previously with the development of the predictive multifactorial scoring systems – Ranson,[24] Glasgow[25] and APACHE II[26] – which rather than predicting the subsequent development of organ failure, more accurately identified established multisystem organ dysfunction. Their principal use is to remind the inexperienced of the multisystem nature of the disease process, or as a method of stratifying patients within a study protocol.

Single biochemical measures

C-reactive protein (CRP)

The major advantage of CRP is its routine availability in clinical practice. Patients with clinically severe pancreatitis usually have a CRP >200 mg/L, with a practical cut-off being 150 mg/L, but its serum peak is not reached for 36–48 h. Its major use is in monitoring the clinical course during the recovery phase.

Interleukin-6 (IL-6)

Peak levels of IL-6 occur within 24 h and this has aroused interest in its use as a predictor of outcome. IL-6 is a pro-inflammatory cytokine induced by stimuli such as tumour necrosis factor (TNF) and interleukin-1 (IL-1), and two studies have indicated the likely benefit of IL-6 when compared with CRP or phospholipase A. Its major disadvantage is that it is only currently measured in the research setting.

Trypsinogen activation peptide (TAP)

When trypsinogen is activated to form trypsin a small peptide molecule is split off (TAP). A pilot study in 1990 indicated the potential for the measurement of urinary TAP levels as an early predictor of severe acute pancreatitis. More recently a commercially developed enzyme assay has been produced and the initial clinical study of this was encouraging. Unfortunately, a follow-up study looking primarily at admission levels of urinary TAP did not find this to be a clinically useful test.[27]

Leucocyte polymorph neutrophil (PMN) elastase

Raised levels of PMN elastase may occur in acute pancreatitis as a manifestation of leucocyte activation. Once again pilot studies in both Spain and Germany confirmed an association with disease severity,[28] but this is not yet a practical approach.

Intra-abdominal hypertension (IAH)

IAH is recognised as a contributing factor to organ dysfunction in the context of a variety of acute abdominal processes. Most of the literature to date focuses on trauma patients, but there is increasing interest in its role in patients with severe acute pancreatitis (SAP). There are data to suggest that raised intra-abdominal pressure (IAP) may be associated with disease severity,[29] organ failure and mortality in SAP.[30] There are, however, no data to suggest improved outcome following surgical decompression for raised IAP in acute pancreatitis, and indeed this may be harmful. At present we cannot advocate monitoring IAP out with a clinical trial.

Repeated clinical assessment

In the absence of clinically useful predictive systems, our own practice is to monitor patients for the development of systemic organ dysfunction by repeated clinical and biochemical assessment. The presence of a systemic inflammatory response syndrome (SIRS; defined as two or more of the following: fever, tachycardia, tachypnoea or leucocytosis) identifies patients at risk of multiple organ dysfunction syndrome (MODS), particularly when three or four SIRS criteria are present or when SIRS persists for 48 h or more after admission. Patients without SIRS at admission are at very low risk. The development of systemic organ dysfunction (usually clinically manifest as hypoxaemia) mandates careful monitoring in a high-dependency or intensive care unit (ICU) environment and worsening respiratory dysfunction or involvement of other systems is associated with a poor prognosis.

Imaging

Role of ultrasound (US)

All patients with acute pancreatitis should have an ultrasonic assessment of the biliary tree within 24 h of admission.[31]

In those with gallstones, the majority will have mild disease, and this will facilitate definitive treatment of cholelithiasis prior to discharge. In the emergency situation, ultrasonography can be difficult due to a number of factors including the presence of intraluminal bowel gas, or lack of patient cooperation. Therefore, in patients with a negative initial US, and no other obvious aetiological factor,

the US should be repeated prior to discharge before a diagnosis of idiopathic acute pancreatitis is made.

Role of CT

CT scanning is a useful adjunct to clarify the diagnosis. In patients with severe acute pancreatitis, particularly when complicated by MODS, early CT helps to exclude other pathology such as intestinal perforation, gut ischaemia or dissecting aortic aneurysm. Dynamic contrast-enhanced CT can be used to assess disease severity (**Fig. 13.2**) and predict the potential for complications.[32] Although not widely used for this purpose clinically in Britain, it is more popular in the USA, Germany and Finland, and can be useful in comparing patient groups in studies. The CT Severity Index (CTSI)[32] combines a score for the radiological pancreatic and peri-pancreatic abnormalities with a weighting for the extent of necrosis. More recently there are reports of perfusion CT, which may be a useful modality for detecting early, subclinical ischaemic changes in the pancreas which then lead to pancreatic necrosis.

Role of magnetic resonance (MR)/magnetic resonance cholangiopancreatography (MRCP)

Magnetic resonance imaging (MRI) offers a realistic alternative to contrast-enhanced CT[33] in the assessment of patients with acute pancreatitis. The avoidance of cumulative radiation exposure, potentially nephrotoxic iodinated contrast media, and the excellent contrast sensitivity and spatial resolution would make it an attractive alternative. Axial T1- and T2-weighted scans produce images analogous to those of CT. Gadolinium contrast enhancement

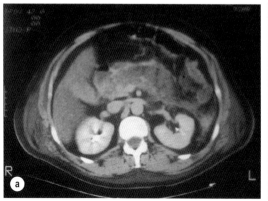
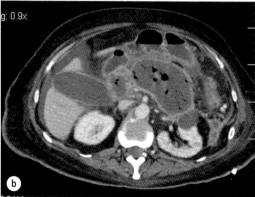

Figure 13.2 • CT scan showing acute pancreatitis with necrosis **(a)** and retroperitoneal gas **(b)**.

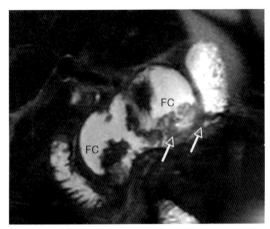

Figure 13.3 • MRI scan showing extensive necrosis (arrowed) within a post-acute fluid collection (FC).

can infer viability and improve anatomical definition. Heavily T2-weighted image acquisition, using a single breath hold and long repetition (TR) and echo (TE) times, results in little signal being produced by solid tissue, and a high signal from static fluid in the biliary and pancreatic ducts, enabling images anatomically comparable to those of ERCP to be produced.

Whilst technically feasible in most centres, the MR environment is unsuitable for patients requiring significant circulatory or respiratory support, and at present few centres have the capability to perform MR-guided intervention. Contrast-enhanced CT therefore remains the imaging modality of choice for assessment and intervention in severe acute pancreatitis. However, MR has a role in the follow-up of acute inflammatory collections, where it is superior to CT in determining the extent of solid material within the collection (**Fig. 13.3**), and the exclusion of choledocholithiasis in suitable patients.

Endoscopic ultrasound (EUS)

EUS has rapidly emerged as an important tool in diagnostic and therapeutic algorithms in patients with acute pancreatitis. Its main areas of use, diagnosis of microlithiasis in idiopathic pancreatitis and the use of linear EUS-guided drainage of peripancreatic collections, are discussed in the relevant sections below.

Management

Initial management

Several guideline documents outlining the management of acute pancreatitis have been published in the last 5 years.[31,34–36]

 The initial management of patients presenting with acute pancreatitis should be directed at the early identification and management of organ failure, most frequently renal and respiratory dysfunction.

At present there are no established end-points of resuscitation to confirm that tissue perfusion and oxygen delivery have been restored adequately in patients with acute pancreatitis. Aggressive fluid resuscitation is often required, and monitoring the response to this relies upon traditional markers, in particular urine output, blood pressure and pulse oximetry. Physiological markers of resuscitation, for example acid–base balance from an arterial blood gas, may be helpful in detecting clinically occult hypoperfusion. Patients who do not respond to initial resuscitation, or who have evidence of organ dysfunction, should be transferred to a critical care environment for more invasive and intensive monitoring with central venous and arterial catheters. Respiratory failure should be treated with humidified oxygen, and this will be guided by continuous pulse oximetry and arterial blood gas analysis. Deteriorating respiratory function is a sign of disease progression and there should be a low threshold for involving the ICU at an early stage. As many as half of all deaths from acute pancreatitis occur in less than 7 days, and the majority of these occur within 72 h of admission.[1] There is evidence that patients managed in specialist institutions have a reduced risk of early death and this may be an indication that management of early MODS could be improved.

Supportive management

 All patients with severe pancreatitis should be managed within a high-dependency/intensive care environment with the potential for organ support.[36]

Where possible, these patients should be managed by a designated multidisciplinary team who have an interest in pancreatico-biliary pathology. Facilities should be available for patients to undergo ERCP/sphincterotomy when indicated (see below). Management of these patients is complex and should be discussed with a specialist unit at an early stage. Specific measures will be determined by the clinical situation. However, therapeutic interventions are aimed at restoring tissue perfusion as rapidly as possible. This is achieved initially with volume resuscitation titrated to haemodynamic and physiological response, rather than the early use of vasopressors or inotropes in patients who are still intravascularly deplete. Acute dialysis for acidosis has not been shown to improve outcome but is required for established renal failure. Currently there is no specific therapy to reverse respiratory failure other than ventilatory support.

Specific medical management

There have been many attempts to introduce specific medical treatments for acute pancreatitis and these broadly fall into the following categories.

Prevention of infection

In patients who survive the early, systemic complications of acute pancreatitis, secondary infection of pancreatic necrosis is the most important late complication. Infection occurs in 30–40% of patients with a minimum 30% pancreatic necrosis[37] and is responsible for the majority of late deaths from acute pancreatitis. Secondary infection manifests as escalating sepsis or a deterioration in organ failure scores, usually in the second (36%) and third (71%) weeks of the illness.[18]

Two meta-analyses from 2006 came to differing conclusions, one supporting prophylaxis, the other showing limited benefit. A Cochrane review[38] of five published studies including 294 patients found a significant reduction in mortality with antibiotic prophylaxis (odds ratio 0.37; 95% CI 0.17–0.83). A reduction in the incidence of infected pancreatic necrosis was only seen with β-lactam antibiotics.

 The most recent meta-analysis,[39] the first to include the results from the Dellinger trial, concluded that prophylactic antibiotics cannot reduce infected pancreatic necrosis and mortality in patients with acute necrotising pancreatitis.

These conflicting conclusions are due to variations in methodology, data inclusion and treatment regimen. At present the decision to use prophylactic antibiotics is based on personal preference rather than evidence base, and further well-designed trials were required.

 Prophylactic antibiotics are not recommended as part of standard management of acute pancreatitis, and where used should be for a defined period.

Nutritional support

There are two main, and very separate, considerations in determining the mode of nutritional support. Acute pancreatitis is a profoundly catabolic and prolonged illness, and there is no doubt that throughout the illness, nutritional integrity should be maintained – the question in these patients is not whether nutritional support is necessary, but rather how it can be best administered.

The second consideration relates to the potential of modulating the disease process by the mode of delivery, either through maintenance of host defences or through the use of immunomodulating feeds. The first issue is a practical problem faced by clinicians on a daily basis, the second remains somewhat speculative, with interesting but inconclusive evidence so far. These will be dealt with separately.

Nutritional delivery in the acute pancreatitis patient

The key study in this regard was the randomised study of Kalfarentzos et al. in 1996, who randomised 38 patients with severe acute pancreatitis to total parenteral nutrition (TPN) or nasojejunal feeding.[40] Six other studies have also shown a benefit for enteral nutrition, a consistent finding being a reduction in TPN associated side-effects and cost, rather than any reduction in pancreas-specific morbidity.

All of these studies utilised enteral feeding distal to the duodeno-jejunal flexure. More recently, three randomised studies, the first from our own group in Glasgow[41] (nasogastric vs. nasojejunal), from Lund (TPN vs. nasogastric), and the most recent from New Dehli (nasogastric vs. nasojejunal), have shown feeding into the stomach, proximal to the ligament of Treitz, to be a practical alternative to jejunal feeding.

 Nutritional support should be by the enteral route where possible.

Disease modulation through content or mode of delivery

There has been interest in the role of the intestine in the pathophysiology of multiple organ failure in critical illness, with loss of gut barrier function potentially leading to endotoxaemia and the systemic inflammatory response syndrome (SIRS). In a small study from Leeds,[42] the authors reported a reduction in the inflammatory response and organ failure showed in those receiving enteral support, but unfortunately there were only 13 patients with severe disease, limiting the validity of the conclusions. There have been several trials comparing so-called 'immunonutrition' with standard enteral feed in critically ill patients, with promising results. Similarly there is great interest in the role of 'probiotics', but enhanced feeding has not been conclusively shown to be associated with improved outcome in patients with acute pancreatitis[43] and until this evidence exists, enhanced feeding should remain within a study context.

Inhibition of pancreatic secretion

Pharmacological attempts to suppress pancreatic function have included intravenous glucagon, somatostatin and, more recently, the somatostatin analogue octreotide. There have now been five randomised trials of octreotide in the management of acute pancreatitis reported in the literature.[44–46] On the basis of the available literature there is no justification for the use of octreotide in acute pancreatitis.

Inhibition of pancreatic enzymes

Several studies evaluated the concept of supporting the endogenous antiprotease defence mechanisms. Double-blind randomised trials of i.v. aprotinin (Trasylol) and gabexate mesilate and a meta-analysis[47] showed no advantage over placebo. Intraperitoneal aprotinin also failed to show any benefit.[48] The use of both low- and high-dose fresh frozen plasma (FFP) proved unhelpful.

Inhibition of the inflammatory response

Following initial promising results with the platelet activating factor antagonist, lexipafant, a multicentre, randomised, placebo-controlled study of anticytokine therapy recruited 1518 patients. This study recruited only those patients with symptoms of less than 48 h duration and was restricted to those with predicted severe attacks. Not only was there no difference in mortality between groups, the incidence of local complications, length of ICU stay, hospital stay and change in organ failure scores were all similar in the three study groups.

The potential for other agents which modify the inflammatory response or to influence outcome in acute pancreatitis has only been assessed in experimental models.

Role of ERCP

There have now been three published randomised trials addressing this issue, and four smaller studies. Contradicting an earlier Cochrane review,[49] the most recent meta-analysis[50] has shown early ERCP in patients with either predicted mild or severe acute biliary pancreatitis without acute cholangitis did not lead to a significant reduction in the risk of overall complications and mortality. There is no role for urgent ERCP in patients with mild disease. All patients with jaundice who exhibit signs of severe acute pancreatitis should undergo urgent ERCP and sphincterotomy as cholangitis may coexist with acute pancreatitis and hyperamylasaemia, but there appears to be little role outside this scenario.

In the non-jaundiced patient there is no role for urgent ERCP and sphincterotomy.

Definitive management issues

The definitive management issues may be considered as being those designed to prevent further attacks once a mild attack has subsided, and secondly those specifically related to the management of early and late complications.

Prevention of recurrent acute pancreatitis

Management of gallstones

The timing of cholecystectomy will obviously depend on the clinical situation. In patients recovering from mild acute biliary pancreatitis, definitive management of the gallstones to prevent a further attack should ideally be achieved during the same admission, and certainly **no later than 4 weeks** following discharge from hospital.[36] This will normally involve a cholecystectomy (laparoscopic or open) **with** intraoperative cholangiography, or alternatively duct imaging by MRCP followed by cholecystectomy. Elderly patients or those with significant medical comorbidity may be managed by an endoscopic sphincterotomy, although this may not be as effective as definitive surgery in preventing further attacks.

In severe acute pancreatitis, interval cholecystectomy should be performed when the inflammatory process has subsided and the procedure is potentially easier.[36]

Definitive management of cholelithiasis should be achieved within 4 weeks of discharge from hospital.

Investigation of non-gallstone-associated pancreatitis

Following resolution of an attack of acute pancreatitis, an assessment of potential aetiological factors is an important aspect of care, and a diagnosis of idiopathic pancreatitis should be made in less than 20% of patients.[36] Evaluation of the initial acute attack should include an adequate history (alcohol/drugs/familial), biochemical (liver function tests/lipids (hypertriglyceridaemia)/calcium) and biliary ultrasound. Patients in whom no cause is identified following these investigations should be considered for EUS, as a cause will be identified in the majority of cases.[51] If these investigations are normal, axial imaging (CT or MR/MRCP) and possibly ERCP may be appropriate to exclude a mechanical cause. A cholecystectomy or biliary sphincterotomy is justified in patients with recurrent idiopathic pancreatitis in whom microlithiasis or biliary sludge is identified. With the increasing use of EUS in these patients, it is increasingly recognised that many of these patients will have changes consistent with early chronic pancreatitis,[51] rather than biliary microlithiasis as suggested by earlier studies. The prevalence of microlithiasis appears to be higher in regions where gallstone disease is the predominant aetiology.

Peripancreatic fluid collections

Management of an early fluid collection

In the early stages of acute pancreatitis, up to 25% of patients with acute pancreatitis will develop a fluid collection in the peripancreatic area identifiable on CT scan. In themselves, these collections are of little significance and require no intervention. There are significant risks associated with aspiration and especially external drainage, in particular the development of secondary infection,[52] and as these interventions are of no benefit they cannot be recommended.

 Simple aspiration of sterile acute fluid collections should be discouraged.

Management of pseudocyst

Management of pseudocysts is determined by an understanding of the anatomy (based on CT), the degree of necrosis (MR/EUS) and the clinical condition of the patient. As a general rule definitive management should be delayed until all organ dysfunction has resolved and can often be performed simultaneously with management of cholelithiasis (see above).

In our experience, it is helpful to characterise pseudocysts associated with acute pancreatitis as either fluid predominant or necrosis predominant.

In each case the collection may be sterile or infected and associated with varying degrees of systemic disturbance. The size of the collection and its relationship to adjacent structures, in particular the stomach, are also important factors to consider when considering treatment options.

Asymptomatic pseudocysts do not require treatment. Acute pseudocysts are most commonly retrogastric, and may or may not link to a disrupted pancreatic duct. Three-quarters will be associated with a mild to moderate hyperamylasaemia. In symptomatic cysts, a conservative policy may be warranted for up to 12 weeks from the onset of acute pancreatitis as up to 50% of these may resolve.[53] This policy is not, however, without risk as pseudocyst rupture or abscess formation may occur. The likelihood of resolution is related, at least in part, to pseudocyst size. Should conservative treatment fail the options are percutaneous, endoscopic or surgical drainage.

Percutaneous drainage

Results of percutaneous drainage suggest wide variation in success (40–96%[54]) and the introduction of infection is a risk that must be considered. In practical terms, the risk of pancreatic fistula limits this approach and there is evidence that it can make subsequent surgical intervention more hazardous if this becomes necessary.[55] In our practice we restrict the use of percutaneous drainage to occasional patients with infected, fluid-predominant collections, particularly where there is a degree of systemic organ dysfunction.

Endoscopic drainage

The technique of endoscopic cystgastrostomy as first described by Baron et al.,[56] initially by blind puncture of a cyst bulging into the stomach wall using side-viewing endoscopes, has been subsequently refined using endoscopic ultrasound guidance. Where disruption of the pancreatic duct has occurred, transpapillary duct stenting can aid resolution. The presence of necrosis should be considered a relative contraindication to simple drainage techniques as drain blockage and secondary infection are common.

Surgical drainage

For patients in whom endoscopic drainage fails, simple surgical drainage is rarely an option and most patients require some form of resection, most commonly a distal pancreatectomy. Primary surgical drainage may be the most appropriate intervention in selected patients, particularly for patients with large, necrosis-predominant collections without infection or systemic organ dysfunction. This can be readily achieved by a laparoscopic, transgastric procedure and allows simultaneous laparoscopic cholecystectomy where appropriate.

Symptomatic or persistent pseudocysts following acute pancreatitis should be managed in a specialist unit where the full range of interventional procedures is available.

 Failure of percutaneous or endoscopic management is associated with the need for complex surgery and should therefore only be undertaken by or following consultation with a pancreatic specialist.[55]

Pancreatic duct fistula

This complication most commonly follows prior intervention for pseudocyst or infected necrosis, and manifests as persistent drainage of amylase-rich opalescent fluid, in the absence of significant sepsis. Management is similar to that of a communicating pseudocyst, initially by transpapillary stenting where possible. Intraperitoneal rupture of a pseudocyst can result in pancreatic ascites or pleural effusion. More invasive management of a persistent fistula, either inaccessible or failing to respond to ductal stenting, should be delayed until the patient has made a full recovery, and often requires surgical resection (distal pancreatectomy) of an isolated functional tail following central glandular necrosis.

Management of necrosis

The management algorithm surrounding necrotising pancreatitis has altered radically in the last 15 years in response to evolving concepts, improved understanding and the development of minimally invasive techniques, including percutaneous necrosectomy, laparoscopic or EUS guided cystgastrostomy as an alternative to conventional open debridement. A multidisciplinary approach has evolved, and it is now common for several techniques to be utilised in a single patient, as the indications and clinical condition of the patient alter during that period.

The development of secondary septic complications is the usual initiator demanding invasive treatment. The choice of intervention technique is underpinned by an understanding of the dynamic evolution of post-acute, necrosis-associated collections in pancreatitis. The aim of intervention is the 'adequate and maintained control of sepsis', and the success of various approaches will be dependent on the anatomical position and particularly the ratio of solid to fluid components within the collection.

The process of maturation or 'organisation', with separation and partial liquefaction of the solid components within a collection, takes in excess of 12 weeks to complete, during which four stages can be recognised:

1. True pancreatic necrosis – minimal separation of devitalised tissue with a high solid/fluid ratio.
2. Transitional pancreatic necrosis with partial but incomplete separation.
3. Organised pancreatic necrosis (OPN) – good separation of devitalised tissue within a fluid-filled cavity and formation of a fibrous wall lined with granulation tissue.
4. Pseudocyst – almost complete resolution of any solid component and a well-formed fibrous wall lined with granulation tissue.

Management of pancreatic or peripancreatic necrosis

The necrotic process associated with pancreatitis tends to involve both the pancreatic parenchyma and surrounding adipose tissue. Indeed, significant quantities of necrotic peripancreatic tissue can be present with an essentially viable gland. Complications relate to the extent of the necrotic

process, and in particular the extent of parenchymal necrosis. Early aggressive debridement in the absence of infection has been advocated. However, mortality in this series was 25% overall, and the only randomised study of early versus late (>12 days) necrosectomy was discontinued as a result of the mortality rate in the early treatment group (56% vs. 27%).[57] The general principle is now to withhold surgery in the early phase of disease, operating for complications ideally once the acute inflammatory insult has subsided.

There is no role for early surgical intervention other than for the management of complications.

Management of sterile necrosis

The development of retroperitoneal necrosis secondary to acute pancreatitis is not in itself an indication for intervention. Both Bradley and Buchler and colleagues have shown that necrosis can be adequately treated by conservative means.[58] There is debate regarding the role of debridement in patients failing to respond to conservative treatment. Early debridement does not improve outcome; however, some specialists advocate debridement in patients with static organ dysfunction after several weeks, but this may also be detrimental.[59] The majority of sterile postinflammatory fluid collections progress into organised pancreatic necrosis, which can be managed with low morbidity and mortality, and our policy is to delay intervention where possible. The management of these patients is discussed in the section dealing with fluid collections associated with necrosis.

Sterile necrosis should initially be treated conservatively where possible, allowing delayed definitive treatment.

Identification of infection/role of fine-needle aspiration

In the 1990s, the identification of secondary infection within necrosis was considered the cornerstone of management,[60,61] as it was thought infected necrosis mandated radical surgical intervention. The presence of a persistent SIRS response made clinical differentiation difficult and this led to CT- or US-guided fine-needle aspiration (FNA) of the pancreatic or peripancreatic collections as a diagnostic test. This remains the policy in some centres.

Our own approach has progressed from one based on the presence or absence of infection to one based on organ dysfunction. Infected collections, even those containing gas, may be observed provided the patient is clinically well and recovering with conservative treatment. Patients with profound organ dysfunction in whom we suspect secondary infection will undergo percutaneous drainage of peripancreatic collections, with later staged percutaneous or open management of the necrosis as clinically appropriate, and we no longer perform diagnostic FNA. Decision-making in these patients is extremely difficult and is best carried out within an experienced multidisciplinary team.

Management of infected necrosis (early phase 2–6 weeks)

Infected pancreatic necrosis has been described as the most feared surgical complication of acute pancreatitis. It occurs in 8–12% of patients with acute pancreatitis, and up to 70% with necrotising pancreatitis and in these patients mortality without intervention approaches 100%.

Methods of necrosectomy

Laparotomy/debridement The technique of pancreatic debridement involves a wide exposure of the abdomen, usually through a bilateral subcostal/rooftop incision. Both colonic flexures are mobilised to expose the retroperitoneum and the lesser sac entered via the gastrocolic omentum, or occasionally the transverse mesocolon. Pus is aspirated from the abscess cavity, leaving the solid component behind, which is then removed by 'blunt finger' dissection (**Fig. 13.4**). Tissue which will not come away by finger teasing should be left in situ to demarcate and subsequent removal at a further procedure. The procedure may also include a cholecystectomy, operative cholangiogram and a feeding jejunostomy.

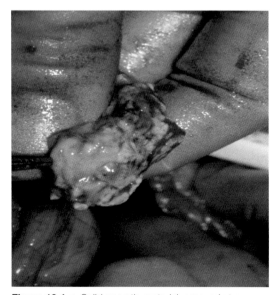

Figure 13.4 • Solid necrotic material removed at open necrosectomy by blunt finger dissection.

Methods for postoperative management of the debridement cavity after laparotomy are as follows:

- **With drainage/'closed packing'.** Simple drainage, often with multiple retroperitoneal tube drains, was the conventional approach to the postoperative management of the debrided pancreatic and peripancreatic bed. Whilst mortality was less than with resective procedures, multiple second-look laparotomies were often required for residual sepsis. The initial results reported by Warshaw and colleagues reported respectable mortality figures of 24% using this technique. Their technique has been modified[62] using multiple soft Penrose drains containing cotton gauze to pack the cavity following completion of the necrosectomy. These are subsequently removed at intervals, allowing the cavity to collapse around the drains. Their reported mortality rate using this technique is the lowest in the literature (6.2%), although the series included patients with sterile necrosis (11%) and pancreatic abscess (39%), and only 14% had both sepsis syndrome and a positive culture requiring early intervention, which is indicative of the difficulties in interpretation of the available literature.

- **With open packing.** Bradley and colleagues from Atlanta have been the principle proponents of the open laparostomy technique.[63] In this, at the conclusion of the debridement, the lesser sac is packed with lubricated cotton gauze and the abdomen left open, allowing planned re-explorations every few days until granulation tissue forms. Enteric fistula and secondary haemorrhage are not uncommon, and the technique is rarely performed as a first option. Surgical packing and planned re-operation is, however, sometimes required to control blood loss from the retroperitoneum following the development of an intraoperative coagulopathy, a lavage system being created, following correction of the coagulopathy, at the time of subsequent pack removal.

- **With closed lavage.** Postoperative closed lavage as described by Beger et al.[64] is the most popular method for postoperative sepsis control following open debridement, the aim of the lavage being the continuous removal of devitalised necrotic material and bacteria. Several (4–6) large-diameter tube drains are inserted in the lesser sac and throughout the abdomen, and the abdomen closed. Continuous lavage is then commenced, our own preference being for CAPD dialysis fluid (Dianil 7, Baxter Healthcare, potassium free, Iso-osmolar) warmed through a blood warmer and delivered at 500 mL/h. The lavage is continued, for around 3–4 weeks on average, until the return fluid is clear and the patient has no residual signs of systemic sepsis. This technique has been adopted with minor variations by centres on both sides of the Atlantic.[16,58,65,66]

Minimally invasive approaches to infected necrosis
Minimally invasive surgery has been shown consistently to be associated with a lesser activation of the inflammatory response than equivalent open surgery and there is experimental evidence suggesting that local sepsis and the inflammatory response may be lessened by a minimally invasive rather than an open technique. It has been suggested that by minimising the massive inflammatory 'hit' of open pancreatic necrosectomy, a minimally invasive approach to the management of infected pancreatic necrosis may lessen the risk of multiple organ failure, and lessen respiratory and wound morbidity in these patients.

- **Percutaneous drainage.** Freeny and colleagues,[67] combining aggressive CT-guided percutaneous drainage with continous post-drainage lavage, showed that nearly half the pancreatic abscesses may resolve. However, more than half of these patients required subsequent surgical intervention for residual sepsis. Drain occlusion is common due to necrotic debris and the use of small-diameter drains.
- **Endoscopic drainage.** In 1996, Baron et al.[56] described a variation on this approach, combining endoscopic cyst-gastrostomy with naso-cyst lavage and reported good results in an initial series of 11 patients. Three-quarters of the patients had pseudocysts rather than abscesses (only 28% were infected at the time of drainage), at a median of 7 weeks following the onset of their illness. Postprocedure infection of the necrotic tissue occurred in 38% of the patients requiring further intervention, highlighting the need for removal of necrotic tissue from the abscess cavity. Solid debris

preventing drainage was again a problem, and 60% of those patients successfully drained developed further collections in the subsequent 2 years. Recent reports of endoscopic necrosectomy for infected pancreatic necrosis suggest a growing enthusiasm for these approaches but so far experience is limited to highly selected cases.[68]

- **Minimally invasive surgery.** Simple percutaneous or endoscopic drainage alone rarely result in complete resolution; however, they may have a useful role as a temporising measure in the hope of finding a 'window of opportunity' in which to perform more definitive intervention. Careful drain management is required to recognise drain blockage early and prevent recurrent sepsis. As a result of the difficulties in maintaining drain patency, we in Glasgow have developed a technique[69] to allow minimally invasive drainage, and in addition removal of the necrotic component. This involves the intraoperative dilatation of a previously placed CT-guided percutaneous drain tract and subsequent necrosectomy using a urological rigid rod lens system (**Fig. 13.5**). Complete resolution of sepsis and necrosis can occur without recourse to further surgery, and the need for postoperative organ support lessened compared to the open procedures,[70] and within our own patient cohort, this technique has significantly reduced mortality. The principle of tract dilatation and minimally invasive necrosectomy has also been used

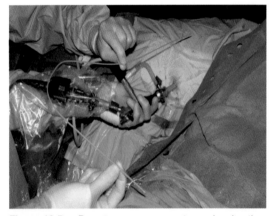

Figure 13.5 • Percutaneous necrosectomy showing the rod lens scope and a guiding catheter to ensure accurate drain placement.

with the endoscopic approach. Seifert et al.[71] have reported the dilatation of the endo-cyst-gastrotomy tract, allowing insertion of the endoscope into the retroperitoneum and subsequent piecemeal debridement, and the VARD variation[72] of the Fagniez technique is another alternative. In this, a small 5-cm incision is made in the left flank, allowing a video-assisted removal of necrotic material, and this technique is currently under comparative evaluation in the PANTER trial – the results are awaited.

Management of pancreatic abscess

A pancreatic abscess by definition is an infected, fluid-predominant acute collection (pseudocyst) with little or no necrosis, and is therefore suitable for minimally invasive drainage. The endoscopic technique of Baron described above has been used in this situation with reasonably good effect, but there is a significant risk of haemorrhage from blind puncture of the abscess wall. An EUS-guided technique has been described, and reported resolution of sepsis in nearly 90%.[73]

Specific late complications

Haemorrhage

Life-threatening haemorrhage may rarely occur acutely into pancreatic necrosis within the first week following presentation and requires mesenteric embolisation or surgical exploration. Haemorrhage is, however, a relatively common problem following prior necrosectomy as a post-operative reactionary haemorrhage due to a combination of a large raw surface, partly controlled sepsis and exposed major vessels, leading to pseudoaneurysm formation (**Fig. 13.6**). Urgent operative intervention and surgical control may be required sometimes necessitating ligation of proximal visceral vessels. However, the combination of haemorrhage and subsequent laparotomy frequently precipitate escalating organ failure and death. Angiography and embolisation, with endovascular metal coils, is therefore the treatment of choice.

Segmental portal hypertension and gastrointestinal haemorrhage

Splenic vein thrombosis is associated with up to 15% patients dying with acute pancreatitis. In those patients with thrombosis that survive the acute attack, the splenic venous drainage diverted through the short gastric vessels may result in patients developing

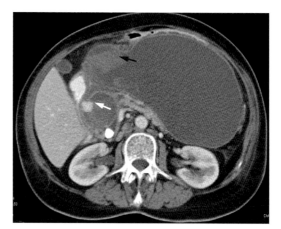

Figure 13.6 • CT scan showing large acute fluid collection with a pseudoaneurysm (indicated by white arrow) and haematoma (black arrow) within the collection.

large venous collaterals. Short gastric and lienocolic varices may make surgery on late complications of an acute pancreatitic episode hazardous. When necessary, splenectomy is curative. Despite the frequency of venous collaterals on follow-up CT, late gastrointestinal haemorrhage through gastric varices is rare in practice.

Pancreatic duct stricture

Pancreatic duct stricture can occur following resolution of an acute attack of acute pancreatitis as a result of local tissue damage and fibrotic repair. It may be present on its own, or in association with a duct disruption causing a pseudocyst or pancreatic fistula. Isolated pancreatic duct stricture can result in recurrent attacks of abdominal pain, sometimes with hyperamylasaemia and with dilatation of the distal duct system. Management of the stricture may be by simple dilatation and temporary stenting, by surgical resection of the stricture along with the pancreatic tail, or by surgical drainage of the pancreatic duct system into a Roux loop.

Gastric outlet obstruction

Gastric outlet obstruction resulting in persistent vomiting or high-volume gastric aspirates from nasogastric suction may complicate up to 10% of patients with severe acute pancreatitis. The recent trend towards nasojejunal intubation has rendered this complication less troublesome and the majority of patients can be treated by nasoenteric feeding until the local oedema/ileus settles. Occasionally a gastroenterostomy is required for longstanding gastric stasis.

References

1. McKay CJ, Evans S, Sinclair M et al. High early mortality rate from acute pancreatitis in Scotland, 1984–1995. Br J Surg 1999; 86:1302–5.

2. Appelros S, Borgstrom A. Incidence, aetiology and mortality rate of acute pancreatitis over 10 years in a defined urban population in Sweden. Br J Surg 1999; 86:465–70.

3. Halvorsen F-A, Ritland S. Acute pancreatitis in Buskerud County, Norway: incidence and etiology. Scand J Gastrol 1996; 31:411–14.

4. Hofbauer B, Saluja AK, Lerch MM et al. Intra-acinar cell activation of trypsinogen during caerulein-induced pancreatitis in rats. Am J Physiol 1998; 275:352–62.

5. Ohshio G, Saluja A, Steer ML. Effects of short-term pancreatic duct obstruction in rats. Gastroenterology 1991; 100:196–202.

6. Steer ML. Early events in acute pancreatitis. Baillière's Best Pract Clin Gastroenterol 1999; 13:213–25.

7. Saluja AK, Bhagat L, Lee HS et al. Secretagogue-induced digestive enzyme activation and cell injury in rat pancreatic acini. Am J Physiol 1999; 276:G835–42.

8. Raraty MGT, Petersen OH, Sutton R et al. Intracellular free ionized calcium in the pathogenesis of acute pancreatitis. Baillière's Best Pract Clin Gastroenterol 1999; 13:241–51.

9. Katz M, Carangelo R, Miller LJ et al. Effect of ethanol on cholecystokinin-stimulated zymogen conversion in pancreatic acinar cells. Am J Physiol 1996; 270:G171–5.

10. Sarles H. Proposal adopted unanimously by the participants of the symposium on pancreatitis at Marseilles, 1963. Bibl Gastroenterol 1965; 7:VII–VIII.

11. Sarner M, Cotton P. Classification of pancreatitis. Gut 1984; 25:756–9.

12. Singer P, Gyr K, Sarles H. Revised classification of pancreatitis. Gastroenterology 1985; 89:683–5.

13. Bradley EL. International Symposium on Acute Pancreatitis AAS1. A clinically based classification system for acute pancreatitis. Arch Surg 1993; 128:586–90.

14. Bollen TL, van Santvoort HC, Besselink MG et al. The Atlanta Classification of acute pancreatitis revisited. Br J Surg 2008; 95:6–21.

15. McKay CJ, Curran F, Sharples C et al. Prospective placebo-controlled randomized trial of lexipafant in predicted severe acute pancreatitis. Br J Surg 1997; 84:1239–43.

16. Isenmann R, Rau B, Beger HG. Early severe acute pancreatitis: characteristics of a new subgroup. Pancreas 2001; 22:274–8.

17. Buter A, Imrie CW, Carter CR et al. Dynamic nature of early organ dysfunction determines outcome in acute pancreatitis. Br J Surg 2002; 89:298–302.

18. Beger HG, Bittner R, Block S et al. Bacterial contamination of pancreatic necrosis. A prospective clinical study. Gastroenterology 1986; 91:433–8.

19. Whitcomb DC, Ulrich CD. Hereditary pancreatitis: new insights, new directions. Baillière's Best Pract Clin Gastroenterol 1999; 13:253–63.

20. Underwood TW, Frye CB. Drug induced pancreatitis. Clin Pharm 1993; 12:440–448.

21. Chari ST. Current concepts in the treatment of autoimmune pancreatitis. JOP 2007; 8:1–3.

22. Hogan WJ, Geenen JE, Dodds WJ. Dysmotility disturbances of the biliary tract: classification, diagnosis, and treatment. Semin Liver Dis 1987; 7:302–10.

23. McKay CJ, Buter A. Natural history of organ failure in acute pancreatitis. Pancreatology 2003; 3:111–14.

24. Ranson HJC, Rifkind KM, Roses DF et al. Prognostic signs and the role of operative management in acute pancreatitis. Surg Gynaecol Obstet 1974; 139:69–81.

25. Blamey SL, Imrie CW, O'Neill J. Prognostic factors in acute pancreatitis. Gut 1984; 25:1340–6.

26. Wilson C, Heath DI, Imrie CW. Prediction of outcome in acute pancreatitis: a comparative study of APACHE II, clinical assessment and multiple factor scoring systems. Br J Surg 1990; 77:1260–4.

27. Johnson CD, Lempinen M, Imrie CW et al. Urinary trypsinogen activation peptide as a marker of severe acute pancreatitis. Br J Surg 2004; 91:1027–33.

28. Uhl W, Beger HG. Prediction of severity in acute pancreatitis. HPB Surg 1991; 5:61–4.

29. Al Bahrani AZ, Abid GH, Holt A et al. Clinical relevance of intra-abdominal hypertension in patients with severe acute pancreatitis. Pancreas 2008; 36:39–43.

30. Zhang WF, Ni YL, Cai L et al. Intra-abdominal pressure monitoring in predicting outcome of patients with severe acute pancreatitis. Hepatobiliary Pancreat Dis Int 2007; 6:420–3.

31. Glazer G, Mann DV. United Kingdom Guidelines in the management of acute pancreatitis. Gut 1998; 42(Suppl 2):S1–13.

32. Balthazar EJ, Robinson DL, Megibow AJ et al. Acute pancreatitis: value of CT in establishing prognosis. Radiology 1990; 174:331–6.

33. Viremouneix L, Monneuse O, Gautier G et al. Prospective evaluation of nonenhanced MR imaging in acute pancreatitis. J Magn Reson Imaging 2007; 26:331–8.

34. Dervenis C, Johnson CD, Bassi C et al. Diagnosis, objective assessment of severity, and management of acute pancreatitis. Santorini consensus conference. Int J Pancreatol 1999; 25:195–210.

35. Uhl W, Warshaw A, Imrie C et al. IAP Guidelines for the surgical management of acute pancreatitis. Pancreatology 1903; 2:565–73.

36. Johnson CD et al. UK guidelines for the management of acute pancreatitis. Gut 2005; 54(Suppl 3):iii1–9.

37. Beger HG, Rau B, Mayer J et al. Natural course of acute pancreatitis. World J Surg 1997; 21:130–5.

38. Villatoro E, Bassi C, Larvin M. Antibiotic therapy for prophylaxis against infection of pancreatic necrosis in acute pancreatitis. Cochrane Database Syst Rev 2006; 4:CD002941.

39. Bai Y, Gao J, Zou DW et al. Prophylactic antibiotics cannot reduce infected pancreatic necrosis and mortality in acute necrotizing pancreatitis: evidence from a meta-analysis of randomized controlled trials. Am J Gastroenterol 2008; 103:104–10.
Most recent meta-analysis of antibiotic prophylaxis.

40. Kalfarentzos F, Kehagias J, Mead N et al. Enteral nutrition is superior to parenteral nutrition in severe acute pancreatitis: Results of a randomized prospective trial. Br J Surg 1997; 84:1665–9.
Key randomised trial since supported by six others.

41. Eatock FC, Chong P, Menezes N et al. A randomized study of early nasogastric versus nasojejunal feeding in severe acute pancreatitis. Am J Gastroenterol 2005; 100:432–9.

42. Windsor ACJ, Kanwar S, Li AGK et al. Compared with parenteral nutrition, enteral feeding attenuates the acute phase response and improves disease severity in acute pancreatitis. Gut 1998; 42:431–5.

43. Pearce CB, Sadek SA, Walters AM et al. A double-blind, randomised, controlled trial to study the effects of an enteral feed supplemented with glutamine, arginine, and omega-3 fatty acid in predicted acute severe pancreatitis. JOP 2006; 7:361–71.

44. Karakoyunlar O, Sivrel F, Tanir N et al. High dose octreotide in the management of acute pancreatitis. Hepato-Gastroenterology 1999; 46:1968–72.

45. McKay C, Baxter J, Imrie C. A randomized, controlled trial of octreotide in the management of patients with acute pancreatitis. Int J Pancreatol 1997; 21:13–19.

46. Uhl W, Buchler MW, Malfertheiner P et al. A randomised double blind multicentre trial of octreotide in moderate to severe acute pancreatitis. Gut 1999; 45:97–104.

47. Messori A, Rampazzo R, Scroccaro G et al. Effectiveness of gabexate mesilate in acute pancreatitis A meta-analysis. Dig Dis Sci 1995; 40:734.

48. Larvin M, Wilson C, Heath D et al. A prospective multcenter randomised trial of intraperitoneal anti-protease therapy for acute pancreatitis. Gastroenterology 1992; 102:274 (abstr).

49. Ayub K, Imada R, Slavin J. Endoscopic retrograde cholangiopancreatography in gallstone-associated acute pancreatitis. Cochrane Database Syst Rev 2004; 4:CD003630.

50. Petrov MS, van Santvoort HC, Besselink MG et al. Early endoscopic retrograde cholangiopancreatography versus conservative management in acute biliary pancreatitis without cholangitis: a meta-analysis of randomized trials. Ann Surg 2008; 247:250–7.
Most recent meta-analysis of the role of ERCP.

51. Yusoff IF, Raymond G, Sahai AV. A prospective comparison of the yield of EUS in primary vs recurrent

idiopathic acute pancreatitis. Gastrointest Endosc 2004; 60:673–8.

52. Imrie CW, Shearer MG. The diagnosis and management of pancreatic pseudocyst. In: Johnson CD, Imrie CW (eds) Pancreatic disease. Springer, 1991; pp. 299–309.

53. Shearer MG, Imrie CW. Spontaneous resolution of pancreatic pseudocysts. Digestion 1990; 46:177–8.

54. Bhattacharya D, Ammori BJ. Minimally invasive approaches to the management of pancreatic pseudocysts: review of the literature. Surg Laparosc Endosc Percutan Tech 2003; 13:141–8.

55. Nealon WH, Walser E. Surgical management of complications associated with percutaneous and/or endoscopic management of pseudocyst of the pancreas. Ann Surg 2005; 241:948–57.

56. Baron TH, Thaggard WG, Morgan DE et al. Endoscopic therapy for organised pancreatic necrosis. Gastroenterology 1996;755–64.

57. Meir J, Luque-de Leon E, Castillo A et al. Early versus late necrosectomy in severe necrotising pancreatitis. Am J Surg 1997; 173:71–5.

The only randomised trial of early surgery.

58. Buchler MW, Gloor B, Muller CA et al. Acute necrotizing pancreatitis: treatment strategy according to the status of infection. Ann Surg 2000; 232:619–26.

59. Uomo G, Visconti M, Manes G et al. Nonsurgical treatment of acute necrotizing pancreatitis. Pancreas 1996; 12:142–8.

60. Rau B, Pralle U, Mayer JM et al. Role of ultrasonographically guided fine-needle aspiration cytology in the diagnosis of infected pancreatic necrosis. Br J Surg 1998; 85:179–84.

61. Gerzof SG, Banks PA, Robbins AH et al. Early diagnosis of pancreatic infection by computer tomography aspiration. Gastroenterology 1987; 93:1315–20.

62. Fernandez-Del CC, Warshaw AL, Rattner DW. Closed packing and drainage following debridement for necrotizing pancreatitis. Problems Gen Surg 1996; 13:126–30.

63. Bradley EL III. Management of infected pancreatitis necrosis by open drainage. Ann Surg 1987; 206:542–50.

64. Beger HG, Buchler M, Bittner R et al. Necrosectomy and postoperative local lavage in necrotizing pancreatitis. Br J Surg 1988; 75:207–12.

65. Branum G, Galloway J, Hirchowitz W et al. Pancreatic necrosis: results of necrosectomy, packing, and ultimate closure over drains. Ann Surg 1998; 227(6):870–7.

66. Larvin M, Chalmers AG, Robinson PJ et al. Debridement and closed cavity irrigation for the treatment of pancreatic necrosis. Br J Surg 1989; 76:465–71.

67. Freeny PC, Hauptmann E, Althaus SJ et al. Percutaneous CT-guided catheter drainage of infected acute necrotizing pancreatitis: techniques and results. Am J Roentgenol 1998; 170:969–75.

68. Charnley RM, Lochan R, Gray H et al. Endoscopic necrosectomy as primary therapy in the management of infected pancreatic necrosis. Endoscopy 2006; 38:925–8.

69. Carter CR, McKay CJ, Imrie CW. Percutaneous necrosectomy and sinus tract endoscopy in the management of infected pancreatic necrosis: an initial experience. Ann Surg 2000; 232:175–80.

70. Connor S, Ghaneh P, Raraty M et al. Minimally invasive retroperitoneal pancreatic necrosectomy. Dig Surg 2003; 20:270–7.

71. Seifert H, Faust D, Schmitt T et al. Transmural drainage of cystic peripancreatic lesions with a new large-channel echo endoscope. Endoscopy 2001; 33:1022–6.

72. Horvath KD, Kao LS, Wherry KL et al. A technique for laparoscopic-assisted percutaneous drainage of infected pancreatic necrosis and pancreatic abscess. Surg Endosc 2001; 15:1221–5.

73. Giovannini M, Pesenti C, Rolland AL et al. Endoscopic ultrasound-guided drainage of pancreatic pseudocysts or pancreatic abscesses using a therapeutic echo endoscope. Endoscopy 2001; 33:473–7.

74. Bone RC, Balk RA, Cerra FB et al. Definitions for sepsis and organ failure and guidelines for the use of innovative therapies in sepsis. The ACCP/SCCM Consensus Conference Committee. American College of Chest Physicians/Society of Critical Care Medicine. Chest 1992; 101:1644–55.

14

Chronic pancreatitis

Philippus C. Bornman

Incidence

The incidence of chronic pancreatitis is on the rise in countries where alcohol is the predominant aetiological factor and where the annual consumption per capita is on the increase. However, accurate epidemiological studies on the frequency of the disease are sparse due to the difficulties in confirming the diagnosis during the early stages of the disease, differences in classification and lack of systematic post-mortem data. In one prospective study performed in the city of Copenhagen,[1] the incidence was 13 per 100 000 inhabitants, which is in keeping with reports from Europe and North America.

Aetiology (Box 14.1)

Alcohol

Alcohol accounts for 60–70% of cases of chronic pancreatitis in the Western world. The precise level of daily alcohol consumption at which patients are at risk for developing chronic pancreatitis has not been clearly established but it is estimated at 60–80 g per day, although individual sensitivity to the toxic effects of alcohol varies. Women are at greater risk as are non-Caucasians when compared to their Caucasian counterparts.[2] Tobacco smoking is now recognised as a compounding factor[3] and also accelerates the progression of the disease.[4]

Labelling patients as having 'alcohol-induced' pancreatitis may have serious implications for medical benefit cover and life insurance policies. Robust criteria should therefore be used before implicating alcohol as the dominant aetiological factor.[5] A number

of objective criteria can be used, ranging from the simpler Paddington Alcohol Test (PAT)[6] to the more complex WHO AUDIT questionnaire (www.who-int/sustance_abuse/publications/alcohol/en/). When they cannot be applied, a serum carbohydrate-deficient transferrin (CDT) measurement may be performed.[7]

 Alcohol remains the most common cause of chronic pancreatitis in Western countries. These patients should be strongly advised to abstain from its use as well as tobacco smoking, which enhances progression of the disease. It is important to use objective criteria before implicating alcohol as the cause of pancreatitis.

Idiopathic chronic pancreatitis

In 10–30% of patients, no obvious aetiological factor is identified, but recent evidence suggests that cystic fibrosis transmembrane conductance regulator (CFTR) gene mutations occur in 20–33% of these patients. Patients with these gene mutations may be more susceptible to alcohol-induced pancreatitis.

Tropical pancreatitis

This form of pancreatitis is noted for the calcific changes in the pancreas which are prevalent in a number of countries situated within 15° of the Equator. These include Indonesia, Asia, Africa, South America and the south-western state of Kerala in India.[8] Protein-calorie malnutrition or childhood kwashiorkor was thought to be the main aetiological factor, but malnutrition is more likely to be the result of the disease. Cyanogenetic glycosides in

Alcohol 60–70%
Idiopathic 20–30%
Tropical
Obstructive
Autoimmune
Miscellaneous

cassava agents (*Manihot esculenta*)[9] deficient in methionine and trace elements such as zinc and selenium have been implicated as the possible damaging substances which interfere with the action of free radical scavengers such as superoxide dismutase.

Hereditary chronic pancreatitis

Hereditary diseases of the pancreas are divided into those presenting with mainly exocrine pancreatic insufficiency and those with acute or chronic pancreatitis as the first manifestation. Associated diseases include cystic fibrosis, α-antitrypsin deficiency and inborn errors of metabolism, and these have an autosomal dominant trait with apparently complete penetrance but variable expression.[10] These patients have a 53-fold increased risk of developing pancreatic ductal adenocarcinoma,[11] which is greatest after 40 years of age.

Patients with unexplained acute or chronic pancreatitis for which no causative factor has been identified or with a history in a first- or second-degree relative should undergo genetic studies.

Obstructive pancreatitis

Obstruction to the pancreatic duct is now recognised as a distinct form of chronic pancreatitis, and is seen in patients with duct disruption from an acute attack of pancreatitis, trauma, ductal adenocarcinoma and, now increasingly recognised, intraductal papillary mucinous neoplasia (IPMN). Congenital anomalies such as pancreas divisum have also been implicated but the causal relationship remains tenuous at best in chronic pancreatitis.[12]

Autoimmune pancreatitis

In recent years, a form of chronic pancreatitis with associated elevated IgG levels and/or detected auto-antibodies has been recognised.[13] The autoimmune nature of this condition is supported by the good response to steroid therapy.

Miscellaneous

Hypercalcaemia associated with hyperparathyroidism and chronic renal failure can rarely give rise to both acute and chronic pancreatitis. Other rare causes include drugs such as phenacetin, antihypertensive and anticonvulsant drugs. Stress, caused by increased energy expenditure during work amongst low social classes, has also been implicated.[8]

Pathobiology of alcohol-induced pancreatitis

The mechanism by which alcohol induces pancreatitis remains uncertain and has recently been extensively reviewed.[14,15] There is increasing evidence that alcohol causes damage to the pancreatic acinar cells via different and complex pathways, one of which is through the transient formation of fatty acid ethanol esters (FAEEs). The precise mechanism is not well established yet, but possibilities include the generation of oxygen-derived free radicals from acetaldehyde, the formation of protein-rich secretory plugs leading to duct obstruction and disruptions of the calcium signalling, to name but a few.

The most widely accepted hypothesis is the so-called 'necrosis–inflammation–fibrosis' sequence[14] (**Fig. 14.1**). An important factor is an intracellular inflammatory response by way of upregulation signalling systems that mediate the production of inflammatory cytokines/chemokines and other inflammatory molecules. The inflammatory response involving mainly macrophages and T lymphocytes appears to play a major role in causing pancreatic tissue destruction. Genetic abnormalities, such as those regulating trypsinogen activation/inactivation and CFTR, have also been implicated.[16]

The main contributing factor in the fibrotic process seen in chronic pancreatitis is the activation of pancreatic stellate cells[17] by alcohol similar to that seen in the liver. Fibrosis is stimulated by cytokines which can be produced and secreted by pancreatic parenchymal cells, inflammatory cells and the pancreatic stellate cells themselves. Alcohol may also cause fibrosis by proteolytic enzymes breaking down extracellular matrix protein through the plasminogen system.

In addition to alcohol and smoking, diets high in protein and fat appear to exacerbate the cause of pancreatitis, while saturated fats and vitamin E may have a protective effect.[18]

With respect to pancreatic stone formation in the calcific form of the disease, it is believed to be the result of decreases in pancreatic bicarbonate and

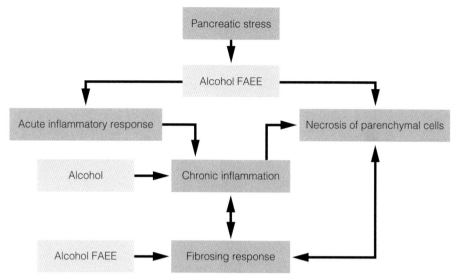

Figure 14.1 • Pathobiological pathways in alcohol-induced pancreatitis. Reproduced from Pandol SJ, Raraty M. Pathobiology of alcoholic pancreatitis. Pancreatology 2007; 7:105–14. With permission from S Karger AG.

water secretion, which in turn results in an increase in protein secretion. There is a disturbed diffusion barrier with increased permeability between interstitial spaces[19] with enhanced diffusion of calcium and proteins into the ducts,[20] where calcium precipitates in the alkaline juice.

Pathology

According to the Marseille classification,[21] chronic pancreatitis is characterised morphologically by irregular sclerosis with destruction and permanent loss of exocrine parenchyma, which may be focal, segmental or diffuse. Oedema and acute inflammation often coexist during acute flare-ups with or without associated necrosis. These changes may be associated with varying degrees of dilatation of the main and side ducts associated with protein plugs and calcification. Intrapancreatic and peripancreatic cysts are common and frequently communicate with the ductal system. There is a general belief that duct dilatation is the result of obstruction by fibrotic strictures and intraductal stones, but the causal relationship remains difficult to prove. It is possible that duct ectasia may develop simultaneously with progressive parenchymal destruction.

There is a subgroup of patients in whom the pancreas is densely sclerosed without duct dilatation.[22] Focal (segmental) pancreatitis is also a recognised entity, sometimes associated with pancreas divisum or groove pancreatitis,[23] where the inflammatory process is confined to the groove between the duodenum, common bile duct and head of the pancreas. These may mimic carcinoma of the pancreas.

Calcification usually indicates advanced disease, and in an appreciable proportion of cases (20–30%) there is an inflammatory mass of the head complicated by bile duct and/or duodenal obstruction (**Fig. 14.2**). Splenic vein thrombosis with segmental portal hypertension is also a recognised complication.

Perineural disintegration and eosinophilic infiltration are typical features and are associated with an increase in mean nerve diameter.[24] These changes and the presence of abnormally large amounts of serotonin and calcitonin gene-related peptide[25] are implicated as important contributing factors to pain.

 There is some conflicting evidence whether patients with non-hereditary chronic pancreatitis and in particular alcohol-induced pancreatitis are at increased risk of developing pancreatic cancer. Lowenfels et al.[26] showed a 16-fold increased risk, while a more recent Swedish cohort study[27] could not provide strong support for a causal association between pancreatitis and pancreatic cancer.

Clinical features

History

Pain is the most important cause of disability in chronic pancreatitis and is responsible for most of the poor quality of life in these patients. The pain presents a heterogeneous pattern ranging from relapsing episodes to persistent pain of varying intensity. There is also a small subgroup of

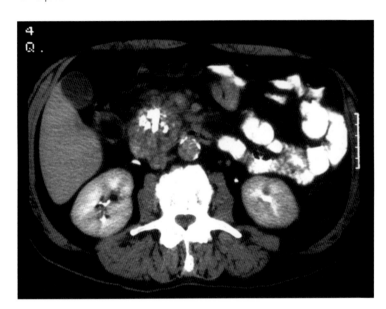

Figure 14.2 • CT scan showing a grossly enlarged and calcified pancreas head.

patients in whom the disease is painless throughout its course, and in these the clinical emphasis is on pancreatic insufficiency. Initially the pain is episodic in nature, with pain-free intervals of varying periods. In alcohol-induced pancreatitis, the recurrent attacks are closely linked to alcohol binges, but with time the pain becomes more persistent and the beneficial effect of alcohol withdrawal becomes less evident.[28]

The pathogenesis of pain in chronic pancreatitis remains an enigma. The cause of pain is multifactorial and may vary at different stages of the disease process.

Causal factors may include:

- the release of excessive oxygen-derived free radicals
- tissue hypoxia and acidosis
- inflammatory infiltration with influx of pain transmitter substances (calcitonin gene-related peptide, substance P and growth-associated protein-43) into damaged nerve ends
- development of pancreatic ductal and tissue fluid hypertension due to morphological changes of the pancreas – the so-called 'compartmental syndrome'
- pancreas-independent, brain-mediated mechanisms in refractory cases,[29] which may explain why some patients continue to experience pain after resection, including those who had a total pancreatectomy.

While there is a tendency for pain to decrease with time,[30] this is by no means predictable nor does this necessarily parallel the development of endocrine and exocrine insufficiency. As with idiopathic pancreatitis,[31] alcohol-induced pancreatitis appears to comprise mild and severe types.[32] Those with mild pain experience intermittent attacks with pain-free intervals responding to conservative treatment and tend to improve with time, whereas those with severe and persistent pain often require surgery for pain relief and complications.

 The so-called burnout syndrome (pain relief with progressive pancreatic insufficiency) is not generally accepted.

Pain is usually felt centrally in the epigastric region or subcostally with radiation to the back or shoulder tip, and is often eased by leaning forward or lying down to one side with knees pulled up, the so-called 'jack-knife' position. Some patients note that the pain is exacerbated by meals or the ingestion of certain foods such as those high in fat. Loss of sleep, time off work and the need for admission to hospital are useful pointers to severity, and it is important to establish whether the pain does significantly impair the patient's quality of life. Assessment of pain can be difficult in these patients, some of whom remain addicted to alcohol and have manipulative personalities.

Progressive pancreatic insufficiency (dysfunction) is a frequent late manifestation of the disease, presenting usually 10–15 years after the clinical onset of the disease. Endocrine and exocrine insufficiency may contribute to the weight loss often observed in these patients, although anorexia, nausea and vomiting may be implicated. Steatorrhoea is recognised as the passage of pale bulky or oily stools, which may be offensive in smell and difficult to flush away. Some patients are incapacitated socially because of this symptom. Patients with diabetes mellitus and chronic pancreatitis are less inclined to the development of retinopathy and diabetic neuropathy, probably due to their shorter life expectancy. Vascular diseases, however, are common with heavy smoking as a major contributing factor.

Pseudocysts are often responsible for exacerbation of pain and may mimic a recurrent acute attack. They may also be responsible for biliary obstruction with jaundice or gastric outlet obstruction. More commonly, jaundice is caused by an inflammatory mass in the head of the pancreas, which may resolve in 30–40% of cases. Duodenal obstruction due to inflammation in the head of the pancreas is uncommon. Rarely, haemorrhage from gastro-oesophageal varices may arise as a consequence of splenic vein thrombosis, or major bleeding may occur from a false aneurysm due to erosion of a pancreatic vessel by adjacent pancreatic enzyme-rich fluid collections. When these collections communicate with the pancreatic duct, haemorrhage will occur via the pancreatic duct and present as an upper gastrointestinal haemorrhage, haemosuccus pancreaticus. There is often a delay in diagnosis of this condition; many patients present with recurrent episodes of upper gastrointestinal bleeding with repeated negative forward-viewing upper gastrointestinal endoscopies. The diagnosis should be suspected when pain is associated with an upper gastrointestinal bleeding against a background of chronic pancreatitis. A side-viewing duodenoscope may detect blood coming from the ampulla but computed tomography (CT) angiography (**Fig. 14.3**) is the most definitive investigation, which may be followed by selective angiography and embolisation of the bleeding site.[33]

Examination

Evidence of weight loss and malnutrition may be present, and mottled burn marks, so-called erythema ab igne, may be associated with the use of heat pads or hotwater bottles (**Fig. 14.4**). Jaundice, a palpable abdominal mass (indicating a pseudocyst) or splenomegaly (pointing to splenic vein thrombosis) may be present. Stigmata of chronic liver disease are unusual in patients with known alcohol-associated pancreatitis. Pancreatic ascites and an isolated pleural effusion are uncommon but typically have an insidious onset. These are often incorrectly attributed to liver decompensation or chronic lung disease respectively. The diagnosis is confirmed when the amylase levels are raised significantly in the ascitic and pleural fluids.

Clinical features of non-alcoholic chronic pancreatitis

Tropical pancreatitis

This is a disease of the young with a male preponderance. Its main clinical features include abdominal pain with distension, calcified pancreatic duct stones, diabetes mellitus, steatorrhoea related to exocrine insufficiency, and early death. The main pancreatic duct is usually grossly dilated and contains large stones (**Fig. 14.5**). There is a higher incidence of pancreatic cancer amongst these patients, with an average age of onset of 45 years.

Idiopathic chronic pancreatitis

As apposed to alcohol, there is an equal gender distribution in idiopathic chronic pancreatitis. There are two distinct forms of idiopathic chronic pancreatitis, namely early-onset (<35 years), which pursues

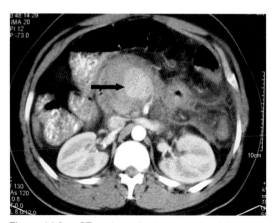

Figure 14.3 • CT angiography demonstrating false aneurysm in the pancreas head.

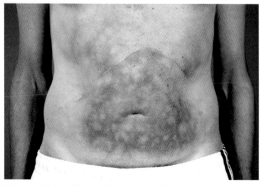

Figure 14.4 • Typical hotwater bottle marks (erythema abigne) in the lower lumbar region.

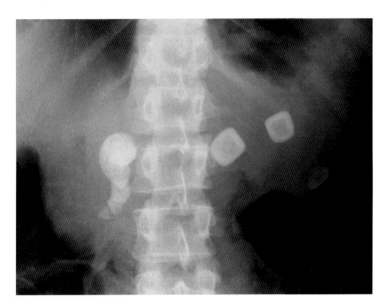

Figure 14.5 • Plain abdominal radiograph showing large pancreatic duct calculi in a patient with tropical pancreatitis.

a long and often severe painful clinical course with slow development of morphological and functional pancreatic damage, and a late-onset type with a mild and often painless clinical course with associated weight loss, exocrine and endocrine insufficiency, and pancreatic calcification.[31] Pancreatic atrophy, functional impairment and morphological change (including calcification) are accepted features of ageing, but it remains unclear whether some patients with late-onset chronic pancreatitis represent an exaggeration of this process.

Hereditary pancreatitis

Hereditary pancreatitis does not normally become manifest until the age of 5–15 years. The onset of the disease may be delayed to the third and fourth decades of life in some patients. The diagnosis should be suspected if several members of a family develop chronic pancreatitis without obvious reason. With their substantial increased risk of developing pancreatic cancer, patients should enter a closer surveillance programme.

Autoimmune pancreatitis

Most patients with this form of pancreatitis are in their sixth decade with a male preponderance. Pain is seldom the dominant symptom and most patients present with painless obstructive jaundice mimicking pancreatic malignancy. Approximately 2% of pancreatic masses resected for suspected malignancy are due to autoimmune pancreatitis.[13] Recent-onset diabetes mellitus occurs in up to 76% of patients. Other associated autoimmune diseases such as Sjogren's syndrome, inflammatory bowel disease and retroperitoneal fibrosis have been reported ranging from 12% to 50%, and may not be detected at the time of the diagnosis of autoimmune pancreatitis.

Investigations

Biochemical and haematological investigation

Serum amylase levels in chronic pancreatitis are usually normal or may be only slightly raised. With biliary tract obstruction liver function tests may demonstrate an obstructive jaundice pattern or, not infrequently, an isolated and disproportionate increase of serum alkaline phosphatase levels. The presence of leucopenia and thrombocytopenia suggests that splenic vein thrombosis may have resulted in hypersplenism. The prothrombin time should be assessed in patients with cholestasis and a random blood glucose level measured to exclude diabetes mellitus.

Patients in whom alcohol is not a clear aetiological factor should undergo extensive investigations before being labelled as idiopathic.[34] In patients with autoimmune pancreatitis, the IgG and in particular its subtype IgG4 will be raised, the latter having a sensitivity and specificity as high as 95–97% respectively. CA19-9 is indicated in patients with suspected pancreatic cancer but it should be noted that levels may be significantly raised in chronic pancreatitis, particularly when associated with jaundice.[35]

With improved imaging, pancreatic function tests[36] are now seldom used in the diagnostic work-up of patients with suspected chronic pancreatitis. Function tests are now mostly reserved when imaging studies are normal or show minimal change.

However, the sensitivities of function tests are insufficient to exclude the diagnosis of chronic pancreatitis when negative.

Imaging studies

Plain abdominal radiography may demonstrate the presence of calcification within the pancreas. The diagnosis is seldom in doubt when there is diffuse calcification but, when localised, other conditions such as pancreatic cancer should be considered. While ultrasound may be useful to detect the presence of biliary dilatation, pancreatic enlargement with duct dilatation or pseudocysts, CT provides better definition of parenchymal and pancreatic

duct morphological changes (**Fig. 14.6**). CT also remains the best imaging modality to define the type and position of cysts and their relationship to adjacent structures (**Fig. 14.7**). Endoscopic retrograde cholangiopancreatography (ERCP) is the most effective method of detecting early chronic pancreatitis and, when combined with ultrasound and CT, a sensitivity of 95–97% and specificity of 100% are obtained to differentiate between chronic pancreatitis and pancreatic cancer.[37] However, in practice it may be difficult to confirm the diagnosis of cancer. Brush cytology at ERCP and fine-needle aspiration cytology have been disappointing and there is an increasing tendency to resect in doubtful cases.[38]

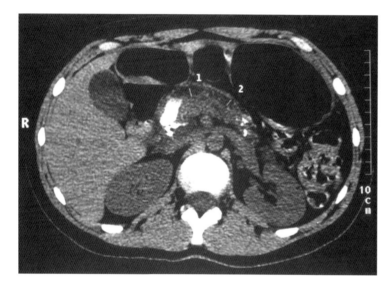

Figure 14.6 • CT scan showing a dilated main pancreatic duct with a large staghorn calculus (labels 1 and 2) in the pancreas head.

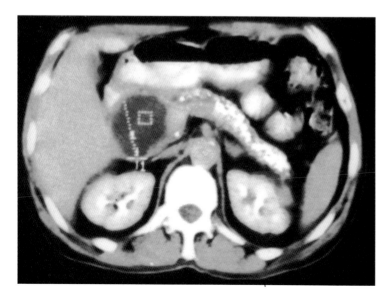

Figure 14.7 • CT scan showing an intrapancreatic cyst in the pancreas head with diffuse calcification in the body and tail.

Endoscopic ultrasound with guided fine-needle aspiration (EUS-FNA) has been used increasingly in specialist centres in patients with suspicious pancreatic lesions. While this test has a high sensitivity (89–95%) in those patients with focal lesions with normal parenchyma, the specificity in those with chronic pancreatitis is disappointingly low.[39]

CT angiography is indicated in cases with suspected bleeding from a false aneurysm and when confirmed should be followed with selective angiography with the view to embolise the bleeding source. Barium studies are usually confined to patients with suspected duodenal stenosis or colonic obstruction. Magnetic resonance cholangiopancreatography (MRCP) (**Fig. 14.8**) is about to replace ERCP (**Fig. 14.9**) as the investigation of choice for demonstrating pancreatic and biliary morphological changes, although detection of minimal ductal changes still eludes the current generation scans.

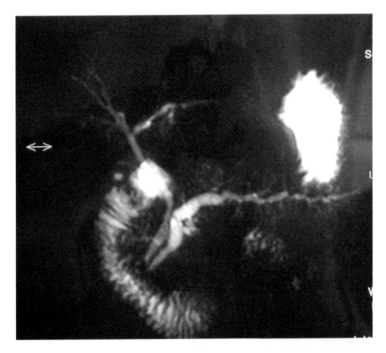

Figure 14.8 • Magnetic resonance cholangiopancreatogram showing clear delineation of both pancreatic and bile ducts.

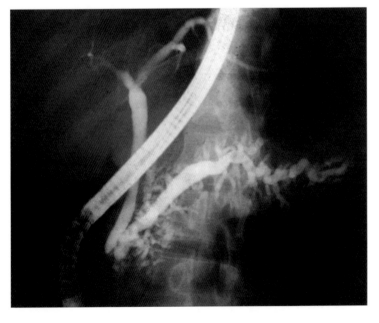

Figure 14.9 • Endoscopic retrograde pancreatogram in a patient with chronic pancreatitis showing irregular areas of narrowing and gross dilatation of the pancreatic duct system.

CT scan and MRCP have become the most appropriate means of demonstrating ductal and morphological abnormalities associated with chronic pancreatitis. While ERCP is now reserved mostly for interventional procedures, it remains the most effective method of detecting early chronic pancreatitis and, when combined with CT scan, will differentiate between chronic pancreatitis and pancreatic cancer in most cases.

Management

Pain control

The selected referral of severe cases to surgical practices may skew the perception that patients with chronic pancreatitis inevitably follow an intractable course with the emphasis on pain. On the contrary, in the majority of patients, symptoms can be managed conservatively for long periods and in some cases indefinitely. Nonetheless, in about half the patients with established chronic pancreatitis, medical treatment, including alcohol withdrawal, fails to control pain by non-narcotic analgesics or prevent the development of complications necessitating surgical intervention. Acute exacerbations of chronic inflammation may produce episodes of severe abdominal pain, often necessitating admission to hospital. The surgeon should resist the temptation to abandon conservative treatment in favour of operation in the face of such acute exacerbations. In the majority of cases, symptoms can be brought under control by hospitalisation and with adequate pain control and enteral or intravenous nutritional support.

Alcohol withdrawal

Patients will require considerable support, which may include counselling, self-help groups and, where necessary, psychiatric treatment. Some patients will attempt to conceal continuing alcohol abuse but it should be noted that while alcohol plays an important role in precipitating acute attacks during the early stages of the disease,[40] the association is less clear among patients with advanced disease[41] and that, in these patients, attacks or persistence of pain may continue despite alcohol withdrawal.

Dietary modifications and pancreatic replacement therapy

In theory, avoidance of a high-fat, high-protein diet should restrict cholecystokinin release and physiological stimulation of the pancreas, but there is no hard evidence that this reduces pain. There has been considerable debate as to whether luminal proteases reduce pancreatic exocrine secretion by a negative feedback mechanism and whether oral enzyme supplements reduce pancreatic pain in addition to combating steatorrhoea.

 Unfortunately, the initial optimism regarding pancreatic replacement therapy has not been substantiated by two placebo-controlled randomised trials.[42,43] Furthermore, similar disappointing results have been reported with the use of octreotide,[44] the most potent suppressing agent of pancreatic secretion. There is little evidence to support this treatment approach in managing chronic pancreatic pain.

Medication

Analgesic requirements vary greatly and there is a plethora of non-opioid and opioid options to choose from which varies from country to country. In principle, opioids should be avoided as this may lead to further addiction. Continuous use of non-steroidal anti-inflammatory drugs (NSAIDs) is also discouraged to avoid their ulcerogenic complications. Input from a multidisciplinary pain clinic is often required with psychiatric and social support. When opioids are required it is advisable to avoid those which are highly addictive such as pethidine. Morphine in one form or another remains the best opioid for long-term pain relief.

Coeliac plexus block

Series on imaging-guided percutaneous coeliac plexus blockade, using a variety of neurolysis agents (e.g. ethanol or phenol), have reported disappointing results for pain control.[45] Endoscopic ultrasound (EUS)-guided coeliac plexus blockade via the posterior wall of the stomach is a recent addition to the list of image-guided techniques and is purported to be safer. In a larger prospective audit on EUS-guided coeliac plexus block,[46] significant improvement in overall pain scores was achieved in 50 (55%) of 90 patients. The follow-up, however, was less than a year, and patients younger than 45 years and those who had previously had pancreatic surgery did not benefit from this treatment.

Video thoracoscopic splanchnicectomy

The emergence of minimal access surgery has rekindled interest in splanchnicectomy for pain control in chronic pancreatitis, particularly in patients with small-duct disease. It has been argued that, unlike coeliac ganglion blocks, splanchnicectomy provides a more complete interruption of the sympathetic nerves that constitute the main pathways for afferent transmission of pancreatic pain. Bilateral thoracoscopic splanchnicectomy is usually recommended, with division of the greater and lesser splanchnic nerves. The procedure is done under general anaesthesia using either a standard or

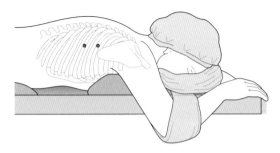

Figure 14.10 • Patient positioned in prone position with port placement in seventh and fifth intercostal spaces, posterior axillary line.

double-lumen endotracheal tube. The patient is placed in the prone position (**Fig. 14.10**). A pneumothorax is introduced with a Veress needle, keeping the pressure below 5 mmHg. This is usually sufficient to expose the operating field. Two ports are used, with the camera port placed in the seventh intercostal space in the posterior axillary line. The dissection port is placed in the fifth intercostal space in the posterior axillary line. The parietal pleura is dissected medial to the main sympathetic chain from the fifth intercostal space to the diaphragmatic recess. All branches along this course are isolated and divided with a hook-diathermy dissector (**Fig. 14.11**). The pneumothorax is evacuated with a combination of suction and positive end-expiratory pressure. The procedure is then repeated on the contralateral side. Postoperative chest radiograph is done when there is any doubt about a residual pneumothorax.

Morbidity and mortality for this procedure are low, but recent series with short- to medium-term follow-up have reported pain relief with variable and sometimes conflicting results.[47–49] For example,

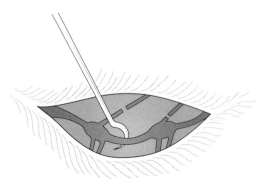

Figure 14.11 • Incision of parietal pleura and division of all sympathetic branches coming off medially from the sympathetic chain.

some reports claim good overall results including patients with dilated pancreatic ducts and an inflammatory mass in the pancreatic head,[48] while others[49] have had disappointing results in these patients. Interpretation of the results is also difficult due to the heterogeneity of the patients (e.g. alcoholic and non-alcoholic), criteria used for successful outcome and variations in technique. It should also be noted that while initial pain relief is encouraging, with time there is often a steady decline in the success rate[48] and a large percentage of patients remain dependent on opioids. Not many studies provide long-term results, which are the ultimate test for success in the treatment of chronic pancreatitis.

Coeliac blockade and thoracoscopic splanchnicectomy have yet to find a niche in the long-term control of pain in chronic pancreatitis.

Management of complications

Biliary obstruction

Obstruction of the biliary tree is common in cases of advanced disease with calcification and when an inflammatory mass is present in the head. The stenosis is usually the tapering type rather than the abrupt cut-off seen in malignant obstruction (**Fig. 14.12**). Obstruction can be caused by oedema, an intrapancreatic pseudocyst or fibrosis, but is seldom complete. The natural history of the obstruction will vary according to the underlying pathology. Jaundice is usually transient when caused by oedema during acute flare-ups. About 20% of patients will present with asymptomatic common duct stenosis, detected only by an isolated raised alkaline phosphatase level or during imaging when patients are investigated for pain. In such patients, deterioration of liver function and the development of secondary biliary cirrhosis is exceptional.[35] Nevertheless, if biliary obstruction persists for longer than 4 weeks, relief should be sought before hepatic sequelae result. Endoscopic insertion of a stent is indicated only as a temporary measure in high-risk patients when associated with cholangitis, since prolonged stenting leads to recurrent blockage, sepsis and possible secondary sclerosing cholangitis. Metal stents in particular should be avoided unless surgery is contraindicated, although newer developments with a removable expandable stent might broaden the indication for endoscopic therapy.

If biliary obstruction is the only complication of chronic pancreatitis, some form of bilioenteric bypass is indicated. Cholecysto-jejunostomy is a poor option as a long-term drainage procedure. Choledocho-duodenostomy or hepatico-jejunostomy utilising a long Roux-en-Y loop can be undertaken although most surgeons prefer the

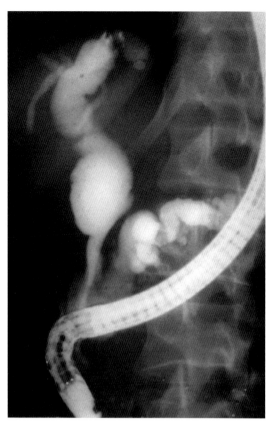

Figure 14.12 • Endoscopic retrograde pancreatogram showing tapering-type stricture of the distal bile duct and a grossly dilated main pancreatic duct.

latter, since this will avoid the possible risk of reflux of enteric contents into the biliary tree and the so-called sump syndrome. It remains uncertain whether isolated biliary obstruction is an important cause of pain, since most patients who require biliary drainage will also undergo a pancreatic drainage procedure for pain, usually in the form of Frey procedure. Some surgeons, however, favour a pylorus-preserving pancreatico-duodenectomy (PPPD) when pain is associated with an inflammatory mass of the pancreas head without pancreatic duct dilatation. PPPD is also indicated when there is concern about an underlying malignancy.

 A proposed management algorithm based on severity of pain, pancreatic parenchymal and ductal abnormalities, and concern for malignancy is outlined in **Fig. 14.13**.

Duodenal obstruction

Some degree of duodenal obstruction is commonly found in chronic pancreatitis during endoscopy or in upper gastrointestinal radiology, but this is seldom a cause of overt gastric outlet obstruction. If isolated duodenal obstruction occurs, this is managed by mobilisation of the duodenum by Kocher's manoeuvre and division of periduodenal fibrosis. Failing this, a duodeno-duodenostomy rather than a gastro-jejunostomy and vagotomy should be undertaken to avoid its attendant sequellae. A resection should be considered when a duodenal obstruction is associated with biliary obstruction, particularly in the presence of an inflammatory mass in the head.

Pseudocyst

Pancreatic and peripancreatic collections occur in some 25–30% of patients with chronic pancreatitis and are frequently associated with gross pancreatic duct abnormalities. Postnecrotic peripancreatic collections rarely occur in patients with established chronic pancreatitis. Cysts when present in the head are mostly intrapancreatic, or located extrapancreatically in the lesser sac region as a complication of duct disruption. In both instances there is a high incidence of communication with the pancreatic duct system. Most of these cysts are mature by the time the diagnosis is made and spontaneous resolution is much less likely than in cases of acute postnecrotic collections. Pancreatic disruption in the tail region may extend in the subcapsular plain of the spleen (**Fig. 14.14**).

Non-operative treatment options and in particular an endoscopic drainage procedure have enjoyed increasing support in the management of pseudocysts. In the context of chronic pancreatitis, simple aspiration or the placement of external drainage catheters is usually inappropriate due to a high failure rate and the potential for development of an external fistula.

Various endoscopic techniques have been employed including transgastric or transduodenal drainage with a needle knife papillotomy with the placement of a stent, or transpapillary stent drainage. The overall success rates are encouraging (65–95%), with a relatively low associated complication rate of 10%.[50] However, long-term results are awaited in terms of recurrence and the need for more formal surgical drainage for pain from associated morphological abnormalities of the pancreas. Nonetheless, this relatively simple method is a worthwhile first option before surgery is contemplated.

It should be stressed that the indications for endoscopic drainage of pseudocysts should not differ from those for surgery. Selection for endoscopic drainage should adhere to the following strict guidelines. Only cysts which are clearly bulging into the bowel lumen and with a wall thickness of less than 10 mm are suitable for endoscopic drainage. Using these criteria, 30–40% of cysts in chronic pancreatitis are suitable for this treatment. CT scanning is essential to determine cyst wall thickness, the

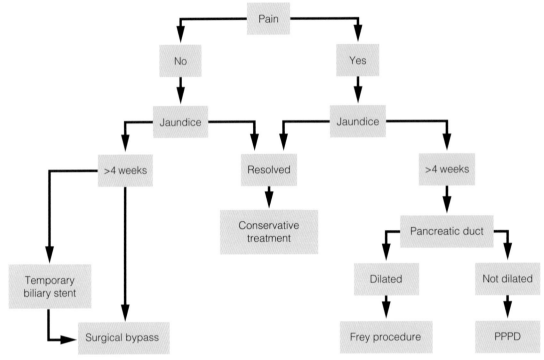

Figure 14.13 • Treatment algorithm for biliary obstruction.

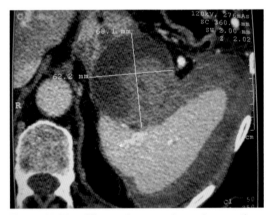

Figure 14.14 • CT scan demonstrating peripancreatic fluid collection extending into the subcapsular plain of the spleen.

relationship of the cyst to the bowel wall and the presence of ascites, which may indicate communication with the peritoneal cavity. CT may also be helpful in excluding the possibility of a cystic tumour. EUS may provide useful additional information in selecting the site of drainage when a bulge is less prominent.[51] ERCP during endoscopic drainage may be difficult due to distortion of the stomach and duodenum. While providing useful information regarding ductal morphology for future

management, the demonstration of a leak or pancreatic duct obstruction has no relevance to the immediate management of the cyst. A diathermy needle knife is used to create a fistula between the gut lumen and the cyst. Using an exchangeable system the needle knife is replaced by a guidewire while the sheath remains within the cyst cavity to avoid losing access. Some authors recommend dilating the tract before placing a pigtail stent. If the cyst cavity is large and contains necrotic material, it is advisable to place several stents to reduce the risk of secondary infection. It is recommended that the stent should remain in place for about 2–3 months to avoid recurrent pseudocyst formation.

The transpapillary route for pseudocyst drainage is usually reserved for pseudocysts in the region of the head but away from the bowel wall. The stent is placed either within the cavity or past the site of the leak. The risk of bleeding and perforation is less than for the transmural approach but secondary infection remains a potential problem.

Surgical drainage is achieved by anastomosing the stomach, duodenum or a Roux-en-Y limb of jejunum at the lowest point of the cyst wall. This latter method has been most popular in Europe. For cysts situated near the tail of the pancreas, resection is often considered, particularly when the spleen is involved. Resection should always be performed when there is a concern about the possibility of a cystic neoplasm.

While endoscopic drainage has become a viable alternative treatment for pseudocysts, surgery remains the most definitive treatment and, when necessary, allows additional drainage procedures or resection.

Pancreatic ascites

Pancreatic ascites and pleural effusion, resulting from rupture of a pseudocyst or pancreatic duct, are rare but potentially serious complications of chronic pancreatitis. Such patients are generally malnourished and hypoalbuminaemia is invariably present, due in part to massive protein losses into the peritoneal cavity. Treatment consists of paracentesis, pleural aspiration and intravenous or enteral nutritional support. There is no convincing proof that the administration of a somatostatin analogue adds to the success of conservative treatment.[52] Resolution on conservative treatment is of the order of 50–60% and usually occurs within 2–3 weeks. When conservative treatment fails, ERCP should be undertaken to identify the site of the leak and successful placement of an endoscopic stent may facilitate resolution of the ascites and pleural effusions.[53] Surgical treatment is now reserved for failures of conservative or endoscopic treatment, which will usually entail a Roux-en-Y jejunostomy limb with or without a pancreatic duct drainage procedure or a distal pancreatic resection when the leak is towards the tail of the pancreas.

Gastrointestinal bleeding

Portal hypertension

Some involvement of the portal venous system is encountered in about 10% of patients presenting with chronic pancreatitis. Involvement ranges from compression to frank occlusion with thrombosis. Splenic vein thrombosis causes segmental portal hypertension and the formation of gastric and oesophageal varices. It has been recommended that thrombosis confined to the splenic vein should be dealt with by distal pancreatectomy and splenectomy before bleeding occurs, but it should be noted that major bleeding from gastric varices in this setting is a rare occurrence. Portal or superior mesenteric venous thrombosis resulting in portal hypertension is considered to be a contraindication to surgical intervention.

Pseudoaneurysms

Erosion of arteries adjacent to pancreatic or peripancreatic enzyme-rich fluid collections may lead to false aneurysms, which may rupture directly into the pancreatic duct, peritoneum or retroperitoneum. When this is suspected, CT angiography will usually demonstrate the false aneurysm, in which case selective angiography with an attempt at embolisation is recommended as the first step in the management. When the head of the pancreas is involved, angiographic embolisation is the treatment of choice to avoid the hazards of major pancreatic resection. This is usually successful for smaller feeding vessels but collateral circulation or large vessel involvement may hamper successful embolisation.[33] When angiographic embolisation fails, a Frey-type procedure (which allows direct access to the bleeding site) is preferred over a resection for aneurysms in the head of the pancreas, while a distal pancreatectomy and splenectomy is recommended for aneurysms in the body and tail region.

Surgical options for pain

Patient selection is as important as the choice of the operative procedure. The decision to undertake surgery should only be made when a full and thorough evaluation of the patient has been made, and the surgeon should not be pressurised into offering surgery until after all factors have been considered. The patient must understand the risks of intervention and be aware that pain may not be relieved. It should also be emphasised that surgical intervention will not reverse the progressive loss of endocrine and exocrine pancreatic function. The timing of surgery is particularly problematic and it is often difficult to find the balance between early operations, which may compromise pancreatic function, and the risk of opioid addiction when conservative treatment is prolonged.

Surgical treatment has, to a large extent, been tailored according to parenchymal and pancreatic ductal morphological changes of the pancreas, and can be divided into pancreatic drainage procedures and some form of resection. Modern imaging, in particular CT scan, has facilitated the selection of the appropriate operation.

Since the 1950s numerous surgical approaches have been devised, ranging from transduodenal sphincteroplasty to total pancreatectomy. Some have fallen into disrepute (e.g. transduodenal sphincteroplasty, caudal pancreatico-jejunostomy and total pancreatectomy) while, more recently, pylorus- or duodenal-preserving resections of the head or the Frey procedure have taken preference to preserve exocrine and endocrine function.

Pancreatic duct drainage procedures

Most surgeons will select some form of drainage procedure when the pancreatic duct is dilated. It is generally recommended that the operation should be performed in patients with pancreatic ducts larger than 7–8 mm in diameter, although others have challenged this restriction. More recently, Izbicki et al.[54] have introduced a modified V-shaped excision of the ventral pancreas with a pancreatico-jejunostomy for ducts smaller than 3 mm in size. In a long-term follow-up study (median 83 months), complete relief of pain was achieved in 22 of 42 patients.[55]

The most commonly performed drainage operation is a lateral pancreatico-jejunostomy, as described by Partington and Rochelle, whereby the drainage is extended well towards the tail and the spleen is preserved (**Fig. 14.15**). The duct should be opened to within 1–2 cm of the splenic hilus, and extended to the head of the gland and, where necessary, into the uncinate process. Intraoperative ultrasonography may be used to locate the duct. Mucosa-to-mucosa apposition can be used as a one-layer continuous suture if the gland overlying the anterior aspect of the duct is thin. However, for most cases, anastomosis to the cut edge is performed when the duct is deeply embedded in an enlarged and inflamed pancreatic parenchyma. It is important to orientate the Roux limb so that its blind end is placed towards the tail of the pancreas, allowing the possibility of using the same limb for anastomosis to the biliary system when this is obstructed. Pseudocysts can also be drained into the same Roux limb without any increase in morbidity or mortality.

Although several series have shown encouraging results, with pain relief in up to 93%, there are other studies where the success rate is appreciably less.[56] Drainage procedures in chronic pancreatitis are based on the concept that ductal obstruction leads to ductal hypertension due to fibrotic strictures, obstructions or stones.[57] A number of studies, however, have shown poor correlation between pain, pancreatic duct obstruction and pressures.[28] This may in part be due to residual tissue pressure from obstructed side ducts which are not relieved by this operation, particularly when there is an inflammatory mass in the head. Thus, in cases with an enlarged inflammatory mass in the head of the pancreas, it is now generally recommended that a Frey procedure[58] (**Fig. 14.16**) should be carried out which will alleviate side-duct obstruction by removal of stones and areas of necrosis. A rim of pancreatic tissue is left between the superior mesenteric vein and the core incision. A similar sliver of pancreatic tissue is preserved along the inner aspect of the duodenum and retroperitoneally. Once this core-out process is complete, the entire open pancreas is anastomosed to a Roux limb of jejunum.

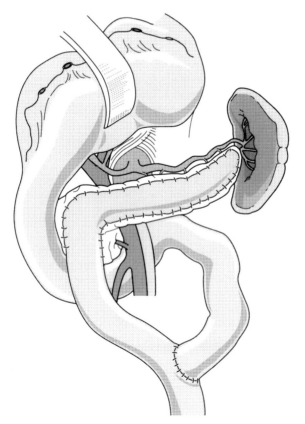

Figure 14.15 • Longitudinal pancreatico-jejunostomy. The pancreatic duct system is opened as widely as possible and anastomosed to a Roux limb of jejunum. Intestinal continuity is restored by an end-to-end jejuno-jejunal anastomosis. The same Roux limb can also be used to drain cystic collections or an obstructed bile duct, and to bypass an obstructed duodenum.

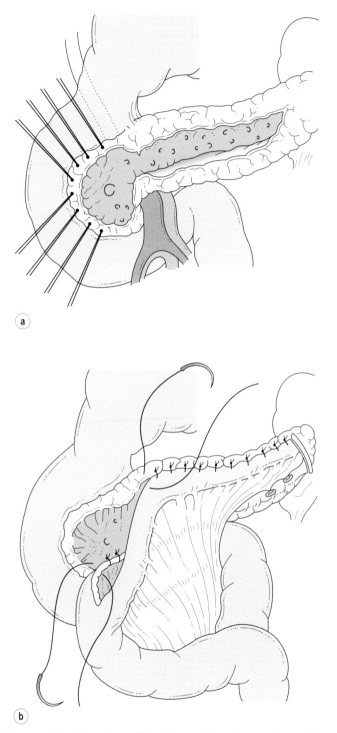

Figure 14.16 • Extended pancreatico-jejunostomy with coning out of head as described by Frey and Mikura.[58]

There are no controlled data available to determine whether this more extensive drainage procedure is better than the standard lateral pancreatico-jejunostomy operation, but when compared to the duodenal-preserving pancreatic head resection operation (Beger procedure) in a controlled study, the results were similar after a 9-year follow-up period.[59]

Pancreatic resection

Chronic pancreatitis generally affects the entire gland, but the temptation to perform a major resection has to be tempered by complications associated with brittle insulin-dependent diabetes and loss of exocrine function. When pancreatitis is confined to the body and tail of the gland a distal pancreatectomy would be appropriate. This procedure would be indicated for the presence of a pseudocyst behind ductal strictures in the body and tail region, and when associated with a false aneurysm or segmental portal hypertension. Distal pancreatectomy has not enjoyed a good reputation because of some series reporting poor pain relief, and the higher risk of developing diabetes mellitus postoperatively is a concern with more extensive resections. Less than an 80% distal pancreatectomy is associated with a 19% incidence of new-onset diabetes mellitus, whereas this rises to 50–80% for an 80–95% distal pancreatectomy.[60] Up to 38% of patients will be troubled by overt steatorrhoea on late follow-up. However, the results seem to be no different from other resections when patients are carefully selected based on ERCP and CT scanning.[61]

The head of the gland will be grossly enlarged by an inflammatory mass in up to 30% of patients with chronic pancreatitis, and is often associated with bile duct and duodenal stenosis.[62] In these patients a Frey procedure or some form of pancreatic head resection is indicated even in the presence of gross pancreatic duct dilatation. The standard Whipple operation has now, to a large extent, been replaced by less radical resections, such as the pylorus-preserving pancreatico-duodenectomy (**Fig. 14.17**) and duodenum-preserving (Beger) pancreatic resection (**Fig. 14.18**). Early reports on the pyloric-preserving resection raised concern about prolonged gastric outlet obstruction and increased risk of duodenal ulceration, but these fears have now been largely allayed.[63]

The duodenal-preserving pancreatic resection popularised by the Ulm group[62] was proposed to cause the least functional disturbances. However, one controlled study[64] and a recent review on the subject[65] were unable to show a clear advantage over

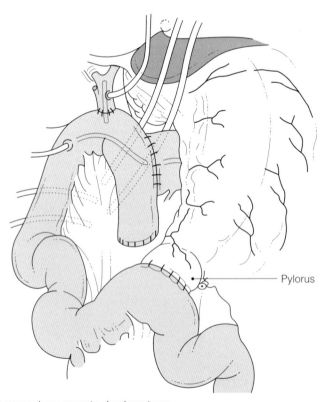

Pylorus

Figure 14.17 • Pylorus-preserving pancreato-duodenectomy.

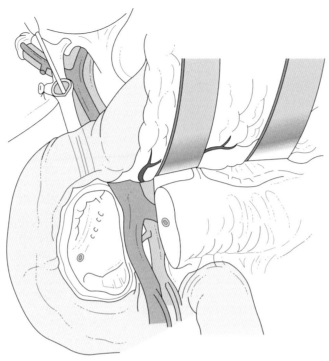

Figure 14.18 • Duodenal-preserving resection of pancreatic head as described by Beger and Imaizumi.[62]

the pylorus-preserving pancreatico-duodenectomy. Long-term results for the lesser resection operations appear to achieve similar pain relief with a tendency to less functional impairment and weight loss.[66]

Generally, patients from lower socio-economic backgrounds tolerate extensive resections and in particular total pancreatectomy poorly, with serious long-term complications due to brittle diabetes, gross steatorrhoea and severe loss of weight rendering them nutritional cripples.

 Surgical strategy is mostly governed by the size of the main pancreatic duct and the presence or absence of an inflammatory mass in the head of the pancreas. There is a paradigm shift away from major pancreatic resections towards the Frey procedure and pyloric- or duodenal-preserving resections to avoid morbidity, long-term sequellae and shortened life expectancy. Pancreatic resection is reserved for localised disease and when there is a suspicion of cancer.

Endoscopic treatment

There have been conflicting reports on the efficacy of endoscopic treatment (sphincterotomy and stenting) with or without extracorporeal lithotripsy in relieving pain in patients with pancreatic duct obstruction due to fibrotic stenosis or stones. Kozarek and Traverso[67] have recently analysed collected experiences of major publications from expert centres and indicated that symptomatic improvement varied greatly from 50% to 85% at 15–25 months.

A recent publication on a large multicentre study by specialised centres has reported encouraging results with a mean follow-up period of almost 5 years.[68] The study included 1018 patients treated for mainly strictures (47%), stones (18%) or a combination (32%). A long-term success rate of 86% was claimed, although this figure was reduced to 65% in an intention-to-treat analysis. While there was no clear difference in the outcome in terms of morphological changes, those patients with intermittent pain fared better than those who had persistent pain. In contrast, another study of 80 patients with chronic pancreatitis found that only 43 (56%) could be treated successfully by extracorporeal lithotripsy followed by endoscopic intervention.[69] Only patients with single stones had successful treatment, but after a mean follow-up of 40 months (24–92) there was no discernible benefit in terms of either pain relief or prevention of progressive glandular insufficiency. In a recent randomised controlled trial, extracorporeal shock-wave lithotripsy (ESWL) provided similar good results to a combination of ESWL and endoscopic treatment, with a significant reduction in cost.[70]

Endoscopic therapy is labour intensive, requires a high degree of expertise and complications occur frequently. These include ERCP-induced acute pancreatitis, bleeding and perforation associated with endoscopic sphincterotomy, and stent-related complications such as occlusion, migration and sepsis. There is also the concern that prolonged stenting may cause ductal and parenchymal injury.[71] Interpreting the results of endoscopic treatment remains problematic. Most studies are retrospective, and assessments of pain severity are often poorly defined. Indeed, in several of the studies pain was intermittent and not severe, suggesting that the outcome may have been similar to conservative treatment.[72]

There are two randomised controlled trials comparing surgery with endoscopic therapy.[73,74] The results of surgery seem to be superior but the interpretation of these two studies is made difficult by the low percentage of patients eligible for inclusion in the studies. Furthermore, in the first study,[73] benefit was only shown in the total group and not in the subgroup of patients who were randomised.

While endoscopic therapy does not provide better results than surgery, it would seem reasonable to offer this less invasive treatment in selected patients with dilated ducts, particularly in those with localised strictures and/or stones.

Steatorrhoea

Fat malabsorption is the most important sequel of exocrine insufficiency in chronic pancreatitis, and as a general rule enzyme replacement is necessary when daily fat excretion exceeds 15 g and/or the patient is losing weight and/or has diarrhoea.[75] The treatment consists of a fat-reducing diet and pancreatic enzyme replacement therapy.

There are numerous pancreatic enzyme preparations available in the form of powder, tablets or capsules. All of the currently available pancreatic enzyme supplements consist of crude extracts of porcine pancreas, known in many countries as pancreatin. The enzymes are inactivated rapidly and irreversibly below pH 5, but more recently enteric-coated microspheres have been developed in which hundreds of individually coated microspheres are contained in a gelatine capsule. Capsules containing microspheres have the advantage of better mixing with the chyme. Under optimal conditions approximately 300 000 IU of lipase is required for each meal. Failure to respond may be due to poor compliance, incorrect diagnosis, incorrect prescription or choice of pancreatic enzyme preparations.

Gastric acid secretion may also influence absorption as lipase activity is inactivated in an acid milieu. This can be prevented by acid reduction with H_2 receptor antagonists, or proton pump inhibitors, or by the use of enteric-coated preparations.

As a general recommendation, pancreatic enzymes should be given in the form of multi-unit acid-protected dosages in patients with proven exocrine insufficiency and normal gastric acid secretion. In those patients who have had previous gastric resections, enzyme substitution should be with granules to ensure adequate mixing and simultaneous transport of enzymes with the chyme. A suggested treatment schema for exocrine pancreatic insufficiency is outlined in **Fig. 14.19**.[75]

Diabetic control may be difficult for patients on oral hypoglycaemic drugs or insulin, particularly if food intake is variable. Lack of endogenous glucagon contributes to a greater sensitivity to insulin and risk of hypoglycaemia, which is a major cause of death in the alcoholic group. Blood glucose control with insulin should therefore be monitored carefully and kept above normoglycaemic levels. However, diabetic ketoacidosis is uncommon in the patient with chronic pancreatitis, since there is usually sufficient insulin secretion to prevent the release of fatty acids from adipose tissue and their subsequent metabolism to ketone bodies in the liver.

Conclusion

Chronic pancreatitis has a mortality rate approaching 50% over 20–25 years. Up to 20% of patients die of complications of the disease, whereas the remainder succumb to problems associated with alcohol abuse, tobacco smoking, malnutrition, infection, diabetes mellitus, insulin overdose and suicide. These patients are at greater risk of death from malignancies, many of which are related to smoking.

It is difficult to interpret the results of the various treatment options for chronic pancreatitis, and in particular that of surgical and endoscopic interventions. Pancreatico-jejunostomy carries a lower operative mortality and morbidity than operations involving major resection of the pancreas. However, it should be recognised that the severity of the disease varies, and those patients who come to some form of resection usually have the more severe form of disease. The generally quoted satisfactory control of pain in up to 75% of patients undergoing pancreatic surgery is similar to claims made in selected cases for endoscopic treatment. The results of all forms of treatment should be interpreted with caution as most studies do not provide sufficient data

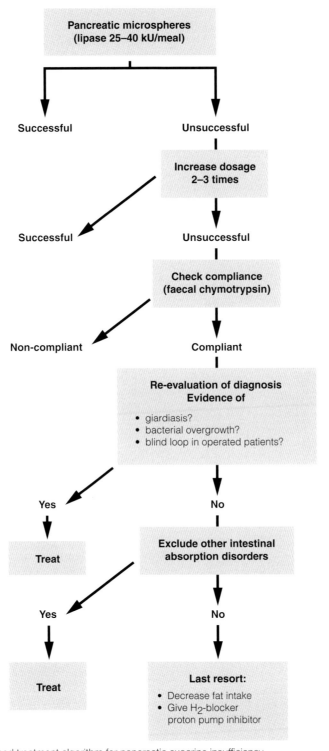

Figure 14.19 • Proposed treatment algorithm for pancreatic exocrine insufficiency.

on objective measurements of success, with few addressing the important aspect of improving quality of life.

Considering the complexity of the disease process in chronic pancreatitis it is not surprising that lack of progress in the understanding of the pathogen-esis of pain and the management thereof have frus-trated the clinician in devising rational medical and surgical treatment strategies. There is a need for standardising basic and clinical research methods to overcome the slow progress in the management of this debilitating disease.

Key points

- Alcohol is the most common causative agent in the development of pancreatitis and abstinence is associated with a more favourable prognosis. Smoking should also be discouraged as this appears to enhance progression of the disease.
- Chronic pancreatitis is associated with a shortened life expectancy mainly due to complications of the disease, poor diabetic control and diseases associated with malnutrition and smoking.
- While endoscopic and radiological interventions have gained an increasing role in the management of complications associated with chronic pancreatitis, their role in controlling pain in uncomplicated cases is limited.
- Minimal access techniques such as thoracoscopic splanchectomy for control of pain have yet to gain widespread acceptance.
- Surgery remains the most definitive treatment for intractable pain, and is governed in the main by the size of the main pancreatic duct and whether an inflammatory mass is present in the head, the goal being to preserve endocrine and exocrine function.
- There is a need to reach agreement on rational medical and surgical strategies for this debilitating disease.

References

1. Copenhagen Pancreatitis Study. An interim report from a prospective epidemiological multicenter study. Scand J Gastroenterol 1981; 16:305–12.

2. Lowenfels AB, Maisonneuve P, Grover H et al. Racial factors and the risk of chronic pancreatitis. Am J Gastroenterol 1999; 94:790–4.

3. Bourliere M, Barthet M, Berthezene P et al. Is tobacco a risk factor for chronic pancreatitis and alcoholic cirrhosis? Gut 1991; 32:1392–5.

4. Maisonneuve P, Lowenfels AB, Müllhaupt B et al. Cigarette smoking accelerates progression of alco-holic chronic pancreatitis. Gut 2005; 54:510–14.

5. Nordback I, Sand J, Andrèn-Sandberg A. Criteria for alcoholic pancreatitis. Results of an International Workshop in Tampere, Finland, June 2006. Pancreatology 2007; 7:100–4.

6. Patton R, Hilton C, Crawford MJ et al. The Paddington alcohol test: a short report. Alcohol Alcoholism 2005; 39:266–8.

7. Jaakkola M, Sillanaukee P, Lof K et al. Blood tests for detection of alcoholic cause of pancreatitis. Lancet 1994; 343:1328–9.

8. Breuer-Katschinski BD, Bracht J, Tietjen-Harms S et al. Physical activity at work and the risk of chronic pancreatitis. Eur J Gastroenterol Hepatol 1996; 8:399–402.

9. Pitchumoni CS. Chronic pancreatitis: a historical and clinical sketch of the pancreas and pancreatitis. Gastroenterologist 1998; 6:24–33.

10. Madrazo-de la Garza GA, Hill ID, Lebenthal E. Hereditary pancreatitis. In: Go VLM, DiMagno EP, Gardner JD et al. (eds) The pancreas: biology, pathobiology and disease, 2nd edn. New York: Raven Press, 1993; pp. 1095–101.

11. Lowenfels AB, Maisonneuve P, DiMagno EP et al. Hereditary pancreatitis and the risk of pancreatic cancer. J Natl Cancer Inst 1997; 89:442–6.

12. Delhaye M, Engelholm L, Cremer M. Pancreas divisum: congenital anatomic variant or anomaly? Contribution of endoscopic retrograde dorsal pan-creatography. Gastroenterology 1985; 89:951–8.

13. Toomey DP, Swan N, Torreggiami W et al. Autoimmune pancreatitis. Br J Surg 2007; 94:1067–74.

14. Pandol SJ, Ratay M. Pathobiology of alcoholic pancreatitis. Pancreatology 2007; 7:105–14.

15. Witt H, Apte MV, Keim V, Wilson JS. Chronic pancreatitis: challenges and advances in pathogenesis, genetics, diagnosis, and therapy. Gastroenterology 2007; 132:1557–73.

16. Cohn JA, Friedman KJ, Noone PG et al. Relation between mutations of the cystic fibrosis gene and idiopathic pancreatitis. N Engl J Med 1998; 339:653–8.

17. Mews P, Phillips P, Korsten M et al. Pancreatic stellate cells respond to inflammatory cytokines: potential role in chronic pancreatitis. Gut 2002; 50:535–41.

18. Lin Y, Tamakoshi A, Hayakawa T et al. Associations of alcohol drinking and nutrient intake with chronic pancreatitis: findings from a case–control study in Japan. Am J Gastroenterol 2001; 96:2622–7.

19. Reber HA, Roberts C, Way LW. The pancreatic duct mucosal barrier. Am J Surg 1979; 137:128–34.

20. Layer P, Hotz J, Schmitz-Moormann HP et al. Effects of experimental chronic hypercalcemia on feline exocrine pancreatic secretion. Gastroenterology 1982; 82:309–16.

21. Singer MW, Gyr K, Sarles H. Revised classification of pancreatitis. Report of the Second International Symposium on the Classification of Pancreatitis in Marseille, France, 28–30 March 1984. Gastroenterology 1985; 89:683–5.

22. Walsh TN, Rodes J, Theis BA et al. Minimal change chronic pancreatitis. Gut 1992; 33:1566–71.

23. Stolte M, Weib W, Vokholz H et al. A special form of segmental pancreatitis: 'groove pancreatitis'. Hepatogastroenterology 1982; 29:198–208.

24. Brokman D, Buchler M, Malfertheiner P et al. Analysis of nerves in chronic pancreatitis. Gastroenterology 1988; 94:1459–69.

25. Di Sebastiano P, Fink T, Weihe E et al. Immune cell infiltration and growth-associated protein 43 expression correlate with pain in chronic pancreatitis. Gastroenterology 1997; 112:1648–55.

26. Lowenfels AB, Maisonneuve P, Cavallini G et al. Pancreatitis and the risk of pancreatic cancer. N Engl J Med 1993; 328:1433–7.

27. Karlson BM, Ekbom A, Josefsson S et al. The risk of pancreatic cancer following pancreatitis: an association due to confounding? Gastroenterology 1997; 587–92.

28. Bornman PC, Marks IN, Girdwood AH et al. Pathogenesis of pain in chronic pancreatitis – an ongoing enigma. World J Surg 2003; 27:1175–82.

29. Fregni F, Pascual-Leone A, Freedman SD. Pain in chronic pancreatitis: a salutogenic mechanism or a maladaptive brain response? Pancreatology 2007; 7:411–22.

30. Ammann RW, Akovbiantz A, Largadier F et al. Course and outcome of chronic pancreatitis.

31. Layer P, Hironori Y, Kalthoff L et al. The different courses of early- and late-onset idiopathic and alcoholic chronic pancreatitis. Gastroenterology 1994; 107:1481–7.

32. Ammann RW, Muellhaupt B and Zurich Pancreatitis Study Group. The natural history of pain in alcoholic chronic pancreatitis. Gastroenterology 1999; 116:1132–40.

33. Gallagher PJ, McLauchlin G, Bornman PC et al. Diagnostic pitfalls and therapeutic strategies in the treatment of pancreatic duct haemorrhage. HPB Surg 1997; 10:293–7.

34. Draganov P, Forsmark CE. "Idiopathic" pancreatitis. Gastroenterology 2005; 756–63.

35. Abdallah AA, Krige JEJ, Bornman PC. Biliary tract obstruction in chronic pancreatitis. HPB 2007; 9:421–8.

36. Lankisch PG. Function tests in the diagnosis of chronic pancreatitis. Int J Pancreatol 1993; 14:9–20.

37. Gilinsky NH, Bornman PC, Girdwood AH et al. The diagnostic yield of ERCP in the diagnosis of pancreatic carcinoma. Br J Surg 1986; 73:539–43.

38. Carter DC. Cancer of the head of pancreas or chronic pancreatitis? A diagnostic dilemma. Surgery 1992; 111:602–3.

39. Fritscher-Ravens A, Brand L. Comparison of endoscopic ultrasound-guided fine needle aspiration for focal pancreatic lesions in patients with normal parenchyma and chronic pancreatitis. Am J Gastroenterol 2002; 97(11):2768–75.

40. Bornman PC, Girdwood AH, Marks IN et al. The influence of continued alcohol intake, pancreatic duct hold-up and pancreatic insufficiency on the pain pattern in chronic non-calcific and calcific pancreatitis: a comparative study. Surg Gastroenterol 1982; 1:5–9.

41. Gullo L, Barbara W, Labó G. Effect of cessation of alcohol use on the course of pancreatic dysfunction in alcoholic pancreatitis. Gastroenterology 1988; 95:1063–8.

42. Mossner J, Secknus R, Meyer J et al. Treatment of pain with pancreatic extracts in chronic pancreatitis: results of a prospective placebo-controlled multicentre trial. Digestion 1992; 53:54–66.

43. Malesci A, Gaia E, Fioretta A et al. No effect of long-term treatment with pancreatic extract on recurrent abdominal pain in patients with chronic pancreatitis. Scand J Gastroenterol 1995; 30:392–8.

Initial enthusiastic response for the use of pancreatic replacement therapy for pain has not been supported by the disappointing results of these two randomised controlled trials.

44. Malfertheiner P, Mayer D, Büchler M et al. Treatment of pain in chronic pancreatitis by

inhibition of pancreatic secretion with octreotide. Gut 1995; 36:450–4.

Octreotide therapy provided no benefit in pain relief.

45. Myhre I, Hilstedt I, Troimier B et al. Monitoring of celiac plexus block in chronic pancreatitis. Pain 1989; 38:269–74.

46. Gress F, Schmitt C, Sherman S et al. Endoscopic ultrasound-guided celiac plexus block for managing abdominal pain associated with chronic pancreatitis: a prospective single center experience. Am J Gastroenterol 2002; 96:409–16.

47. Moodley J, Singh B, Shaik AS et al. Thorascopic splanchnicectomy: effects on pancreatic pain and function. Ann Surg 1999; 23:785–91.

48. Buscher HCJL, Jansen JBMJ, van Dongen R et al. Long-term results of bilateral thoracoscopic splanchnicectomy in patients with chronic pancreatitis. Br J Surg 2002; 89:158–62.

49. Cuschieri A, Shimi SM, Crosthwaite G et al. Bilateral endoscopic splanchnicectomy through a posterior thorascopic approach. J R Coll Surg Edin 1994; 39:44–7.

50. Beckingham IJ, Krige JEJ, Bornman PC et al. Endoscopic management of pancreatic pseudocysts. Br J Surg 1997; 84:1638–45.

51. Wiersma MJ. Endosonography-guided cyst-duodenostomy with therapeutic ultrasound endoscope. Gastrointest Endosc 1996; 44:611–17.

52. Gomes-Cerezo J, Barbado Cano A, Suarez I et al. Pancreatic ascites: study of therapeutic options by analysis of case reports and case series between the years 1975 and 2000. Am J Gastroenterol 2003; 93(3):568–77.

53. Kozarek RA. Endoscopic therapy of complete and partial pancreatic duct disruption. Gastrointest Endosc Clin North Am 1998; 8:39–53.

54. Izbicki JR, Bloechle C, Broering DC et al. Longitudinal V-shaped excision of the ventral pancreas for small duct disease in severe chronic pancreatitis. Prospective evaluation of a new surgical procedure. Ann Surg 1998; 227(2):213–19.

55. Yekebas EF, Bogoevski D, Honarpisheh H et al. Long-term follow-up in small duct chronic pancreatitis: a plea for extended drainage by "V"-shaped excision of the anterior aspect of the pancreas. Ann Surg 2006; 244:940–8.

56. O'Neil SJ, Aranha GV. Lateral pancreatico-jejunostomy for chronic pancreatitis. Word J Surg 2003; 27:1196–1202.

57. Karanjia ND, Widdison AL, Leung F et al. Compartment syndrome in experimental chronic obstructive pancreatitis: effects of decompressing the main pancreatic duct. Br J Surg 1994; 81:259–64.

58. Frey CF, Mikura K. Local resection of the head of the pancreas combined with longitudinal pancreaticojejunostomy in the management of

patients with chronic pancreatitis. Ann Surg 1994; 220:492–507.

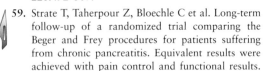

59. Strate T, Taherpour Z, Bloechle C et al. Long-term follow-up of a randomized trial comparing the Beger and Frey procedures for patients suffering from chronic pancreatitis. Equivalent results were achieved with pain control and functional results. Ann Surg 2005; 241:591–8.

60. Howard TJ, Maiden CL, Smith HG et al. Surgical treatment of obstructive pancreatitis. Surgery 1995; 118:727–34.

61. Saforafas GH, Sarr MG, Rowlands CM et al. Post-obstructive chronic pancreatitis. Results with distal resection. Arch Surg 2001; 136:643–7.

62. Beger HG, Imaizumi T. Duodenum-preserving head resection in chronic pancreatitis. J Hepatobil Pancreat Surg 1995; 2:13–18.

63. Martin RF, Rossi RL, Leslie KA. Long-term results of pylorus preserving pancreatoduodenectomy for chronic pancreatitis. Arch Surg 1996; 131:247–52.

64. Buchler M, Friess H, Muller MW et al. Randomised trial of duodenum-preserving pancreatic head resection versus pylorus preserving Whipple in chronic pancreatitis. Am J Surg 1995; 169:65–9.

Duodenal preservation did not yield better results than the pylorus-preserving pancreatico-duodenectomy. Randomised trial showing no obvious benefit when a duodenum-preserving operation is performed.

65. Jimenez RE, Castillo CF, Rattner DW et al. Pylorus-preserving pancreatico-duodenectomy in the treatment of chronic pancreatitis. World J Surg 2003; 27:1211–16.

66. Frey CF, Mayer KL. Comparison of local resection of the head of the pancreas combined with longitudinal pancreatico-jejunostomy [Frey procedure] and duodenal preserving resection of the pancreatic head [Beger procedure]. World J Surg 2003; 27:1217–30.

67. Kozarek RA, Traverso LW. Endoscopic treatment of chronic pancreatitis: an alternative to surgery? Dig Surg 1996; 13:90–100.

68. Rosch T, Daniel S, Scholtz M et al. Endoscopic treatment of chronic pancreatitis: a multicenter study of 1000 patients with long-term follow-up. Endoscopy 2002; 34(10):765–71.

69. Adamek HE, Jakobs R, Buttmann A et al. Long-term follow-up of patients with chronic pancreatitis and pancreatic stones treated with extracorporeal shock wave lithotripsy. Gut 1999; 45:402–5.

70. Dumonceau J-M, Costamangna G, Tringali A et al. Treatment of painful calcified chronic pancreatitis: extracorporeal shock wave lithotripsy versus endoscopic treatment: a randomized controlled trial. Gut 2007; 56:545–52.

Extracorporeal shock-wave lithotripsy alone provides similar pain relief than when combined with endoscopic treatment at a significantly reduced cost.

71. Sherman S, Hawes RH, Savides TJ et al. Stent-induced pancreatic ductal and parenchymal changes: correlation of endoscopic ultrasound with ERCP. Gastrointest Endosc 1996; 44:276–82.

72. Di Magno EP. Towards understanding and management of painful chronic pancreatitis. Gastroenterology 1991; 116:1252–7.

73. Dite P, Ruzicka M, Zoril V et al. A prospective, randomized trial comparing endoscopic and surgical therapy for chronic pancreatitis. Endoscopy 2003; 35:553–8.

74. Cahen DL, Gouma DJ, Nio Y et al. Endoscopic versus surgical drainage of the pancreatic duct in chronic pancreatitis. N Eng J Med 2007; 356:676–84.

Two randomised trials showed superior long-term results with surgery compared to endoscopic therapy.

75. Lankish PG, Banks PA. Chronic pancreatitis: treatment of pancreatic insufficiency. Berlin: Springer-Verlag, 1998; pp. 316–25.

15

Pancreatic adenocarcinoma

Iqbal Z. Khan
Kevin C.P. Conlon

Pancreatic ductal adenocarcinoma is the second most common cause of death from cancer of all gastrointestinal (GI) malignancies. The disease has an insidious onset and most patients have incurable disease by the time they present with symptoms. The overall survival rate is less than 5% at 5 years and is unchanged over the last 25 years. However, recent improvements in preoperative imaging and staging strategies, coupled with improvements in perioperative care, have led to a resurgence of interest in this deadly cancer. A degree of optimism is also seen in the role and efficacy of adjuvant therapies combined with better understanding of the molecular basis of the disease.

Around 95% of pancreatic tumours are adenocarcinoma, originating from the exocrine part of the pancreas. Nearly all of these are ductal adenocarcinomas, and they will form the focus of this chapter.

Epidemiology

An estimated 30 700 new cases of adenocarcinoma of the pancreas will occur in the USA each year, with 30 000 ensuing disease-related deaths.[1] The UK figures mirror this, with 3795 women and 3603 men diagnosed with the disease in 2004. This confers a 1 in 96 risk for males (11th commonest) and 1 in 95 risk for females (eighth commonest).[2] Peak incidence for the disease occurs between the seventh and eighth decades of life, this form of cancer being very rare under the age of 30. In American populations, African and Hawaiian ethnicities confer a higher incidence than Caucasian, whereas Hispanic and Asian appear to be at lower risk of developing the disease.[3] The incidence of pancreatic cancer is rising, particularly in Europe, although this observation is subject to reporting bias related to improved diagnostics. In the USA, the incidence increased threefold over the first three-quarters of the 20th century but has stabilised since.[4]

Risk factors

Smoking

Smoking is estimated to cause 25–30% of pancreatic cancers in the UK and is the only established preventable risk factor.[5] In 1986, the International Agency for Research on Cancer (IARC) classified smoking as a proven carcinogen with respect to cancer of the pancreas. Observational studies suggest that a dose-dependent relationship exists, necessitating long-term exposure.[5] While the chemical cause is unclear, it is possible that N-nitroso compounds in tobacco are carried to the pancreas in the blood.[6] The time in which cigarette smoking exerts its negative influence is also subject to debate; however, observational studies seem to point towards the latter stages of carcinogenesis, particularly in the 15 years preceding development.

Diet and alcohol

The evidence of chronic heavy alcohol consumption as a risk factor is inconsistent and has been questioned.[7] Diets high in saturated fat have a suggested contributing role in cancer development,[8] although data are not robust. Total energy intake has been also suggested,[9] although there are confounding issues such as increased body mass index (BMI) and over-reporting. Obesity has a positive association, with a relative risk of 1.72.[10] Height also has a proposed increased risk, although this may simply represent a surrogate for diet as a child.[10] Other associations include vitamin C (protective),[10] fibre (protective)[8] and caffeine (negative),[11] but these are disputed and probably play minimal roles at best. Carcinogenic substances related to meat preparation methods might be responsible for the positive association to red and processed meat intakes.[12]

Occupation

Workers exposed to ionising radiation, insectisides, aluminium, nickel, acrylamide[13] and halogenated hydrocarbons[14] have been reported to have an increased risk of developing pancreatic adeno-carcinoma.[2] There is evidence of increased risk in people exposed to chlorinated hydrocarbon solvents (metal degreasing workers and dry cleaners),[15] and those working in the paint and varnish industry and the textiles industry.[15] A study of recorded occupation in Finnish women reported significant trends for occupational exposure to lead, iron and chromium,[16] but these data are considered weak overall and particular associations are controversial.

Past medical history

Chronic pancreatitis patients have up to 18-fold higher risk of pancreatic cancer compared to the general population. It has been suggested that increased risk is at its maximum shortly after diagnosis.[17] Whether these conditions have similar causal factors, represent precursors or are directly implicated in the carcinogenesis pathway is uncertain. In the case of pancreatitis, the risk of cancer approximates to normality after 10 years; with diabetes a positive association lasts beyond the 5-year mark. There is a a relative risk of 1.8 for pancreatic cancer in people with type II (non-insulin-dependent) diabetes.[18] Other conditions linked with pancreatic cancer include Gardner's syndrome and multiple endocrine neoplasia type 1 (neuroendocrine cancers).

Hereditary pancreatic cancer

Previously, despite various reports of pancreatic cancer families,[19] the disease was not thought to have a significant familial preponderance. Silverman et al.[20] demonstrated a significantly increased risk of developing pancreatic cancer where a first-degree relative suffered the disease, in particular if the index case smoked. This was confirmed in a large US cohort study suggesting an odds ratio of 1.5 among first-degree relatives.[21] Seven percent of pancreatic cancers (over and above controls) are now thought to have some genetic relationship.[22] There exist known familial conditions such as Peutz–Jeghers syndrome[23] and the STK11/LLLLKB1 gene, BRCA2 expression,[24] and atypical multiple mole syndrome (p16 inactivated in 95% of sporadic cancers) may predispose to pancreatic cancer.[24] Links with familial adenomatous polyposis, BRCA1 and von Hippel–Lindau have been suggested but not confirmed as conferring increased risk. Patients suffering from hereditary pancreatitis have a risk ratio of at least 50[25] and an estimated lifetime risk of pancreatic cancer of 40–70%.[26]

Precursor lesions

Defining precursor lesions and identifying factors with respect to pancreatic cancer development has proven difficult, due in part to the lack of a robust animal model for the disease. However, molecular pathways characterising change to the neoplastic phenotype have been better elucidated in recent times. The advent of microarray chip analysis of normal and pathological pancreatic tissue represents a significant step forward not only in the efficiency of investigation, but also in identifying novel patterns for study. Tumour suppressor gene p16 has received much interest as over 95% of pancreatic cancers demonstrate a loss of function. This is usually due to homozygous deletions, loss of heterozygosity or promoter methylation.[27,28] Occasionally this can be an inherited defect. The K-ras gene product mediates signal transduction in the growth factor receptors, and mutations to this pathway are present in over 90% of ductal lesions.[29] Alteration in cell-cycle regulation, in particular inhibition of entry in S phase, accomplished by p53 protein, is lost in over 50% of cases.[29] Other targets include transforming growth factor-β (TGF-β) receptor genes, BRCA2, HER-2/NEU, DPC4, MKK4 and EBER-1.

Three common precursor lesions of pancreatic adenocarcinoma have been proposed: pancreatic intraepithelial neoplasia, intraductal papillary mucinous neoplasm and mucinous cystic neoplasm. Each of these precursor lesions harbours a unique repertoire of clinicopathological and genetic characteristics that has an impact on natural history and prognosis of these lesions.[30]

Workers in Johns Hopkins University have recently proposed pancreatic intraepithelial neoplasms (PanIN; 1A → 1B → 2 → 3)[31] as the precursor lesions to invasive carcinoma in the pancreas. The model is analogous to that of ductal carcinoma in situ (DCIS) of the breast or adenomatous polyps in colorectal cancer. The lesions display atypical mucinous epithelium replacing the physiological

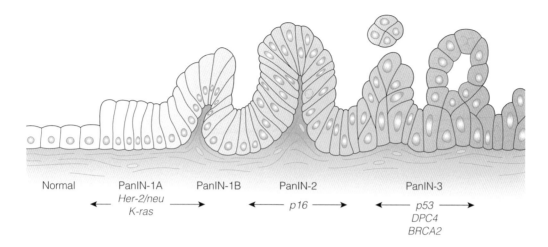

Normal | PanIN-1A | PanIN-1B | PanIN-2 | PanIN-3

Her-2/neu ⟶ ← p16 ⟶ ← p53 ⟶
K-ras DPC4
BRCA2

Figure 15.1 • Diagrammatic representation of PanIN progression to invasive carcinoma. Reproduced from Wilentz RE, Iacobuzio-Donahue CA, Argani P et al. Loss of expression of Dpc4 in pancreatic intraepithelial neoplasia: evidence that DPC4 inactivation occurs late in neoplastic progression. Cancer Res 2000; 60:2002–6. With permission from the American Association for Cancer Research.

cuboidal epithelium. The evidence for PanIN being true premalignant states is largely circumstantial although pressing. These lesions were first described adjacent to resected adenocarcinoma[32] more commonly than in non-neoplastic pancreas. The more atypical PanIN-2 and -3 were seen exclusively in neoplastic pancreas. These lesions also display similar genetic aberrations to the frankly invasive samples. In particular, the percentage of p16 and K-*ras* mutations increases the more atypical the PanIN. These data have heralded development of a tumorigenesis model[33] involving sequential progression from PanIN 1a to invasive adenocarcinoma (**Fig. 15.1**). Similarly to breast DCIS, the natural progression and history of these lesions remain to be elucidated.

Presentation

The majority of patients present with symptoms that are vague and non-specific (Box 15.1). As a result, disease is commonly widespread at diagnosis, and reports suggest in the region of 80% continue to present with irresectable disease.[34]

Tumours in the body and tail present late, pain being the most consistent symptom. Painless jaundice is seen in 13% of patients, 34% present with only pain and 46% present with both pain and jaundice. Weight loss and anorexia are observed in 7% of patients. Tumour invasion into stomach or duodenum might present as haematemesis and malaena. Patients may also present with late-onset diabetes mellitus and acute pancreatitis.[35] While there is currently insufficient

Box 15.1 • Symptoms/signs suggestive of pancreatic neoplasm

- Obstructive jaundice (with or without pain)
- Unexplained weight loss
- Endoscopy-negative epigastric/back symptoms
- Late-onset diabetes without antecedent risks
- Signs of malabsorption without defined cause
- None

evidence to support the introduction of population screening for pancreatic cancer[36] there may be a place for secondary (targeted) screening for high-risk groups in the future.[37]

The classical Courvoisier syndrome (palpable gallbladder in the presence of painless jaundice) occurs in less than 25%. Jaundice may represent either primary disease causing biliary obstruction or advanced disease in the porta hepatis nodes. Pain is a more common symptom than physicians usually appreciate.[38] This may occur due to involvement of the visceral afferent nerves (and may be a portent of irresectability) or be related to an induced local pancreatitis. Weight loss is not necessarily a metastatic feature as in other epithelial tumours and, with pain, form the most tangible symptom and sign. Body and tail lesions tend to present insidiously and are therefore frequently advanced by the time symptoms appear.

Virchow's node (left supraclavicular node associated with upper GI malignancy), thrombophlebitis migrans (non-specific paraneoplastic sign named after Trousseau) and Sister Mary Joseph nodule (umbilical metastatic lesion via the falciform ligament) are well-described features of advanced disease. Hepatomegaly seen in 65% of patients may indicate liver metastasis. Blumer's shelf (rectally palpable rectovesical or rectovaginal mass) occurs exceptionally and is not usually sought as part of routine examination.

The most useful aid in disease diagnosis is an index of suspicion. Vague epigastric symptoms and weight loss in the presence of normal endoscopy and preliminary radiology should initiate further detailed investigation.

Investigation

Serology

Haematological and hepatic biochemical measurements are largely unhelpful in diagnosis. A mild normochromic anaemia may be present secondary to occult loss and thrombocytosis is also sometimes observed. Elevated serum bilirubin and alkaline phosphatase confirm obstructive jaundice, and amylase and lipase may be elevated in patients presenting with pancreatitis (5%). A raised prothrombin time suggests hepatic dysfunction secondary to metastases. Hyperglycaemia is non-specific and occurs in at least 20% of patients. The exact aetiology of this is unclear as glucose homeostasis is usually preserved until less than 10% of islet function remains. However, peripheral glucose resistance is present in >50% and may account for the abnormal glucose tolerance tests in the majority of patients. Patients with malnutrition have hypoalbuminaemia and low cholesterol level.

Markers

There is no ideal tumour marker for pancreatic carcinoma. The most valuable is a glycoprotein, carbohydrate antigen 19-9 (CA19-9; 0–37 U/mL). Initially it was based on a monoclonal antibody to colorectal cancer cell lines. As with all markers it has sensitivity and specificity issues. Falsely elevated CA19-9 is documented in non-malignant conditions such as pancreatitis, hepatic dysfunction and jaundice (failure to excrete). Levels higher than 200 U/mL confer a 90% sensitivity, and levels in the thousands are associated with high specificity (but also irresectability). Patients expressing Lewis blood group antigens (a and b) may have elevated levels.[39] CA19-9 is related to prognosis and, in particular, if it is elevated pre-resection, it can be used to predict recurrence postoperatively.[40,41] Levels exceeding a median of 243 U/mL for those undergoing primary chemoradiotherapy for locoregionally advanced

disease also signify poorer median survival (7.1 vs. 12.3 months).[42] Although CA19-9 is primarily a marker of ductal adenocarcinoma, certain endocrine pancreatic tumours with ductal differentiation may also express the marker.[43] CA19-9 is probably not useful as a screening test in asymptomatic populations.[44]

Other markers, namely carcinoembryonic antigen (CEA), CA242, CA50, SPAN-1, DU-PAN2 and CAM-17.1, are proposed as having application in pancreatic neoplasms, although relative insensitivity or unavailability limits their usefulness in practice.[45] CA242 shows promise as a marker of tumour load and CA494 may play a role in immunotherapy.[46]

Diagnosis

Imaging studies

Transabdominal (TA) ultrasound (US) is obtained commonly in the jaundiced patient. It is often the first investigation in the jaundiced patient as its sensitivity for determining cholelithiasis is superior to that of computed tomography (CT). Common bile duct dilatation (>7 mm; >10 mm in cholecystectomised patients) is an indirect sign, together with pancreatic duct dilatation (>2 mm). The primary pancreatic lesion is often visible together with liver metastases and ascites if present. TAUS is operator dependent and is not as sensitive as CT at detecting smaller lesions.[47] Echo-enhanced ultrasound may have an emerging role in evaluating pancreatic masses.[48]

Thin-cut intravenous contrast-enhanced multidetector CT (MDCT) is the radiological investigation of choice (**Figs. 15.2–15.4**). Oral contrast is often omitted with the patient taking 1000 mL water by mouth, and scans are performed in three phases (noncontrast, pancreatic parenchymal and portal venous phase (PVP)). Combination of pancreatic parenchymal phase and PVP imaging efficiently assesses pancreatic adenocarcinoma.[49] Postprocessing imaging can give excellent images of the pancreatic duct and peripancreatic vasculature. It is approximately 90% sensitive for lesions greater than 2 cm, although this drops to approximately 60% for smaller lesions. Good-quality CT has advanced imaging to the point where it is useful in determining resectability. Direct evidence of a tumour is often seen as a hypodense mass but more subtle signs may be present such as pancreatic atrophy, deformity of the glandular contour or dilatation of the common bile and pancreatic ducts. Metastatic lesions can be demonstrated, and portal vein or superior mesenteric artery involvement can be determined. It is noteworthy, however, that small-volume liver and peritoneal disease is missed frequently.

The predilection of **magnetic resonance imaging** (MRI) for defining soft tissue has seen it overtake CT in many areas. Although this has not yet happened for the pancreas, the combination of

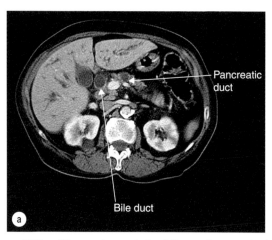
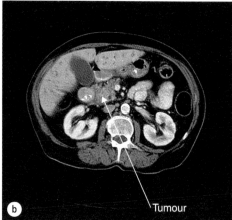

Figure 15.2 • CT scan demonstrating biliary and pancreatic duct obstruction **(a)** caused by a carcinoma of the head of the pancreas **(b)**.

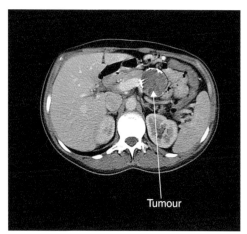

Figure 15.3 • CT scan of a 42-year-old woman with a solid pseudopapillary tumour in the body of her pancreas. Diagnosis was made after an incidental calcification was noted on routine abdominal radiograph.

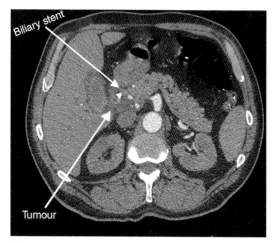

Figure 15.4 • MDCT showing obstructive pancreatic adenocarcinoma with biliary stent for decompression.

T1/T2-weighted imaging with magnetic resonance cholangiopancreatography (MRCP) is useful as the primary tumour can be visualised together with its relationship to biliary and pancreatic ducts, as well as peripancreatic vasculature. T1-weighted images demonstrate the lesion with decreased signal, and on T2 the signal can be variable. The main use of T2 images is in MRCP after the intravenous injection of gadolinium-based contrast.

Endoscopic retrograde cholangiopancreatography (ERCP) is reserved mainly to characterise obstructive intraductal lesions and to relieve biliary obstruction in selected cases. Non-invasive MRCP is replacing ERCP as a diagnostic modality in this area. **Endoscopic ultrasound** (EUS) is useful in determining lesions that are equivocal on CT, allowing fine-needle aspiration if diagnosis is required. EUS-guided fine-needle aspiration (FNA) has similar sensitivity and specificity to CT-guided FNA (Fig. 15.8).

Positron emission tomography (PET) has variable sensitivities (71%) and specificities (64%) for demonstrating the pancreatic primary,[50] it does not define anatomical detail. Its main use is in demonstrating occult metastases, although it is important to remember that hyperglycaemia (present in 15%) may induce false negatives. PET–computed tomography fusion may improve the staging accuracy for pancreatic cancer.[48]

Cytology/histology

High-quality thin-slice pancreas CT forms the mainstay of diagnosis. Many tertiary referral centres forego histological or cytological confirmation prior

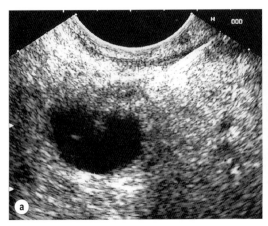
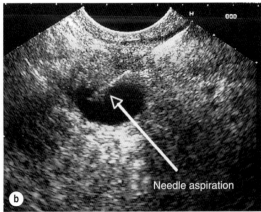

Figure 15.5 • Endoscopic ultrasound diagnosing pancreatic cyst **(a)** and fine-needle aspiration for cytology **(b)**.

to embarking on resection. The need for preoperative pathological confirmation depends in part on the radiological experience as well as the therapeutic philosophy and experience of the treating institution's surgeons. However, in such cases patients should be specifically counselled of a 10% rate of resection for benign disease. Conversely, due to the sclerotic nature of the adenocarcinomas a negative fine-needle aspirate should not deter the attending surgeon when there is robust CT evidence of neoplasia.

If neoadjuvant therapy is considered, histological confirmation is mandatory. This can be accomplished by transabdominal biopsy (US/CT) or endoscopy (ERCP/EUS + fine-needle aspiration cytology (FNAC); **Fig. 15.5**).

 It is accepted that thin-cut contrast-enhanced multidetector CT (MDCT) is the radiological investigation of choice in the diagnosis and staging of pancreatic cancer.

Advanced staging techniques

Laparoscopy

Laparoscopic strategies for staging of cancers have become increasingly relevant in recent times. Both laparoscopy and laparoscopic ultrasound (**Figs. 15.6 and 15.7**) have proven roles in assessing those suffering from selected pancreatic neoplasms.[51,52] Laparoscopy may be performed immediately before conversion[53,54] to laparotomy or as an interval staging measure.[55] The added value of laparoscopy over state-of-the-art dynamic multislice CT remains up to 20%.[55,56]

The main aim of staging laparoscopy is to mimic the open procedure with the minimum of access-related trauma. There exists some considerable controversy

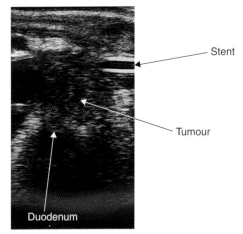

Figure 15.6 • Laparoscopic ultrasound characterising an ampullary carcinoma.

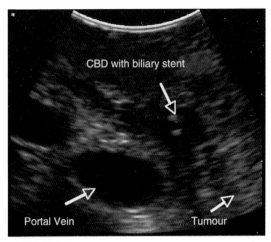

Figure 15.7 • Laparoscopic ultrasound showing pancreatic cancer, adjacent portal vein and a biliary stent.

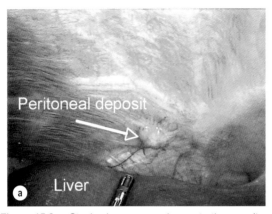
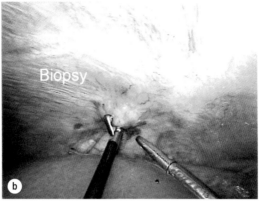

Figure 15.8 • Staging laparoscopy demonstrating a peritoneal deposit being biopsied.

regarding its employment. Although in specialist hands it appears to correctly stage in the region of 20% more cases, critics extrapolate from open data suggesting that laparoscopy should only influence 10% of cases. These data include ampullary lesions, where laparoscopy classically only affects management where small-volume liver or rarely peritoneal disease is discovered (**Fig. 15.8**).

Those who oppose minimal access staging suggest that a significant proportion of patients require surgical bypass and therefore laparoscopic staging should only be used if this would not be contemplated at laparotomy.[57]

Single-centre studies suggest that need for subsequent operative palliation is less than 5%.[57] However, two randomised prospective studies have reported that approximately 20% of patients randomised to no prophylactic gastroenterostomy at the time of their initial surgery required subsequent operative intervention for duodenal obstruction.[58,59]

It is helpful to mark the definitive incision, thus allowing ports to be placed along the planned bilateral subcostal wound. A 5-mm/10-mm port is placed in the right upper quadrant after induction of the pneumoperitoneum via the infraumbilical port site. A further 5-mm port is placed left of the midline. General laparoscopy is performed with an angled (usually 30°) lens looking for small-volume peritoneal and liver metastases. The liver is examined systematically and usually all but segment 7 can be viewed. Biopsy of hepatic or peritoneal deposits for frozen section histology is taken and the procedure is terminated if positive. Should there be no evidence of metastases, the hepatico-duodenal ligament is inspected for nodal disease. The lesser sac is opened by incising the gastrocolic omentum. This is achievable in approximately 80%. Once the sac is open it is inspected for tumour, and biopsies of the primary may be performed. In certain centres, mobilisation of the duodenum is performed but in the majority of cases this is unnecessary. When neo-adjuvant therapies become more efficacious, there is no doubt that laparoscopic strategies will become increasingly important to define a group that may be suitable for downstaging similar to advanced rectal lesions. Laparoscopic ultrasound (LUS) can depict accurately vascular involvement and thus may aid determination of resectability.[60] Peritoneal cytology taken at the time of laparoscopic staging may also improve the accuracy of laparoscopic staging. In a prospective study of 150 consecutive patients with pancreatic carcinoma unexpected metastases were found in 5–10%.[61] Positive cytology is associated with advanced disease; it predicts unresectability of pancreatic adenocarcinoma and a decreased survival. Antecedent FNA is not associated with an increased incidence of positive cytology.[62]

Other staging techniques

Where CT or MRI suggests portal vein involvement, endoscopic ultrasound may be useful to characterise further the presence and degree of invasion. EUS may also help define benign conditions mimicking cancer such as sclerosing pancreatitis or atypical choledocholithiasis. Using the stomach or duodenal wall as a sonic window, it can give fine anatomical detail including pancreas, gallbladder, common bile duct, coeliac axis and liver. While it is operator dependent, it has been reported to pick up lesions as small as 5 mm, while CT and MRI are less sensitive below 2 cm. EUS is extremely useful in defining small periampullary lesions[63] and has similar efficacy to ERCP. Vertical arrays can facilitate placement of fine needles for biopsy. EUS accuracy is affected by the presence of biliary stents. Angiography to stage pancreatic cancer is no longer used routinely. ERCP for staging is reserved primarily for lesions involving the common bile duct to assess tumour extent but has largely being replaced by MRCP.

There is a strong evidence that laparoscopy provides additional beneficial information in staging of pancreatic cancer over conventional radiological investigation; however, debate continues regarding its impact on quality of survival in centres favouring operative palliative techniques.

Pathology

Pathologically, the adenocarcinomas may be classified as follows:

- duct cell origin;
- duct cell adenocarcinoma;
- giant cell carcinoma;
- giant cell carcinoma (epulis-osteoid);
- adenosquamous carcinoma;
- microadenocarcinoma;
- mucinous (colloid) carcinoma;
- cystadenocarcinoma (mucinous);
- acinar cell origin;
- acinar cell carcinoma;
- cystadenocarcinoma (acinar cell).

Ductal adenocarcinomas account for 90–95% of all tumours and can occur anywhere in the gland; however, the pancreatic head is the predominant site (75%). Microscopically there is intense stromal fibrosis. The presence of perineural invasion is an independent poor prognostic factor.[64] Metastatic spread is usually to liver, peritoneum and lungs. Case reports of cutaneous metastases are also documented.

Treatment

Treatment strategy in pancreatic cancer is defined by stage (Table 15.1, **Fig. 15.9**). The major decision point is whether the patient is suitable for resectional therapy requiring some form of pancreatectomy. Unfortunately, less than 20% are in this group at presentation.

Resection

Surgical resection offers the only chance of long-term survival, yet prognosis is poor even with resection.

If jaundice is a presenting symptom it is controversial whether biliary decompression should be undertaken. Available evidence suggests an increased risk of perioperative sepsis, pancreatic fistula and wound infections.[65,66] The authors' practice is not to decompress the bile duct preoperatively, unless symptoms and signs of cholangitis or secondary signs of hyperbilirubinaemia are present. Coagulopathy, if present, is treated 3 days prior to resection with vitamin K.

Patient selection is paramount since, despite surgery with curative intent, median survival ranges between 11 and 18 months, with less than 10% alive at 5 years. Cardiovascular and respiratory performance must be fully evaluated, and age in itself is not a contraindication.[67] Leaving aside the oncological aspects, which are difficult to use as quality measures when ultimate prognosis is relatively poor, pancreatic resections previously were associated with significant mortality; however, recently they have been shown to be safe with acceptable mortality risks. Retrospective analysis of 39463 patients undergoing pancreatic resections for neoplastic disease from 1998 to 2003

Table 15.1 • American Joint Committee on Cancer TNM staging, 2002

Tumour (T)	Node (N)	Metastasis (M)
T1: <2 cm within pancreas	N0: no nodes	M0: no metastases
T2: >2 cm within pancreas	N1: positive nodes	M1: spread to distant organs or non-regional nodes (e.g. aortocaval)
T3: adjacent extrapancreatic spread (duodenum, bile duct)		
T4: non-adjacent spread (stomach, colon, large vasculature)		
Stage I: T1, 2, N0, M0		
Stage II: T3, N0, M0		
Stage III: T1, 2, 3, N1, M0		
Stage IVA: T4, any N, M0		
Stage IVB: any T, any N, M1		

Data from American Joint Committee on Cancer. AJCC cancer staging manual, 6th edn. Springer-Verlag, 2002.

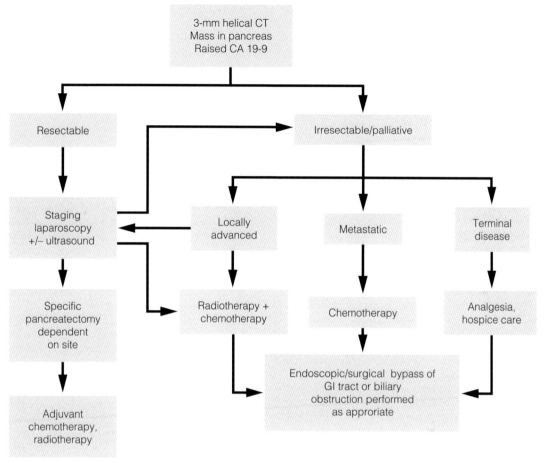

Figure 15.9 • Treatment algorithm for patients with pancreatic cancer.

showed a decrease in mortality from 7.8% to 4.6%. Resections done at high-volume centres (more than 18 procedures/year) had low mortality in comparison to centres with low (<5 procedures/year)- and medium (5–18 procedures/year)-volume centres.[67] The regionalisation of pancreatic surgery may have partially contributed to the observed decrease in mortality rates and probably represents the development of medical, nursing and radiological skill based on repetition and familiarity in dealing with these patients.

Pancreatico-duodenectomy

In 1935, Whipple described, to the American Surgical Association, three cases where ampullary cancers were treated by two-stage pancreatico-duodenectomy.[68] Later, in the 1940s, it was described as a one-stage procedure and although technical variations have since been described, it remains the mainstay of surgical therapy for tumours of the pancreatic head and neck.

Under general anaesthesia and antibiotic prophylaxis, standard laparotomy through a bilateral subcostal 'rooftop' is performed to confirm laparoscopic findings. The right colon is mobilised exposing the third and fourth parts of the duodenum and an extended Kocherisation is performed. This allows a tumour in the head of the pancreas to be palpated and views of the left renal vein. The aortocaval and portal vein (PV) nodal packages are dissected and the respective vessels are skeletonised. Resectability is finally assessed as extensive involvement of the confluence of the PV/superior mesenteric vein (SMV) may herald termination of the procedure. Trial dissection allows this assessment to be made by passing one finger along the PV from above, the other along the SMV to establish the plane. It is important to remember that short segments of the PV can be resected if necessary and therefore an involved PV does not necessarily denote irresectability.

The remaining porta hepatis is dissected and nodes are cleared. Cholecystectomy facilitates higher ligation of the bile duct which is transected just proximal to the insertion of the cystic duct. It is our practice to send a biliary aspirate for routine culture and sensitivity as postoperative infective complications tend to involve biliary organisms.[66] The common bile duct is mobilised distally and the hepaticoduodenal ligament is dissected along its length, taking care to identify and preserve the common hepatic artery and PV. The gastroduodenal artery is ligated while care is taken not to damage an aberrant right hepatic artery.

In a conventional Whipple operation the distal stomach is resected. This is the authors' favoured approach as resection includes the nodes along the greater and lesser curves, reduces stomach-emptying dysfunction postoperatively, diminishes the density of parietal cells and theoretically reduces the risk of gastritis. The stomach is transected at the antrum along with the attached omentum. The proximal jejunum along with its mesentery is transected and the mobilised duodenum and jejunum is delivered back under the ligament of Treitz.

The pancreas is transected between four stay sutures (to facilitate haemostasis in the marginal arteries) after the uncinate process is dissected from the superior mesenteric vessels. Retroperitoneal dissection allows the tumour and nodal package to be delivered en bloc. If any doubt exists regarding the adequacy of tumour clearance, the pancreatic resection margin should be sent for frozen section histology.

Reconstruction is undertaken with the biliary anastomosis followed by the pancreatic and finally the gastric. The pancreatic anastomosis has been the subject of research interest fuelled by desire to decrease pancreatic leaks and fistulas. Pancreatico-gastrostomy has been compared against the pancreatico-jejunostomy in a number of trials.[69,70] These suggest a marginal decrease in fistula rates with the former, although differences are not clinically significant and have not induced a change in operative strategy, with jejunal reconstruction still favoured.

The nature of the pancreatic reconstruction is subject to individual variation. The authors favour a two-layered pancreatico-jejunal anastomosis with mucosa-to-mucosa reconstruction. Choledocho-jejunostomy is performed in a similar manner (end to side), leaving gastro-jejunostomy until the end. We perform washout with warmed water for the theoretical hypotonic tumoricidal action. Abdominal drains are not placed routinely, based on the evidence supplied by the randomised New York experience[71] in which drains failed to decrease the rate of intra-abdominal collections and fistulas.

Complications following pancreatic resection include wound infection (10%), delayed gastric emptying (20%) and intra-abdominal collections/fistulas (12.5–15%). Mostly these complications can be dealt with either conservatively or using interventional radiologically placed drains.[71] Less than 5% require re-operation.

Pylorus-preserving pancreatico-duodenectomy (PPPDR)

It is attractive to preserve the distal stomach and duodenum to diminish nutritive, dumping and bile reflux sequelae.[72] Watson described the first PPPDR in 1944.[73] However, this procedure did not become popular until the last two decades. Both pancreatico-duodenectomy and PPPDR have similar perioperative adverse events; however, in overall analysis PPPDR has decreased operating times, fewer blood transfusions, lower mortality and improved long-term patient survival.[74] Detractors of PPPDR point to delayed gastric emptying as a potential cause for concern with this procedure.[75]

The procedure dictates conventional mobilisation up to where the stomach requires transection. In PPPDR the right gastric artery is preserved and the duodenum is transected at least 2 cm distal to the pylorus. Reconstruction is usually accomplished by duodeno-jejunostomy or gastro-jejunostomy, both probably equivalent in terms of postoperative function.[76]

Extended lymph node dissection

It is the authors' practice to perform extended lymphadenectomy in the majority of cases. At the time of presentation most tumours have involved lymph nodes beyond the gland.[77] Even 50% of the sub-2-cm tumours have lymph node involvement.[78] Ishikawa et al. were the first to demonstrate increased median (but not long-term) survival following extended lymph node dissection.[79] Others suggest that due to the propensity for pancreatic cancer to demonstrate perineural spread, resection should also include the neural tissue.[80] Outside Japan, findings of increased survival have not been proven statistically. These studies fail to demonstrate the increased morbidity that one would expect with the radical operation, although in our experience there is invariably increased ascites in those who undergo extended lymphadenectomy. A subsequent trial from Johns Hopkins Hospital[81] demonstrated extended lymphadenectomy to be comparable with standard resection in terms of morbidity and early mortality. There was no difference in survival. A follow-up study[81] with expanded numbers suggested a slightly increased morbidity in the radical group coupled with protracted hospital stay. We believe that clearance of the left gastric and aortocaval nodes increases the specificity of staging and therefore predicted prognosis and increases the likelihood of a negative surgical margin, although this lethal aspect is difficult to prove and remains controversial.

Distal pancreatectomy

Distal pancreatectomy is performed for resectable tumours of the body and tail of the pancreas. This operation is used rarely for carcinoma as almost always the tumour is irresectable due to direct involvement of the middle colic vessels or metastases. Hence, the procedure is reserved usually for more benign lesions.

Through a bilateral subcostal incision the pancreatic neck is dissected from the portal vein and the splenic flexure of the colon is taken down. It is standard to resect with the spleen, although in certain circumstances (and hence all patients are vaccinated prophylactically against encapsulated organisms, *Haemophilus influenzae* B, meningococcus C and pneumococcus) it is possible to resect while leaving the spleen.[82] If the spleen is to be taken, then early posterior mobilisation and sequential artery and vein ligation are performed to minimise blood loss. The residual gland is oversewn once resection has been performed between stay sutures.

Laparoscopic distal pancreatectomy has been shown to be a safe and effective treatment but should only be undertaken by a surgeon experienced in laparoscopic and pancreatic surgery. It is associated with a higher likelihood of splenic preservation, increased operative time, decreased blood loss and decreased length of stay.[83]

Total pancreatectomy

Some suggest that pancreatic cancer is a multicentric disease and therefore advocate total pancreatectomy, which was first performed by Rockey in 1943.[84] Support in the 1970s for the procedure was probably related to the inadequacies of standard pancreatico-duodenectomy as opposed to benefits of total resection.[85] Although total pancreatectomy can be performed safely, the outcome is so dismal in cases of adenocarcinoma[86] as to call into question the indication for the operation.

 Resectional surgery is possible in less than 20% of all cases but there is increasing evidence that operative mortality is reduced when patients are managed in high-volume institutions.
Pylorus-preserving pancreatico-duodenectomy has similar morbidity and mortality rates to Whipple's operation and there is insufficient evidence to favour one procedure over the other. The role of extended lymph node dissection remains controversial but there is no evidence that extended lymphadenectomy prolongs duration of survival.

Surgical palliation

With efficacious laparoscopic staging, the role of surgical bypass is giving way to endoscopic biliary and GI tract stenting. Nevertheless, surgical bypass techniques are still used occasionally.

Obstructive jaundice

Obstructive jaundice and its secondary symptoms of nausea, anorexia, pruritus and progressive malnutrition may require surgical palliation. Hyperbilirubinaemia causes hepatic, coagulation and myocardial dysfunction and can lead to early death. Pruritus may be debilitating and resistant to medical therapies such as antihistamines and the bile salt binder, cholestyramine. Stenting at ERCP is now favoured for low lesions whereas percutaneous radiologically placed stents are reserved for higher common hepatic obstructions.

Surgical options include choledocho-duodenostomy, choledocho-jejunostomy, cholecysto-jejunostomy and hepatico-jejunostomy. Choledocho-jejunostomy is the procedure of choice in patients with a median life expectancy of 6 months or more since cystic duct obstruction may arise from tumour progression over time. The short-term mortality, morbidity and efficacy of operative and non-operative interventions are equivalent.[87] In-hospital stay is longer in the surgery group but clinical pathways in high-volume centres may serve to diminish morbidity and in-hospital stay.[88]

Upper GI tract outflow obstruction

Gastric and duodenal outlet obstruction is said to occur in 20% of patients. Once jaundice has been addressed, persistent nausea and vomiting should alert the attending physician that upper GI obstruction is present. If biliary obstruction is being dealt with at open operation, prophylactic duodenal bypass should be considered. It is estimated by meta-analysis that 13% would require subsequent bypass if not performed at that time, with a further 20% dying with duodenal outlet symptoms.[89] Randomised data suggest comparable figures (19%)[77] requiring bypass. These data have been criticised by some centres where laparoscopic staging is routine, suggesting that only 2–3% require surgical bypass, which may be accomplished laparoscopically.[57] Minimal access laparoscopic gastro-jejunostomy is probably the management of choice where the local expertise exists. Luminal endoscopic stent placement is associated with more favourable short-term results, whereas gastro-jejunostomy may be a better treatment option in patients with a more prolonged survival.[58]

Pain

Back pain is a feature seen in up to 90% of pancreatic cancers and despite improved palliative care, analgesic regimens may not meet the patient's requirements. In a randomised placebo-controlled trial, Lillemoe et al.[90] reported significantly improved long-term pain scores as well as a survival advantage in patients who received chemical splanchnicectomy.

Adjuvant therapies

Surgery with curative intent still has a disappointing 5-year survival rate of 10–15% and median survival of 11–18 months. Therapy failure must represent progression of micrometastases present at the time of surgery.[77] Even in lymph node-negative tumours, survival is rare beyond 40 months.[91] Thus chemoradiotherapy treatment was considered an attractive proposition. The Gastrointestinal Tumor Study Group (GITSG)[92,93] reported a 20- versus 11-month median survival after adjuvant chemoradiotherapy based on 5-fluorouracil, adriamycin (doxorubicin) and mitomycin C (FAM). This study was criticised based on the delay in entering the treatment arm of up to 10 weeks postsurgery, suggesting that only the fit patients were entered into the study. It is difficult to equivocate regarding the longer-term survival, where 19% were still living at 10 years versus none in the surgery-alone group.

The European Study Group for Pancreatic Cancer 1 trial demonstrated a median 5.7-month increased survival when the chemotherapy groups were compared to the observational postoperative group.[94] This translated to only a 1.5-month trend when analysed separately and suggested a detrimental effect on survival with radiotherapy. The ESPAC-3 trial has recruited more than 1500 patients in over 150 centres in 17 countries to compare adjuvant gemcitabine and 5-fluorouracil/folinic acid, improve survival compared to no treatment and the difference between them.

The Radiation Therapy Oncology Group trial showed gemcitabine to be superior to 5-fluorouracil as an addition to chemoradiotherapy; however, it did not allow value of radiation in the combined modality approach.[95] The CONKO-1 trial compared adjuvant gemcitabine with postoperative observation alone. It did not show a difference in overall survival; however, postoperative gemcitabine was significantly delayed the development of recurrent disease (13.9 months vs. 6.9 months) after R0 or R1 resection.[96]

Regine et al., in a randomised controlled phase 3 trial of 451 patients, analysed effects of adding gemcitabine to conventional 5-fluorouracil chemoradiotherapy and compared the two groups. Results showed a 3.6-month increase in median survival and a 9% improvement in 3-year survival.[97] There has been disappointment[98] with antiangiogenic, metalloprotease inhibitors[99] and hormonal-based therapies,[100] as well as immunotherapy, which has largely stalled in early phase trials.

Neoadjuvant therapy

Intuitively, neoadjuvant multimodal strategies should represent a significant area of interest, as 80% are unresectable at presentation. Chemoradiation therapy should be efficacious since it works best on well-oxygenated tissue, and pretreatment may diminish the chance of tumour seeding at laparotomy. Patients inappropriate for resection may also be selected on the evidence of disease progression at the time of restaging (affecting 15–25%). Some prospective evidence exists suggesting a small response rate in terms of downstaging (10–25%)[101] without any increase in postoperative complication rates.[102] In a recent study, feasibility and efficacy of neoadjuvant chemotherapy and radiation in locally unresectable disease were evaluated. Patients with unresectable disease received GTX (gemcitabine, docetexal and capecitabine); 75% of these also received radiation. Median survival was increased for the inoperable disease with acceptable morbidity and mortality.[103]

Future areas of interest

The last decade has seen considerable improvements in diagnosis as well as advances in minimally invasive and endoscopic management of pancreatic cancer. The surgical questions regarding pylorus preservation and extended lymph node dissection are well advanced, and elective resection can be performed safely. It is therefore disappointing that neoadjuvant strategies appear to confer little or no survival advantages, thus identifying the area where most investigation is needed. Immunotherapies held great promise, although delivery systems and potency have undermined the failure of standard therapies to materialise. Today, complete surgical therapy with adjuvant chemoradiation represents the best available therapy for this disease, and lifetime survival rates of 5% remain a challenge for the future.

Key points

- Pancreatic cancer is associated with poor prognosis despite surgery with curative intent.
- Pancreatic cancer is strongly associated with cigarette smoking.
- Pancreatic protocol CT forms the mainstay of imaging.
- Preoperative staging is enhanced by focused laparoscopy, although this is controversial.
- Resectional surgery is only possible in 20% of cases.
- There is increasing evidence to justify postoperative adjuvant therapy.

References

1. Jemal A, Murray T, Samuels A et al. Cancer statistics, 2003. CA Cancer J Clin 2003; 53:5–26.

2. Cancer Research UK. Cancer statistics. London: CRUK, 2007.

3. Miller BA, Kolonel LN, Bernstein I et al Racial/ethnic patterns of cancer in the United States 1988–92. Bethesda, MD: NIH, 1996.

4. Lillemoe KD, Yeo CJ, Cameron JL. Pancreatic cancer: state-of-the-art care. CA Cancer J Clin 2000; 50:241–68.

5. Lowenfels AB, Maisonneuve P. Epidemiology and prevention of pancreatic cancer. Jpn J Clin Oncol 2004; 34:238–44.

6. Risch HA. Etiology of pancreatic cancer, with a hypothesis concerning the role of N-nitroso compounds and excess gastric acidity. J Natl Cancer Inst 2003; 95:948–60.

7. Olsen GW, Mandel JS, Gibson RW et al. A case control study of pancreatic cancer and cigarettes, alcohol, coffee and diet. Am J Public Health 1989; 79:1016–19.

8. Howe GR, Burch JD. Nutrition and pancreatic cancer. Cancer Causes Control 1996; 7:69–82.

9. Silverman DT, Schiffman M, Everhart J et al. Diabetes mellitus, other medical conditions and familial history of cancer as risk factors for pancreatic cancer. Br J Cancer 1999; 80:1830–7.

10. Michaud DS, Giovannucci E, Willett WC et al. Physical activity, obesity, height, and the risk of pancreatic cancer. JAMA 2001; 286:921–9.

11. MacMahon B, Yen S, Trichopoulos D et al. Coffee and cancer of the pancreas. N Engl J Med 1981; 304:630–3.

12. Nöthlings U, Wilkens LR et al. Meat and fat intake as risk factors for pancreatic cancer: the multiethnic cohort study. J Natl Cancer Inst 2005; 97:1458–65.

13. Marsh GM, Lucas LJ, Youk AO et al. Mortality patterns among workers exposed to acrylamide: 1994 follow up. Occup Environ Med 1999; 56:181–90.

14. Ojajarvi IA, Partanen TJ, Ahlbom A et al. Occupational exposures and pancreatic cancer: a meta-analysis. Occup Environ Med 2000; 57:316–24.

15. Blair A, Stewart PA, Tolbert PE et al. Cancer and other causes of death among a cohort of dry cleaners. Br J Ind Med 1990; 47:162–8.

16. Weiderpass E et al. Occupational exposures and gastrointestinal cancers among Finnish women. J Occup Environ Med 2003; 45:305–15.

17. Everhart J, Wright D. Diabetes mellitus as a risk factor for pancreatic cancer. A meta-analysis. JAMA 1995; 273:1605–9.

18. Huxley R et al. Type-II diabetes and pancreatic cancer: a meta-analysis of 36 studies. Br J Cancer 2005; 92:2076–83.

19. Ehrenthal D, Haeger L, Griffin T et al. Familial pancreatic adenocarcinoma in three generations. A case report and a review of the literature. Cancer 1987; 59:1661–4.

20. Ahlgren JD. Epidemiology and risk factors in pancreatic cancer. Semin Oncol 1996; 23:241–50.

21. Coughlin SS, Calle EE, Patel AV et al. Predictors of pancreatic cancer mortality among a large cohort of United States adults. Cancer Causes Control 2000; 11:915–23.

22. Ghadirian P, Boyle P, Simard A et al. Reported family aggregation of pancreatic cancer within a population-based case control study in the Francophone community in Montreal, Canada. Int J Pancreatol 1991; 10:183–96.

23. Giardiello FM, Welsh SB, Hamilton SR et al. Increased risk of cancer in the Peutz–Jeghers syndrome. N Engl J Med 1987; 316:1511–14.

24. Ozcelik H, Schmocker B, Di Nicola N et al. Germline BRCA2 6174delT mutations in Ashkenazi Jewish pancreatic cancer patients. Nat Genet 1997; 16:17–18.

25. Lowenfels AB, Maisonneuve P, Whitcomb DC. Risk factors for cancer in hereditary pancreatitis. International Hereditary Pancreatitis Study Group. Med Clin North Am 2000; 84:565–73.

26. Maisonneuve P, Lowenfels AB. Chronic pancreatitis and pancreatic cancer. Dig Dis 2002; 20:32–7.

27. Goldstein AM, Fraser MC, Struewing JP et al. Increased risk of pancreatic cancer in melanoma prone kindreds with p16INK4 mutations. N Engl J Med 1995; 333:970–4.

28. Schutte M, Hruban RH, Geradts J et al. Abrogation of the Rb/p16 tumor-suppressive pathway in virtually all pancreatic carcinomas. Cancer Res 1997; 57:3126–30.

29. Pellegata NS, Sessa F, Renault B et al. K-ras and p53 gene mutations in pancreatic cancer: ductal and nonductal tumors progress through different genetic lesions. Cancer Res 1994; 54:1556–60.

30. Singh M, Maitra A. Precursor lesions of pancreatic cancer: molecular pathology and clinical implications. Sol Goldman Pancreatic Cancer Research Center, Johns Hopkins University School of Medicine, Baltimore, MD. USA Pancreatology 2007; 7:9–19.

31. Hruban RH, Adsay NV, Albores-Saavedra J et al. Pancreatic intraepithelial neoplasia: a new nomenclature and classification system for pancreatic duct lesions. Am J Surg Pathol 2001; 25:579–86.

This paper provides a description of the new classification system for pancreatic cancer.

32. Cubilla AL, Fitzgerald PJ. Morphological lesions associated with human primary invasive non-endocrine pancreas cancer. Cancer Res 1976; 36:2690–8.

33. Wilentz RE, Iacobuzio-Donahue CA, Argani P et al. Loss of expression of Dpc4 in pancreatic intraepithelial neoplasia: evidence that DPC4 inactivation occurs late in neoplastic progression. Cancer Res 2000; 60:2002–6.

34. Singh SM, Longmire WP Jr, Reber HA. Surgical palliation for pancreatic cancer. The UCLA experience. Ann Surg 1990; 212:132–9.

35. Gullo L et al. Do early symptoms of pancreatic cancer exist that can allow an earlier diagnosis? Pancreas 2001; 22:210–13.

36. Wong T et al. Molecular diagnosis of early pancreatic ductal adenocarcinoma in high-risk patients. Pancreatology 2001; 1(5):486–509.

37. Vimalachandran D et al. Genetics and prevention of pancreatic cancer. Cancer Control 2004; 11:6–14.

38. Kelsen D. Neoadjuvant therapy for upper gastrointestinal tract cancers. Curr Opin Oncol 1996; 8:321–8.

39. Safi F, Schlosser W, Kolb G et al. Diagnostic value of CA 19-9 in patients with pancreatic cancer and nonspecific gastrointestinal symptoms. J Gastrointest Surg 1997; 1:106–12.

40. Safi F, Roscher R, Beger HG. Tumor markers in pancreatic cancer. Sensitivity and specificity of CA 19-9. Hepatogastroenterology 1989; 36: 419–23.

An important paper that summarises well the role of CA19-9 in pancreatic cancer.

41. Fujioka S, Misawa T et al. Preoperative serum carcinoembryonic antigen and carbohydrate antigen 19-9 levels for the evaluation of curability and resectability in patients with pancreatic adenocarcinoma. J Hepatobiliary Pancreat Surg 2007; 14:539–44.

42. Micke O, Bruns F, Kurowski R et al. Predictive value of carbohydrate antigen 19-9 in pancreatic cancer treated with radiochemotherapy. Int J Radiat Oncol Biol Phys 2003; 57:90–7.

43. Kamisawa T, Tu Y, Egawa N et al. Ductal and acinar differentiation in pancreatic endocrine tumors. Dig Dis Sci 2002; 47:2254–61.

44. Kim JE, Lee KT, Lee JK et al. Clinical usefulness of carbohydrate antigen 19-9 as a screening test for pancreatic cancer in an asymptomatic population. J Gastroenterol Hepatol 2004; 19:182–6.

45. Moossa AR, Gamagami RA. Diagnosis and staging of pancreatic neoplasms. Surg Clin North Am 1995; 75:871–90.

46. Chung M, Chang H. Clinical use of tumor markers in pancreatic carcinoma. Semin Surg Oncol 1995; 11:103–7.

47. Ishiguchi T, Maruyama K, Fukatsu H et al. Radiologic diagnosis of pancreatic carcinoma. Semin Surg Oncol 1998; 15:23–32.

48. Nichols MT, Russ PD, Chen YK. Pancreatic imaging: current and emerging technologies. Pancreas 2006; 33:211–20.

49. Ichikawa T, Erturk SM et al. MDCT of pancreatic adenocarcinoma: optimal imaging phases and multiplanar reformatted imaging. Am J Roentgenol 2006; 187:1513–20.

50. Sendler A, Avril N, Helmberger H et al. Preoperative evaluation of pancreatic masses with positron emission tomography using ^{18}F-fluorodeoxyglucose: diagnostic limitations. World J Surg 2000; 24: 1121–9.

51. van Dijkum EJ, de Wit LT, van Delden OM et al. Staging laparoscopy and laparoscopic ultrasonography in more than 400 patients with upper gastrointestinal carcinoma. J Am Coll Surg 1999; 189:459–65.

52. Pisters PW, Lee JE, Vauthey JN et al. Laparoscopy in the staging of pancreatic cancer. Br J Surg 2001; 88:325–37.

53. Conlon KC, Dougherty E, Klimstra DS et al. The value of minimal access surgery in the staging of patients with potentially resectable peripancreatic malignancy. Ann Surg 1996; 223:134–40.

The author's seminal paper describing the role and value of minimal access surgery in staging of peripancreatic cancer.

54. Holzman MD, Reintgen KL, Tyler DS et al. The role of laparoscopy in the management of suspected pancreatic and periampullary malignancies. J Gastrointest Surg 1997; 1:236–44.

55. Jimenez RE, Warshaw AL, Rattner DW et al. Impact of laparoscopic staging in the treatment of pancreatic cancer. Arch Surg 2000; 135:409–14; discussion 414–15.

56. Catheline JM, Turner R, Rizk N et al. The use of diagnostic laparoscopy supported by laparoscopic ultrasonography in the assessment of pancreatic cancer. Surg Endosc 1999; 13:239–45.

57. Espat NJ, Brennan MF, Conlon KC. Patients with laparoscopically staged unresectable pancreatic adenocarcinoma do not require subsequent surgical biliary or gastric bypass. J Am Coll Surg 1999; 188:649–55; discussion 655–7.

58. Jeurnink SM, Eijck C, Steyerberg EW et al. Stent versus gastrojejunostomy for the palliation of gastric outlet obstruction: a systematic review. BMC Gastroenterol 2007; 7:18.

59. Lillemoe KD, Cameron JL, Hardacre JM et al. Is prophylactic gastrojejunostomy indicated for unresectable periampullary cancer? A prospective randomized trial. Ann Surg 1999; 230:322–8; discussion 328–30.

Two key papers arguing the role for and against prophylactic gastroenterostomy in palliation of pancreatic cancer.

60. Piccolboni D, Ciccone F et al. The role of echo-laparoscopy in abdominal surgery: five years' experience in a dedicated center. Surg Endosc 2008; 22:112–17.

61. Schmidt J, Fraunhofer S et al. Is peritoneal cytology a predictor of unresectability in pancreatic carcinoma? Hepatogastroenterology 2004; 51(60):1827–31.

62. Merchant NB, Conlon KC et al. Positive peritoneal cytology predicts unresectability of pancreatic adenocarcinoma. J Am Coll Surg 1999; 188:421–6.

63. Legmann P, Vignaux O, Dousset B et al. Pancreatic tumors: comparison of dual-phase helical CT and endoscopic sonography. Am J Roentgenol 1998; 170:1315–22.

64. Nagakawa T, Mori K, Nakano T et al. Perineural invasion of carcinoma of the pancreas and biliary tract. Br J Surg 1993; 80:619–21.

65. Pisters PW, Hudec WA, Hess KR et al. Effect of preoperative biliary decompression on pancreatico-duodenectomy-associated morbidity in 300 consecutive patients. Ann Surg 2001; 234:47–55.

66. Povoski SP, Karpeh MS Jr, Conlon KC et al. Association of preoperative biliary drainage with postoperative outcome following pancreatico-duodenectomy. Ann Surg 1999; 230:131–42.

A paper highlighting the contribution of biliary stenting to operative morbidity.

67. McPhee JT, Hill JS, Whalen GF et al. Perioperative mortality for pancreatectomy: a national perspective. Ann Surg 2007; 246:246–53.

68. Whipple AO, Parson WB, Mullins CR. Treatment of carcinoma of the ampulla of Vater. Ann Surg 1935; 102:763–79.

69. Yeo CJ, Cameron JL, Maher MM et al. A prospective randomized trial of pancreatico-gastrostomy versus pancreatico-jejunostomy after pancreatico-duodenectomy. Ann Surg 1995; 222:580–8; discussion 588–92.

A trial showing no difference in outcome for pancreatic anastomotic techniques employed at pancreatico-duodenectomy.

70. Takano S, Ito Y, Watanabe Y et al. Pancreatico-jejunostomy versus pancreatico-gastrostomy in reconstruction following pancreatico-duodenectomy. Br J Surg 2000; 87:423–7.

71. Conlon KC, Labow D, Leung D et al. Prospective randomized clinical trial of the value of intraperitoneal drainage after pancreatic resection. Ann Surg 2001; 234:487–93; discussion 493–4.

The author's own report showing no benefit for continuing drainage following pancreatic resection.

72. Klinkenbijl JH, van der Schelling GP, Hop WC et al. The advantages of pylorus-preserving pancreatoduodenectomy in malignant disease of the pancreas and periampullary region. Ann Surg 1992; 216:142–5.

73. Watson K. Carcinoma of the ampulla of Vater. Successful radical resection. Br J Surg 1944; 31:368–73.

74. Iqbal N, Lovegrove RE, Tilney HS et al. A comparison of pancreaticoduodenectomy with pylorus preserving pancreaticoduodenectomy: A meta-analysis of 2822 patients. Eur J Surg Oncol 2008.

75. Cooperman AM, Kini S, Snady H et al. Current surgical therapy for carcinoma of the pancreas. J Clin Gastroenterol 2000; 31:107–13.

76. Konishi M, Ryu M, Kinoshita T et al. Pathophysiology after pylorus-preserving pancreatoduodenectomy: a comparative study of pancreatogastrostomy and pancreatojejunostomy. Hepatogastroenterology 1999; 46:1181–6.

77. Fortner JG, Klimstra DS, Senie RT et al. Tumor size is the primary prognosticator for pancreatic cancer after regional pancreatectomy. Ann Surg 1996; 223:147–53.

78. Birk D, Fortnagel G, Formentini A et al. Small carcinoma of the pancreas. Factors of prognostic relevance. J Hepatobiliary Pancreat Surg 1998; 5:450–4.

79. Ishikawa O, Ohigashi H, Sasaki Y et al. Adjuvant therapies in extended pancreatectomy for ductal adenocarcinoma of the pancreas. Hepatogastroenterology 1998; 45:644–50.

80. Hiraoka T, Uchino R, Kanemitsu K et al. Combination of intraoperative radiation with resection of cancer of the pancreas. Int J Pancreatol 1990; 7:201–7.

81. Yeo CJ, Cameron JL, Lillemoe KD et al. Pancreatico-duodenectomy with or without distal gastrectomy and extended retroperitoneal lymph-adenectomy for

periampullary adenocarcinoma, part 2: Randomized controlled trial evaluating survival, morbidity, and mortality. Ann Surg 2002; 236:355–66; discussion 366–8.

Report of a trial showing no benefit for extended lymphadenectomy at the time of pancreatico-duodenectomy for pancreatic cancer.

82. Shoup M, Brennan MF, McWhite K et al. The value of splenic preservation with distal pancreatectomy. Arch Surg 2002; 137:164–8.

83. Melotti G, Butturini G, Piccoli M et al. Laparoscopic distal pancreatectomy: results on a consecutive series of 58 patients. Ann Surg 2007; 246:77–82.

84. Rockey EW. Total pancreatectomy for carcinoma: case report. Ann Surg 1943; 118:603–11.

85. Ihse I, Anderson H, Andren S. Total pancreatectomy for cancer of the pancreas: is it appropriate? World J Surg 1996; 20:288–93; discussion 294.

86. Karpoff HM, Klimstra DS, Brennan MF et al. Results of total pancreatectomy for adenocarcinoma of the pancreas. Arch Surg 2001; 136:44–7; discussion 48.

87. Watanapa P, Williamson RC. Surgical palliation for pancreatic cancer: developments during the past two decades. Br J Surg 1992; 79:8–20.

88. Pitt HA, Murray KP, Bowman HM et al. Clinical pathway implementation improves outcomes for complex biliary surgery. Surgery 1999; 126:751–6; discussion 756–8.

89. Sarr MG, Cameron JL. Surgical management of unresectable carcinoma of the pancreas. Surgery 1982; 91:123–33.

90. Lillemoe KD, Cameron JL, Kaufman HS et al. Chemical splanchnicectomy in patients with unresectable pancreatic cancer. A prospective randomized trial. Ann Surg 1993; 217:447–55; discussion 456–7.

91. Warshaw AL, Fernandez-del Castillo C. Pancreatic carcinoma. N Engl J Med 1992; 326:455–65.

92. Kalser MH, Ellenberg SS. Pancreatic cancer. Adjuvant combined radiation and chemotherapy following curative resection. Arch Surg 1985; 120:899–903.

93. Gastrointestinal Tumor Study Group. Further evidence of effective adjuvant combined radiation and chemotherapy following curative resection of pancreatic cancer. Cancer 1987; 59:2006–10.

94. Neoptolemos JP, Dunn JA, Stocken DD et al. Adjuvant chemoradiotherapy and chemotherapy in resectable pancreatic cancer: a randomised controlled trial. Lancet 2001; 358:1576–85.

95. Regine WF, Winter KW, Abrams R et al. RTOG 9704 a phase III study of adjuvant pre and post chemoradiation (CRT) 5-FU vs. Gemcitabine (G) for resected pancreatic adenocarcinoma. J Clin Oncol 2006; 24:4007.

96. Oettle H, Post S, Neuhaus P et al. Adjuvant chemotherapy with gemcitabine vs. observation in patients undergoing curative-intent resection of pancreatic cancer: a randomized controlled trial. JAMA 2007; 297:267–77.

97. Regine WF, Winter KA et al. Fluorouracil vs gemcitabine chemotherapy before and after fluorouracil-based chemoradiation following resection of pancreatic adenocarcinoma. JAMA 2008; 299:1019–26.

A randomised trial showing significant benefit for gemcitabine in advanced pancreatic cancer.

98. Bramhall SR, Rosemurgy A, Brown PD et al. Marimastat as first-line therapy for patients with unresectable pancreatic cancer: a randomized trial. J Clin Oncol 2001; 19:3447–55.

99. Burris HA 3rd, Moore MJ, Andersen J et al. Improvements in survival and clinical benefit with gemcitabine as first-line therapy for patients with advanced pancreas cancer: a randomized trial. J Clin Oncol 1997; 15:2403–13.

100. Sherman WH, Fine RL. Combination gemcitabine and docetaxel therapy in advanced adenocarcinoma of the pancreas. Oncology 2001; 60:316–21.

101. Farrell TJ, Barbot DJ, Rosato FE. Pancreatic resection combined with intraoperative radiation therapy for pancreatic cancer. Ann Surg 1997; 226:66–9.

102. Snady H, Bruckner H, Cooperman A et al. Survival advantage of combined chemoradiotherapy compared with resection as the initial treatment of patients with regional pancreatic carcinoma. An outcomes trial. Cancer 2000; 89:314–27.

103. Allendorf JD, Lauerman M, Bill A et al. Neoadjuvant chemotherapy and radiation for patients with locally unresectable pancreatic adenocarcinoma: feasibility, efficacy and survival. J Gastrointest Surg 2008; 12:91–100.

16

Non-adenocarcinoma of the pancreas

Saxon Connor

Introduction

Although pancreatic ductal adenocarcinoma accounts for the majority of patients with neoplastic disease of the pancreas, over the last two decades there has been an increasing recognition of cystic and neuroendocrine pancreatic neoplasms.[1] In addition, other non-epithelial neoplasms can also arise within the pancreas.[2] The aim of this chapter is to examine these tumours in more detail, and where possible provide evidence-based recommendations for the investigation and management of these tumours.

Intraductal papillary mucinous neoplasms

Intraductal papillary mucinous neoplasms (IPMNs) have only been recognised as separate entities to ductal adenocarcinoma of the pancreas since 1982,[3] subsequent to which the World Health Organisation clarified their definition.[4] They are defined as a grossly visible, mucin-producing epithelial neoplasm of the pancreas, which arises from within the main pancreatic duct (main-duct IPMN) or one of its branches (branch-duct IPMN), and most often but not always has a papillary architecture. They are distinguished from mucinous cystic neoplasms by the absence of ovarian-type stroma.[5]

The incidence and aetiology are not well understood. McDonald et al.[6] extrapolated the incidence from the number of patients who underwent resection for IPMNs, estimating an incidence of 1 per 281 000 patients. In contrast to this, an autopsy study of 300 elderly patients identified cystic lesions in 24% of patients, of which 3.4% contained carcinoma in situ.[7] The precise aetiology remains unknown, although an association with extrapancreatic primaries (10%), most commonly colorectal, breast and prostate, has been reported, but this is not significantly different to that seen with primary pancreatic adenocarcinoma.[8]

Clinical presentation

IPMNs most commonly present with symptoms related to pancreatic duct obstruction. The Johns Hopkins group reported their experience comparing the presentation and demographics to those patients presenting with pancreatic adenocarcinoma.[9,10] Although the mean age of presentation was similar to that of pancreatic adenocarcinoma (seventh decade), the clinical presentation was significantly different. Of the 60 patients with IPMN, 59% presented with abdominal pain but only 16% presented with obstructive jaundice, compared to 38% and 74% of patients with pancreatic adenocarcinoma respectively.[9] This is in spite of the fact that only 5 of the 60 patients with IPMNs had tumours within the body or tail.[9] In addition, those with IPMNs were more likely to have been smokers and 14% had had previous attacks of acute pancreatitis (compared to 3% of those with pancreatic ductal adenocarcinoma).[9] Weight loss was a prominent factor reported in 29% of patients with IPMN.[10] Symptoms reported to be associated with invasive malignancy included the presence of jaundice, weight loss, vomiting[10] and diabetes.[11] Patients with invasive IPMN were a mean of 5 years older (68 vs. 63 years) compared to those with non-invasive IPMN.[10] This led the authors to conclude that IPMN would appear to be a slow-growing tumour with a significant latency to develop invasive disease.[10] Increasingly, an important presentation is the incidental finding due to cross-sectional imaging for other medical indications. IPMN was the final diagnosis in 36% of pancreatic 'incidentalomas' that underwent pancreaticoduodenectomy.[12]

Investigation

Computed tomography (CT) and magnetic resonance (MR) imaging form the mainstay of non-invasive radiological imaging of suspected IPMN. The classical features of main-duct IPMN are of a grossly dilated main pancreatic duct (**Fig. 16.1**), while branch-type IPMN can present with small cystic lesions which may appear in a 'grape-like' configuration.[13] Although MR and CT have been shown to identify accurately tumour location and communication with the pancreatic duct, the detection of invasive malignancy remains problematic.[14–16] Radiological features associated with malignancy include the presence of a solid mass, biliary dilatation >15 mm and increasing size of either the tumour for branch-type IPMN or main pancreatic duct diameter for main-duct IPMN.[16] Differentiating IPMNs from other cystic neoplasms

(particularly branch-type IPMNs from mucinous cystic neoplasms (MCNs)) can be difficult and the importance of considering the clinical picture cannot be underestimated, particularly the patient's age, gender and history of pancreatitis or genetic syndromes.[17] Radiologically, localisation within the uncinate process, detection of non-gravity-dependent luminal filling defects (papillary projections) or grouped gravity-dependent luminal filling defects (mucin), and upstream dilatation of ducts (MCN ducts are normal) all favour the diagnosis of branch-type IPMN.[18] Differentiating diffuse main-duct IPMN from chronic obstructive pancreatitis can be challenging radiologically[18] (clinically, patients with IPMN tend to be 20 years older and lack a history of heavy alcohol use), but high-quality cross-sectional imaging looking for endoluminal filling defects (either mucin or papillary proliferations), cystic dilatation of collateral branches (particularly within the uncinate process), communication of dilated ducts with normal ducts without evidence of an obstructing lesion or a widely open papilla (Fig. 16.1) all favour IPMN.[18]

Endoscopic ultrasound (EUS) has the advantage of being able to sample cystic fluid and biopsy solid lesions at the time of assessment. Features seen at

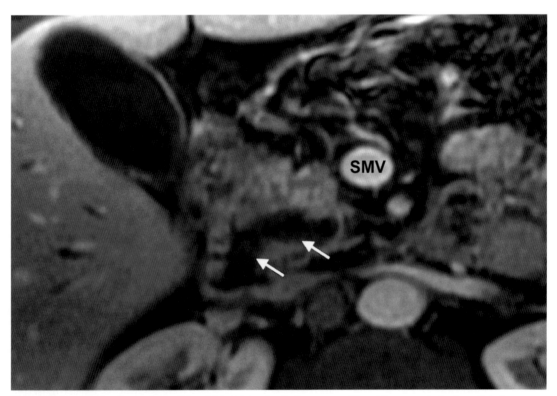

Figure 16.1 • MRI (post-gadolinium, T1-weighted, fat-saturated) pancreas. The white arrows indicate a dilated pancreatic duct with a widely open ampulla consistent with a main-duct intraductal papillary neoplasm. SMV, superior mesenteric vein. Histology is shown in Fig. 16.2.

EUS suggestive of malignancy include main duct >10 mm (for main-duct IPMN), while suspicious features for branch-type IPMN include tumour diameter greater than 40 mm associated with thick irregular septa and mural nodules >10 mm.[19] In a series of 74 patients with IPMN of which 21 (28%) had invasive carcinoma, the sensitivity, specificity and accuracy of EUS fine-needle aspiration in predicting invasive carcinoma were 75%, 91% and 86% respectively.[20] In this particular study, the elevated levels of carcinoembryonic antigen (CEA) and carbohydrate antigen (CA) 19-9 within cyst fluid did not predict the presence of malignancy.[20] Importantly, the absence of mucin does not exclude IPMN.[21] While the presence of necrosis is the only feature which is strongly suggestive of invasive carcinoma, abundant background inflammation and parachromatin clearing are suspicious for carcinoma in situ.[21]

Endoscopic retrograde cholangiopancreatography (ERCP) can be used in the diagnosis of IPMN, although MR imaging (including the use of gadolinium) is increasingly replacing it (Fig. 16.1). The observation at ERCP of mucin protruding from a widely open papilla is diagnostic.[22] Biopsies and aspiration of ductal contents can be obtained; however, the yield is less than 50%.[22]

Although there are no tumour markers specific to IPMN, serum CA19-9 but not CEA has been shown to be an independent predictor of malignancy.[11] Fujino et al.[11] have proposed a new clinicoradiological scoring system for predicting the presence of invasive malignancy in patients with both branch and main-duct IPMN (based on an analysis of 64 patients who underwent resection). It consists of seven factors (Table 16.1), each with an assigned score. A cut-off of 3 or more predicts malignancy with a sensitivity, specificity, positive predictive value, negative predictive value and overall accuracy of 95%, 82%, 91%, 90% and 91% respectively. No patients with a score of >4 had benign lesions, while no patient with a score of <2 had malignancy. Clearly, if this system is validated and further refined with larger numbers of patients, this may prove a very simple and useful predictor of underlying malignancy.

Pathology

Overwhelmingly, the majority of IPMNs involve the head of the gland (70%), while 5–10% are spread diffusely throughout the gland, with the rest located within the body and tail.[23] On sectioning, the involvement can be diffuse or segmented with projections of papillary epithelium (**Fig. 16.2**) and tenacious thick mucin within the involved dilated ducts. The projections and mucin can extend along the ducts and into the surrounding structures, including the ampulla, duodenum and bile duct. Communication of the main pancreatic duct with the cystic lesion can usually be established. IPMNs are subclassified into main duct, branch type or mixed depending on site of origin. This is important as branch-type neoplasms are less likely to be

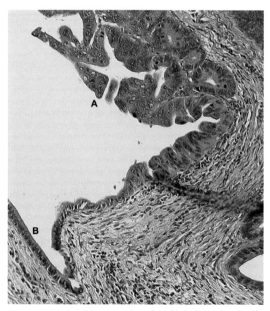

Figure 16.2 • H&E-stained section from the pancreaticoduodenectomy specimen of the patient in Fig. 16.1. Label A is in the lumen of the proximal pancreatic duct with adjacent proliferation of severely dysplastic glandular epithelium with intraluminal papillary growth, but no stromal invasion in this area. Elsewhere in the specimen focal stromal invasion was identified. Label B indicates remnant low columnar non-neoplastic epithelium of the duct.

Table 16.1 • Proposed scoring system[11] to predict malignancy in patients with suspected intraductal papillary mucinous neoplasms of the pancreas

Variable	Score
Patulous papilla	1
Jaundice	1
Diabetes mellitus	1
Tumour size ≥42 mm	1
Main-duct type	2
Main duct ≥6.5 mm	3
CA19-9 ≥35 units/mL	3

A cut-off of 3 or more predicts malignancy with a sensitivity, specificity, positive predictive value, negative predictive value and overall accuracy of 95%, 82%, 91%, 90% and 91% respectively.

associated with malignancy.[22] Surrounding pancreatic parenchyma may appear firm and hard due to scarring and atrophy from obstructive chronic pancreatitis secondary to the tumour.[23] The presence of gelatinous or solid nodules should raise the suspicion of an invasive component.[23] Microscopically, the most typical appearance is of mucin-secreting columnar epithelium with variable atypia (low-, moderate-, high-grade dysplasia or invasive carcinoma).[23] The growth pattern varies from flat ducts (ectasia) through to prominent papillae. The tumour tends to follow the pancreatic ducts and can be multifocal in 20–30% of patients.[23] IPMNs can contain intestinal, gastric or less commonly pancreaticobiliary type differentiation.[23] The gastric type are more often associated with branch-type IPMNs and would seem to be associated with a different (lower) malignant potential, growth pattern and type of mucin production compared to the intestinal type.[24] Invasive carcinoma occurs focally and is thought to result from a stepwise progression through increasingly dysplastic lesions.[23] The invasive growth pattern can be muconodular (colloid) or a conventional ductal pattern and would appear to be related to the underlying cellular differentiation (intestinal vs. pancreatico-biliary respectively).[23]

Pathologically differentiating IPMN from other cystic neoplasms of the pancreas is important. The absence of ovarian stroma helps to separate IPMN from MCN.[5] For lesions between 0.5 and 1 cm differentiating pancreatic intraepithelial neoplasia (PanIN) from IPMN is difficult. IPMNs tend to have taller and more complex papillae and are associated with abundant luminal mucin.[23] While the presence of coarse and stippled chromatin with a smooth nuclear membrane will differentiate cystic pancreatic endocrine neoplasms from IPMNs.[23]

Management

In determining the most appropriate management of patients with IPMNs, the following should be considered. Given the preponderance for these to present in older patients and the fact the majority will be located within the head of the pancreas, it is important to assess the patient's comorbidities and fitness for major pancreatic surgery. If the patient is not fit enough for surgery, then simple medical management of the patient's symptoms is appropriate. Equally, in the event of an incidental diagnosis, intensive follow-up regimens are not indicated if any progression in the tumour will not lead to surgical intervention. Presuming the patient is a suitable candidate for surgery (if required) then appropriate staging to determine surgical resectability (criteria equivalent to that for pancreatic adenocarcinoma) should be performed.

For main-duct IPMNs, a recent consensus document (International Association of Pancreatology (IAP) guidelines)[5] recommended that all such patients should undergo resection. This was based on reviewing available evidence which concluded the following: the incidence of malignancy (in situ or invasive disease) in main-duct tumours is between 60% and 92%; it is thought that most main-duct IPMNs will undergo transformation into malignant disease if left untreated; a significant survival advantage is seen for those who are resected with in situ or benign disease compared to those with invasive disease; the ability to exclude malignancy on clinico-radiological criteria is limited.

The same IAP guidelines[5] recommended that all symptomatic branch-duct IPMNs underwent resection on the basis that it would alleviate symptoms and because the literature would suggest that there is a higher rate of malignancy within patients who are symptomatic (risk of invasive malignancy 30%).[5] For asymptomatic patients[5] it was recommended that patients with tumours ≥30 mm or with mural nodules underwent resection due to the increased risk of malignancy. Although risk factors for malignancy have been identified by more than one study using multivariate analysis,[11,25] these have been based on small numbers of patients. Nagai et al.[26] have challenged this approach, advocating aggressive surgical resection for branch-type IPMNs, arguing the identified risk factors do not have a high enough negative predictive value, that survival is significantly compromised in those with invasive disease, and that pancreatic surgery can be performed with a low morbidity and mortality in experienced centres.

Since publication of the IAP guidelines,[5] a large dual-centre study[27] consisting of 145 patients with branch-duct IPMNs who underwent resection has been reported. Of these 145 patients, 22% had malignant disease (in situ or invasive) and 40% of patients were asymptomatic. Although symptoms per se were not found to be a predictor of malignancy, on univariate analysis, jaundice and abdominal pain were more likely to be associated with malignancy. Radiologically malignant tumours were larger and on pathological analysis the presence of a thick wall, nodularity and size ≥30 mm were all associated significantly with malignancy. It is important to note, however, that other than size these factors were not assessed radiologically. In addition, there was a significant size discrepancy between radiologically and pathologically measured size (radiological measurement was consistently 15% greater). The authors concluded that their results supported the IAP guidelines, particularly with regard to non-surgical management of those which were asymptomatic with no concerning features of malignancy.

Given that even branch-duct IPMN would appear to be a pre-malignant lesion, albeit a slow-growing one, one has to know the outcome from long-term follow-up if conservative management is to be successful. In a large prospective contemporary study[28] of branch-duct IPMNs, 109 patients were allocated to a surgical or intensive follow-up arm. The decision to operate was based on symptoms (all were resected) or features suggestive of malignancy (radiological (size >3.5 cm, thick walls, mural nodules), CA19-9 >25 U/mL, new onset or worsening diabetes). Only 20 of the 109 patients met the criteria for surgery at initial presentation. Of these patients the final histology was malignant (in situ or invasive disease) in only three patients but the two with invasive disease subsequently succumbed to metastatic disease. Of the 89 asymptomatic patients who underwent intensive follow-up (6-monthly for the first 2 years and then yearly contrast-enhanced ultrasound and MR imaging (with or without secretin) with CA19-9 and glucose levels), only five patients progressed (for a mean increase in tumour size of 1 cm) to surgery at a median of 18 months. All five patients had benign pathology. The remaining 84 patients were followed for a median of 32 (24–71) months with no significant change in their lesion. There were no deaths attributable to their disease.

The methodology of the follow-up regimen of this study[28] raises further questions. It uses state-of-the-art imaging at a frequency which many health systems may struggle to provide. Additionally, given the lack of progression of any of the tumours to significant pathology, it is debatable that such an intensive regimen can be justified. It is likely that further large or multicentre studies with longer follow-up will be required before definite recommendations can be made.

The authors concluded that this approach supported the IAP guidelines,[5] yet even for those patients operated on, only 3 of 20 had malignant disease, and therefore future studies should focus on whether other more specific indicators of malignancy can be used to identify high-risk patients.[29]

 For branch-duct IPMNs a selective approach to resection should be undertaken based on symptoms, CA19-9 >25 U/mL, tumour size >3.5 cm, presence of mural nodules or thick walls.[5,27,28]

For those patients in whom surgery is indicated, the decision regarding the extent of pancreatic resection and nodal dissection needs to be decided. Fujino et al.[30] reviewed the outcome for 57 patients who underwent surgical resection for IPMNs. Their approach was to perform a localised resection where pre-resection imaging revealed localised disease (including intraoperative ultrasound (IOUS) to determine the point of pancreatic transection), while for diffuse disease a total pancreatectomy was performed. Frozen section was performed and for patients with invasive carcinoma a radical resection was performed. Where non-invasive disease was detected a tumour-free margin was sufficient. Of the 33 patients with main-duct IPMNs, 14 met the pre-resection criteria for total pancreatectomy. All 24 branch-duct tumours underwent partial resections, although two subsequently required completion pancreatectomy for complications. Correlating the final pathological assessment with the IOUS indicated an accuracy of ductal spread of 74% for main-duct tumours and 96% for branch-duct tumours. Frozen section was performed in 30 of the patients who underwent partial resection and in 29 it correlated with the final result. Only one patient had invasive malignancy at the transected surface, while a further two patients who did not have a frozen section assessment had invasive malignancy at the resection margin.

In reviewing the final histology of the 16 patients undergoing total pancreatectomy, resection was found to be appropriate (frankly or potentially malignant tissue throughout all segments of the pancreas) in 12 of the patients. Importantly, six of these 16 patients had severe long-term problems with hypoglycaemia, two of whom died as a result of this complication. For those 41 patients undergoing partial pancreatectomy, five patients had an involved margin (three with invasive carcinoma, two with dysplasia). The three patients with invasive carcinoma all died from metastatic disease. Of the patients with clear margins, 7 of 34 died from metastatic disease, while two developed metachronous pancreatic disease at 2 and 12 years. The results of this study[30] led the authors to conclude that if possible partial pancreatectomy should be performed and that the risk of recurrent malignancy in the remnant is outweighed by the severe long-term complications from total pancreatectomy.

Although Fujino et al.[30] report frozen section to be very accurate, it can be a challenging undertaking for the pathologist. However, not all positive margins require resection. Current recommendations from the IAP guidelines[5] are that in the presence of adenoma or borderline atypia, no further resection is required, but if in situ or invasive carcinoma is present then further resection should be performed. However, what has not yet been addressed in the literature is the effect of potentially spilling invasive carcinoma cells (i.e. cutting through invasive tumour) during surgery and the effect this has on long-term outcomes. This is particularly important as increasingly limited resections are being reported for low-grade lesions within the pancreas[31] with good long-term outcomes. Yet for main-duct IPMNs, the authors[31] have advised caution for exactly this reason given the risk of a positive resection margin and subsequent recurrence.

For those undergoing resection, partial pancreatectomy is preferred to total pancreatectomy and intraoperative frozen section should be performed to ensure clear margins.[30]

Outcome

The main determinant of survival following resection is the presence of invasive disease (Table 16.2). The 5-year survival for those with non-invasive disease is 77–100%[10,26,28,30,32,33] vs. 13–60%[1,10,26,28,30,32,33] for those with invasive disease. Other factors associated with a poor survival include presence of jaundice,[34] tumour type (tubular worse than colloid),[10,34] vascular invasion,[34] percentage of tumour which was invasive[34] and positive lymph node involvement,[10,32,34] which has been reported in up to 41%[32] of patients with invasive disease. Invasive branch-type tumours have been shown to have similar survival to those with main-duct disease[34] and margin status has not been associated with worse long-term outcome.[10,34] It should be noted that only one study[34] has performed a multivariate analysis and did so with 30

patients comparing six variables, and therefore it should be interpreted with caution. In addition, most studies are too small to confidently exclude a type II error in identifying truly independent predictors of survival. Invasive IPMN would still appear to have a better prognosis than pancreatic ductal adenocarcinoma.[26,32] The role of adjuvant therapy for those with invasive disease has not yet been addressed, yet a small study[35] has reported its use. Of particular concern within this study was the number of patients who received both chemo- and radiotherapy for non-invasive disease after their pathology was re-reviewed and subsequently downgraded.

Recurrence following resection can be classified as disseminated (including peritoneal disease) or local (within the pancreatic remnant). White et al.[36] have reported on 78 patients who underwent resection for non-invasive IPMNs over a 13-year period. The median follow-up was 40 months. Only six (7.7%) patients developed local recurrence, of whom three underwent further resection and remained under active follow-up. Importantly, time to recurrence was extremely variable with a range of 8–62 months, indicating that long-term surveillance of the pancreatic remnant is required. There was a significant association of recurrence with positive margins,[36] although this has not been shown elsewhere.[10] Given the significant morbidity and late mortality associated with total pancreatectomy,[30] the authors[36] favoured follow-up of the remnant as opposed to total pancreatectomy.

Table 16.2 • Survival following resection for intraductal papillary mucinous neoplasms by presence of invasion

Author	Number of patients	Five-year survival (%)	
		Non-invasive	Invasive
Sohn et al.[10]	84	77	–
	52	–	43
Hardacre et al.[33]	24	90	–
	13	–	22
Wada et al.[32]	75	100	–
	25	–	46
Salvia et al.[28]	80	100	–
	58	–	60
D'Angelica et al.[34]	32	95	–
	30	–	60
Fujino et al.[30]	19	91	–
	38	–	13
Winter et al.[1]	90	–	48
Nagai et al.[26]	42	100	–
	30	–	58

In a large series[27] of 145 patients who underwent resection for branch-type IPMNs, 6.9% of patients developed recurrence. Four of 139 patients with non-invasive disease developed local recurrence at a mean follow-up of 34 months,[27] while 6 of 16 patients with invasive carcinoma developed distant disease (three also had local recurrence) at a mean follow-up of 24 months (all died within 2 years of recurrence).[27] In a small series of 12 patients[37] who underwent resection for invasive IPMNs, six developed recurrence. All six developed recurrence within the pancreatic remnant while two had evidence of distant disease (peritoneal, liver). Interestingly, time to recurrence varied between 18 and 63 months. However, few were operable and survival following recurrence for these patients was often very short (<6 months for 3 of 6 patients). Similar figures have been reported by Raut et al.[35]

 In terms of what follow-up regimens are recommended following resection there is a lack of reliable evidence. The IAP guidelines[5] acknowledge this, but feel it is reasonable to perform yearly CT or MRI and space it out once the patient has shown no signs of change after several years. They do not routinely support the use of tumour markers.

Given that recurrence would seem to occur most commonly within the pancreatic remnant, Tomimaru et al.[38] have proposed performing a pancreatico-gastrostomy to allow easy endoscopic follow-up of the duct. Additionally, the association of IPMNs with other gastrointestinal (GI) malignancies[5] should alert physicians to investigate new GI symptoms promptly.

Pancreatic neuroendocrine tumours

Pancreatic neuroendocrine tumours (PNETs) are rare tumours with a reported incidence of 0.2–0.4 per 100 000, although post-mortem studies have reported a rate of PNETs in up to 10% of the population.[39] Eighty-five percent of PNETs are non-syndromic (non-functional), with the rest comprised of syndromic tumours[40] of which carcinoid, insulinoma and gastrinoma are the most common.[41] The aetiology is poorly understood and although the majority of tumours are sporadic there are associations with several hereditary syndromes, including Von Hippel–Lindau, multiple endocrine neoplasia-1 (MEN-1), neurofibromatosis type 1 and tubular sclerosis.[42]

Clinical presentation

The mode of presentation is dependent on the functional state of the tumour. For non-functioning tumours presentation may be incidental or if symptomatic is usually related to mass effect or the presence of metastatic disease. For those tumours associated with a syndrome it is obviously related to the specific hormone production (Table 16.3).

Investigations

The order of investigations will be dependent on presentation. The general principle for functional tumours is to confirm the diagnosis (biochemically) prior to localisation (radiologically).

Biochemical

For functional tumours specific fasting gut hormones can be measured.[41] For insulinoma and carcinoid, fasting glucose, insulin, C-peptide and 24-hour urinary 5-hydroxyindoleacetic acid (5-HIAA), for the latter tumour, can be measured.[41] In addition, in the majority of PNETs, including in non-functional tumours,[41] serum chromogranin A (protein produced from cells arising from the neural crest) will be elevated.

Other investigations such as calcium, parathyroid hormone, calcitonin and thyroid function tests should also be considered, particularly if there is a history that may suggest MEN-1.[41] For those in whom a hereditary component is suspected, referral to an appropriate genetic service for further investigation should be initiated.

Radiology

For non-functioning tumours, where localisation is often not an issue, a high-quality arterial and portal venous phase CT will be sufficient to direct therapy, particularly in determining if surgery is indicated. Features suggestive of a PNET on CT include the presence a hypervascular or hyperdense lesion within the pancreas; however, they can also appear cystic or contain calcifications.[43] The presence of a large incidental mass within the pancreas, particularly without vascular encasement or desmoplastic reaction, should also alert the clinician to the possibility of a PNET.[43]

Although somatostinomas, VIPomas and glucagonomas tend to be large and easily identified and staged by contrast-enhanced CT, often this is not so for insulinomas and gastrinomas, unless there is widespread metastatic disease. Most insulinomas are under 2 cm and solitary. On CT they tend to be hypervascular (**Fig. 16.3**) with either uniform or

Table 16.3 • Presentation, diagnosis and initial medical management of functional pancreatic neuroendocrine tumours

Tumour type	Syndrome	Symptoms	Diagnosis	Medical options for initial symptom control
Insulinoma	Whipple's triad	Neuroglycaemic or neurogenic symptoms relieved with eating	1) Insulin:glucose ratio >0.3 in presence of hypoglycaemia 2) C-peptide suppression test	Overnight feeding Diazoxide titrated to symptom resolution Somatostatin analogue
Gastrinoma	Zollinger–Ellison	Complicated peptic ulceration or gastro-oesophageal reflux, diarrhoea, abdominal pain	1) Serum fasting gastrin >1000 pg/mL (if gastric pH <2.5) 2) Secretin stimulation test	High-dose proton pump inhibition (may require up to 60 mg b.d.)
Glucagonoma	Glucagonoma syndrome	Necrolytic migratory erthyma, weight loss, diabetes mellitus, stomatitis, diarrhoea, thromboembolism	Plasma glucagon >1000 pg/mL	Somatostatin analogue Hyperalimentation Thrombosis prophylaxis
VIPoma	Verner–Morrison syndrome	Profuse watery diarrhoea, hypokalaemia	Plasma VIP >1000 pg/mL	Somatostatin analogue
Somatostatinoma		Gallstones, steatorrhoea, hypochlorhydria, glucose intolerance	Raised plasma somatostatin	
Carcinoid	Carcinoid syndrome	Abdominal pain, If metastases then flushing, palpitations, rhinorrhoea, diarrhoea, bronchospasm, pellagra	24-hour urinary 5-HIAA	Somatostatin analogue

target enhancement; however, given that they are often non-contour conforming, detection of the vascular blush is essential to localise them (the chance of detection can be maximised by timing the images 25 seconds after contrast injection).[43] MR features include low signal intensity on T1-weighted images; they are particularly well seen on fat-suppressed (T1- and T2-weighted) images.[43] In contrast to insulinoma, gastrinoma can be multiple and extrapancreatic (located within the gastrinoma triangle, the junction between neck and body of the pancreas medially, junction of the second and third parts of the duodenum inferiorly and the junction of the common bile duct and cystic duct superiorly).[44] On radiological examination, they tend to be less vascular than insulinoma.[43] There is a high rate (70–80%) of lymph node and hepatic metastases.[43] The sensitivity of CT in the detection of gastrinoma is related to size and can be as low as 30–50%.[44] Although slightly better figures have been reported for insulinomas, this can be increased to 94% with the use of thin formats and with the addition of endoscopic ultrasound sensitivities of 100% have been reported.[44]

Endoscopic ultrasound is particularly useful for imaging the duodenal wall, regional lymph nodes and the pancreatic head, and has reported sensitivities of 79–100%, but is obviously operator dependent.[44] Equally the use of intraoperative ultrasound has also been shown to be useful, particularly in gastrinomas, by identifying occult multiple primaries or metastatic disease. The sensitivity for detecting small lesions in the pancreatic head is reported to be as high as 97%.[44]

PNET hepatic metastases often appear as low attenuation lesions on pre-contrast CT and hypervascular lesions on post-contrast imaging.[44] It is, however, important to perform a hepatic arterial phase as they can be isointense with normal parenchyma on portal venous imaging.[44] MRI appearances of hepatic metastases are usually of low signal intensity lesions on T1 and high signal intensity on T2-weighted images.[44] Importantly, 15% of hepatic metastases were only seen on immediate post-gadolinium imaging.[44]

In addition to standard radiological imaging, somatostatin receptor scintigraphy (SRS) is also very

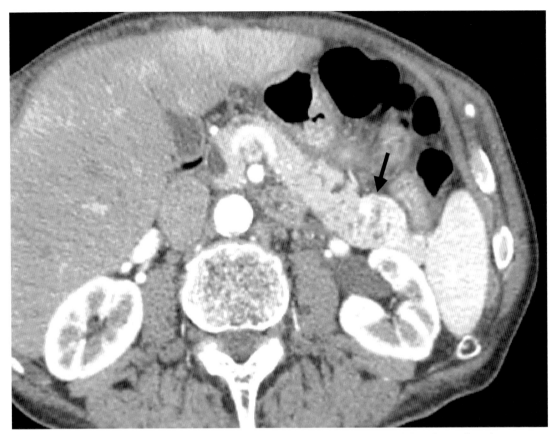

Figure 16.3 • A 78-year-old man presented with neuroglycaemic symptoms. Biochemical testing confirmed an insulinoma. Arterial phase computed tomography revealed a hypervascular lesion in the tail of the pancreas (black arrow). Laparoscopic spleen-preserving distal pancreatectomy was performed. Histology confirmed malignant, node-positive neuroendocrine tumour consistent with an insulinoma. Patient remains well, symptom free at 10 months follow-up.

useful in the staging and treatment of PNETs (with the exception of insulinomas[45]). This works on the principle that PNETs express somatostatin receptors. The use of a somatostatin analogue labelled with a radioactive isotope (of which there are several) allows a functional image to be obtained but it requires somatostatin analogues to be stopped prior to the scan. As a single investigation, it is probably the most sensitive for the detection of PNETs; however, equivalence can be achieved with a combined approach of standard radiology (particularly MRI and EUS), which has the advantage of providing a detailed anatomical analysis.[46] SRS does, however, offer the advantage of reflecting functionality which is important if treatment doses of radiolabelled somatostatin analogues or meta-iodobenzylguanidine (MIBG) are to be used. ^{18}F-labelled deoxyglucose positron emission tomography has not been shown to be useful for the majority of PNETs; however, the development of newer alternatives to ^{18}F-labelled deoxyglucose would appear to be promising.[46] Invasive investigations such as selective arterial calcium (insulinoma) and secretin (gastrinoma) stimulation with hepatic/portal venous sampling are not used routinely and limited to those where there is a high suspicion but non-invasive imaging has failed to localise the tumour.[45,47]

Treatment

Once the diagnosis of a functioning tumour is established, control of the hormonal excess is the first priority in minimising symptoms and complications. Medications used for each individual tumour are shown in Table 16.3. Somatostatin analogue infusions are recommended pre- and intraoperatively for carcinoid tumours to prevent carcinoid crisis.[41]

Surgery offers the only chance of cure for those with localised disease for PNETs. The approach is dependent on tumour type and the presence or absence of an inherited syndrome. The specific management of hereditary PNETs is beyond the remit of this chapter and readers are referred to more detailed reviews[42,45,47] for an in-depth discussion.

Over 80% of localised sporadic insulinoma will be solitary, benign and under 2 cm in size, making them ideal candidates for consideration for enucleation and laparoscopic resection.[45] Enucleation is considered possible if the lesion can be clearly localised pre- or intraoperatively and that the relationship to the pancreatic duct has been clearly identified.[41] Intraoperative ultrasound has been shown to be particularly valuable in helping to assess these factors.[45] Postoperatively, histological conformation of the benign nature must be confirmed.[41] For tumours where malignancy is suspected (hard, infiltrating tumour, duct obstruction or lymph node involvement), there is major vascular involvement or the presence of a large tumour resection will be required.[45] Patients should be assessed for resection as for any pancreatic tumour. However, if a distal pancreatectomy is being performed attempts to preserve the spleen should be made.[45] Blind pancreatic resection should be avoided.[45] Not surprisingly given the rare nature of the tumour, data in support of laparoscopic resection remain limited to small case series; however, early results indicate that although it can be performed safely a significant conversion, re-exploration and morbidity rate remain.[48]

For localised sporadic gastrinoma, surgery has been shown to increase survival.[49]

Duodenotomy and intraoperative ultrasound combined with palpation (sensitivity 91–95%) are the key to successful intraoperative localisation.[47] For duodenal gastrinomas, small tumours (<5 mm) can be enucleated from the submucosa while larger tumours require full-thickness excision.[47] For pancreatic gastrinomas intraoperative assessment for suitability for enucleation (similar to that described above for insulinomas) should be performed. However, if the tumour is not suitable, a formal pancreatic resection (pancreaticoduodenectomy) should be performed. If enucleation is performed consideration to peripancreatic nodal sampling should be undertaken given the high rate of metastatic disease.[50]

For localised non-functioning tumours most will be detected at such a size that enucleation is not feasible. Given the discrepancy between the clinical and autopsy incidence of PNETs and the increasing use of cross-sectional imaging, this is likely to become a more frequent possibility. The size at which patients with asymptomatic suspected benign, non-functioning PNETs should undergo resection is not clear.[51] Although the risk of malignancy is related to size, tumours between 1 and 3 cm can harbour malignant potential[51] (**Fig. 16.4**). Currently, patients should be assessed for fitness for surgery and an

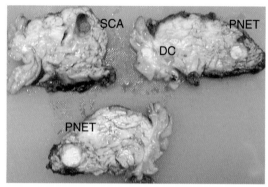

Figure 16.4 • A 30-year-old female with Von Hippel–Lindau disease underwent pancreatic screening. Radiological imaging revealed five neuroendocrine tumours within the pancreatic head. Pancreaticoduodenectomy was performed. Pathological sectioning of the pancreatic head revealed multiple neuroendocrine tumours (PNET) including at least one well-differentiated pancreatic endocrine carcinoma (node positive) and a well-differentiated duodenal endocrine carcinoma (DC). All tumours were 12–18 mm in diameter. An incidental serous cyst adenoma (SCA) was also identified.

informed decision made with the patient regarding resection or observation. Central pancreatectomy has also been shown to be feasible for selected tumours and has the advantage of reducing the risk of postoperative diabetes.[31] For suspected malignant tumours a formal resection with lymphadenectomy should be performed as lymph node metastases are common (27–83%).[51]

Resection is the treatment of choice for symptomatic patients with localised disease.[51] The median survival for those who underwent resection was significantly longer for those with metastatic disease and locally advanced unresectable disease (7.2 years vs. 2.1 and 5.2 years respectively).[51] Importantly, however, 48% of patients who underwent resection for localised disease developed recurrence at a median follow-up of 2.7 years.[51] Because of the long natural history of these tumours and given that many are symptomatic and difficult to palliate without resection (e.g. tumour bleeding), the criteria for what determines unresectable disease may not be the same as those for adenocarcinoma of the pancreas. The MD Anderson experience[51] would suggest that in high-volume centres major venous reconstruction can be performed safely, but only rarely would they perform arterial reconstruction (isolated hepatic artery involvement) or upper abdominal exenteration due to the associated high long-term morbidity. In addition, a recent report has also indicated that an incomplete resection (R2) is associated with a high perioperative mortality and may in fact be detrimental to the patient's survival.[52]

Metastatic disease

Only 10% of patients with hepatic metastases will be suitable for potential curative resection.[41] For patients with non-functioning unresectable metastatic disease there is no evidence to support palliative or 'debulking' resections, with possibly the only exception being those who have significant local symptoms from the primary and low-volume hepatic metastases.[51]

> For patients with hormonal excess and hepatic metastases a cytoreductive (surgery or ablative therapies) approach has been advocated if 90% of tumour bulk can be removed, although randomised trials are lacking.[41,45,47] Other options assessed by recent UK guidelines[41] on the management of PNETs included somatostatin analogues (short and long acting), interferon-α, hepatic artery embolisation, radiolabelled analogues (MIBG and somatostatin), liver transplantation and radiofrequency ablation.

The role of chemotherapy for PNETs has been based around streptozocin and 5-flurouracil after a randomised trial in 1980 showed a survival advantage for those receiving combination chemotherapy.[53] Whether subsets of PNETs are more likely to respond is yet to be determined.[41,51]

Pathology and outcome

PNETs are classified into four groups based on a combination of clinical, histological and molecular features.[41] Tumours confined to the pancreas are classified as well-differentiated endocrine tumours which can be subdivided into those of benign behaviour (<2 cm size), <2 mitoses per 10 high-power fields (HPFs), Ki67 index <2% (and no vascular invasion) or uncertain behaviour (if above criteria not met). Tumours not confined to the pancreas (gross local invasion or metastases) or that exhibit evidence of small-cell carcinoma are considered endocrine carcinoma, which are further subdivided into well differentiated (well to moderately differentiated, mitotic rate 2–10 per 10 HPFs, Ki67 index >5%) or poorly differentiated (small-cell carcinoma, necrosis, >10 mitoses per 10 HPFs, Ki67 >15% index, prominent vascular and perineural invasion). Importantly, the diagnosis of functional tumours is not made histologically but clinically as immunohistochemical staining of specific hormones does not correlate with the clinical picture.[41] Although no specific staging system exists for PNETs, Bilimoria et al.[53] applied the American

Joint Committee on Cancer (AJCC) 6th edition for pancreatic adenocarcinoma to a population-based PNET database. In 4793 patients with PNETs, the median and 5-year survival for patients who underwent resection was 9.3 years and 61% for stage 1, 5.3 years and 52% for stage 2, 3 years and 41.4% for stage 3, and 1.2 years and 15.5% for stage 4 respectively. Interestingly, patients who underwent resection had an improved stage-specific survival. Whether a more accurate one can be devised remains to be determined.

Other tumours

The other two main types of cystic neoplasms are serous (SCA) and mucinous (MCN) cystic neoplasms. Because of the difference in malignant potential, the management of these two tumours differs, yet clinically and radiologically there is considerable overlap. It is therefore useful to contrast and compare them. The exact incidence of serous and mucinous cystic tumours is unknown; however, in a retrospective review of 24 039 patients undergoing radiological imaging, 0.7% had pancreatic cystic neoplasms. Of the 49 (0.2%) who underwent surgery, 10 and 16 patients had a final diagnosis of SCA and MCN respectively.[54] SCAs are more common in men (2:1) with a peak incidence in the seventh decade and evenly distributed throughout the pancreas with up to a third being asymptomatic.[55] In contrast, MCNs are predominantly found in women with a peak incidence in the fifth decade and more likely to be located within the tail.[56] SCAs are also commonly associated with Von Hippel–Lindau[42] (Fig. 16.4) and young patients presenting with multiple cystic lesions involving the pancreas and kidneys should be genetically assessed.[55]

On cross-sectional imaging, the typical appearances of an SCA are of a microcystic (>6 cysts, each cyst <2 cm individual diameter) lesion with or without central calcification (so-called sunburst calcification).[17,57] When the classic features are present, differentiation from other tumours is not difficult; however, a rare solid type exists that radiologically can be mistaken for neuroendocrine tumour.[13] MRI may be useful in this setting.[17] The presence of a uni- or oligolocular macrocystic (>2 cm) lesion is more difficult to diagnose and a wide differential exists. Both SCAs (oligocystic type) and MCNs can fall into this group, although MCNs are less likely to be multilocular and if calcification occurs, it does so peripherally and may be a marker of underlying malignancy.[17] The presence of solid components within a cystic lesion indicates the presence of or a high risk of malignancy and therefore surgical resection should be considered.[17] Included within this differential would be PNET, solid pseudopapillary neoplasm (young women) or mucinous cyst adeno-carcinoma.[17] It is unusual for either SCAs or MCNs to communicate with the pancreatic duct, but it has been reported.[17]

The ability of non-interventional imaging to obtain an accurate diagnosis is limited. In a recent report of 100 SCAs from Bassi and colleagues,[58] the correct diagnosis was achieved in 53%, 54% and 76% by ultrasound (US), CT and MRI respectively. The incorrect diagnosis was made in 31%, 34% and 26%, and the investigation was non-diagnostic in 16%, 12% and 0% of US, CT and MRI respectively.

In a recent study[59] of solitary cystic (IPMNs were excluded) neoplasms, 71 patients underwent EUS and fluid aspiration (for mucin, viscosity, amylase, lipase, CEA, CA19-9, cytology) followed by surgery to assess its accuracy. The authors[59] concluded that an accurate algorithm using measurement of viscosity, lipase and CEA can be used to determine the diagnosis of cystic lesions. If the viscosity is ≥1.6 then this indicates an MCN and the patient should be offered resection. If it is <1.6 and the lipase is <6000 U/mL this indicates an SCA. If the viscosity is <1.6 and lipase is >6000 U/mL then a CEA measurement should be performed, and if this value is less than 480 U/mL the diagnosis is a pseudocyst. If it is >480 U/mL, a repeat EUS and fine-needle aspiration should be performed in 3–6 months. Using this algorithm, only 2 of the 71 patients underwent resection for suspected MCN but the final histology was a pseudocyst.

The management of SCAs and MCNs differs on their malignant potential. It is currently recommended that all suspected MCNs undergo resection because of their malignant potential[5] but for SCA malignant transformation is very rare and for asymptomatic lesions no intervention is required.[58] Symptomatic lesions should be resected.

Pathologically SCAs demonstrate monomorphous cuboidal-shaped epithelium. The cells are glycogen rich with cellular cytoplasm and small regular nuclei. There is a lack of mitotic activity. The cysts appear 'empty' on microscopy. In contrast, the cyst content of MCNs is turbid and tenacious.[55] Microscopically (unlike SCAs) the cyst lining can be highly variable. The cells are mucin producing, which can be a single cell layer of flattened cuboidal epithelium or contain papillary tufting.[55] The tumours are classified as benign, borderline or malignant depending on the nuclear features of the cells.[55] It is important to examine the whole tumour as malignant invasion can occur without the presence of a mass.[55] The unique feature of MCNs, however, is the presence of ovarian stroma (highly cellular, densely packed, plump spindle cells). Current recommendations require the presence of this for a tumour to be classified as MCN.[5] This is particularly important when the differential includes IPMN, in which this type of stroma is not seen.[5]

Key Points

- As the use of cross-sectional imaging has become more frequent, there has been an increase in the diagnosis of cystic neoplasms within the pancreas.
- Main-duct intraductal papillary mucinous neoplasms should be resected due to the high incidence of underlying malignancy; however, a selective approach to intervention for side-branch intraductal papillary mucinous neoplasms should be taken (dependent on the presence of symptoms, tumour markers and tumour characteristics).
- Investigation and follow-up of cystic lesions of the pancreas requires a multimodal approach, of which endoscopic ultrasound with biopsy is becoming an increasingly important component.
- While asymptomatic serous cyst adenomas do not require intervention, mucinous cystic neoplasms should be resected due to their underlying malignant potential.
- The management of pancreatic neuroendocrine tumours will be dependent on the presence or absence of an underlying genetic syndrome, whether the tumour is hormonally active, and stage of disease.

References

1. Winter JM, Cameron JL, Campbell KA et al. 1423 pancreaticoduodenectomies for pancreatic cancer: a single-institution experience. J Gastrointest Surg 2006; 10:1199–210.

2. Pauser U, Kosmahl M, Sipos B et al. Mesenchymal tumors of the pancreas. Surprising, but not uncommon [in German]. Pathologie 2005;26:52–8.

3. Ohashi K, Murakami Y, Maruyama M et al. Four cases of mucin producing cancer of the pancreas on specific findings of the papilla of Vater [in Japanese]. Prog Dig Endosc 1982; 20:348–51.

4. Longnecker DS, Adler G, Hruban RH et al. Intraductal papillary mucinous neoplasm of the pancreas. In: Hamilton SR, Aaltonen LA (eds) World Health Organisation classification of tumours, pathology and genetics of tumours of the digestive system. Lyon: IARC Press, 2000; pp. 237–41.

5. Tanaka M, Cahri S, Adsay V et al. International consensus guidelines for management of intraductal papillary mucinous neoplasms and mucinous cystic neoplasms of the pancreas. Pancreatology 2006; 6:17–32.

6. McDonald JM, Williard W, Mais D et al. The incidence of intraductal papillary mucinous tumors of the pancreas. Curr Surg 2000; 57:610–14.

7. Kimura W, Nagai H, Kuroda A et al. Analysis of small cystic lesions of the pancreas. Int J Pancreatol 1995; 186:197–206.

8. Riall TS, Stager VM, Nealon WH. Incidence of additional primary cancers in patients with invasive intraductal papillary mucinous neoplasms and sporadic pancreatic adenocarcinomas. J Am Coll Surg 2007; 204:803–13.

9. Sohn TA, Yeo CA, Cameron JL et al. Intraductal papillary mucinous neoplasms of the pancreas: an increasingly recognized clinicopathologic entity. Ann Surg 2001; 234:313–21.

10. Sohn TA, Yeo CA, Cameron JL et al. Intraductal papillary mucinous neoplasms of the pancreas: an updated experience. Ann Surg 2004; 239:788–97.

11. Fujino Y, Matsumoto I, Ueda T et al. Proposed new score predicting malignancy of IPMN of the pancreas. Am J Surg 2007; 194:304–7.

12. Winter JM, Cameron JL, Lillemoe KD et al. Periampullary and pancreatic incidentaloma: a single institution's experience with an increasingly common diagnosis. Ann Surg 2006; 243:673–80.

13. Irie H, Yoshimutu K, Tajima T et al. Imaging spectrum of cystic pancreatic lesions: learn from atypical cases. Curr Probl Diagn Radiol 2007; 36:213–26.

14. Yamada Y, Mori H, Matsumoto S. Intraductal papillary mucinous neoplasms of the pancreas: correlation of helical CT and dynamic MR imaging features with pathologic findings. Abdom Imaging 2008; PMID:17680299, August (E-pub ahead of print).

15. Pilleul F, Rochette A, Partensky C et al. Preoperative evaluation of intraductal papillary mucinous tumors performed by pancreatic magnetic resonance imaging and correlated with surgical and histopathologic findings. J Magn Reson Imaging 2005; 21:237–44.

16. Kawamoto S, Lawler LP, Horton KM et al. MDCT of intraductal papillary mucinous neoplasm of the pancreas: evaluation of features predictive of invasive carcinoma. AJR 2006; 186:687–95.

17. Figuerias RG, Martin CV, Figuerias AG et al. The spectrum of cystic masses of the pancreas. Imaging features and diagnostic difficulties. Curr Probl Diagn Radiol 2007; 36:213–26.

18. Procacci C, Carbognin G, Biasiutti C et al. Intraductal papillary mucinous tumours of the pancreas: spectrum of CT and MR findings with pathologic correlation. Eur Radiol 2001; 11:1939–51.

19. Kubo H, Chijiiwa Y, Akahoshi K et al. Intraductal papillary-mucinous tumors of the pancreas: differential diagnosis between benign and malignant tumors by endoscopic ultrasonography. Am J Gastroenterol 2001; 96:1429–34.

20. Pais SA, Attasaranya S, Leblanc JK et al. Role of endoscopic ultrasound in the diagnosis of intraductal papillary mucinous neoplasms: correlation with surgical histopathology. Clin Gastroenterol Hepatol 2007; 5:489–95.

21. Michaels PJ, Brachtel EF, Bounds BC et al. Intraductal papillary mucinous neoplasm of the pancreas: cytologic features predict histologic grade. Cancer 2006; 108:163–73.

22. Tanaka M, Kobayashi K, Mizumoto K et al. Clinical aspects of intraductal papillary mucinous neoplasm of the pancreas. J Gastroenterol 2005; 40:669–75.

23. Hruban RH, Pitman MB, Klimstra DS (eds). AFIP atlas of tumour pathology. Tumors of the pancreas. Washington, DC: ARP Press, 2007.

24. Ban S, Naitoh Y, Mino-Kenudson M et al. IPMN of the pancreas: its histopathological difference in 2 types. Am J Surg Pathol 2006; 30:1561–9.

25. Sugiyama M, Izumisato Y, Abe N et al. Predicitive factors for malignancy in IPMN of the pancreas. Br J Surg 2003; 90:1244–9.

26. Nagai K, Doi R, Kida A et al. Intraductal papillary mucinous neoplasms of the pancreas: clinicopathological characteristics and long term follow up after resection. World J Surg 2008; 32:271–8.

27. Rodriguez JR, Salvia R, Crippa S et al. Branch-duct intraductal papillary mucinous neoplasms: observations in 145 patients who underwent resection. Gastroenterology 2007; 133:72–9.

28. Salvia R, Crippa S, Falconi M et al. Branch-duct intraductal papillary mucinous neoplasms of the pancreas: to operate or not to operate? Gut 2007; 56:1086–90.

29. Ghaneh P, Neoptolemos JP. A new approach to managing IPMN. Gut 2007; 56:1041–4.

30. Fujino Y, Suzuki Y, Yoshikawa T et al. Outcomes of surgery for IPMN of the pancreas. World J Surg 2006; 30:1909–14.

31. Crippa S, Bassi C, Warshaw AL et al. Middle pancreatectomy: indications, short- and long-term operative outcomes. Ann Surg 2007; 246:69–76.

32. Wada K, Kozarek RA, Traverso LW. Outcomes following resection of invasive and non invasive IPMN of the pancreas. Am J Surg 2005; 189:632–5.

33. Hardacre JM, McGee MF, Stellato TA et al. An aggressive surgical approach is warranted in the management of cystic pancreatic neoplasms. Am J Surg 2007; 193:374–9.

34. D'Angelica M, Brennan MF, Suriawinata AA et al. Intraductal papillary mucinous neoplasms of the pancreas. An analysis of clinicopathological features and outcome. Ann Surg 2004; 239:400–8.

35. Raut CP, Cleary KR, Staerkel GA et al. IPMN of the pancreas; the effect of invasion and pancreatic margin status on recurrence and survival. Ann Surg Oncol 2006; 13:582–94.

36. White R, D'Angelica M, Katabi N et al. Fate of the remnant pancreas after resection of non-invasive IPMN. J Am Coll Surg 2007; 204:987–95.

37. Sho M, Nakajima Y, Kanehiro H et al. Patterns of recurrence after resection for IPMN of the pancreas. World J Surg 1998; 22:874–8.

38. Tomimaru Y, Ishikawa O, Ohigashi H et al. Advantage of pancreaticogastrostomy in detecting recurrent intraductal papillary mucinous carcinoma in the remnant pancreas: a case of successful re-resection after pancreaticoduodenectomy. J Surg Oncol 2006; 93:511–5.

39. Kimura W, Kurda A, Morioka Y. Clinical pathology of endocrine tumours of the pancreas: analysis of autopsy cases. Dig Dis Sci 2004; 36:933–42.

40. Bilimoria KY, Tomlinson JS, Merkow RP et al. Clinicopathologic features and treatment trends of pancreatic neuroendocrine tumors: analysis of 9,821 patients. J Gastrointest Surg 2007; 11:1460–7.

41. Ramage JK, Davies AHG, Ardill J et al. Guidelines for the management of gastroenteropancreatic neuroendocrine tumours. Gut 2005; 54:1–16.

42. Alexakis N, Connor S, Ghaneh P et al. Hereditary pancreatic endocrine tumours. Pancreatology 2004; 4:417–33.

43. Rha SE, Jung SE, Lee KH et al. CT and MR imaging of endocrine tumour of the pancreas according to WHO classification. Eur J Radiol 2007; 62:371–7.

44. Rockall AG, Reznek RH. Imaging of neuroendocrine tumours. Best Pract Clin Endocr Metab 2007; 21:43–68.

45. Tucker ON, Crotty PL, Conlon KC. The management of insulinoma. Br J Surg 2006; 93:264–75.

46. Sundin A, Garske U, Orlefors H. Nuclear imaging of neuroendocrine tumours. Best Pract Clin Endocr Metab 2007; 21:69–85.

47. Fendrich V, Langer P, Waldmann J et al. Management of sporadic and multiple endocrine neoplasia type 1 gastrinomas. Br J Surg 2007; 94:1331–41.

48. Mabrut JY, Fernandez-Cruz L, Azagra JS et al. Laparoscopic pancreatic resection; results of a multi-centre European study of 127 patients. Surgery 2005; 137:597–605.

49. Norton JA, Fraker DL, Alexander HR et al. Surgery increases survival in patients with gastrinoma. Ann Surg 2006; 244:410–19.

   In a study of 160 patients with gastrinomas, 35 patients (with similar staged localised disease) who did not undergo resection were compared to those who underwent resection. After 12 years follow-up, 29% of those who did not undergo surgery had developed hepatic metastases compared to 5% in the resected group ($P < 0.001$).

50. Akerstrom G, Hellman P. Surgery on neuroendocrine tumours. Best Pract Clin Endocr Metab 2007; 21:87–109.

51. Kouvaraki MA, Solorzano CC, Shapiro SE et al. Surgical treatment of non functioning pancreatic islet cell tumours. J Surg Oncol 2005; 89:170–85.

52. Bloomston M, Muscarella P, Shah MH et al. Cytoreduction results in high perioperative mortality and decreased survival in patients undergoing pancreatectomy for neuroendocrine tumors of the pancreas. J Gastrointest Surg 2006; 10:1361–70.

53. Bilimoria KY, Bentrem DJ, Merkow RP et al. Application of pancreatic adenocarcinoma staging system to PNETs. J Am Coll Surg 2007; 205:558–63.

54. Spinelli KS, Fromwiller TE, Daniel RA et al. Cystic pancreatic neoplasms: observe or operate. Ann Surg 2004; 239:651–9.

55. Compton CC. Histology of cystic tumours of the pancreas. Gastroint Endosc Clin N Am 2002; 12:673–96.

56. Sarr MG, Kendrick ML, Nagorney DM et al. Cystic neoplasms of the pancreas. Surg Clin N Am 2001; 81:497–509.

57. Megibow AJ, Lavelle MT, Rofsky NM. Cystic tumours of the pancreas. The radiologist. Surg Clin N Am 2001; 81:489–95.

58. Bassi C, Salvia R, Molinari E et al. Management of 100 consecutive cases of pancreatic serous cystadenoma: wait for symptoms and see at imaging or vice versa? World J Surg 2003; 27:319–23.

59. Linder JD, Geenen JE, Catalano MF. Cyst fluid analysis obtained by EUS guided FNA in the evaluation of discrete cystic neoplasms of the pancreas: a single centre experience. Gastroint Endosc 2006; 64:697–702.

17

Hepatobiliary and pancreatic trauma

Rowan W. Parks

Introduction

Despite its relatively protected location, the liver is the most frequently injured intra-abdominal organ, although splenic injuries are more common following blunt abdominal trauma. Associated injuries to other organs, uncontrolled haemorrhage from the liver and subsequent development of septic complications contribute significantly to morbidity and death.

This chapter will address the presentation, initial assessment and management of patients with liver, non-iatrogenic biliary and pancreatic injuries. The selection criteria for conservative management will be discussed together with the indications for operative intervention. The factors guiding operative decision-making and the available therapeutic options at operation will be examined. The spectrum of complications and likely outcomes following trauma will also be reviewed. It is not always possible in clinical practice to separate these injuries into clearly distinct categories; however, practical guidance based on the evidence available will be presented.

Liver trauma

Mechanisms of liver injury

Blunt and penetrating trauma are the two principal mechanisms of liver injury. Road traffic accidents account for the majority of blunt injuries, whereas knife and gunshot wounds constitute the major cause of penetrating injuries. In the UK, blunt trauma predominates by a ratio of approximately 2:1 as documented in a large Scottish epidemiological study.[1] Whilst this is typical for other European centres,[2] it differs from the experience in South Africa, where penetrating injuries account for 66% of liver trauma,[3] and in North America, where up to 86% of liver injuries are penetrating wounds.[4,5]

Two types of blunt liver trauma have been described – deceleration (shearing) trauma and crush injury. Deceleration injuries occur in road traffic accidents and in falls from a height where there is movement of the liver relative to its diaphragmatic attachments.[6] Crush injuries are caused by direct trauma to the liver area. The two types of injury may coexist but tend to produce somewhat different types of liver injury. Deceleration or shearing injuries create lacerations in the hepatic parenchyma, typically between the right posterior section (segments 6 and 7) and the right anterior section (segments 5 and 8), which can extend to involve major vessels. In contrast, a direct blow to the abdomen may lead to a crush injury, with damage to the central portion of the liver (segments 4, 5 and 8). Compression between the right lower ribs and the spine may also cause bleeding from the caudate lobe (segment 1). Blunt trauma can rupture Glisson's capsule and can also lead to subcapsular or intraparenchymal haematoma formation. Penetrating injuries are usually associated with gunshot or stab wounds, with the former usually resulting in more tissue damage due to the cavitation effect as the bullet traverses the liver substance.

Injury to the hepatic veins and juxtahepatic vena cava can occur as a result of shearing stress in blunt trauma. It is worth noting that there may not be initial exsanguinating haemorrhage as the weight of the liver may provide some compression.

Classification of liver injury

The severity of liver trauma ranges from a minor capsular tear, with or without parenchymal injury, to extensive disruption involving both lobes of the liver with associated hepatic vein or vena caval injury. The American Association for the Surgery of Trauma has adopted for general use the classification of liver injury described initially in 1989 by Moore and colleagues, and revised subsequently in 1994[7] (Table 17.1). The hepatic injury grade is calculated from assessment of the liver injury using information derived from radiological study, operative findings or autopsy report. Where there are multiple injuries to the liver the grade is advanced by one stage. Grade I or II injuries are considered minor; they represent 80–90% of all cases and usually require minimal or no operative treatment. Grade III–V injuries are generally considered severe and may require surgical intervention, while grade VI lesions are regarded as incompatible with survival. Schweizer and colleagues have described a protocol-based liver trauma management system employing this classification system that permits lesser injuries to be treated non-operatively and allows more appropriate selection of patients for operative treatment.[8]

The initial assessment and management of an injured patient should proceed according to the Advanced Trauma Life Support (ATLS) guidelines of the American College of Surgeons Committee on Trauma. The initial focus of attention is on the patient's airway, breathing and circulation. The airway is secured, intravenous access established and fluid resuscitation commenced.

The role of 'aggressive' high-volume fluid replacement in trauma victims has been questioned, with evidence suggesting that excessive fluid replacement is associated with adverse outcome.[9] As this evidence came from an American series that included a large proportion of relatively young, previously fit adults suffering from penetrating trauma to the torso, with ready access to trauma centres, the results may not necessarily be applicable to practice in other countries.

Diagnosis of liver injury

In penetrating abdominal trauma, hepatic injury should be considered in any patient with a wound to the abdomen. Hepatic injury should also be considered in patients with penetrating low thoracic wounds and also in posterior penetrating wounds below a coronal plane at the tips of the scapulae.

Patients with major hepatic injury may present with profound clinical shock and abdominal distension. Hypotension resistant to fluid resuscitation combined with gross abdominal distension is an indication for immediate laparotomy. The operative management options for patients in this situation will be discussed in detail subsequently. Emergency room thoracotomy with cross-clamping of the descending thoracic aorta is a dramatic intervention, but even in centres where this technique is advocated the outcome is poor.

In Feliciano's series of 1000 patients with liver trauma treated during a 5-year period, 45 patients underwent emergency room thoracotomy for control of haemorrhage related to their liver injury and all died.[4] Similarly, in an 11-year review of 783 patients who sustained liver trauma in Scotland, 11 patients underwent an unsuccessful laparotomy or thoraco-laparotomy in the emergency room.[1]

Table 17.1 • Hepatic injury scale used by the American Association for the Surgery of Trauma

Grade		Description
I	Haematoma	Subcapsular, <10% surface area
	Laceration	Capsular tear, <1 cm parenchymal depth
II	Haematoma	Subcapsular, 10–50% of surface area
	Laceration	Intraparenchymal <10 cm in diameter
		1–3 cm parenchymal depth, <10 cm in length
III	Haematoma	Subcapsular, >50% surface area or expanding; ruptured subcapsular or parenchymal haematoma; intraparenchymal haematoma >10 cm or expanding
	Laceration	>3 cm parenchymal depth
IV	Laceration	Parenchymal disruption involving 25–75% of hepatic lobe or 1–3 Couinaud segments within a single lobe
V	Laceration	Parenchymal disruption involving >75% of hepatic lobe or > 3 Couinaud segments within a single lobe
	Vascular	Juxtahepatic venous injuries – retrohepatic cava, major hepatic veins
VI	Vascular	Hepatic avulsion

Note: advance one grade for multiple injuries up to grade II.

Emergency room surgery remains a potentially life-saving manoeuvre in patients with significant intrathoracic injury who may have a coexistent liver injury. However, there is little place for this intervention in patients with a predominant abdominal injury. These patients are better served by rapid assessment and transport to the operating theatre.

In less dramatic situations, with a patient who is haemodynamically stable or responds to fluid resuscitation, appropriate investigations can be employed to obtain more information regarding the liver injury and to ascertain whether there is coexisting intra-abdominal visceral injury. During the initial survey a detailed clinical history is taken. Particular attention is paid to the mechanism of a road traffic accident, with supplemental information from ambulance crew, witnesses or police being used to piece together a picture of the accident. Speed of vehicle, position of occupant in vehicle, use of seatbelts, employment of airbag restraint systems and a history of ejection of the patient from the vehicle are important items of information. Conscious patients may complain of abdominal pain. Shoulder tip pain may arise from blood in the subdiaphragmatic space causing phrenic nerve irritation.

As resuscitation proceeds, a detailed physical examination is carried out. On inspection, attention is paid to the presence of anterior abdominal wall bruising, which may indicate compression from a seatbelt, and flank bruising, which may indicate retroperitoneal extravasation of blood. Signs of localised or generalised peritonitis are recorded in the conscious patient. In this context it should be noted that although there is evidence that the use of opiate analgesia will not significantly obscure physical signs in patients with acute abdominal pain, these findings have not been confirmed in abdominal trauma patients where the situation may be complicated by head injury, alcohol intoxication or the requirement for assisted ventilation.

Baseline investigations consist of a full blood count (for haemoglobin and haematocrit), serum urea and electrolytes, serum amylase, a coagulation screen, and blood for crossmatching. An erect chest radiograph and a plain abdominal film can be taken if the patient is sufficiently stable. In the context of diagnosing liver injury, features that may be of relevance include fractures of the lower ribs, elevation of the right hemidiaphragm and loss of the psoas shadow suggesting retroperitoneal bleeding. Retroperitoneal perforation of the duodenum may give rise to soft tissue shadowing in the right upper quadrant, loss of the psoas shadow and occasionally extraluminal gas may be noted.

Following initial assessment, patients who are conscious but have haemodynamic instability resistant to fluid resuscitation and with clinical signs of peritonitis should undergo laparotomy. In patients who are haemodynamically stable and have suspected liver injury, further diagnostic tests may be undertaken at this stage to define the nature of the injuries. An ideal test will establish the presence and extent of any liver injury together with providing information on concomitant visceral injury.

Diagnostic peritoneal lavage (DPL) has been advocated in patients with impaired conscious levels and equivocal physical signs.[10] DPL may help in the diagnosis of hollow visceral injury. However, a DPL that yields a positive result for blood will provide no information regarding either the site or the nature of the injury, and in the context of liver injury may lead to patients undergoing surgery where they may be better treated non-operatively.

An alternative test that may be used in the emergency department is abdominal ultrasonography. Several recent prospective studies have reported that ultrasonography can be performed with a sensitivity of 82–88% and a specificity of 99% in detecting intra-abdominal injuries, but it remains critically dependent on the skill of the operator. Recognising this, the multicentre North American FAST study (Focused Assessment for the Sonographic examination of the Trauma patient) attempted to increase the reliability of ultrasound scanning in abdominal trauma by adhering to an agreed protocol for scanning that sequentially surveyed for haemopericardium and then the right upper quadrant, left upper quadrant and pelvis for haemoperitoneum in patients with potential truncal injuries.

The FAST study demonstrated a significant correlation between haemoperitoneum in the right upper quadrant and injury to the liver, and suggested that adherence to a pre-agreed protocol increased the reliability of ultrasound assessment of abdominal trauma.[11] Other centres have also reported that ultrasound is a reliable 'first' test for the assessment of a patient with suspected liver trauma.[12] However, an important cautionary note comes from the study carried out by Richards and colleagues.[13] In a series of 1686 abdominal ultrasound scans for trauma, 71 patients had bowel or mesenteric injury and 30 patients had a negative ultrasound scan (43% false-negative rate).

Computed tomography (CT) is the 'gold standard' investigation for the evaluation of a patient with suspected liver trauma (**Fig. 17.1**). The use of intravenous contrast may help in the detection of non-viable parenchyma. CT has high sensitivity and specificity for detecting liver injuries; these attributes increase as the time between injury and scanning increases, as haematomas and lacerations become better defined. Specific CT features of liver trauma have been reported by a number of authors. Fang and colleagues described intraparenchymal 'pooling'

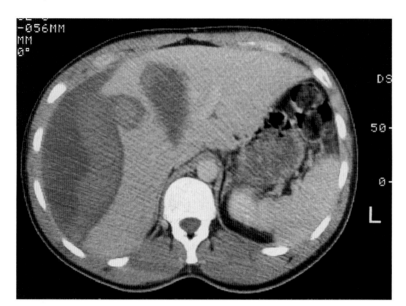

Figure 17.1 • CT of a 25-year-old male who sustained a blunt injury to the right chest wall but was admitted to hospital haemodynamically stable. The scan shows a substantial subcapsular haematoma associated with an intraparenchymal laceration. This patient was managed successfully without operation.

of intravenous contrast that correlated strongly to the presence of ongoing haemorrhage.[14] Yokota and Sugimoto documented 'periportal tracking' to consist of a circumferential area of low attenuation around the portal triad.[15] Periportal tracking is thought to represent blood or fluid within the condensation of the Glissonian sheath around the portal structures and indicates the presence of injury to structures in the portal triad. If the sign is present in the periphery of the liver it may alert the clinician to the presence of a peripheral bile duct injury that in turn may present as a bile leak. Addition of oral contrast medium does not appear to add to the diagnostic yield of CT in the assessment of liver injury.[16]

In order to maintain a balanced perspective, it is worthwhile considering some of the limitations of CT in the assessment of liver trauma. The CT-defined grade of injury may differ from the grade of liver injury found at operation, with the predominant tendency being to overdiagnose the grade of injury on CT as compared with subsequent operative findings. Croce and colleagues concluded that CT should not be used in isolation to estimate blood loss and that CT may not provide an accurate assessment of the extent of a liver laceration in some areas of the liver – specifically in the vicinity of the falciform ligament.[17]

Bearing the above limitations in mind, CT will help define the extent of the liver injury and will be of value in the detection of injury to other intra-abdominal viscera, in particular pancreatic injury. CT will allow the liver injury to be graded and thus will provide objective information that is mandatory if non-operative treatment is to be contemplated. Further refinements now permit accurate three-dimensional image reconstruction, and technical modifications such as helical

CT combined with intravenous contrast allow demonstration of the biliary tree (CT cholangiography) or vascular anatomy (CT angiography).

Other diagnostic modalities for the assessment of liver injury

Non-invasive imaging techniques such as magnetic resonance imaging (MRI) have the advantage of being free of ionising radiation, but increased cost aside, the time taken to produce a scan means that this technique is not yet widely used in the trauma setting. Angiography may be used as a complementary investigation to CT.[18] In this context, it is of value in patients with high-grade liver injury and may be combined with therapeutic angiographic embolisation for ongoing blood loss or haemobilia.[19]

Other diagnostic modalities may be used in specific situations. Endoscopic retrograde cholangiopancreatography (ERCP) may help in delineation of the biliary tree in patients with liver trauma, and endoscopic transpapillary stents may be used as a therapeutic modality to treat biliary leaks.[20]

Diagnostic laparoscopy has been used successfully in patients with abdominal trauma, and therapeutic laparoscopic techniques for managing liver injuries using fibrin glue have also been described. However, in the specific context of liver trauma, concerns have been raised about the use of laparoscopy because general anaesthesia, muscle relaxation and the creation of a pneumoperitoneum may decompress a stable perihepatic haematoma. Furthermore, laparoscopic assessment of the injured liver may not provide sufficient detail concerning parenchymal injury. For these reasons, the role of laparoscopy has yet to be established in the assessment of liver injuries.

In the initial management of suspected liver trauma there is little evidence to support the use of emergency room thoracotomy. Ultrasound is reliable for the initial assessment of a patient with suspected liver trauma but CT remains the gold standard to define the extent of injury in a stable patient.

Management of liver injury: selection of patients for non-operative management

The feasibility of non-operative management of patients with intra-abdominal solid organ injury was first established in paediatric surgery and has extended gradually to adult practice. Richie and Fonkalsrud described successful conservative management of four patients with liver injury in an era before the availability of CT.[21] Further indirect evidence for the feasibility of a non-operative approach came from a report published by White and Cleveland[22] in the same year. They reported a consecutive series of 126 patients with liver trauma, all of whom underwent laparotomy. Interestingly, 67 patients in this series (53%) had placement of a drain to the subhepatic space as their only liver-related surgical intervention at laparotomy. Subsequent studies have recognised that 50–80% of liver injuries stop bleeding spontaneously and this has led to a non-operative approach for blunt liver trauma in selected patients.

Non-operative management of liver trauma is now a well-established treatment option. Trunkey's group in Portland, Oregon, first defined in 1985 the following criteria for the selection of patients for non-operative management:

- haemodynamic stability
- absence of peritoneal signs
- availability of good-quality CT
- an experienced radiologist
- ability to monitor patients in an intensive care setting
- facility for immediate surgery (and by implication, availability of an experienced liver surgeon)
- simple liver injury with <125 ml of free intraperitoneal blood
- absence of other significant intra-abdominal injuries.[23]

Farnell and colleagues extended the threshold of haemoperitoneum to 250 mL and described specific liver injuries suitable for non-operative management.[24] Feliciano suggested subsequently that any blunt hepatic injury, regardless of its magnitude, should be managed without operation if the patient was haemodynamically stable and had a haemoperitoneum of less than 500 mL.[25] The degree of liver injury amenable to successful non-operative management has gradually extended over recent years, and most authors now believe that the ultimate decisive factor in favour of non-operative management is haemodynamic stability of the patient at presentation or after initial resuscitation, irrespective of the grade of liver injury on CT or the amount of haemoperitoneum.[26,27]

A 22-month prospective study from Memphis of the initial non-operative treatment of haemodynamically stable blunt hepatic trauma patients compared outcome to a matched cohort of blunt hepatic trauma patients treated operatively.[28] The study reported that of 136 patients with blunt trauma, 24 (18%) underwent emergency surgery. Of the remaining 112 patients, 12 (11%) failed conservative management (for causes not related to the liver injury in seven) and the remaining 100 patients were treated successfully without operation. Of these, 30% had minor injuries (grades I–II) but 70% had major injuries (grades III–V). This study concluded that non-operative management was safe for haemodynamically stable patients and that this was independent of the CT-delineated grade of the liver injury. The blood transfusion requirement and the incidence of abdominal complications were lower in the non-operatively treated group.

Reporting a single institutional experience, Boone and colleagues stated that 46 (36%) of 128 consecutive patients with blunt liver trauma were successfully treated non-operatively, including 23 patients with grade III and IV injuries.[26] A review of 495 patients from the published literature noted a success rate for non-operative treatment of 94%.[29] This was accomplished with a mean transfusion rate of 1.9 units, a complication rate of 6% and a mean hospital stay of 13 days. There were no liver-related deaths, nor were there any missed enteric injuries.

The current consensus view is that successful selection of patients for conservative treatment after blunt abdominal trauma cannot be carried out by CT scanning alone, but that an overall assessment of suitability for such an approach must take into account the findings of careful repeated clinical examination and the results of close monitoring of haemodynamic and haematological parameters. If non-operative management is selected, haemodynamic instability is the predominant indication for intervention early in the clinical course whilst intervention (often radiological or endoscopic) may be required later for management of bile leak or intrahepatic collections.

If a non-operative strategy is selected it should be borne in mind that the risk of hollow organ injury increases in proportion to the number of solid organs injured[30] and that there is a small but significant risk of delayed haemorrhage. However, it appears that the natural course of liver injuries is more analogous to that of lung or kidney injuries, rather than splenic injuries, in that any deterioration is usually gradual, with a fall in haemoglobin level or an increase in fluid requirement, rather than acute haemodynamic decompensation. Therefore, with close supervision, patients who fail with an initial non-operative approach can be detected early and treated appropriately.

Although non-operative management of haemodynamically stable patients with liver trauma has become the standard of care over the past decade, the role of in-hospital follow-up CT to monitor the injury remains controversial. Demetriades and colleagues reported that follow-up CT at a mean of 10 days after surgical intervention showed a 49% incidence of liver-related complications, most of which required subsequent intervention.[31] However, other authors suggest there is little evidence that follow-up CT provides additional information and rarely changes management.[32] In the author's practice, routine in-hospital follow-up scan is not employed routinely unless the patient develops symptoms or signs suggestive of hepatic abnormality, but a follow-up scan 4–6 weeks later is undertaken to ensure resolution of the injury.

The management policy for abdominal gunshot injuries in most centres continues to be a mandatory laparotomy, regardless of the clinical presentation;[33] however, several studies have reported successful non-operative management of selected liver gunshot injuries.[34,35] In the study by Omoshoro-Jones and colleagues, 26.6% of patients who presented with liver gunshot injuries were managed non-operatively with an overall success rate of 94% and a morbidity rate of 36%, of which 3% was liver-related.[34] This approach is associated with the risk of failure to detect concomitant intra-abdominal visceral injury and therefore should only be considered in specialist centres with experience in management of liver trauma and appropriate facilities to deal with any complications that arise.

Non-operative management is safe for haemodynamically stable patients with CT evidence of liver injury.

Operative management of liver injury

General strategy

Primary operative intervention is indicated for liver injury if the patient is haemodynamically unstable despite adequate initial resuscitation. Important prerequisites for a successful outcome are: adequate blood, platelets, fresh frozen plasma and cryoprecipitate; an intensive care unit; the necessary diagnostic facilities to monitor and detect potential complications; and an experienced liver surgeon. Although this is the ideal, patients with liver trauma often present initially to surgeons without specialist hepatobiliary experience and without the facilities available in liver surgery units. The surgeon operating on a patient in this situation should therefore attempt to control bleeding without causing further complications.

Choice of incision

A long midline incision is widely employed for an emergency laparotomy. It has the advantages that it can be made rapidly, extended proximally (to enter the chest after median sternotomy) or distally as required. Access to the liver can be improved by converting the incision into a 'T' by adding a right transverse component or to a 'Y' by adding a right lateral thoracotomy, although extension of the incision into the chest is exceptional. In situations where an operation is being carried out after initial conservative management, for example to treat bile leakage or perform delayed resectional debridement, a subcostal incision with fixed costal margin retraction affords excellent access to the liver.

Intraoperative assessment

Once the abdomen has been entered, blood and clots should be removed and packs inserted into each quadrant of the abdomen. A thorough laparotomy is performed in a systematic manner to identify all intra-abdominal injuries. Any perforations in the bowel should be sutured immediately to minimise contamination. Significant liver haemorrhage can usually be controlled initially by direct pressure using packs, although additional techniques that may be employed include: temporary digital compression of the free edge of the lesser omentum (Pringle manoeuvre; **Fig. 17.2**); bimanual compression of the liver; or manual compression of the aorta above the coeliac trunk. At this point, further evaluation of the extent of liver injury should be delayed until the anaesthetist has replenished adequately the intravascular volume and stabilised the blood pressure. Attempts to evaluate the liver injury before adequate resuscitation may result in further blood loss, with worsening hypotension and acidosis.

The packs can subsequently be gently removed to allow a detailed evaluation of the type and extent of the liver injury. It should be borne in mind that a subcapsular haematoma may cover an area of ischaemic tissue and that parenchymal lacerations may be associated with damage to segmental bile ducts. Many liver injuries will have stopped bleeding spontaneously by the time of surgery. However, if there is active bleeding, a Pringle manoeuvre can be used

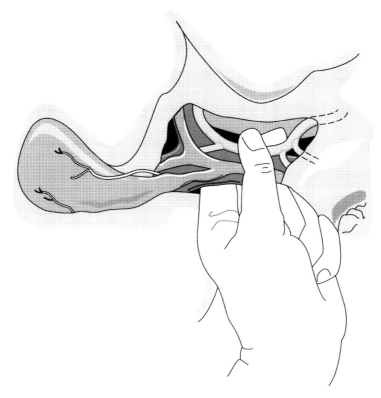

Figure 17.2 • Manual occlusion of the structures of the portal triad – the Pringle manoeuvre. From Garden OJ. Liver Trauma. In: Carter D, Russell RCG, Pitt H, Bismuth H (eds) Hepatobiliary and pancreatic surgery (Rob & Smith's operative surgery), 5th edition. London: Hodder Arnold, 1998, Reproduced by permission of Edward Arnold (Publishers) Ltd.

diagnostically and compression can be maintained with an atraumatic vascular clamp if haemorrhage decreases (**Fig. 17.3**). The clamp should be occluded only to the degree necessary to compress the blood vessels and not to injure the common bile duct. A normal liver can tolerate inflow occlusion for up to 1 hour; however, the ability of a damaged liver to tolerate ischaemia may be impaired. If haemorrhage is unaffected by portal triad occlusion, major vena cava injury or atypical vascular anatomy should be suspected. Hepatic outflow control may also be required. Access to the suprahepatic cava can be gained by an experienced liver surgeon, and slings may be placed around the hepatic veins following mobilisation of the liver from its peritoneal attachments. Total vascular occlusion of the liver requires control of the inferior vena cava below the liver in addition to the suprahepatic cava but is likely to be poorly tolerated by an injured liver.

Perihepatic packing

In situations where it is thought that definitive control of haemorrhage cannot be obtained, the liver injury should be packed, the incision closed and the patient transferred to the care of a specialist hepatobiliary surgeon for definitive treatment.[36] Packing can also be employed as a holding manoeuvre in patients who are critically unstable, coagulopathic or acidotic and therefore would not tolerate a prolonged operative procedure. As packing is thus a widely applicable procedure, some attention should be devoted to technical considerations. The packs should not be inserted into the liver substance itself, as this will tend to distract the edges of the parenchymal tear and encourage continued bleeding. Rather, the technique of packing involves manual closure or approximation of the parenchyma, followed by sequential placing of dry abdominal packs or a single rolled gauze around the liver and directly over the injury in an attempt to provide tamponade to a bleeding wound (**Fig. 17.4**). Most surgeons employ skin closure only, leaving the fascia for primary closure at the subsequent procedure for pack removal. The presence of packs, combined with massive oedema of the bowel, may lead to difficulties in wound closure. If this is encountered, a mesh can be inserted to prevent further compromise of ventilation and bowel viability, and to avoid pressure necrosis of the liver.[37]

The principal complications and limitations of perihepatic packing can be considered as 'early' or 'late'. Early complications include failure to control

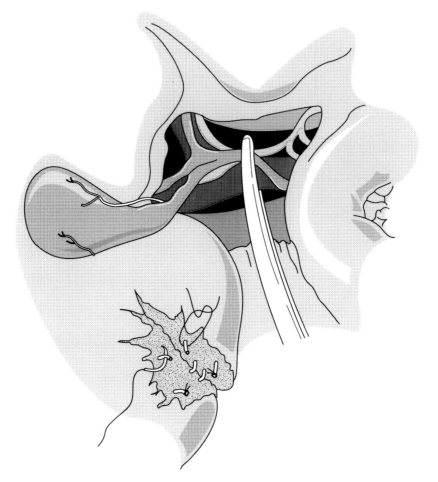

Figure 17.3 • Occlusion of the structures in the portal triad using a soft non-crushing clamp. From Garden OJ. Liver Trauma. In: Carter D, Russell RCG, Pitt H, Bismuth H (eds) Hepatobiliary and pancreatic surgery (Rob & Smith's operative surgery), 5th edition. London: Hodder Arnold, 1998, Reproduced by permission of Edward Arnold (Publishers) Ltd.

haemorrhage. However, this is relatively uncommon as even in patients with caval or hepatic venous injuries, packing may control haemorrhage. Concerns may also be raised about the potential for compromise of caval blood flow by packing, although this may be avoided by monitoring caval pressure if this technique is available. The principal late complications of packing are infection and multiple organ dysfunction. The risk of septic complications has led to the recommendation that liver packs should be removed as soon as possible. However, Nicol and colleagues reported in a series of 93 patients requiring liver packing that an early re-look laparotomy at 24 hours rather than at 48 hours or later was associated with a higher incidence of rebleeding necessitating re-packing without any difference in the incidence of liver-related complications or intra-abdominal collections.[38] Perihepatic packing is an indication for intravenous antibiotic administration.

 The first re-look laparotomoy following packing for a liver injury should only be performed after 48 hours when hypotension, hypothermia, coagulopathy and acidosis have been corrected.

Techniques for surgical haemostasis

Exposed bleeding vessels can be suture-ligated, clipped or repaired to achieve haemostasis. The ultrasonic dissector is useful in removing damaged and non-viable hepatic parenchyma whilst exposing blood vessels. Diathermy coagulation can also be used and in this context the argon beam coagulator, which 'sprays' the diathermy current on an argon beam, is invaluable as it produces surface eschar without the diathermy probe becoming adherent to the liver surface. The argon beam coagulator also has the advantage of producing less hepatic tissue necrosis than conventional diathermy, which is an advantage in a potentially contaminated operative field. Fibrin glue

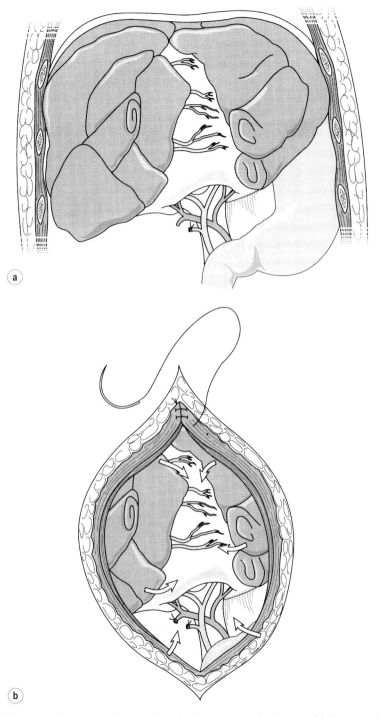

Figure 17.4 • (a) Placement of gauze packs around the liver to compress the fracture. **(b)** Closure of the incision provides additional compression. Reproduced from Berne TV, Donovan AJ. Section 10. Injury and haemorrhage. In: Blumgart LH, Fong Y (eds) Surgery of the liver and biliary tract, 3rd edn, Vol. 2. Edinburgh: Churchill Livingstone, 1994. With permission from Elsevier.

has been used as an adjunctive measure in some centres; however, there are concerns regarding the use of fibrin glue in humans. Fatal hypotension following application of fibrin glue into a deep hepatic laceration has been reported.[39] Recently, recombinant factor VIIa has been reported as a potential adjunct in the management of liver injuries;[40] however, further controlled studies are warranted to evaluate the safety and efficiency of this drug.

Liver sutures are absorbable sutures on a large curved blunt-tipped needle often used in conjunction with a bolster of haemostatic material. These can be used to approximate a fissured parenchymal injury and thus control haemorrhage as an alternative to exploration of the depths of the injury. The disadvantages of this technique are that vessels may continue to bleed resulting in a cavitating haematoma, bile duct injuries may not be detected, and the suture itself may cause further bleeding, ischaemia or intrahepatic bile duct injury (**Fig. 17.5**).

Stone and Lamb reported that the greater omentum could be employed as a pedicled flap to fill a defect in the liver parenchyma and may help stop oozing from the low-pressure venous system of the liver parenchyma.[41] The use of an absorbable polyglactin perihepatic mesh, particularly for major parenchymal disruptions, has also been reported.[42] This technique is not indicated where juxtacaval or hepatic vein injury is suspected. Advocates of mesh wrapping claim that it can provide the benefits of packing without the disadvantages. In particular, a second laparotomy is not required routinely and, as mesh wrapping does not increase intra-abdominal volume or pressure, abdominal closure is much easier and respiratory or renal function is less compromised. However, there is some concern about the amount of time needed to apply the mesh wrap in a haemodynamically unstable patient who might be best treated with rapid insertion of perihepatic packs, and as yet there is insufficient general experience with this technique.

Resectional debridement

This technique involves removal of devitalised liver tissue down to normal parenchyma using the lines of the injury, rather than anatomical planes, as the boundaries of the resection.[43] The optimum timing may be to combine debridement with pack removal, as necrotic tissue will be well demarcated at 48 h post-injury. Resectional debridement is by definition 'non-anatomical' and may expose segmental bile ducts (**Fig 17.6**). Disrupted bile ducts exposed in the periphery of the liver should be sutured or ligated in order to prevent postoperative bile leaks, as this troublesome complication will not necessarily be treatable by endoscopic transampullary biliary stenting. It is better to anticipate and avoid this complication.

Anatomical liver resection

The practical difficulties of undertaking formal anatomical liver resection in a patient with a significant liver injury, who will frequently have associated shock, coagulopathy and concomitant injury, are such that this type of treatment is not used widely. It is generally accepted that anatomical resections should be reserved for situations in which no other procedure adequately achieves haemostasis, such as with deep liver lacerations involving major vessels and/or bile ducts, where there is extensive devascularisation or if there is major hepatic venous bleeding.

Strong et al. reported a single-centre series of 37 patients undergoing anatomical resection for liver trauma from an institutional experience of 287 patients with liver injury treated over a 13-year period.[44] Twenty-seven of these patients underwent right hemihepatectomy and overall there were three postoperative deaths (8% mortality rate). However, these excellent results achieved by a technically skilled liver surgeon and his unit may not be reproduced if the technique were more widely used.

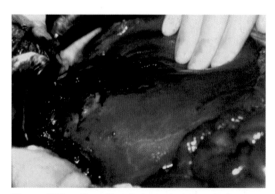

Figure 17.5 • Operative photograph demonstrating a liver injury with necrosis at the site of previously inserted liver sutures which had been applied in an attempt to arrest haemorrhage.

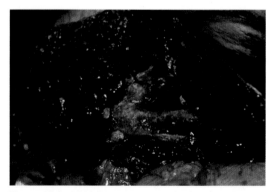

Figure 17.6 • Debridement of a liver injury managed 3 days before by packing has left the branches of the right portal pedicle exposed.

Selective ligation of the hepatic artery

Selective ligation of the hepatic artery is no longer a commonly used technique and is not mentioned frequently in contemporary reports. It may be used when intrahepatic manoeuvres have failed and when persistent re-bleeding occurs on unclamping the hepatic pedicle. In a series of 60 patients,[45] Mays reported ligation of the right hepatic artery in 36 patients, the left hepatic artery in 15 patients and the main hepatic artery in the remaining nine patients. No cases of liver failure or necrosis were observed but it seems likely that modern liver surgical approaches have rendered ligation an uncommon manoeuvre in liver injury. Hepatic arterial ligation to control haemorrhage should only be performed when other manoeuvres have failed, when selective ligation has failed and when pedicle clamping has been demonstrated to arrest haemorrhage. Acute gangrenous cholecystitis is a well-recognised complication of hepatic artery ligation, and cholecystectomy should be performed if the main hepatic artery or right hepatic artery is ligated.

Management of hepatic venous and retrohepatic caval injury

Suspicion that one of these serious injuries is present should be raised if the Pringle manoeuvre fails to arrest haemorrhage. In this situation it is vital that a systematic approach be adopted. Injudicious mobilisation of the liver can cause exsanguination or embolisation of air or detached fragments of liver parenchyma. Therefore it is important to exclude anatomical vascular variants as a source of persistent bleeding. For example, there may be bleeding from the left liver due to the presence of a left hepatic artery arising from the left gastric artery or there may be bleeding from the right liver due to an aberrant right hepatic artery. The commonest anatomical variation in the origin of the right hepatic artery (occurring in approximately 15% of cases) is the persistence of the right primordial hepatic artery where the right hepatic artery arises from the superior mesenteric artery and runs just to the right and slightly posterior to the structures in the porta hepatis. These anatomical variants should be considered and excluded. During this process, active bleeding can be reduced or arrested by perihepatic packing. Persistent bleeding despite exclusion of anatomical variants may then indicate the presence of hepatic venous or retrohepatic caval injury. These injuries account for about 10% of liver trauma cases, and there is no clear consensus on an optimal management strategy. Total vascular exclusion (clamping of the inferior vena cava and suprahepatic cava in addition to the Pringle manoeuvre) may be used. However, clamping the vena cava will seriously compromise venous return in a situation of major trauma and seems unwise. Veno-venous bypass (shunt from common femoral vein to left internal jugular or axillary vein) has the advantage of preserving venous return. Atriocaval shunting has also been described and, combined with a Pringle manoeuvre, allows total vascular isolation of the liver. Chen and colleagues reported on a series of 19 patients with blunt juxtahepatic venous injury from a group of 92 patients with blunt liver trauma over a 2-year period.[46] Five patients with isolated left hepatic vein injuries were treated with the use of veno-venous bypass with no mortality. Ten of the 20 patients with isolated right hepatic vein injury were treated using an atriocaval shunt but the mortality in these 20 patients was 18 (80%), with one survivor in both the shunted and non-shunted groups. Of four patients with combined right and left hepatic vein injury, one was treated by liver transplantation but all four patients in this group died. The overall mortality rate in patients with juxtahepatic vein injury was 63%. The opportunity to optimise the outcome in patients with these serious injuries probably lies in packing followed by transfer to a specialist liver surgery unit.

Ex vivo surgery and liver transplantation

Ringe and Pichlmayr[47] reported a consecutive series of eight patients with severe liver trauma treated by total hepatectomy followed by liver transplantation. These patients had all undergone prior surgery for trauma, which had been followed by severe complications – uncontrollable bleeding in four and massive necrosis in four. Where a donor liver was not immediately available a temporary portacaval shunt was used as a bridging procedure. There was a high mortality in this group, with six out of eight patients dying from multiple organ failure or sepsis. The authors conclude that total hepatectomy can be a potentially life-saving procedure in exceptional emergencies in patients with major liver injuries. Heparinised coated tubes such as the Gott shunt can be used to bridge caval defects if total hepatectomy and excision of a caval segment is required in order to obtain haemostasis.[48] The shunt acts as a temporary bridge during the anhepatic phase and has been reported to remain patent over an 18-h period. Whilst experience of this sort of surgery is extremely infrequent, awareness of the therapeutic potential is useful and small series continue to report encouraging results.[49]

Complications of liver trauma

Complications of non-operative management

Complications of non-operative management of liver trauma can be considered in three main categories. First, it should be borne in mind that complications can arise as a result of inappropriate selection of a patient for conservative management. If a patient has continued bleeding this may present as episodes of hypotension requiring fluid and blood replacement, impaired renal function, impaired respiratory function (due to diaphragmatic splinting by intra-abdominal haematoma) and there may be evidence of coagulopathy. These features represent not so much a 'complication' as the natural progression of a patient with continued active intra-abdominal bleeding, and in such a case the policy of non-operative intervention will require reappraisal.

The second group of complications are those relating to coexisting injuries that have not been recognised at the time of initial presentation or become apparent after initial delay. Bile leaks may manifest as biliary peritonitis or as a localised bile collection. ERCP is useful in diagnosing the source of a bile leak in patients with liver trauma treated non-operatively and also in postoperative patients. Perforations of the intestine are also at risk of being missed as the signs of abdominal tenderness may be attributed to intra-abdominal blood from the liver injury. The risk of missing this type of injury can be minimised by regular careful clinical observation. Intestinal perforation may become apparent on serial ultrasound or CT by the presence of free intraperitoneal fluid or gas. In Sherman's series of patients with liver trauma treated non-operatively, 4 of 30 (13%) patients initially treated without operation required subsequent laparotomy.[27] These were due to splenic injury in three patients and renal injury in one patient. Although the grade of injury to these organs is not specified, in all cases the injuries became apparent after a period of clinical observation. However, the authors concluded that this risk of missed solid organ injury does not obviate the benefits of initial non-operative management.

The third category of complication relates to the late complications of liver injury. Liver injury may give rise to a transient increase in liver transaminase enzymes. Their persistent elevation suggests significant liver injury. Septic complications such as intra-abdominal abscess and bile leak are recognised late complications and may require radiological, endoscopic or surgical intervention.

Postoperative complications after surgery for liver trauma

The complications after liver surgery for trauma are similar to those encountered after any form of hepatic surgery. Haemorrhage in the immediate postoperative period may be due to coagulopathy related to large-volume transfusion and may require correction with fresh frozen plasma and platelet concentrates. If there is no evidence of a significant coagulopathy and bleeding continues, CT angiography may provide diagnostic information. Selective mesenteric angiography may permit therapeutic embolisation,[50] but if this is unsuccessful, re-laparotomy will be

indicated to assess and control the source of bleeding and to remove retained blood and clot. Bleeding in the later postoperative period may be due to haemobilia or bleeding from the biliary tree into the gut. It has been reported to occur in 1.2% of patients with liver trauma.[51]

Postoperative sepsis may be due to infected collections of bile or blood, or related to devitalised segments of liver parenchyma. Ultrasound and CT are of value in diagnosis and these modalities may be used to guide placement of drains. Bile leakage from a drain site is not uncommon and usually ceases spontaneously; however, if it persists, ERCP may be all that is required to define the site of the leak and allow temporary stent placement. Arteriovenous fistula is not an uncommon complication after liver injury and can manifest as an arterioportal fistula resulting in portal hypertension.

Outcome after liver injury

The outcome after liver trauma is related not only to the severity of the injury but also to the severity of any associated injury. Most series report mortality rates of approximately 10–15%; however, the large variation in case mix between different centres makes comparison difficult. In a large series of 1000 cases of liver trauma from Houston, an overall mortality of 10.5% was reported.[4] White and Cleveland documented a similar mortality rate, with eight deaths occurring in a consecutive series of 126 patients (6.3%).[22] The results in the series reported by Schweizer and colleagues reported an overall mortality rate of 12% (21 deaths in 175 patients), with a progressively higher mortality rate associated with an increasing grade of liver injury.[8] In a series of 337 patients, Kozar and colleagues reported 37 hepatic-related complications in 25 patients; 63% (5 of 8) of patients with grade V injuries developed complications, 21% (19 of 92) of patients with grade IV injuries, but only 1% (1 of 130) of patients with grade III injuries.[52] The mechanism of injury has an important bearing on the mortality rate, with blunt trauma carrying a higher mortality rate (10–30%) than penetrating liver trauma (0–10%). While most early deaths seem to be due to uncontrolled haemorrhage and associated injuries, most late deaths result from head injuries and sepsis with multiple organ failure.

Extrahepatic biliary tract trauma

Non-iatrogenic injury to the extrahepatic biliary tract is uncommon and encountered only rarely by surgeons outside specialist hepatobiliary centres. Most injuries are due to penetrating rather than blunt abdominal trauma. Biliary tract injury is diagnosed infrequently before operation and is often only recognised incidentally at laparotomy. Extrahepatic bile duct injury due to blunt trauma is only rarely associated with injury to the portal vein or hepatic artery. This may be explained by the increased length, tortuosity and elasticity of the vascular structures. Furthermore, a vascular injury, especially portal vein rupture, is likely to be associated with a high immediate mortality.

Incidence of biliary injury

The reported incidence of injury to the extrahepatic biliary system varies between 1% and 5% of patients who sustain abdominal trauma.[53] In a review of 5070 patients who sustained blunt and penetrating abdominal trauma, Penn reported a 1.9% incidence of gallbladder injury.[54] Soderstrom and colleagues identified 31 patients (2.1%) with gallbladder injury in a group of 1449 patients who sustained blunt abdominal trauma and underwent exploratory laparotomy.[55] In a further review of 949 patients undergoing laparotomy for acute trauma, there were 32 injuries to the gallbladder (3.4%) and five to the common bile duct (0.5%).[56] Burgess and Fulton reported that, over a 5-year period, 24 of 184 patients with abdominal trauma had extrahepatic bile duct or gallbladder injury as well as liver injury.[57] They reported that this injury was often seen with severe hepatic trauma and in association with multiple organ injury. Dawson and colleagues reviewed the results of treatment of all patients with porta hepatis injuries presenting to a level I trauma centre in Seattle over an 11-year period.[58] A total of 21 patients (0.21% of 10 500 admissions) had injuries to the portal triad, of whom 11 (52%) died. Isolated extrahepatic bile duct injury occurred in four of these patients. Injuries to the portal vein or hepatic artery, either in isolation or in association with extrahepatic bile duct injury, were associated with the worst prognosis. Of note is the fact that in none of the 21 cases was the diagnosis of the injury made preoperatively. The male to female ratio is usually reported as approximately 5:1.[59] However, Bade and colleagues reported a male to female ratio of 25:1, which may reflect the higher number of injuries from stab wounds seen in a South African population.[60] Most series report a median age of approximately 30 years and there are many reports in children.

Classification of biliary injury

The gallbladder is the most frequently injured part of the extrahepatic biliary tract. The largest reported series of extrahepatic biliary tract injuries consists of 53 patients, of whom 45 (85%) sustained injury to the gallbladder and eight (15%) had an injury to the bile duct.[60] Kitahama and colleagues reported the gallbladder to be involved in 32 (80%) of 40 patients, while ductal injury occurred in 12 (30%), some patients having multiple injuries.[59]

Injury to the gallbladder resulting from blunt trauma can be classified as contusion, avulsion or perforation. In addition to these three main types of injury, Penn added traumatic cholecystitis as a pathological entity.[54] The most common type of gallbladder injury is perforation. Avulsion of the gallbladder may refer to the organ being partially or completely torn from the liver bed, while still attached to the bile duct, or it may signify complete separation from all attachments with the organ lying free in the abdomen. Contusion is probably under-reported, as it will be recognised only if laparotomy is performed. The natural course of an untreated gallbladder contusion is not known, although it is likely that the majority resolve without further complication. It has been speculated that an intramural haematoma might result in necrosis of the gallbladder wall and result in a subsequent perforation. There have been a number of reports of delayed rupture of the gallbladder, and it is plausible that unrecognised contusion of the gallbladder might lead to such a delayed presentation.

Bile duct injury is classified according to the site of injury and according to whether the transection is partial or complete. Partial duct injuries are often referred to as 'tangential' wounds. Penetrating injuries can affect any part of the extrahepatic biliary system; however, the commonest sites of injury due to blunt trauma are at the point where the common bile duct enters the pancreas and where the biliary confluence exits from the liver. These sites are at points of maximum fixation, which accounts for their propensity to injury.

Isolated injury to the extrahepatic biliary tract is very uncommon. The liver is the organ most commonly injured in association with biliary tract trauma (approximately 80% of cases), with the duodenum, stomach, colon and pancreas being the next most frequently reported. Associated vascular injuries are relatively rare; however, inferior vena cava and portal vein injuries are more commonly reported than those to the hepatic artery, renal vessels or aorta.

Presentation and diagnosis of biliary injury

Clinical presentation of the vast majority of bile duct injuries can be divided into two broad categories. The first contains patients in whom clinical signs or associated injury lead to laparotomy with early diagnosis and surgical management (early presentation); these patients generally present with hypovolaemic shock or signs of an acute abdomen.

The second category of patient has a delay (greater than 24 h) in diagnosis and definitive therapy (delayed presentation). These patients comprised over half the cases (53.2%) in a review of combined series.[61] In addition, a third category of patient, representing a very small proportion of those who sustain a bile duct injury, may present with obstructive jaundice months or even years after the initial trauma (late presentation). In these patients, the bile duct injury is always isolated. Compromise of the blood supply to the duct may occur either at the time of the primary injury or at operation during the Pringle manoeuvre, and this may contribute to the development of a late biliary stricture. Bourque and colleagues reported that the delay between clinical presentation and surgical intervention for isolated bile duct injury averaged 18 days, with a range from several hours to 60 days.[62] Michelassi and Ranson reported that biliary injury was not recognised at initial operation in 11 (12%) of 91 patients with extrahepatic biliary tract trauma,[61] whereas Dawson and Jurkovich reported that 41% of bile duct injuries were missed at initial laparotomy.[63]

If a non-operative course of management for abdominal trauma is adopted, suspicion of an extrahepatic bile duct injury may be raised by CT evidence of a central liver injury involving the porta hepatis or the head of the pancreas, the presence of fluid collections in the subhepatic space, or evidence of periportal tracking of haematoma.[15] The diagnostic procedure of choice is ERCP, and if a duct injury is identified, this may be treated by endoscopic stenting.[64]

Intraoperative recognition of biliary tract injury requires a high index of suspicion. The presence of free bile in the peritoneal cavity, or the presence of bile staining in the hepatoduodenal ligament or retroperitoneum, is a sign of injury to the extrahepatic biliary tract. Biliary tract injury must also be suspected if there is profuse bleeding from the hepatic artery or portal vein, particularly following blunt trauma, as the bile duct is also likely to be injured. Penetrating wounds near the porta hepatis require careful examination. If routine dissection does not reveal the location of the injury, fine-needle intraoperative cholangiography via the gallbladder or common bile duct may identify the site. Cystic duct cholangiography should be considered after cholecystectomy for traumatic gallbladder injury to avoid missing an associated bile duct injury.

It is possible for a patient who has sustained blunt abdominal trauma to be discharged from hospital only to return days or weeks later with a combination of symptoms and signs, including jaundice, abdominal distension, nausea, vomiting, anorexia, abdominal pain, low-grade fever or weight loss – a clinical picture similar to that seen in patients with intraperitoneal bile leakage following cholecystectomy. When jaundice develops after abdominal trauma, missed extrahepatic biliary injury must be considered.

Operative management of biliary injury

Many patients with extrahepatic biliary tract injury present in shock due to associated haemorrhage, and the priority at laparotomy is to identify and control haemorrhage. The report of Dawson and colleagues demonstrates that these patients are at risk of exsanguinating on the operating table.[58] Injuries to the gallbladder are best treated by cholecystectomy. Primary repair of a clean and simple partial or complete transection of the common duct using absorbable sutures such as 4/0 polydioxanone over a T-tube inserted through a separate choledochotomy has been described. However, this type of repair is not appropriate if there is any evidence of duct contusion, loss of ductal tissue or possible injury to the hepatic artery as this may increase the risk of late development of an ischaemic stricture. In general, it is therefore safer to recommend that most injuries should be managed by fashioning a Roux-en-Y hepatico-jejunostomy as in the management of iatrogenic bile duct injuries.

Outcome after biliary injury

Injuries of this nature are associated with a mortality rate of 10% from concomitant injuries.[59] Septic complications and bile leakage account for most of the early morbidity and may require operative intervention. Late morbidity after repair of a traumatic biliary tract injury is unusual; however, jaundice or episodes of ascending cholangitis suggest a stricture of the ductal system.

Pancreatic trauma

Injuries to the pancreas are uncommon, accounting for 1–4% of severe abdominal injuries and usually occur in young men.

Mechanisms of pancreatic injury

Deceleration injury is a major mechanism of blunt pancreatic trauma with the neck of the gland being at risk of transection across the vertebral column. The deep location of the pancreas means that considerable force is needed to cause an injury and this level of force may often be sufficient to damage other organs.

Diagnosis of pancreatic injury

Pancreatic injury should be suspected in any patient with penetrating trauma to the trunk, particularly if the entry site is between the nipples and the iliac crest, and in any patient with blunt compression trauma of the upper abdomen.

In an early study, Moretz and colleagues found that there was no reliable correlation between serum amylase and pancreatic injury.[65] In a later report, Takashima and colleagues retrospectively studied admission serum amylase values in a series of 73 patients with blunt pancreatic trauma treated in a single institution over a 16-year period.[66] Sixty-one (84%) of these patients had a raised serum amylase level. Of interest, the serum amylase level was found to be abnormal in all patients admitted more than 3 hours after trauma.

Bearing in mind the practicality that patients with pancreatic injury will simultaneously be undergoing evaluation to exclude concomitant intra-abdominal visceral injury, contrast-enhanced CT has been the investigation of choice. Reported CT features of pancreatic injury include free intraperitoneal fluid, localised fluid in the lesser sac, retroperitoneal fluid, pancreatic oedema or swelling and changes in the peripancreatic fat. The presence of fluid in the lesser sac between the pancreas and the splenic vein is reported by Lane and colleagues to be a reliable sign in blunt pancreatic injury.[67] However, Sivit and Eichelberger reported that this radiological sign was rarely the only abnormal CT finding in pancreatic injury.[68] It should be borne in mind that many of these CT features are also seen in acute pancreatitis (and furthermore that acute pancreatitis may occur as a result of blunt abdominal trauma). There is also evidence that CT tends to underdiagnose pancreatic injury. Akhrass and colleagues evaluated the clinical course of 72 patients with pancreatic injury admitted over a 10-year period.[69] Seventeen of these patients underwent CT as part of their initial assessment and this was reported as normal in nine. Eight of these patients underwent laparotomy (principally for suspected associated splenic injury) and three were found to have pancreatic injury requiring distal pancreatectomy. Newer, non-invasive imaging modalities such as magnetic resonance pancreatography have been reported in the assessment of patients with suspected pancreatic trauma.[70] Increased sophistication with the use of this technique may allow for accurate assessment of pancreatic ductal integrity.

Classification of pancreatic injury

Of the various proposed classification schemes, Lucas suggested in an early report that appropriate treatment be formulated according to the type of injury.[71] This classification system divides pancreatic injuries into three groups:

- grade I – superficial contusion with minimal damage

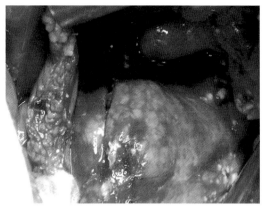

Figure 17.7 • Operative photograph of a transection injury along the neck of the pancreas resulting from a direct blow to the abdomen. This injury was managed by distal pancreatectomy and splenectomy.

- grade II – deep laceration or transection of the left portion of the pancreas
- grade III – injury of the pancreatic head (**Fig. 17.7**).

A more complex system of classification taking into account the frequent coexistence of duodenal and pancreatic injuries was proposed by Frey and Wardell[72] (Table 17.2). The most common site of injury is the neck of the pancreas. The relative frequency of pancreatic injuries reported in collected reviews is represented in **Fig. 17.8**.

Initial management of pancreatic injury

In a major retrospective clinical casenote review of pancreatic trauma from six hospitals, Bradley and colleagues demonstrated a significant association between pancreas-related morbidity and injury to the main pancreatic duct.[73] Delayed intervention (due to delay in recognition of main pancreatic duct injury) was associated with high morbidity. CT was unreliable for the assessment of main pancreatic ductal integrity and an accurate assessment required ERCP.

 Assessment of the integrity of the main pancreatic duct is critical to the treatment of pancreatic injury. In patients with a suspected pancreatic injury (who are haemodynamically stable), ERCP is indicated to assess major duct integrity. Demonstration of an intact main pancreatic duct at ERCP in a patient with suspected isolated pancreatic injury may allow for a trial of non-operative management.

Table 17.2 • Classification of pancreatic injury proposed by Frey and Wardell

Pancreatic injury	
Class I	Capsular damage, minor gland damage (P_1)
Class II	Body or tail pancreatic duct transection, partial or complete (P_2)
Class III	Major duct injury involving the head of the pancreas or the intrapancreatic common bile duct (P_3)
Duodenal injury	
Class I	Contusion, haematoma or partial-thickness injury (D_1)
Class II	Full-thickness duodenal injury (D_2)
Class III	Full-thickness injury with >75% circumference injury or full-thickness duodenal injury with injury to the extrahepatic common bile duct (D_3)
Combined pancreatico-duodenal injuries	
Type I	P_1D_1, P_2D_1, or D_2P_1
Type II	D_2P_2
Type III	D_3P_{1-2} or P_3D_{1-2}
Type IV	D_3P_3

Reproduced from Frey CF, Wardell JW. Injuries to the pancreas. In: Trede M, Carter DC (eds) Surgery of the pancreas. Edinburgh: Churchill Livingstone, 1993 with permission from Elsevier.

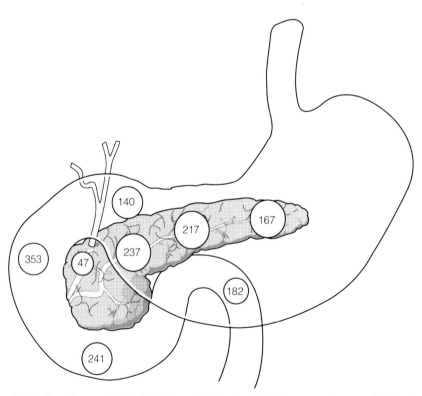

Figure 17.8 • Distribution of pancreatic injuries in the world literature. Note the preponderance of injuries in the junctional area of the neck of the gland. Reproduced from Frey CF, Wardell JW. Section 9. Injuries to the pancreas. In: Trede M, Carter DC (eds) Surgery of the pancreas. Edinburgh: Churchill Livingstone, 1993. With permission from Elsevier.

Operative management of pancreatic injury

The mainstay of treatment remains operative as pancreatic injuries are usually diagnosed at laparotomy. The important principles at operation are to gain good access to allow thorough inspection of the gland. Access to the lesser sac is best done by creating a window in the gastrocolic omentum outside the gastroepiploic arcade to allow examination of the body of the pancreas. A Kocher manoeuvre is necessary to permit palpation of the head of the pancreas between the thumb and fingers. A thorough inspection of the base of the transverse mesocolon is also undertaken. Injury to the pancreas is suspected if retroperitoneal haemorrhage can be seen through the base of the mesocolon or the lesser omentum. Absence of any sign of haemorrhage over the pancreas and duodenum makes injury unlikely.

Experience of patients with pancreatic injury from Durban led to the recommendation for operative treatment of patients with penetrating or gunshot injury and signs of peritoneal irritation.[74] In this large series of 152 patients with pancreatic trauma presenting during a 5-year period, 63 patients had been shot, 66 stabbed and 23 had blunt trauma. The mainstay of treatment was exploratory laparotomy followed by drainage of the pancreatic injury site. Large-bore soft silastic drains were used to minimise the risk of drain erosion into a major vessel. The mortality rates in these groups were 8% after gunshot injury, 2% after stab wounds and 10% after blunt trauma. The majority of these deaths were attributed to damage of other organs. The proportions of patients developing pancreatic fistulas in the three groups were 14%, 9% and 13% respectively. The authors concluded that 'conservative' surgical drainage (avoiding pancreatic resection) was justified after pancreatic injury. This large contemporary report lends weight to the treatment plan proposed by Lucas for grade I injuries, which consists of passive closed drainage using a wide-bore drain.

Simplified management guidelines based on the treatment protocols developed during the treatment of 124 pancreatic injuries at the University of Tennessee[75] also advocate simple drainage alone for proximal pancreatic injuries. There were 37 (30%) patients with proximal injuries. The 'pancreas-related' morbidity was 11% – principally the sequelae of pancreatic fistulas. Of 87 distal pancreatic injuries, the integrity of the main pancreatic duct was not established in 54 (62%). Patients thought to have a high probability of duct transection were treated by distal pancreatectomy. A concern with simple drainage for injuries in the head of the pancreas is persistent pancreatic fistula, and thus a surgical alternative is to drain the head of the pancreas into a Roux-en-Y limb of jejunum.

Moncure and Goins described their experience over a 6-year period with a consecutive series of 44 patients with pancreatic injury,[76] of which penetrating abdominal trauma accounted for the majority of cases. Class I pancreatic injuries occurred in 55% of patients and the majority were managed by simple drainage. Grade II injuries occurred in 18% and grade III injuries in 21%. Coexistent duodenal injuries were treated by primary closure in 21% and more complex duodenal exclusion techniques were used in 20%. The most frequent complications were intra-abdominal abscesses (31%) and pancreatic fistulas (16%).

Severe Lucas grade III injuries involving the head of the pancreas, duodenum and distal bile duct represent a major challenge, but fortunately are relatively rare, occurring in approximately 5% of all duodenal injuries.[77] The principles of treatment are to ensure that haemorrhage from concomitant injuries is dealt with first, as this is likely to be the major source of mortality. Similarly a prolonged operative procedure should be avoided in a potentially unstable patient and the involvement of an experienced pancreatic surgeon is desirable. Duodenal injuries can be closed primarily or drained into a Roux loop. Bile duct injuries may be repaired primarily over a T-tube or drained into a Roux limb of jejunum. The large variety of operative procedures described for these complex injuries suggests that treatment has to be tailored to the individual injury complex and that no single procedure is likely to be uniformly applicable or successful. Very rarely, pancreatico-duodenectomy may be required for complex, severe pancreatic injuries with concomitant duodenal and distal bile duct injuries. Clearly, this sort of resection should not be undertaken lightly in an individual suffering from shock and its sequelae, but rather like liver transplantation for trauma it is useful to have an index of awareness of the available therapeutic options.

Complications of pancreatic injury

The most common post-traumatic complications include necrotising pancreatitis, pseudocyst formation, pancreatic abscesses and pancreatic fistula. Cerwenka and colleagues reported the incidence of these complications to be 15%, 9%, 6% and 4% respectively.[78] The principles regarding management are similar to those for treating these complications when they arise as a result of pancreatitis or pancreatic surgery. Inflammation of the pancreas after trauma behaves in much the same way as acute biliary or acute alcohol-induced pancreatitis with the possible exception that there is a higher incidence of development of local complications such as pseudocyst – possibly relating to the nature of duct disruption in trauma. The Cape Town group reported that, of a series of 64 patients with pancreatic trauma, pseudocysts developed in 15 patients (23%), of whom eight had a duct injury demonstrated by endoscopic retrograde pancreatography.[79] Patients with pseudocysts related to distal duct injury were treated successfully by percutaneous aspiration. Three patients with duct injuries in the neck/body region underwent distal pancreatectomy. Pseudocysts related to ductal injury in the head of the pancreas were drained internally by Roux-en-Y cyst-jejunostomy. The authors concluded that traumatic pancreatic pseudocysts associated with a peripheral duct injury may resolve spontaneously whereas those associated with injuries to the proximal duct wound more likely require surgical intervention. Alternative treatment strategies include endoscopic transpapillary or transmural drainage of the pseudocyst.

The incidence of pancreatic fistula after surgery for trauma is dependent on the type of procedure, with some evidence that the fistula rate is higher after drainage procedures than after resection. Successful insertion of pancreatic duct stents has been reported for management of major pancreatic duct disruption; however, the incidence of long-term ductal stricture is high and therefore the role of pancreatic duct stenting needs to be further defined.[80]

Management of post-traumatic pseudocysts and fistulas will depend on the time from injury, presence of ongoing ductal leak, site of leak and presence of debris within a pseudocyst cavity. The optimal treatment strategy should involve a multidisciplinary approach in a specialist unit employing similar principles to those of managing these complications following an attack of acute pancreatitis.

Conclusion

The contemporary management of patients with suspected liver, biliary or pancreatic injury involves detailed clinical assessment and resuscitation followed, in haemodynamically stable patients, by imaging investigations. If surgical intervention is required, the mainstay of treatment is to control haemorrhage. In European healthcare systems, the optimum care of the patient may consist of packing followed by transfer to a regional hepato-pancreatico-biliary unit. A paper by Hoyt and colleagues examining preventable causes of death in 72 151 admissions with abdominal trauma to North American level I trauma centres identified abdominal injury as the cause of death in 287, with liver injury being responsible for 92.[81] Delays in packing were highlighted as a preventable cause of death, as was a need for better understanding of the end-points to be achieved by packing. The conclusion of this large survey was that the management of liver injury remains a major technical challenge.

Key points

- Management of patients with suspected liver, biliary or pancreatic injury involves detailed clinical assessment and resuscitation.
- Haemodynamic instability resistant to fluid resuscitation associated with clinical signs of peritonism is an indication for immediate laparotomy.
- Patients who are haemodynamically stable or who respond to initial fluid resuscitation should undergo further imaging investigations.
- Laparotomy is generally required for patients with an abdominal gunshot wound.

Liver trauma

- Non-operative management of liver trauma is now a well-established treatment option.
- Significant liver haemorrhage can initially be controlled at operation by manual compression of the liver parenchyma, a Pringle manoeuvre or by compression of the aorta above the coeliac trunk. Perihepatic packing is a highly effective technique to control bleeding from the liver or juxtahepatic veins.
- Resectional debridement of non-viable hepatic parenchyma may be undertaken, but anatomical resection is rarely indicated.

- Other techniques to control haemorrhage include suture ligation of vessels, mesh wrapping of a liver lobe and selective hepatic arterial ligation.
- Postoperative complications include bile leakage or sepsis, and may require radiological, endoscopic or surgical intervention.

Extrahepatic biliary tract trauma

- This uncommon injury is more likely to be due to penetrating rather than blunt abdominal trauma.
- It is rarely diagnosed before operation and is usually recognised incidentally at laparotomy.
- Concomitant vascular injury of the portal vein or hepatic artery is rare.
- ERCP may demonstrate bile leakage and allow therapeutic insertion of a biliary stent.
- Definitive operative intervention for gallbladder trauma is cholecystectomy.
- Roux-en-Y hepatico-jejunostomy is the operation of choice for most injuries to the bile duct.

Pancreatic trauma

- This is most commonly diagnosed by CT; however, ERCP may be undertaken to assess pancreatic duct integrity and may allow therapeutic stenting if leakage of contrast is identified.
- Exploratory laparotomy and drainage of the pancreatic region remains the mainstay of surgical treatment.
- Selected injuries may be managed by distal pancreatectomy, pancreatico-duodenectomy or pancreatico-jejunostomy Roux-en-Y.

References

1. Scollay JM, Beard D, Smith R et al. Eleven years of liver trauma: the Scottish experience. Br J Surg 2004; 91(Suppl 1):24.

2. Talving P, Beckman M, Haggmark T et al. Epidemiology of liver injuries. Scand J Surg 2003; 92:192–4.

3. Krige JE, Bornman PC, Terblanche J. Liver trauma in 446 patients. S Afr J Surg 1997; 35:10–15.

4. Feliciano DV, Mattox KL, Jordan GL et al. Management of 1000 consecutive cases of hepatic trauma (1979–84). Ann Surg 1986; 204:438–54.

5. Fabian TC, Croce MA, Stanford GG et al. Factors affecting morbidity following hepatic trauma. A prospective analysis of 482 injuries. Ann Surg 1991; 213:540–7.

6. Parks RW, Chrysos E, Diamond T. Management of liver trauma. Br J Surg 1999; 86:1121–35.

7. Moore EE, Cogbill TH, Jurkovich GJ et al. Organ injury scaling: spleen and liver (1994 revision). J Trauma 1995; 38:323–4.

8. Schweizer W, Tanner S, Baer HU et al. Management of traumatic liver injuries. Br J Surg 1993; 80:86–8.

9. Bickell WH, Wall MJ Jr, Pepe PE et al. Immediate versus delayed fluid resuscitation for hypotensive patients with penetrating torso injuries. N Engl J Med 1994; 331:1105–9.

10. Reed RL II, Merrell RC, Meyers WC et al. Continuing evolution in the approach to severe liver trauma. Ann Surg 1992; 216:524–38.

11. Rozycki GS, Ochsner MG, Feliciano DV et al. Early detection of hemoperitoneum by ultrasound examination of the right upper quadrant: a multi-center study. J Trauma 1998; 45:878–83.

12. McKenney MG, Martin L, Lentz K et al. 1000 consecutive ultrasounds for blunt abdominal trauma. J Trauma 1996; 40:607–12.

13. Richards JR, McGahan JP, Simpson JL et al. Bowel and mesenteric injury: evaluation with abdominal US. Radiology 1999; 211:399–403.

14. Fang JF, Chen RJ, Wong YC et al. Pooling of contrast material on computed tomography mandates aggressive management of blunt hepatic injury. Am J Surg 1998; 176:315–19.

15. Yokota J, Sugimoto T. Clinical significance of periportal tracking on computed tomographic scan in patients with blunt liver trauma. Am J Surg 1994; 168:247–50.

16. Shankar KR, Lloyd DA, Kitteringham L et al. Oral contrast with computed tomography in the evaluation of blunt abdominal trauma in children. Br J Surg 1999; 86:1073–7.

17. Croce MA, Fabian TC, Kudsk KA et al. AAST organ injury scale: correlation of CT graded liver injuries and operative findings. J Trauma 1991; 31:806–12.

18. Hagiwara A, Yukioka T, Ohta S et al. Non-surgical management of patients with blunt hepatic injury: efficacy of transcatheter arterial embolization. Am J Roentgenol 1997; 169:1151–6.

19. Forlee MV, Krige JEJ, Welman CJ et al. Haemobilia after penetrating and blunt liver injury: treatment with selective hepatic artery embolisation. Injury 2004; 35:23–8.

20. Carrillo EH, Spain DA, Wohltmann CD et al. Interventional techniques are useful adjuncts in the non-operative management of hepatic injuries. J Trauma 1999; 46:619–22.

21. Richie JP, Fonkalsrud EW. Subcapsular haematoma of the liver: non-operative management. Arch Surg 1972; 104:780–4.

22. White P, Cleveland RJ. The surgical management of liver trauma. Arch Surg 1972; 104:785–6.

23. Meyer AA, Crass RA, Lim RC et al. Selective non-operative management of blunt liver injury using computed tomography. Arch Surg 1985; 120:781–4.

24. Farnell MB, Spencer MP, Thompson E et al. Non-operative management of blunt hepatic trauma in adults. Surgery 1988; 104:748–56.

25. Feliciano DV. Continuing evolution in the approach to severe liver trauma. Ann Surg 1992; 216:521–3.

26. Boone DC, Federle M, Billiar TR et al. Evolution of management of major hepatic trauma: identification of patterns of injury. J Trauma 1995; 39:344–50.

27. Sherman HF, Savage BA, Jones LM et al. Non-operative management of blunt hepatic injuries: safe at any grade? J Trauma 1994; 37:616–21.

28. Croce MA, Fabian TC, Menke PG et al. Nonoperative management of blunt hepatic trauma is the treatment of choice for hemodynamically stable patients. Results of a prospective trial. Ann Surg 1995; 221:744–53.

29. Pachter HL, Hofstetter SR. The current status of nonoperative management of adult blunt hepatic injuries. Am J Surg 1995; 169:442–54.

30. Nance ML, Peden GW, Shapiro MB et al. Solid viscus injury predicts major hollow viscus injury in blunt abdominal trauma. J Trauma 1999; 43:618–22.

31. Demetriades D, Karaiskakis M, Alo K et al. Role of postoperative computed tomography in patients with severe liver injury. Br J Surg 2003; 90:1398–1400.

32. Cox JC, Fanian TC, Maish GO et al. Routine follow-up imaging is unnecessary in the management of blunt hepatic injury. J Trauma 2005; 59:1175–80.

33. Cogbill TH, Moore EE, Jurkovich GJ et al. Severe hepatic trauma: a multicenter experience with 1335 liver injuries. J Trauma 1988; 28:1433–8.

34. Omoshoro-Jones JAO, Nicol AJ, Navsaria PH et al. Selective non-operative management of liver gunshot injuries. Br J Surg 2005; 92:890–5.

35. Demetriades D, Hadjizacharia P, Constantinou C et al. Selective nonoperative management of penetrating abdominal solid organ injuries. Ann Surg 2006; 244:620–8.

36. Calne RY, McMaster P, Pentlon BD. The treatment of major liver trauma by primary packing with transfer of the patient for definitive treatment. Br J Surg 1978; 66:338–9.

37. Cue JI, Cryer HG, Miller FB et al. Packing and planned reexploration for hepatic and retroperitoneal hemorrhage: critical refinements of a useful technique. J Trauma 1990; 30:1007–13.

38. Nicol AJ, Hommes M, Primrose R et al. Packing for control of haemorrhage in major liver trauma. World J Surg 2007; 31:569–74.

39. Berguer R, Staerkel RL, Moore EE et al. Warning: fatal reaction to the use of fibrin glue in deep hepatic wounds. Case reports. J Trauma 1991; 31:408–11.

40. Vick LR, Islam S. Recombinant factor VIIa as an adjunct in nonoperative management of solid organ injuries in children. J Pediatr Surg 2008; 43:195–9.

41. Stone HH, Lamb JM. Use of pedicled omentum as an autogenous pack for control of haemorrhage in major injuries of the liver. Surg Gynecol Obstet 1975; 141:92–4.

42. Brunet C, Sielezneff I, Thomas P et al. Treatment of hepatic trauma with perihepatic mesh: 35 cases. J Trauma 1994; 37:200–4.

43. Cox EF, Flancbaum L, Dauterieve AH et al. Blunt trauma to the liver. Analysis of management and mortality in 323 consecutive patients. Ann Surg 1988; 207:126–34.

44. Strong RW, Lynch SV, Wall DR et al. Anatomic resection for severe liver trauma. Surgery 1998; 123:251–7.

45. Mays ET. Hepatic trauma. Curr Probl Surg 1976; 13:6–73.

46. Chen RJ, Fang JF, Lin BC et al. Surgical management of juxtahepatic venous injuries in blunt hepatic trauma. J Trauma 1995; 38:886–90.

47. Ringe B, Pichlmayr R. Total hepatectomy and liver transplantation: a life-saving procedure in patients with severe hepatic trauma. Br J Surg 1995; 82:837–9.

48. Lin PJ, Jeng LB, Chen RJ et al. Femoro-arterial bypass using Gott shunt in liver transplantation following severe hepatic trauma. Int Surg 1993; 78:295–7.

49. Ginzburg E, Shatz D, Lynn M et al. The role of liver transplantation in the subacute trauma patient. Am Surg 1998; 64:363–4.

50. Wagner WW, Lundell CJ, Donovan AJ. Percutaneous angiographic embolisation for hepatic arterial hemorrhage. Arch Surg 1985; 120:1241–9.

51. Maurel J, Aouad K, Martel B et al. Post-traumatic hemobilia. How to treat? Ann Chir 1994; 48:572–5.

52. Kozar RA, Moore FA, Cothren CC et al. Risk factors for hepatic morbidity following nonoperative management: multicentre study. Arch Surg 2006; 141:451–9.

53. Parks RW, Diamond T. Non-surgical trauma to the extrahepatic biliary tract. Br J Surg 1995; 82:1303–10.

54. Penn I. Injuries of the gallbladder. Br J Surg 1962; 49:636–41.

55. Soderstrom CA, Maekawa K, DuPriest RW Jr et al. Gallbladder injuries resulting from blunt abdominal trauma: an experience and review. Ann Surg 1981; 193:60–6.

56. Posner MC, Moore EE. Extrahepatic biliary tract injury: operative management plan. J Trauma 1985; 25:833–7.

57. Burgess P, Fulton RL. Gall bladder and extrahepatic biliary duct injury following abdominal trauma. Injury 1992; 23:413–14.

58. Dawson DL, Johansen KH, Jurkovich GJ. Injuries to the portal triad. Am J Surg 1991; 161:545–51.

59. Kitahama A, Elliott LF, Overby JL et al. The extra-hepatic biliary tract injury: perspective in diagnosis and treatment. Ann Surg 1982; 196:536–40.

60. Bade PG, Thomson SR, Hirshberg A et al. Surgical options in traumatic injury to the extrahepatic biliary tract. Br J Surg 1989; 76:256–8.

61. Michelassi F, Ranson JHC. Bile duct disruption by blunt trauma. J Trauma 1985; 25:454–7.

62. Bourque MD, Spigland N, Bensoussan AL et al. Isolated complete transection of the common bile duct due to blunt trauma in a child, and review of the literature. J Paediatr Surg 1989; 24:1068–70.

63. Dawson DL, Jurkovich GJ. Hepatic duct disruption from blunt abdominal trauma: case report and literature review. J Trauma 1991; 31:1698–702.

64. Jenkins MA, Ponsky JL. Endoscopic retrograde cholangiopancreatography and endobiliary stenting in the treatment of biliary injury resulting from liver trauma. Surg Laparosc Endosc 1995; 5:118–20.

65. Moretz JA III, Campbell DP, Parker DE et al. Significance of serum amylase in evaluating pancreatic trauma. Am J Surg 1975; 130:739–41.

66. Takashima T, Sugimoto K, Hirata M et al. Serum amylase level on admission in the diagnosis of blunt injury to the pancreas: its significance and limitations. Ann Surg 1997; 226:70–6.

67. Lane MJ, Mindelzun RE, Sandhu JS. CT diagnosis of blunt pancreatic trauma: importance of detecting fluid between the pancreas and the splenic vein. Am J Roentgenol 1994; 163:833–5.

68. Sivit CJ, Eichelberger MR. CT diagnosis of pancreatic injury in children: significance of fluid separating the splenic vein and the pancreas. Am J Roentgenol 1995; 165:921–4.

69. Akhrass R, Kim K, Brandt C. Computed tomography: an unreliable indicator of pancreatic trauma. Am Surg 1996; 62:647–51.

70. Nirula R, Velmahos GC, Demetriades D. Magnetic resonance cholangiopancreatography in pancreatic trauma: a new diagnostic modality? J Trauma 1999; 47:585–7.

71. Lucas CE. Diagnosis and treatment of pancreatic and duodenal injury. Surg Clin North Am 1977; 57:49–65.

72. Frey CF, Wardell JW. Injuries to the pancreas. In: Trede M, Carter DC (eds) Surgery of the pancreas. Edinburgh: Churchill Livingstone, 1993; pp. 565–89.

73. Bradley E, Young PR Jr, Chang MC et al. Diagnosis and initial management of pancreatic trauma: guidelines from a multi-institutional review. Ann Surg 1998; 227:861–9.

74. Madiba TE, Mokoena TR. Favourable prognosis after surgical drainage of gunshot, stab or blunt trauma of the pancreas. Br J Surg 1995; 82:1236–9.

75. Patton JH Jr, Lyden SP, Croce MA et al. Pancreatic trauma: a simplified management guideline. J Trauma 1997; 43:234–9.

76. Moncure M, Goins WA. Challenges in the management of pancreatic and duodenal injuries. JAMA 1993; 85:767–72.

77. Feliciano DV, Martin TD, Cruse PA et al. Management of combined pancreatoduodenal injuries. Ann Surg 1987; 205:673–80.

78. Cerwenka H, Bacher H, El-Shabrawi A et al. Management of pancreatic trauma and its consequences – guidelines or individual therapy ? Hepato-Gastroenterology 2007; 54:581–4.

79. Lewis G, Krige JEJ, Bornman PC et al. Traumatic pancreatic pseudocysts. Br J Surg 1993; 80:89–93.

80. Lin BC, Liu NJ, Fang JF et al. Long-term results of endoscopic stent in the management of blunt major pancreatic duct injury. Surg Endosc 2006; 20:1551–5.

81. Hoyt DB, Bulger EM, Knudson MM et al. Death in the operating room: an analysis of a multicenter experience. J Trauma 1994; 37:426–38.

Index

B

F

H